COMPREHENSIVE REVIEW IN TOXICOLOGY

Second Edition

Peter D. Bryson, MD
Assistant Clinical Professor of Surgery
University of Colorado Health Sciences Center
Staff Physician
Emergency Department
St. Anthony Hospital Systems
Denver, Colorado

AN ASPEN PUBLICATION®
Aspen Publishers, Inc.
Rockville, Maryland
Royal Tunbridge Wells
1989

Library of Congress Cataloging-in-Publication Data

Bryson, Peter D.
Comprehensive review in toxicology/ Peter D. Bryson.--2nd.ed.
p. cm.
"An Aspen publication."
Includes bibliographies and index.
ISBN: 0-87189-777-6
1. Toxicological emergencies. 2. Toxicology. 3. Drug abuse. I. Title.
[DNLM: 1. Poisoning. 2. Poisons. QV 600 B915c]
RA1224.5.B79   1988   615.9--dc19
DNLM/DLC
for Library of Congress
88-22297
CIP

The authors have made every effort to ensure the accuracy of the information herein, particularly with regard to drug selection and dose. However, appropriate information sources should be consulted, especially for new or unfamiliar procedures. It is the responsibility of every practitioner to evaluate the appropriateness of a particular opinion in the context of actual clinical situations and with due consideration to new developments. Authors, editors, and the publisher cannot be held responsible for any typographical or other errors found in this book.

Editorial Services: Ruth Bloom

Library of Congress Catalog Card Number: 88-22297
ISBN: 0-87189-777-6

Printed in the United States of America

1 2 3 4 5

Especially To
To G M and G P
and
C.M. and D.H.

Table of Contents

Preface

In this age of specialization, physicians are expected to practice the "state of art." This is especially true for toxicology, where new drugs are being introduced at an astonishing rate—drugs with new mechanisms of action as well as new toxicities. It is almost impossible for the average clinician to keep abreast of new developments in all of the subspecialties without the aid of the most up-to-date information presented in a clear and concise manner.

With the publication of this second edition, I believe I have achieved the goal of a truly comprehensive text that is easy for the clinician to use. This edition has been expanded to more than 50 chapters with a complete update and revision of previous chapters. Comments from readers of the first edition have been seriously considered and because of this, the format of each chapter has remained unchanged as has the use of summary tables. References have been reordered into those specifically cited by number as well as those additionally selected because of their merit. In addition, the index has been expanded and hard-to-find material such as street names for drugs, volumes of distribution for drugs and therapeutic concentrations appear in the appendixes.

Written by a practicing emergency physician who is also a board certified clinical toxicologist, this text is intended to be both a comprehensive review of all toxicological areas and a practical information source on how to evaluate, diagnose, and treat a poisoned patient in an acute care setting.

As in many areas of medicine, there is controversy in the field of toxicology. I have attempted to present these controversial viewpoints and make recommendations based on the published literature.

The model for this textbook came from the comprehensive review in toxicology (CRIT) courses that I have taught for the past several years throughout the United States. The idea of a reference book actually came from many of the course participants who wanted a toxicology reference that would fit their needs. Whereas the courses are limited by time, this text, which does not have that limitation, can present a much more comprehensive amount of useful information in greater detail.

My sincere gratitude to the librarians of St. Anthony Hospital Systems as well as the staff of Aspen Publishers, Inc., for their help and support in making this book a reality.

Peter D. Bryson
September 1988

part I

GENERAL PRINCIPLES OF OVERDOSE MANAGEMENT

chapter 1

General Management of the Overdosed Patient

The field of toxicology is concerned with the chemical and physical properties of poisons and the physiological and behavioral effects of these poisons on living organisms. In addition, toxicology involves the analysis, both qualitative and quantitative, of these agents in biological materials as well as the development of procedures for the treatment of the poisoned patient.

Poisonings and drug overdoses, both accidental and intentional, continue to be a major medical problem. The field of toxicology is constantly expanding and changing, and in the last decade there have been many important advances that aid in both the diagnosis and the treatment of poisoned patients.[1] It is vitally important for the practitioner to be aware of the most up-to-date treatment protocols so as to improve the chances of the patient's survival.

Any drug under certain circumstances can be toxic, and this toxicity can present itself as various signs and symptoms.[2] The poisoned patient may represent a clinical challenge to the emergency department physician, who must be aware of the potential for multisystem involvement. Whenever a patient who appears to be ill presents with a history or symptom complex that is unusual or confusing, purposeful or accidental ingestion or exposure to a toxic chemical should be considered.[3] This may be the critically ill patient who presents with an altered mental status, unexplained cardiotoxicity, unexplained metabolic acidosis, seizures, or head trauma for which there is no satisfactory explanation. Although the most common route for accidental exposure to poisons is the gastrointestinal tract, toxic effects may also be produced by accidental absorption of the toxin through the skin, inhalation through the lungs, or parenteral administration.[4] This chapter is a general overview of the patient who has ingested or been exposed to a toxic material and who may or may not be manifesting toxic symptoms.

There is often no difference between the mechanism of action of a drug and that of a poison, only an extension of effect. A drug may be administered in dosages that alter physiological function to produce a desired therapeutic effect. When a drug is administered in greater than therapeutic quantities, toxic effects may be noted. It may be difficult to diagnose drug toxicity when the poisoning is of a chronic nature, especially when a relevant history is unavailable.

INITIAL EVALUATION

The initial evaluation of the patient should include obtaining as reliable a history as possible and performing a thorough but quick physical examination.[5–7] In conjunction with appropriate laboratory analyses, these provide essential data for appropriate patient management (Table 1-1).

Table 1-1 Items in the Initial Patient Evaluation

History
- Patient history
- Corroborative history
- Worst possible scenario

Physical Examination
- Vital signs
    Blood pressure
        Hypertension (see Table 1-2)
        Hypotension (see Table 1-3)
    Pulse
        Tachycardia
        Bradycardia (see Table 1-4)
        Dysrhythmia
    Respiratory rate
        Tachypnea (see Table 1-5)
            Respiratory alkalosis
            Metabolic acidosis
    Temperature
        Hyperthermia (see Table 1-6)
        Hypothermia
- Skin and mucous membranes
    Burns
    Cyanosis
    Bullous lesions (see Table 1-7)
    Diaphoresis (see Table 1-8)
    Jaundice (see Table 1-9)
- Odors (see Table 1-10)
- Neurologic examination (see Table 1-11)
- Emesis
    ? Pill fragments
    ? Amount
    ? Hematemesis

History

A history may not always be easy to obtain and may be inaccurate, especially if the patient is a toddler who cannot relate a good and accurate history or an adult intent on causing himself or herself harm who will purposely not give an accurate account.[8] In addition, poisoning as a manifestation of child abuse has been reported and should be considered, especially in the very young or in children who repeatedly "overdose."[9,10] In the infant, poisoning is largely a result of therapeutic overdosing.[11] In children 1 to 5 years old, ingestions are most often accidental. A child older than 6 or 7 years at the time of overdose must be evaluated for psychological dysfunction, because in this age group overdose is rarely an accident.[11]

It is wise in all cases of overdose to obtain a separate history from a friend, a relative, or the person who brought the patient to the emergency department to corroborate the patient's history. The family, friends, or paramedical personnel should be asked about any known prescription or over-the-counter medications found in the house or known to be used by the patient.[12] It is also wise to consider the history as the worst possible scenario so as not to minimize the effect of the potential toxin.[13]

Physical Examination

A brief physical examination should be performed shortly after the patient arrives. This will determine what immediate treatment may be necessary as well as provide clues to the practitioner as to what was ingested or the extent of toxicity when the ingested agent is known.[14] Particular attention should be paid to the following areas.

Vital Signs

A clue as to what was ingested may be discovered by a critical examination of the patient's vital signs. An accurate measurement of each parameter, including the respiratory rate and temperature, should be obtained.

Heart rate and blood pressure: tachycardia and hypertension. Persistent tachycardia and hypertension, if drug induced, may be caused by a sympathomimetic agent, anticholinergic drug, or phencyclidine or by acute withdrawal from a central nervous system (CNS) depressant, alcohol, clonidine, or β-adrenergic blocking agents (Table 1-2).[8,15] Hypertension and tachycardia may also result from late ganglionic stimulation during organophosphate insecticide intoxication. Drugs that cause initial stimulation resulting in hypertension or tachycardia may be followed by generalized depression.

Hypertension, when caused primarily by intense α-receptor–mediated vasoconstriction, is frequently accompanied by reflex bradycardia. This may be noted with phenylephrine, phenylpropanolamine, and other α-stimulatory agents.[15]

Table 1-2 Substances Causing Hypertension and Tachycardia

Anticholinergics
  Antihistamines
  Antipsychotics
  Mushrooms
  Over-the-counter medicines
  Plants
  Tricyclic antidepressants
Phencyclidine
Substances Associated with Withdrawal Syndromes
  Alcohol
  Aldomet⑨
  β-Blocking agents
  Central nervous system depressants
  Clonidine
  Sedative-hypnotics
Sympathomimetics
  Amphetamines
  Caffeine
  Cocaine
  Lysergic acid diethylamide (LSD)
  "Look-alikes" (phenylpropanolamine, caffeine, ephredrine)
  Monoamine oxidase inhibitors
  Nicotine
  Phencyclidine
  Theophylline

Table 1-3 Substances Associated with Hypotension

Hypotension and Tachycardia
  Carbon monoxide
  Cyanide
  Disulfiram
  Iron
  Narcotics
  Nitrites
  Phenothiazines
  Sedative-hypnotics
  Theophylline
  Tricyclic antidepressants
Hypotension and Bradycardia
  β-Adrenergic blockers
  Calcium channel blockers
  Clonidine
  Digoxin
  Organophosphate insecticides

Table 1-4 Substances Associated with Bradycardia

α-Adrenergics
β-Adrenergic blockers
Calcium channel blockers
Cardiac glycosides
Cholinergics
Clonidine
Cyanide
Hypertensives
Insecticides (organophosphates)
Local anesthetics
Mushrooms (cholinergic)
Nicotine
Parasympathomimetics
Tricyclic antidepressants (late)

Heart rate and blood pressure: hypotension and tachycardia. Hypotension accompanied by tachycardia may be due to fluid loss, third spacing, or direct depression of cardiac contractility with peripheral vascular collapse.[8] Hypotension may be due to α-receptor blockade or β-adrenergic stimulation and has been seen in overdoses with cyanide, iron, the sedative-hypnotics, theophylline, and carbon monoxide.

Heart rate and blood pressure: hypotension and bradycardia. Hypotension associated with bradycardia may be due to calcium channel blockers, central depression of sympathetic output, overdose with membrane depressant drugs or digitalis, or peripheral blockade of β-adrenergic receptors (Table 1-3).[15]

Bradycardia. Bradycardia may be caused by digitalis preparations, β-adrenergic blockers, calcium channel blockers, clonidine, and acetylcholinesterase inhibitors (parasympathomimetic agents). Bradycardia may also occur as a response to hypertension caused by α-adrenergic drugs.[15] Additional agents are listed in Table 1-4.

Respiratory Rate. The respiratory rate and depth may be increased by sympathomimetics such as amphetamine, cocaine, or caffeine. The respiratory rate and pattern may also be the first clue that the patient has an acid-base disorder (Table 1-5). As an example, tachypnea may represent primary respiratory alkalosis (from salicylates or dinitrophenol) or a compensation for an underlying and potentially dangerous metabolic acidosis (ethylene glycol, methanol, and others).

Hypoventilation associated with respiratory depression may result from an overdose of any central nervous system depressant. It is usually due to depression of the reticular activating system and the respiratory drive center in the brain, and endotracheal intubation may be required to protect the patient.

Temperature. Hyperthermia secondary to drug overdose may be an immediate threat to life and must be quickly recognized and treated (Table 1-6). Hyperthermia caused by any drug can lead to extensive muscle breakdown and renal failure as well as direct brain injury. It may result from impaired thermoregulatory mechanisms, muscle hyperactivity, or increased metabolic rate.[15] Hypothermia is a common problem seen with a substantial overdose. It is frequently caused by a central nervous system depressant and may be the result of exposure to a cool ambient temperature in a patient with inadequate physiological responses to body cooling due to the ingested drug.

Skin and Mucous Membranes

The skin should be examined for evidence of needle marks, skin lesions, or rash or if the patient had dermal contact with a toxin. It should

be thus ascertained whether decontamination is necessary.

Bullous lesions may be a clue to the examiner that a sedative-hypnotic was ingested, that the patient was exposed to carbon monoxide, that the patient was bitten by an insect or a snake, or that the patient may have come in contact with a chemical that, owing to its caustic nature, has caused a burn (Table 1-7).[15] Diaphoresis may be profuse and may be the clue to the agent ingested (Table 1-8). Jaundice is not an immediate effect of a toxin but may also be noted 48 to 72 hours after exposure to a hepatotoxin (Table 1-9).

Table 1-5 Substances Associated with Tachypnea

Carbon monoxide
Cyanide
Dinitrophenol
Drug-associated metabolic acidosis
Drug-associated hepatic failure
Pentachlorophenol
Salicylates

Table 1-6 Substances Associated with Hyperthermia

Anticholinergics
Dinitrophenol
Monoamine oxidase inhibitors
Metal fumes
Pentachlorophenol
Phencyclidine
Phenothiazines
Salicylates
Sympathomimetics
Thyroid hormone
Withdrawal of substances of abuse

Table 1-7 Substances Causing Bullous Lesions

Caustic Agents
  Acids
  Alkalis
Environmental Hazards
  Carbon monoxide
  Snake bite toxin
  Insect bite toxin (spider, scorpion)
Sedative-Hypnotic Agents
  Barbiturates
  Diphenoxylate (Lomotil®)
  Glutethimide (Doriden®)
  Meprobamate (Equanil®, Miltown®, Equagesic®)
  Methaqualone (Quaalude®)

Table 1-8 Substances Causing Diaphoresis

Acetaminophen
Acetylcholinesterase inhibitor insecticides
Drugs causing hypoglycemia
Mushrooms (cholinergic)
Nicotine
Salicylates
Withdrawal of substances of abuse
Sympathomimetics

Table 1-9 Substances Causing Jaundice

Acetaminophen
Amanita phalloides and related mushrooms
Arsenic
Carbon tetrachloride
Iron
Toluene

Odors

Odors on the breath and body may help indicate the nature of the ingested toxin.[16] For example, the odor of alcohol is frequently encountered in the emergency department and is well recognized. Alcohol, however, is associated with many drug ingestions and may only indicate that the patient is intoxicated with alcohol in addition to an overdose of another substance.

The odor of garlic may suggest the ingestion of arsenic (or arsine gas inhalation), organophosphate insecticide, or phosphorus rodenticide or the topical application of dimethylsulfoxide. Cyanide may have the odor of bitter almonds or macaroons, and the odor of rotten egg may indicate hydrogen sulfide gas. Other odors that may be helpful in diagnosing an unknown overdose are noted in Table 1-10. Although the presence of certain odors may aid the diagnosis, their absence is not a reliable means of excluding intoxication.

Table 1-10 Substances Causing Characteristic Odors

Odor	Substance
Acetone	Ethyl alcohol
	Isopropyl alcohol
	Lacquer
Bitter almond	Amygdalin
	Apricot pits
	Cyanide
	Laetrile
Burned rope	Marijuana
Carrot	Cicutoxin
Garlic	Arsenic
	Arsine gas
	Dimethylsulfoxide
	Organophosphates
	Phosphorus
	Selenium
	Thallium
Mothballs	Naphthalene
	Paradichlorobenzene
Peanuts	Rodenticides
Pear	Chloral hydrate
	Paraldehyde
Pungent aromatic	Ethchlorvynol
Rotten egg	Hydrogen sulfide
	Mercaptans
	Sewer gas
Shoe polish	Nitrobenzene
Violets	Turpentine
Wintergreen	Methyl salicylate

Emesis

History of emesis should be ascertained and documented on the patient's chart. Emesis before arrival in the emergency department may explain why a patient remains asymptomatic after having ingested what appeared to be a toxic amount of substance. Further questioning concerning approximate amount of emesis and whether there was accompanying hematemesis should also be documented.

Neurologic Examination

A brief neurologic examination (Table 1-11) should include evaluating the patient's mental status, looking for evidence of previous seizure activity (Table 1-12), evaluating the size and reactivity of the pupils (Table 1-13), observing for the presence of nystagmus, and testing for the presence or absence of the gag reflex.[17]

Seizure activity. Seizure is a relatively common feature of poisoning by many drugs and toxins. The most common causes of toxin-induced seizures are theophylline, isoniazid, sympathomimetics, and withdrawal from alcohol or sedative-hypnotics.[15] The acronym "WITH L.A. COPS" is presented for the drug causes of seizure (Table 1-12). Seizures may result in pulmonary aspiration, hypoxia, and lactic acidosis and may ultimately cause rhabdomyolysis and acute renal failure.

Eye changes. There are many classes of compounds that cause changes in the eyes, such as mydriasis, miosis (Table 1-13), or nystagmus

Table 1-11 Items in the Neurologic Examination of the Overdosed Patient

Focal signs
Gag reflex
Mental status
  Affect
  Behavior and appearance
  General intellectual functioning
  Perceptual disorders
  Thought content
  Thought process
Nystagmus (see Table 1-13)
Pupil size/reactivity (see Table 1-13)
Seizure activity (see Table 1-12)

(Table 1-14). Pupil size is controlled by the autonomic nervous system and is determined by the relative balance between the parasympathetic and sympathetic systems. Dilation is mediated by α_1-adrenoceptors, and constriction is mediated by muscarinic cholinergic receptors.[15] Anticholinergic drugs would therefore be expected to cause mydriasis. Although phenothiazines have some anticholinergic side effects, they frequently cause miosis because of a predominant α-blocking action.[15]

Sympatholytic agents, narcotics, and cholinergics usually cause miosis. Although phencyclidine is considered a sympathomimetic agent, its cholinergic properties predominate and miosis may be frequently noted.[15] The acronym "SALEM TIP" is presented for drugs that cause nystagmus (Table 1-14).

Radiopacity of Substances

There are a number of pills with different chemical compositions that exhibit varying degrees of radiopacity.[17] Although clinical experience has led to the development of the acronym "CHIPS,"[17] an updated acronym, "BET A CHIP," is suggested to describe the more common radiopaque medications (Table 1-15). For a substance to be radiopaque, it should have stability in the gastric or intestinal contents, low water solubility, and the ability to decrease gastrointestinal motility.

Radiographs are of little use in most ingestions,[17] yet for those pills that are consistently visible on a plain abdominal roentgenogram a radiographic diagnosis may be possible. A postemesis or lavage radiograph may also be used to assess the effectiveness of the gastric emptying procedure.

Table 1-12 Substances Causing Seizure Activity (Acronym: WITH L.A. COPS)

W	Withdrawal
I	Isoniazid
T	Theophylline
H	Hypoglycemic agents, hypoxia
L	Lead
	Lithium
	Local anesthetics
A	Anticholinergics
	Amphetamines
C	Camphor
	Carbon monoxide
	Carbamazepine (Tegretol®)
	Chlorinated hydrocarbons (DDT, lindane)
	Cholinergics
	Cocaine
	Cyanide
O	Organophosphates (malathion, parathion)
P	Phencyclidine
	Phenothiazines
	Phenytoin (Dilantin®)
	Propoxyphene (Darvon®)
S	Salicylates
	Strychnine
	Sympathomimetics

Table 1-13 Substances Causing Characteristic Eye Changes

Mydriasis
    Anticholinergics
    Glutethimide (Doriden®)
    Meperidine (Demerol®)
    Mushrooms (anticholinergics)
    Withdrawal of abused substances
    Sympathomimetics
Miosis
    Cholinergics
    Clonidine (Catapres®)
    Insecticides
    Mushrooms (cholinergic)
    Narcotics
    Nicotine
    Phenothiazines
    Phencyclidine

Table 1-14 Toxins Causing Nystagmus (Acronym: SALEM TIP)

S	Sedative-hypnotics
	Solvents
A	Alcohol
L	Lithium
E	Ethanol
	Ethylene glycol
M	Methanol
T	Thiamine depletion
	Tegretol® (carbamazepine)
I	Isopropanol
P	Phencyclidine
	Phenytoin (Dilantin*)

Table 1-15 Substances That May Be Radiopaque (Acronym: BET A CHIP)

B	Barium
E	Enteric-coated tablets
T	Tricyclic antidepressants
A	Antihistamines
C	Chloral hydrate, cocaine condoms, calcium
H	Heavy metals
I	Iodides
P	Potassium, phenothiazines

Compounds containing iron and other heavy metals are the most radiopaque class of medications. This is not necessarily true for vitamin tablets containing iron, which are not consistently radiopaque. Calcium carbonate is strongly radiopaque, but other calcium compounds may be radiolucent. Potassium preparations are also among the most radiopaque substances. The tricyclic antidepressants and the phenothiazines demonstrate a highly variable degree of radiopacity. Although enteric-coated tablets are part of the acronym, there is variability in the degree of radiopacity of the particular compounds.[15] Antihistamines with and without enteric coating frequently demonstrate radiopacity.

Classification of Coma

Although there are many systems to describe an altered mental status, there is not one description that is universally accepted. Rather than using terms such as lethargy, semicoma, and coma, which may not adequately communicate to another person what the examiner intended, it is more important to describe specific findings, such as response to pain and gag reflex, as well as circulatory or respiratory depression. One such system is divided into five stages as follows.[18]

Stage 0: The patient is asleep but easily aroused and has normal response to pain and an intact gag reflex (this constitutes the majority of patients seen).

Stage 1: The patient is comatose, withdraws from painful stimuli, and has an intact gag reflex

(gastric contents may be evacuated without prior nasotracheal intubation).

Stage 2: The patient is comatose and does not withdraw from pain, but the gag reflex is intact (gastric contents may be evacuated without prior nasotracheal intubation).

Stage 3: The patient is comatose, does not withdraw from pain, and has lost the gag reflex. There is no circulatory or respiratory depression (requires nasotracheal intubation prior to gastric evacuation).

Stage 4: The patient is comatose, does not withdraw from pain, and has lost the gag reflex; cyanosis and circulatory and/or respiratory depression are present (requires ABCs of emergency medicine followed by nasotracheal intubation and gastric lavage).

THERAPEUTIC AGENTS

If the patient enters the emergency department with an altered mental status, it is wise to administer a trial of therapeutic agents that are considered relatively safe: (1) naloxone, (2) dextrose, (3) thiamine, and (4) oxygen.[14]

Since naloxone is a pure narcotic antagonist, in the absence of a narcotic it will not cause any further deterioration of the patient's condition. Glucose, administered with thiamine, will not harm the patient who is hyperglycemic if the diagnosis is made shortly thereafter; at the same time it may be lifesaving to the hypoglycemic patient, and thus its use is strongly encouraged (Table 1-16).

ESSENTIALS OF OVERDOSE MANAGEMENT

There are four essentials of overdose management that should be considered for every patient[14]:

1. Supportive care (the mainstay of care)
2. Prevention of further absorption (see Chapter 2)
3. Enhancement of excretion (see Chapter 3)
4. Administration of an antidote if available

Table 1-16 Suggested Therapy for Patients with Altered Mental Status (Acronym: DONT)

	Drug	Dosage
D	Dextrose	Adult: 50 mL of $D_{50}W$ (25 g)
		Child: 1 mL/kg of same solution
		diluted 1:1
O	Oxygen	As necessary
N	Naloxone	2 mg IV
T	Thiamine	50 to 100 mg IM or IV

Supportive Care

One of the important aspects in the management of the poisoned patient is supportive care.[19] For the most part, patients will detoxify as the ingested compound is metabolized by normal body processes. Support of the vital signs, in addition to good pulmonary hygiene, will enhance any of the other more specific methods. Because the cardiac status is unknown, the patient should be observed on a cardiac monitor until medically cleared.

A large group of acutely poisoned patients can be treated with supportive care, which includes the appropriate treatment of common complications that may occur during intoxication (hypotension, cardiac dysrhythmias, and seizures).[14] The drug will be progressively eliminated over the next 12 to 36 hours in most patients, and many times this is all the care that is necessary. In some cases of poisoning, hypotension should be treated initially with the intravenous infusion of isotonic fluids.[14] In general, seizures should be treated initially with intravenous diazepam.

The poisoned patients may be in shock for a number of reasons. Pooling of blood in an expanded vascular bed caused by vasodilation may have occurred. Hypovolemia from lack of fluid intake during prolonged unconsciousness or from a direct myocardial depressant effect of the drug may also be involved.

Prevention of Absorption

Prevention of absorption of a toxin is another important facet to the care of the poisoned patient. This is due to the fact that once a toxin is absorbed there may be very little that can be done to enhance the excretion of the particular compound. Methods for the prevention of absorption include (1) decontamination of the skin, (2) administration of syrup of ipecac, (3) gastric lavage, (4) administration of activated charcoal, and (5) use of a cathartic. These methods are discussed in detail in Chapter 2.

Enhancement of Excretion

Although there are various methods for enhancing the excretion of drugs and toxins, their use in toxicology is limited. Procedures intended to enhance the excretion of the ingested agent from the body include (1) forced diuresis, (2) alteration of urine pH, (3) dialysis, (4) hemoperfusion, (5) interruption of the enterohepatic circulation, (6) "intestinal dialysis," (7) plasmapheresis, and (8) exchange transfusion. The various methods available for enhancing excretion are listed in Table 1-17 and are discussed in Chapter 3.

Administration of an Antidote

It is essential to be aware that certain patients present to the emergency department with toxic symptom complexes that may respond to the administration of an antidote. The antidote is rarely the essence of the management of a poisoned patient. Antidotal therapy may not be necessary,

Table 1-17 Methods To Enhance Drug Excretion

Diuresis
    Neutral diuresis
    Alkaline diuresis
    Acid diuresis
Dialysis
    Hemodialysis
    Peritoneal dialysis
Hemoperfusion
Multiple doses of activated charcoal
    Interruption of enterohepatic recirculation
    "Intestinal dialysis"
Plasmapheresis
Exchange transfusion

but to have the antidote available and to know when and how to use it may be lifesaving.[20–22] Although there are a number of specific antidotes known for poisoning, their use should not take the place of good general supportive measures. A list of available antidotes is given in Table 1-18.

ANALEPTIC AGENTS

Analeptics act on the central nervous system to stimulate respiration. In the past, analeptics were sometimes advocated for those patients who presented with central nervous system depression. The use of such agents is condemned because they may cause a seizure when the patient is not in control of his or her airway.[23,24] Although analeptic agents may be of some benefit in the operating room, they have no place in emergency medicine and toxicology (Table 1-19).

COMPLICATIONS OF OVERDOSE

There are a number of complications that can occur after an overdose (Table 1-20). These potential complications may arise from overly vigorous fluid replacement with ensuing fluid overload or as a direct result of the toxin, with seizures, hypothermia, rhabdomyolysis,[25] aspiration, and acid-base disorders as consequences. The clinician should be prepared for these complications.

Table 1-18 Antidotes and Their Dosages

Drug/Toxin	Antidote	Antidote Dosage
Acetaminophen	N-Acetylcysteine	140 mg/kg orally (loading) 70 mg/kg every 4 hours, 17 doses (maintenance)
Anticholinergics	Physostigmine	Adult: 1 to 2 mg IV slowly Child: 0.5 mg or 0.02 mg/kg IV slowly
β-Adrenergic blockers	Glucagon	1 to 5 mg IV
Bromide	Sodium chloride	
Carbamate insecticides	Atropine	2 to 4 mg IV as needed
Carbon monoxide	Oxygen	
Cyanide	Amyl nitrite perles	
	Sodium nitrite	Adult: 300 mg Child: 10 mg/kg
	Sodium thiosulfate	Adult: 12.5 g IV Child: 1.5 mL/kg
Cardiac glycosides	Fragment, antigen-binding (Fab) antibody therapy	As necessary
Ethylene glycol	Ethyl alcohol	1 mL/kg of 95% solution, diluted (loading) 0.1 mL/kg/hour, diluted (maintenance)
Gyrimetra mushrooms	Pyridoxine	2 to 5 g IV slowly
Heavy metals	Dimercaprol (BAL) Penicillamine Disodium EDTA	
Isoniazid	Pyridoxine	2 to 5 g IV slowly
Iron	Deferoxamine	10 to 15 mg/kg/hour
Methanol	Ethyl alcohol	As for ethylene glycol
Narcotics	Naloxone	2 mg IV
Nitrites	Methylene blue	1 to 2 mg/kg of 1% solution
Organophosphates	Atropine	1 to 2 mg IV as needed
	Pralidoxime	1 g
Tricyclic antidepressants	Sodium bicarbonate	1 to 3 mEq/kg IV
Warfarin	Vitamin K_1	5 to 25 mg IV or IM

Table 1-19 Analeptic Agents (Contraindicated)

Amphetamine
Bemegride
Caffeine
Nikethamide (Coramine®)
Picrotoxin

Table 1-20 Complications of Overdose

Respiratory
  Airway occlusion
  Aspiration
  Pneumonia
  Pulmonary edema
  Respiratory depression
Cardiovascular
  Dysrhythmias
  Cardiovascular collapse
  Hypotension
Neurologic
  Cerebral edema
  Central nervous system depression
  Seizures
Renal
  Myoglobinuria
  Renal failure
Miscellaneous
  Acid-base disorder
  Decubitus ulcers
  Hypothermia
  Sepsis

THE "NONTOXIC" INGESTION

Toxicity is a matter of degree, so that, in a sense, anything in excess may cause toxicity.[26] The substances listed in Table 1-21 are those that are relatively nontoxic and for which no treatment may be indicated.[27–29] Accidental ingestion of a substance known to be nontoxic may be dealt with by reassurance alone.

Simple antacids are generally nontoxic in a single acute ingestion. Antibiotics may, in general, cause diarrhea or an allergic reaction, but they do not typically cause any more serious medical problems.

Ballpoint pen inks of the black or blue variety contain tannic acid, gallic acid, and ferrous sul-

Table 1-21 Partial Listing of Nontoxic Substances

Pharmaceuticals
  Antacids
  Antibiotics
  Contraceptives
  Corticosteroids
  Laxatives
  Mineral oil
Household Products
  Ballpoint pen inks
  Bathtub floating toys
  Bath oil
  Candles
  Crayons
  Dehumidifying packets (silica gel)
  Deodorants
  Felt-tip pens
  Magic markers
  Matches
  Pencils
  Skin conditioners
  Teething rings
  Thermometers
  Toothpaste
Soaps and Detergents
  Bar soap
  Bath foam
  Bubble bath soap
  Fabric softeners
  Hair conditioners
Cosmetics
  Eye makeup
  Hand lotion
  Lipstick
  Makeup
  Perfume
  Suntan preparations
  Toilet water
Miscellaneous
  Chalk
  Clay
  Lubricating oil
  Motor oil
  Paint (water-based)
  Pistol caps
  Play Doh
  Starch
  Sweetening agents

fate and are nontoxic.[28] Purple, green, and red inks may contain aniline dyes, which are hazardous if taken in large amounts. Household bleach contains approximately 5% sodium hypochlorite and typically causes no more than erythema.[29] Candles contain beeswax or paraffin, which are inert.[27] Toy pistol caps and matches contain potassium chlorate, which in the amount that might be ingested is nontoxic.[27] Chalk contains calcium carbonate.[29] Corticosteroids do not cause toxicity from a single ingestion.[30] Crayons of the AP and CP markings are nontoxic.[29] Dehumidifying packets contain silica gel or charcoal.

Anionic and nonionic detergents are essentially nontoxic but are irritants and may cause vomiting and diarrhea.[30] Dishwasher or laundry detergents may contain surfactants and builders, which may be very toxic. Soaps are mild irritants that may affect the skin, eyes, or gastrointestinal tract; nausea, vomiting, and diarrhea are common after their ingestion, but mucosal erosion or ulceration does not occur. Cationic detergents are the most toxic of the detergents.

Mineral oil may cause diarrhea. Oral contraceptives can be regarded as nontoxic, although withdrawal bleeding may occur. Water-based paints must be distinguished from oil-based paints, in which the hydrocarbon solvents may be dangerous.

Pencils contain no lead but do contain graphite and coloring agents. The ingredients in Play Doh may be nontoxic, but the material may cause physical obstruction.[29] Solvents and most perfumes contain alcohol, but the small amounts ingested are rarely enough to cause harm.[30] Wet shampoos may cause nausea and vomiting, but dry shampoos may contain carbon tetrachloride, trichloroethylene, or other hydrocarbons that may result in systemic toxicity. Most shoe polishes contain no aniline dyes, but the ingestion of shoe polish may result in the development of methemoglobinemia. Teething rings and bathtub floating toys contain water and glycerin, which are not toxic; however, toxicity may develop from any pathogenic organisms that might be present. Toothpaste may contain stannous fluoride, which might cause nausea and vomiting.

PSYCHIATRIC EVALUATION

It is easy for emergency department personnel to become insensitive to the overdosed individual, who may be hard to handle and who may also be intoxicated with alcohol. Often it is forgotten that these individuals are in psychological distress. Although they may be difficult for emergency personnel to care for, these individuals need someone to talk with them and to try to calm them down.[31] If the physician and nurse taking care of the patient can spend that extra time, it might make it easier for all concerned. Medical professionals should regard the event with empathy and as an overreaction to a short-lived crisis that usually resolves.[32]

All patients who overdose should have psychiatric clearance before discharge, even if the overdose is minimal. Patients who overdose on a minimal amount of pills or other toxic substances are still trying to get the attention of someone. This should be investigated before their discharge to avoid the possibility that they will return later after a more successful attempt at massive overdose.

A patient who has attempted suicide may have a number of reasons for this behavior. It may represent a cry for help, the actual intent to die, an expression of anger, a means of conferring guilt on someone else, or an impulsive act of rage.[33] Any patient in whom suicidal ideation or intent is suspected should be questioned directly in this area.[33] Once a patient is assessed as being suicidal, he or she must not be left alone or sent home. Emergently, the patient should be prevented from escaping the emergency department and from hurting himself or herself or others.

Patients who are considered at high risk for suicide are those with a history of previous suicide attempts, older people living alone, individuals who have had a recent loss of employment or a spouse, or a person who has had a fight with a family member. There has been a recent dramatic increase in the rate of suicide among teenagers and young adults, particularly in young men 15 to 24 years old.[32]

The suicidal patient may exhibit certain classic symptoms indicating the intention to die, including leaving a suicide plan or note and giving away property. Suicidal risk is higher if the patient is strongly considering suicide and has thought of a specific way to accomplish it.

A full psychiatric evaluation is necessary to determine the suicidal status of the patient. This should begin with a mental status examination with assessment of orientation to time, place, and person.[34] Memory is also checked, including memory for recent events.[35] Direct questioning of the patient concerning suicidal thoughts and ideation should be attempted. The relatives or friends of the patient should also be questioned thoroughly.

SUMMARY

The overdosed patient many times represents a diagnostic dilemma in that there may be no way to obtain an accurate history of the preceding events. It is therefore important to use the clues obtained from a thorough physical examination. The establishment of an intravenous line and continuous cardiac monitoring in the potentially overdosed patient is considered good prophylactic care should the patient deteriorate or have an underlying dysrhythmia secondary to the ingested compound (Table 1-22).

Table 1-22 Summary of Generalized Treatment of the Overdosed Patient

Peripheral intravenous line
Continuous cardiac monitoring
Vital sign monitoring
History, including route of administration
Physical examination
Appropriate laboratory studies (see Chapter 4)
  Toxicology screen with selected blood levels
  Complete blood count
  Serum electrolytes
  Blood urea nitrogen
  Urinalysis
Administration of therapeutic agents
  Glucose
  Naloxone
  Oxygen
  Thiamine
Evacuation of stomach and intestine (see Chapter 2)
Administration of activated charcoal and cathartic (see Chapter 3)
Administration of an antidote if available
Psychiatric evaluation when medically cleared

REFERENCES

1. Arena J: The clinical diagnosis of poisoning. *Pediatr Clin North Am* 1970;17:477–494.

2. Kaufman R, Levy S: Overdose treatment. *JAMA* 1974;227:411–416.

3. Ficarra B: Toxicologic states treated in an emergency department. *Clin Toxicol* 1980;17:1–43.

4. Sunshine I: Basic toxicology. *Pediatr Clin North Am* 1970;17:509–513.

5. Oderda G, Klein-Schwartz W: General management of the poisoned patient. *Crit Care Q* 1982;4:1–18.

6. Saxena K, Kingston R: Acute poisoning—Management protocol. *Postgrad Med* 1982;71:67–77.

7. Sullivan J, Rumack B, Peterson R: Management of the poisoned patient in the emergency department: Poisonings and overdose. *Top Emerg Med* 1979;1:1–12.

8. Benowitz N, Rosenberg J, Becker C: Cardiopulmonary catastrophes in drug-overdosed patients. *Med Clin North Am* 1979;63:267–296.

9. Dine M, McGovern M: Intentional poisoning of children—An overlooked category of child abuse: Report of seven cases and review of literature. *Pediatrics* 1982; 70:32–35.

10. Gaudreault P, McCormick M, Lacouture P, et al: Poisoning exposures and use of ipecac in children less than 1 year old. *Ann Emerg Med* 1986;15:808–810.

11. Atwood S: The laboratory in the diagnosis and management of acetaminophen and salicylate intoxications. *Pediatr Clin North Am* 1980;27:871–879.

12. Cashman T, Shirkey H: Emergency management of poisoning. *Pediatr Clin North Am* 1970;17:525–534.

13. Nicholson D: The immediate management of overdose. *Med Clin North Am* 1983;67:1279–1293.

14. Goldberg M, Spector R, Park G, et al: An approach to the management of the poisoned patient. *Arch Intern Med* 1986;146:1381–1385.

15. Olson K, Pentel P, Kelley M: Physical assessment and differential diagnosis of the poisoned patient. *Med Toxicol* 1987;2:52–81.

16. Goldfrank L, Weisman R, Flomenbaum N: Teaching the recognition of odors. *Ann Emerg Med* 1982; 11:684–686.

17. Savitt D, Hawkins H, Roberts J: The radiopacity of ingested medications. *Ann Emerg Med* 1987;16:331–339.

18. Reed C, Driggs M, Foote C: Acute barbiturate intoxication: A study of 300 cases. *Ann Intern Med* 1952; 37:290–292.

19. Brett A, Rothschild N, Gray R, et al: Predicting the clinical course in intentional drug overdose. *Arch Intern Med* 1987;147:133–137.

20. Conner C, Robertson N, Murphrey K, et al: Rational use of emergency antidotes: Poisonings and overdose. *Top Emerg Med* 1979;1:27–41.

21. Meredith T, Caisley J, Volans G: Emergency drugs: Agents used in the treatment of poisoning. *Br Med J* 1984;289:742–747.

22. Litovitz T: The anecdotal antidotes. *Emerg Med Clin North Am* 1984;2:145–158.

23. Matthew H: Acute poisoning: Some myths and misconceptions. *Br Med J* 1971;1:519–522.

24. Wright N: Common errors in the management of poisoning. *J R Coll Physicians Lond* 1980;14:114–116.

25. Chaikin H: Rhabdomyolysis secondary to drug overdose and prolonged coma. *South Med J* 1980;73:990–994.

26. Brown J: Incomplete labeling of pharmaceuticals: A list of ''inactive'' ingredients. *N Engl J Med* 1983; 309:439–441.

27. Done A: Poisoning from common household products. *Pediatr Clin North Am* 1970;17:569–581.

28. Mofenson H, Greensher J: The nontoxic ingestion. *Pediatr Clin North Am* 1970;17:583–590.

29. Mofenson H, Greensher J, Caraccio T: Ingestions considered nontoxic. *Emerg Med Clin North Am* 1984; 2:159–174.

30. Henry J, Wiseman H: Non-poisons. *Br Med J* 1984;289:240–241.

31. Wagemaker H, Lippman S, Cade R: Acutely psychotic patients: A treatment approach. *South Med J* 1985;78:833–37.

32. McAlpine D: Suicide: Recognition and management. *Mayo Clin Proc* 1987;62:778–781.

33. Tavani-Petrone C: Psychiatric emergencies. *Primary Care* 1986;13:157–167.

34. Cavanaugh S: Psychiatric emergencies. *Med Clin North Am* 1986;70:1185–1202.

35. Anderson W, Kuehnle J: Diagnosis and early management of acute psychosis. *N Engl J Med* 1981; 305:1128–1130.

ADDITIONAL SELECTED REFERENCES

Barnes J: Toxic substances and the nervous system. *Sci Basis Med* 1969;183–201.

Cereda J, Scott J, Quigley E: Endoscopic removal of pharmacobezoar of slow release theophylline. *Br Med J* 1986;293:1143.

Comstock E, Stewart E: Current literature on medical toxicology. *Clin Toxicol* 1979;15:91–95.

Done A: For particulars on poisons. *Emerg Med* 1982; 14:102–104.

Eriksson M, Catz C, Yaffe S: Drugs and pregnancy. *Clin Obstet Gynecol* 1973;16:199–224.

Fazen L, Lovejoy F, Crone R: Acute poisoning in a children's hospital: A 2-year experience. *Pediatrics* 1986;77:144–151.

Gilles C, Ford P, Lovejoy F, et al: Management of pediatric poisoning. *Pediatr Nurs* 1980;6:33–44.

Gossel T, Wuest J: The right first aid for poisoning. *RN* 1981;44:73–75.

Keller E: Poisoning in children. *Postgrad Med* 1979; 65:177–186.

Walton W: An evaluation of the poison prevention packaging act. *Pediatrics* 1982;69:363–370.

Weisman R, Price D, Wald P: Outpatient management of acute and chronic poisoning. *Primary Care* 1986; 13:151–156.

White L, Driggers D, Wardinsky T: Poisoning in childhood and adolescence: A study of 111 cases admitted to a military hospital. *J Fam Pract* 1980;11:27–31.

Woolf A, Lewander W, Gilippone G, et al: Prevention of childhood poisoning: Efficacy of an educational program carried out in an emergency clinic. *Pediatrics* 1987;80:359–363.

Yaffe S, Sjoeqvist F, Alvan F: Pharmacological principles in the management of accidental poisoning. *Pediatr Clin North Am* 1970;17:495–507.

chapter 2

Methods of Preventing Absorption

Drugs and toxins may be absorbed through the skin, be ingested orally, or go directly into the systemic circulation with parenteral administration. The attempt at preventing absorption of a drug or toxin is of utmost priority in lessening the likelihood that subsequent toxicity will ensue.[1] This chapter discusses the various methods of preventing absorption of drugs and toxins. The major areas of discussion cover the role of skin decontamination, emetics, gastric lavage, activated charcoal, and cathartics in treating the poisoned patient.

SKIN DECONTAMINATION

There are a number of toxins that are absorbed through the skin. Skin decontamination in select cases should therefore not be overlooked because it may be the only method available to prevent further absorption of the toxin. Decontamination may not only be useful but in certain circumstances may be lifesaving. As an example, the organophosphates can be absorbed through the intact skin, and unless decontamination is performed continuous absorption will occur. Other toxins for which decontamination is both necessary and beneficial are listed in Table 2-1.

Skin decontamination may be carried out after attending to life-threatening problems. Decontamination may be performed with at least two soap-and-water washes. For most agents, protective clothing (gloves, gown, and mask) should be used to protect personnel from being contaminated.

GASTROINTESTINAL DECONTAMINATION

In the case of an overdose by ingestion, the generally accepted standard of care for the patient is an attempt at preventing further absorption of the toxin followed by the administration of activated charcoal and a cathartic.[2] Although this regimen has recently been questioned,[3,4] these methods are still advocated by many toxicologists. Other methods of decreasing gastrointestinal absorption have been whole gut lavage and removal of material by surgical or endoscopic intervention. This has occasionally been reported for foreign body removal, bezoars, or gastric concretions.[1,5,6]

EMETICS

Many methods have at one time been advocated to induce vomiting. Most have been discarded because evidence revealed that they were either potentially toxic or unreliable.[7] Although

Table 2-1 Toxins for Which Skin Decontamination Is Effective

Aniline dyes
Caustic agents
Cyanide
Dimethylsulfoxide
Hydrocarbons
Mace (CS, CN gas)
Methanol
Pesticides
Radiation

syrup of ipecac is considered the only acceptable emetic, the relative usefulness of other emetics is also briefly discussed below.

Syrup of Ipecac

Syrup of ipecac is the emetic of choice in both children over the age of 6 months and in adults.[2,7–9] Although ipecac has been known for many years as a potent emetic, its common usage as an antidotal agent in the treatment of accidental ingestion of poisons began in the 1960s.

Ipecac is the dried root of *Cephaelis ipecacuanha*, which is found in South and Central America.[1] The principal alkaloids of ipecac are emetine and cephaline.[10] Emetine, which constitutes more than one-half the total alkaloid, is cardiotoxic, while cephaline causes nausea and vomiting.[10] During the last few years, ipecac syrup has been prepared from powdered ipecac, not from the fluid extract that had been reported as the source of toxicity. The concentration of the alkaloid in the syrup is $1/14$ that of the powdered ipecac, which itself contains approximately 2% of the alkaloids emetine and cephaline. In the United States, ipecac is available without a prescription in 15- and 30-mL bottles. In two-thirds of the countries in Europe, it is available only by prescription.[11]

Mechanism of Action

Ipecac has a dual mechanism by which it causes an emesis; it acts both locally in the stomach and has a delayed effect on the chemoreceptor trigger zone located in the floor of the fourth ventricle.[1,10] The chemoreceptor trigger zone then activates the vomiting center located in the reticular formation, resulting in an emesis.[10,12] Early vomiting is due to the direct local irritant action of ipecac on the gastric mucosa, while late vomiting is a result of central stimulation of the vomiting center.[13,14]

Dosage

The therapeutic dose of syrup of ipecac for an adult is 30 mL. The suggested dose for children 6 months of age and older is 15 mL. This dose may be repeated in 20 to 30 minutes if necessary. Recently it has been shown that an initial dose of 30 mL in children produces an emesis significantly faster than the traditional dose. In addition, when 30 mL of syrup of ipecac is administered no repeat doses of the emetic may be necessary.[8]

Adjunctive Methods

After the initial dose of syrup of ipecac is administered, ingestion of fluids should be encouraged to empty the stomach more adequately: 12 to 16 ounces is recommended for an adult and 4 to 8 ounces for a child.[1,15] Larger volumes of fluids may be counterproductive because they may promote more rapid gastric emptying, placing the ingested toxin beyond retrieval. There also does not appear to be any benefit from walking compared to remaining stationary at bedrest.[16]

There is no difference in the speed at which emesis occurs if the fluid is administered before or after syrup of ipecac.[1] Although almost any available nontoxic liquid may be administered, milk is not recommended because it has been shown to increase significantly the time before onset of vomiting.[1,10,17] Carbonated beverages do not appear to have an adverse effect on the onset or amount of emesis.[18]

Repeating Ipecac

If the patient has received ipecac but has not had an effective emesis in 15 to 20 minutes, it is advisable to attempt to stimulate the gag reflex with a tongue blade before administering a second dose.[1] This stimulation may cause the desired emesis. In general, 60% of patients will have an emesis within the first 15 minutes and 90% will have an emesis within the first 30 minutes.[1,19–21] Although not recommended, even ipecac that is expired produces an emesis in a comparable period and is not accompanied by more severe side effects.[1,22]

Safety of Ipecac in Children

Syrup of ipecac is safe to use in children older than 6 months of age and, when used properly, should not exacerbate the patient's condition.[8,11,12,19] The use of ipecac syrup in infants younger than 6 months of age is generally not advocated because of risk of aspiration, although there are no data to substantiate this concern.[1,23,24]

Ipecac and Antiemetics

Many of the phenothiazine derivatives are effective antiemetics and are believed to act centrally by depression of the vomiting center in the medulla. Ipecac has been shown, however, to be effective for these antiemetics, probably as a result of its direct irritant action on the gastrointestinal tract.[8,10,19,20] Thus the same initial dose should be administered.[1] If the patient has had a documented antiemetic overdose and there has been no effective emesis within a reasonable period of time, the ipecac and the ingested material should be retrieved by means of gastric lavage.

Ipecac and Activated Charcoal

Although it has been assumed that activated charcoal and syrup of ipecac should not be administered at the same time because of the adsorption of ipecac by the charcoal,[1,25] it has been shown that a 10-minute interval between the administration of 60 mL of syrup of ipecac and activated charcoal prevents the inhibition of the emetic properties of ipecac and allows a successful emesis to occur.[26,27] Nevertheless, more documentation as to whether conventional amounts of ipecac would also be effective is necessary before this method is advocated.

Disadvantages of Ipecac

The prolonged time to emesis is the major disadvantage of ipecac syrup because the delay results in continued absorption of the ingested toxin.[1] In addition, it may delay the administration of activated charcoal. Because prolonged vomiting after administration of syrup of ipecac has been a frequent problem, attempts have been made to shorten the time of emesis. In one report the intravenous use of prochlorperazine (Compazine®) as an effective and safe treatment was described.[28] Because experience with this method is lacking, it can be neither advocated nor condemned. One potential disadvantage of this regimen might be the potential side effects associated with this antiemetic.

Specific toxins with rapid absorption that can lead to early central nervous system disturbance or cardiovascular dysfunction are best treated by immediate removal from the gastrointestinal tract. Examples of such toxins are strychnine, tricyclic antidepressants, cyanide, camphor, propoxyphene, the rapidly acting barbiturates, and toxic liquids.[5]

Toxicity of Ipecac

Clinically significant toxicity from the use of syrup of ipecac is unusual, and there are few reports of serious toxicity directly attributable to the use of the emetic in recommended doses.[8,10,15,29,30] Side effects, including diarrhea and mild drowsiness, are minimal with therapeutic doses.[1,15,20,31–34] Rare reports of gastrointestinal side effects from the fluid extract include hemorrhage and ulceration of the small bowel, gastritis, and recently a Mallory-Weiss syndrome.[35] Diarrhea due to increased peristalsis caused by emetine as well as to local irritation of the mucosa of the gastrointestinal tract has been noted.[1]

Chronic Ipecac Toxicity

General Considerations

Ipecac alkaloid toxicity primarily involves the gastrointestinal tract and cardiovascular and neuromuscular systems.[36] In very large doses, when fluid extract was mistakenly given in place of syrup of ipecac, or with chronic administration of the syrup, reports of central nervous system depression and of cardiovascular effects, including tachycardia, hypotension, and electrocardiographic abnormalities have been noted.[12]

Syrup of ipecac may be chronically abused by patients with anorexia nervosa and bulimia nervosa.[15,32] This has resulted in cumulative toxicity from the various alkaloids in ipecac. Syrup of ipecac has been implicated as the causal factor in the deaths of several women with bulimia and anorexia who used it on a long-term basis to induce vomiting after eating binges.[37] This drug is chosen because it is a relatively inexpensive, nonprescription item that is effective in producing an emesis.[15] Patients with these eating disorders may use the drug daily in doses that are higher than recommended and over a long period of time. Because the rate of excretion of emetine is slow, the ingestion of daily oral doses may produce an accumulation that approaches the single fatal parenteral dose.[15]

Neuromuscular Manifestations of Chronic Toxicity

The neuromuscular manifestations of ingestion of emetine are weakness, aching, tenderness, and stiffness of the skeletal muscles, particularly those in the proximal extremities and the neck.[12,32] Myopathy has developed in patients who chronically used excessive doses for weight reduction. This has been found to be reversible unless complicated by cardiovascular toxicity.[17,37,38] Other signs of neuromuscular toxicity include skeletal muscular weakness, tremor, and generalized tonic-clonic seizures. The neuromuscular toxicities may be caused by a block of norepinephrine released by acetylcholine at adrenergic nerve terminals (Table 2-2).[39]

Cardiovascular Manifestations of Chronic Toxicity

Signs of cardiovascular toxicity from emetine include electrocardiographic abnormalities such as alterations in the QRS duration, ST and T wave alterations, prolongation of the PR interval, and atrial prematurity.[32] This is due to decreased metabolic activity, which results in a

Table 2-2 Potential Toxic Effects of Ipecac

Acute Administration
General
  Emesis
  Drowsiness (mild)
Gastrointestinal
  Mallory-Weiss tears
  Diarrhea
  Vomiting
Chronic Administration
Neuromuscular
  Weakness
  Muscle aches
  Muscle tenderness
  Tremor
  Seizure
Cardiovascular
Electrocardiographic abnormalities
  Atrial premature contractions
  ST-T wave changes
  QRS prolongation
  Prolongation of PR interval
Cardiomyopathy

decrease in contractile function in the myocardium.[12,15,40] The delay in clinical signs is attributable to the time required for the inhibition of the biosynthesis of new contractile proteins.

Pneumomediastinum and retropneumoperitoneum have also been reported.[29,37] Both these events occur after prolonged vomiting. Syrup of ipecac, when used in appropriate doses, should not cause any of the above problems.

Methods Not Advocated

There are several methods of inducing emesis that are contraindicated (Table 2-3).

Mechanical Induction

An attempt at mechanical pharyngeal stimulation with a finger or other blunt object is a simple

Table 2-3 Contraindicated Methods To Induce Emesis

Mechanical induction
Salt water
Copper sulfate
Mustard water
Detergents and soaps
Apomorphine

method that may produce an emesis, but the volume produced is small.[1] This method has been ineffective for adequate retrieval of toxin and has the potential of causing physical harm; therefore its use is not recommended.[8,40]

Salt Water

At one time salt water was recommended as an emetic, and although an effective emesis may occur serious side effects have been found with its use.[1] Electrolyte disorders, such as fatal hypernatremia, seizures, and intestinal damage, have occurred. Because of the nonuniformity of the product and the side effects, salt water is considered too dangerous and is therefore contraindicated.

Copper Sulfate

Copper sulfate is an irritant to the gastrointestinal tract and typically will cause an emesis. When absorbed, however, copper sulfate has the ability to produce severe renal and hepatic toxicity.[1,42] Copper sulfate has led to elevated serum copper levels, raising the possibility of copper toxicity. Because of its local corrosive effect, which has caused mucosal erosions and a hemorrhagic gastroenteritis, and its potential for systemic toxicity, its use is also contraindicated.[43]

Mustard Water

Mustard water is difficult to induce patients to drink. In addition it is unreliable as an emetic, and time should not be wasted with its administration.

Detergents and Soaps

The emetic response to soaps is thought to be the result of gastrointestinal irritation rather than stimulation of the chemoreceptor trigger zone. Although anionic detergents (soaps) may be useful in causing emesis and have a rather quick emetic response,[1,14,44] confusion may arise as to what product should be used and the more corrosive detergents may be easily mistaken for anionic soaps. This confusion might lead to a more dangerous detergent being administered. For example, liquid soaps used for dishes (such as Palmolive®) may only cause nausea and

vomiting, while dishwasher soaps (such as Electrosol® and Cascade®) have corrosive properties due to the alkaline builders such as the sodium salts of phosphates, carbonates, metasilicates, and silicates. The general pH ranges of automatic dishwasher detergents is from 10.5 to 12.0.[45] Industrial strength detergents and the new liquid products may have pH values as high as 13.0. This confusion may be even more dangerous now that liquid dishwasher soaps are available. For this reason, the use of soaps as a routine measure for inducing emesis should be avoided.

Apomorphine

Apomorphine is a morphine congener prepared by reacting morphine with a strong mineral acid.[1] It induces emesis in a relatively short period of time by stimulation of the chemoreceptor trigger zone in the medulla oblongata. It is inactive if administered orally.[10]

The advantage of this drug is that it can be administered intramuscularly to an uncooperative patient who would refuse orally administered ipecac. The usual dose is 0.1 mg/kg to a maximum of 6 mg in adults or 0.07 mg/kg in children.[1] It offers a high degree of success, with a latency period averaging 5 minutes, and promotes a forceful emesis with reflux of the proximal small bowel contents.[10] There is also a high incidence of serious side effects relating to the drug's narcotic-like action, however, including CNS depression, apnea, and hypotension in previously nondepressed individuals.[10] In addition, these individuals may have a variable response to the narcotic antagonist naloxone.

Apomorphine is unstable in solution and must be prepared for injection by placing a tablet in a syringe, dissolving it in normal saline, and then sterilizing the solution before use.[1,19] With so many potential dangers and disadvantages, its use is not recommended.[46,47]

GASTRIC LAVAGE

Gastric lavage is another method for removing substances from the stomach. Gastric lavage can be considered essentially equal to the use of syrup of ipecac in the amount of material retrieved,[48] although this has long been an area of controversy, with many studies showing conflicting results.[5,7,19,48–50] If gastric lavage is used, it should be accomplished with the largest tube that can be passed through the oropharynx. An orogastric tube 26F to 28F or larger for children and 32F to 40F for adults should be chosen.[5,51,52] The Ewald tube, a soft rubber tube with a single distal aperture, is considered less effective than other tubes with additional lateral holes.[5] The tube should therefore have a number of lateral holes.[1] Large-bore oral tubes increase the return of pill fragments, decrease the likelihood of tube occlusion, and increase the rapidity with which gastric lavage is performed.

Technique of Lavage

The technique of lavage involves placing the patient in the Trendelenburg, left lateral decubitus position with knees flexed, which should give maximal abdominal wall relaxation and maximal gastric emptying.[1,5,50,53] In addition, this position has been suggested to reduce the risk of aspiration should vomiting occur.

The lavage tube should be advanced gently. After it is inserted, it is essential to determine that it is correctly placed before initiating the lavage. Proper location of the tube in the stomach can be assessed by auscultating the stomach while injecting air into the tube.[5] Coughing, cyanosis, or respiratory distress may indicate that the tube has entered the larynx. Aspiration of the stomach contents confirms its proper location. If the patient has demonstrated an intact gag reflex, lavage may be performed without prior endotracheal intubation. If the patient has lost the gag reflex, and this is associated with CNS depression, then adequate protection of the airway should be performed before lavage.

Typically, a passive lavage system can be used. The stomach should be completely aspirated until no return is obtained.[5] In an adult, tap water can be safely used[54] because there are no resultant changes in serum electrolytes or serum osmolality.[53] Lavage is then begun with 50 mL of warm tap water instilled into the stomach and retrieved. After repeating this procedure, 200-mL to 300-mL aliquots of warm saline or warm tap water are then flushed down the large-bore tube and retrieved either by suction or by lowering the tube to the floor and siphoning out the effluent.[53] For pediatric patients, the amount of saline during each lavage is 10 mL/kg.[1,5] For adults, larger aliquots (300 to 500 mL) are preferable to smaller aliquots (50 mL) in that the distension of the stomach can inhibit stomach contractions, and the larger aliquots tend to open up the rugae in the stomach so that pills, pill fragments, or other toxic substances in the rugal folds are exposed.[1,53] Warm lavage solution is recommended because it can increase the rate of dissolution of pills while also decreasing gastric peristalsis, thereby decreasing the potential loss of medication through the pylorus.[52] The patient is lavaged until there is a clear return, and for a greater margin of safety 1 or 2 L more lavage solution should then be instilled and retrieved.[5,53] Generally, 5 to 20 L of fluid is required.[1]

A left upper quadrant massage is recommended when there is the possibility of a drug that can cause concretions (Table 2-6).[54] The massage is an attempt to loosen existing or potential concretions. Although this method is empiric and anecdotal, there does not appear to be any harm associated with its use, and there is good possibility for benefit.

Complications of Lavage

Although rare, there is the possibility for significant complications from an attempt at lavage.[51,55] Laryngospasm, cyanosis, aspiration of stomach contents, gastric erosion, and esophageal tears may be caused by the lavage tube (Table 2-4).[1,5,56] Epistaxis may occur after gastric lavage if the tube has been placed through the nose. Mediastinitis can be a potentially devastating complication.[5] A case of Legionnaires'

Table 2-4 Complications of Lavage

Aspiration
Cyanosis
Gastric erosion
Epistaxis
Esophageal tears
Laryngospasm
Mediastinitis

---

disease caused by *Legionella pneumophila* was documented after an 18-year-old male aspirated postgastric lavage fluid when tap water was used.[41]

CONTRAINDICATIONS FOR IPECAC OR LAVAGE

In addition to the complications that are possible from the use of lavage or ipecac, there are also contraindications for their use.[11] Neither should be used to retrieve any agent that might burn the gastrointestinal tract because an additional burn may occur. In the absence of other neurologic signs and symptoms, an absent gag reflex should not be considered a contraindication to emesis because a demonstrable gag reflex is not present in a significant percentage of normal people.[1] Ipecac should not be administered, however, to a patient who has *lost* the gag reflex, and the patient should only be lavaged after the airway has been protected with a cuffed endotracheal tube. In addition, hydrocarbons such as kerosene, gasoline, coal oil, fuel oil, paint thinner, cleaning fluid, and furniture polish should, for the most part, be left in the gastrointestinal tract (Table 2-5).

WHOLE GUT LAVAGE

Another method that has been suggested but has not met with wide acceptance is whole gut lavage or whole bowel irrigation.[57–61] This procedure has been successfully used for bowel preparation before major surgical resections of bowel and has also been useful in removing heavy objects (such as lead pellets) and iron pills from the gastrointestinal tract.[61] Nevertheless, a significant fraction of the solution may be absorbed and result in rapid weight gain. This method of cleaning the colon may therefore be dangerous in patients who are unable to excrete salt and water loads normally.

Proponents of this method suggest seating the patient on a commode and instilling lactated Ringer's solution (30 to 300 mL/min) via a nasogastric tube until a total of 4 to 6 L of fluid has been administered. Emptying begins approximately 8 to 10 minutes after the pro-

Table 2-5 Substances for Which Ipecac or Lavage Are Contraindicated

Caustic Agents
Acids
Alkalis
Ammonia
Coffee pot cleaners
Drain cleaners
Automatic dishwasher detergent
Hair bleaches
Lye
Metal cleaners
Mildew removers
Oven cleaners
Rust removers
Toilet bowl cleaners
Wart removers
Petroleum Distillates
Furniture polish
Gasoline
Kerosene
Linseed oil
Lighter fluid
Mineral spirits
Naphtha
Oils
Paint and lacquer thinners
Petroleum solvents
Pine oil cleaners
Turpentine
Wood stains

cedure has begun, and there should be a clear return after 20 to 25 minutes. Such a method is not recommended because of the lack of experience of most physicians in its use and because it appears to be awkward and cumbersome. Another major concern is that a significant fraction of the solution may be absorbed, resulting in fluid overload with a weight gain of 1.5 to 2.5 kg being noted on occasion.[58] A balanced electrolyte solution with added polyethylene glycol has been manufactured for this purpose and has been termed Golytely solution.[58]

CONCRETIONS

Concretions may form from the ingestion of certain drugs and may possibly explain why a patient may have continual absorption when it was thought that the gastrointestinal tract was adequately emptied. The possibility of concretions should always be considered when patients do not respond to adequate therapy or when blood concentrations of the toxin do not diminish as expected. Concretion may also explain why a patient may have a waxing and waning clinical status.

Concretions usually develop after the ingestion of a large number of pills or capsules in a short period of time.[43,52,62] There appears to be little relationship between the drug's chemical nature and the fact that it can cause concretions.[5,6] Drugs that can cause concretions are listed in Table 2-6. The method of massage of the left upper quadrant described above is an attempt to break up these concretions so that they are more easily solubilized and retrieved. That a drug may cause a concretion has no relation to its degree of radiopacity. Gastroscopy and even gastrotomy may be required to remove a toxic concretion.[1,5,63]

ACTIVATED CHARCOAL

General Considerations

There is an incomplete return with the use of either ipecac or lavage. Although this incomplete return may represent material absorbed from the intestine, it also represents material still present in the gastrointestinal tract. Because of this incomplete return, it is important that additional methods be attempted to decrease the absorption of the material still remaining in the gastrointestinal tract. This is accomplished through the use of activated charcoal and a cathartic.[64]

Activated charcoal or activated carbon is a residue from the distillation of various organic materials such as sawdust, wood, paper, and bone. Most carbon-based compounds can be converted to activated charcoal, which is "activated" by heating with steam, oxygen, and acids at temperatures in excess of 600°C in the absence of air.[1,65–67] This activation process not only cleans the charcoal but expands each grain, producing a fine network of external and internal pores that increase the surface area of the material and thereby its adsorptive power. The size and number of pores that develop determine the surface area of the activated charcoal and its adsorptive capacity.[65,67] Activated charcoal adsorbs toxic substances within the gastrointestinal tract, forming an activated charcoal-toxin complex and thus preventing absorption of the toxin.[68,69] The adsorption of a toxin to charcoal is a reversible process, and with prolonged gastrointestinal transit time the process may shift toward desorption.[26]

Activated charcoal is a safe, effective, and inexpensive gastrointestinal adsorbent and is universally advocated for adsorbing a wide range of chemicals, including alkaloids, salicylates, barbiturates, phenothiazines, tricyclic antidepressants, sulfonamides, and selected inorganic compounds in nonionized form (Table 2-7).[3,65,70–74] In general, most drugs and household products are adsorbed well enough for the administration of activated charcoal to be clinically useful. The substance is ineffective for inorganic compounds in ionic form, such as mineral acids and bases, boric acid, cyanide, ferrous sulfate, lithium, and other small ionized molecules (Table 2-8).[1,5,65] In addition, there may be times when an interaction of the charcoal with therapeutic methods may be detrimental, such as with N-acetylcysteine in the treatment of acetaminophen poisoning. There are, however, no absolute contraindications for its use.

Activated charcoal is an inert, fine, black, odorless, tasteless powder with a gritty consistency.[75–77] It is available as a powder, can be supplied as an aqueous charcoal slurry, or can be mixed with water before administration to make an aqueous slurry.[64] In addition, activated charcoal is marketed as a suspension of 20% activated charcoal in 70% sorbitol. This is also a bacteriostatic concentration of sorbitol.[1,78–81] Activated charcoal can be instilled into the stomach through a lavage tube or a nasogastric tube.

Table 2-6 Substances Causing Concretions (Acronym: BIG MESS)

B	Barbiturates
I	Iron
G	Glutethimide
M	Meprobamate
E	Extended-Release Theophylline
SS	Salicylates

Table 2-7 Substances Adsorbed by Activated Charcoal

Acetaminophen	Glutethimide	Phenolphthalein
Aconitine	Hexachlorophene	Phenothiazines
Alcohol	Imipramine	Phenylbutazone
Amphetamines	Iodine	Phenylpropanolamine
Antimony	Ipecac	Phenytoin
Antipyrine	Isoniazid	Phosphorus
Arsenic	Kerosene	Potassium
Atropine	Malathion	Primaquine
Barbiturates	Mefenamic acid	Probenecid
Camphor	Meprobamate	Propantheline
Cantharides	Mercuric chloride	Propoxyphene
Carbamazepine	Methotrexate	Quinacrine
Chlordane	Methyl salicylate	Quinidine
Chloroquine	Methylene blue	Quinine
Chlorpheniramine	Morphine	Salicylamide
Chlorpromazine	Muscarine	Salicylates
Cocaine	Narcotics	Selenium
Colchicine	Nicotine	Silver
Dapsone	Nortriptyline	Stramonium
2,4-Dichlorophenoxyacetic acid	Opium	Strychnine
Digitalis	Oxalates	Sulfonamides
Digitoxin	Paracetamol	Theophylline
Diphenylhydantoin	Parathion	Tricyclic antidepressants
Ergotamine	Penicillin	
Ethchlorvynol	Phenobarbital	

Source: Adapted with permission from *Clinical Pediatrics* (1985;24:678–684), Copyright © 1985, JB Lippincott Company.

If the patient is conscious and cooperative it can be administered orally. Activated charcoal is most effective when administered early in treatment.[24]

Dosage

Activated charcoal is an excellent adsorbent and will adsorb not only the poison but also other substances.[71,72] It does not appear to adsorb sorbitol or magnesium sulfate. For this reason, activated charcoal should be administered after ipecac has induced vomiting,[20] although a recent study suggests that there is no interference with the efficacy of ipecac when 60 mL of the emetic is administered initially.[25]

A dose of activated charcoal that provides a charcoal-to-poison ratio of 10:1 ensures optimal binding. Because estimates of ingested doses of toxin are often inaccurate, an arbitrary dose of 1 to 2 g of activated charcoal per kilogram of body weight is recommended.[1,5,65,78,79,82] In addition, the presence of food in the stomach may actually enhance the adsorption of drugs by

activated charcoal, possibly by giving more time for drugs to be absorbed[1,80]; this is a controversial finding, however.

The activated charcoal slurry should be mixed with 60 to 90 mL of water and should be stirred constantly to ensure uniform distribution and

Table 2-8 Substances with Little or No Adsorption by Activated Charcoal

Alkali
Boric acid
Cyanide
DDT
Ferrous sulfate
Mineral acids
N-Methyl carbamate
Potassium hydroxide
Sodium hydroxide
Sodium metasilicate
Tolbutamide

Source: Adapted with permission from *Clinical Pediatrics* (1985;24:678–684), Copyright © 1985, JB Lippincott Company.

delivery of the full dose to the patient. Because activated charcoal sticks to the walls of a bottle during storage, the bottle should be rinsed.[78] Sealed aqueous suspensions of activated charcoal can be stored for at least 1 year without measurable loss of activity.[83]

Activated charcoal USP, Norit-A®, Nuchar®, Actidose®, and Superchar® are among the many acceptable charcoal preparations (Table 2-9).[1,83] Tablets of activated charcoal are ineffective because once activated charcoal is compressed into a tablet its effective surface area is drastically lowered, the result being a much less effective adsorbent than an equal amount of granular activated charcoal.[1] The adsorptive capacity of the pills is not restored by crushing or chewing the tablets.[84]

Superactivated Charcoal

A superactivated charcoal preparation appears to have a greater adsorption capability in vitro than regular activated charcoal.[65,85] This substance, commercially available as Superchar®, has an extremely large internal surface area, two to three times that of regular activated charcoal.[66] This substance may reduce the quantities of activated charcoal required yet still provide the same adsorptive capacity as regular activated charcoal.[66]

Factors Limiting Use

The factors limiting the use of activated charcoal are inconvenience of admixture and the

---

Table 2-9 Activated Charcoal Preparations by Trade Name

Acta-Char
Actidose
Adsorba
Arm-a-char
Charcoaid
Insta-char
Norit-A
Nuchar
Superchar

---

repugnant and unpalatable physical characteristics of the substance.[67] There may be problems with patient compliance because the black color of the slurry, its gritty texture, and its tendency to adhere to the throat all tend to limit its acceptability. The use of activated charcoal is strongly recommended, however, because it may adsorb much of the compound still remaining in the gastrointestinal tract. Besides acting as an adsorbent, activated charcoal can also serve as a fecal marker, providing evidence that the poison has passed through the gastrointestinal tract. Contrary to popular belief, activated charcoal taken orally does not appear to induce emesis unless syrup of ipecac has been administered earlier.[86]

The time of administration of activated charcoal is influenced by whether ipecac-induced emesis or gastric lavage is used to empty the gastrointestinal tract of poison. In many patients, activated charcoal may not be tolerated for some time after ipecac-induced vomiting, which constitutes a serious drawback to the use of ipecac.

Attempts To Increase Palatability

Thickening agents such as bentonite (2.5 g per 10 g of activated charcoal) and sodium carboxymethylcellulose have been suggested as additives to activated charcoal.[1,87] These agents can provide a smooth yet tasteless consistency that may enhance patient compliance without interfering with the binding capacity of the activated charcoal.[35]

Most attempts at flavoring charcoal or mixing it with ice cream have met with little success because most of these flavoring agents are well adsorbed by the charcoal and thereby decrease its available binding sites.[67,87] The addition of sorbitol appears to improve palatability more than aqueous solutions and does not compromise the efficacy of the activated charcoal.[1,67,81,88]

Safety of Activated Charcoal

Activated charcoal has been investigated for inherent toxicity on skin contact, via inhalation, and during ingestion. No detectable harmful effects have been noted on prolonged skin contact,[76] and inhalation has also produced no significant toxic effects.[77] If charcoal were aspirated into the lungs, the particles would remain inert and would not produce an inflammatory reaction.[72] It can therefore be considered a safe, inert, nontoxic material.

Activated Charcoal As a Sole Agent for Decontamination

The use of activated charcoal as a sole means for preventing absorption of an ingested compound is a subject of much research. Some investigators have questioned the utility of gastric emptying procedures unless performed within 1 hour of ingestion in obtunded patients.[3] Although this should be kept in mind, further studies are needed to confirm this conclusion. There are conflicting reports concerning the role of activated charcoal as the sole agent for preventing absorption of a toxin,[89] and until further work is performed it would not be prudent to limit treatment of the overdosed patient solely to activated charcoal. Until that time, when not contraindicated, emesis or lavage should be induced because the patient's history may be inaccurate, gastric motility may be reduced, or concretions of the drug may have been formed in the stomach. Some investigators believe that gastric emptying has value up to 24 hours after ingestion of certain long-acting compounds.[1,65] In view of the efficacy and safety of activated charcoal, however, it is in the best interests of the patient to begin this treatment as quickly as possible after admission to the emergency department.

Multiple-Dose Activated Charcoal

In addition to the role of activated charcoal as an adsorbent for ingested material, there also appears to be a role for its use with toxins that undergo enterohepatic or enterogastric circulation.[9,90] Drugs such as digitalis, tricyclic antidepressants, and phencyclidine undergo either enterohepatic circulation or secretion into the stomach, and the activated charcoal remaining in the small intestine expedites the removal of the toxic substance from the body by binding the drug within the lumen of the small intestine, thereby making it unavailable for reabsorption.[65] Therefore, repeated doses of activated charcoal without a cathartic,[90] also known as pulse charcoal, may further decrease drug absorption if the drug undergoes enterogastric or enterohepatic recirculation (Table 2-10).[9] Intestinal dialysis can also be used to increase the clearance of certain drugs through repeated doses of activated charcoal.[65,67,80,90–92] This is discussed further in Chapter 3.

"Universal Antidote"

Activated charcoal should not be confused with the "universal antidote," for which there are two preparations: (1) the hospital preparation is a mixture of activated charcoal, magnesium oxide, and tannic acid; (2) the household preparation consists of burnt toast, tea, and Milk of Magnesia.[93] In theory, the "universal antidote" has a three-way action, with (1) adsorption of the toxic substance by the activated charcoal or burnt toast, (2) a neutralization and precipitation of acidic poisons by the magnesium oxide or Milk of Magnesia, and (3) neutralization and precipitation of alkaline poisons by the tannic acid or tea. In actual practice the "universal antidote" is less effective in detoxifying drugs than is activated charcoal alone, and there is the potential for toxicity from the tannic acid. This combination is therefore useless and potentially dangerous and should not be used.[1,93]

Table 2-10 Drugs for Which Multiple-Dose Activated Charcoal May Be of Benefit

---

Carbamazepine (Tegretol®)
Cyclic antidepressants
Dapsone
Digitoxin
Glutethimide (Doriden®)
Meprobamate (Equanil®, Miltown®)
Nadolol (Corgard®)
Phenobarbital
Phenylbutazone (Azolid®, Butazolidin®)
Theophylline

CATHARTICS

The rationale for cathartics is to decrease the toxin's intestinal transit time, thus minimizing the availability of nonabsorbed toxin for gut absorption.

Cathartics are typically categorized as stimulant or osmotic.[94] The stimulant cathartics include cascara, castor oil, bisacodyl, senna, and phenolphthalein; they act by increasing peristalsis and also increase secretion of enteral fluid. The osmotic cathartics are of greater interest and use in toxicology. They are generally classified as saline or saccharide cathartics. Although controlled studies have demonstrated the effectiveness of activated charcoal in decreasing serum levels of many toxins, the use of a cathartic is based primarily on empiric and anecdotal evidence.[90,94] Most toxicologists agree with the use of a cathartic as a method of decreasing gastrointestinal transit time of the toxin and thereby of decreasing the likelihood that the toxin will be absorbed.[94,95]

Saline Cathartics

The saline cathartics include the magnesium and sodium cathartics such as magnesium sulfate, citrate, and hydroxide and sodium sulfate and phosphate (Table 2-11). These agents produce catharsis on an osmotic basis by causing a large volume of fluid to be retained in the stomach, which leads to an increase of small bowel peristalsis, decreases toxin transit time, and causes defecation.[64,69,94]

The intraluminal wall of the small intestine acts as a semipermeable membrane to magnesium and its salts, retaining most of these osmotic ions in the gut.[10] The osmotic character of the saline cathartics draws fluids intraluminally. Theoretically, the extra fluid from the gastrointestinal blood supply creates a "bulk" or diarrheal state. This state activates peristalsis and propulsion.[10] In actuality, the mechanisms may be more complex.[69]

In the past, magnesium sulfate (Epsom salts) has been the cathartic of choice.[96] Its advantages are that it is readily available and that, unless the magnesium ion represents a hazard, it can be given in liberal doses. An adult can be given 15 to 30 g as a 10% solution along with the activated charcoal because there is no significant adsorption of the cathartic to the charcoal. The pediatric dose of magnesium sulfate is 250 mg/kg.[1,90] Hypermagnesemia may be a consequence of using multiple-dose magnesium cathartics in the patient with renal impairment as well as in the patient with normal renal function.[90,96]

It was once thought that phosphate was poorly absorbed from the colon and that phosphate enemas could be safely used as cathartics. Disodium phosphate solutions have produced significant morbidity and mortality, however, including hyperphosphatemia with resultant hypocalcemia when used in excessive amounts in children; their use is therefore not recommended.[95,97]

Saccharide Cathartics

The saccharide cathartics are sorbitol, mannitol, and lactulose.[90] Recently, sorbitol has been shown to be more efficacious than some of the other available cathartics.

Sorbitol, a hexahydric alcohol that is 50% to 60% as sweet as sucrose, has been suggested as an additive to activated charcoal to make it more palatable.[80] Although in the past saline cathartics were recommended, many toxicologists are now preferring sorbitol as the cathartic of choice because the combination of sorbitol and acti-

Table 2-11 Saline and Saccharide Cathartics and Their Dosages

Drug	Dosage
Sorbitol	Adult: 100 to 150 mL of 70% solution
	Child: 1 to 2 mL/kg of 70% solution
Magnesium sulfate (Epsom salts)	Adult: 15 to 30 g
	Child: 250 mg/kg
Magnesium citrate	Adult: 15 to 30 g
	Child: 250 mg/kg
Sodium sulfate (Glauber's solution)	Adult: 15 to 30 g
	Child: 250 mg/kg
Disodium phosphate (Fleets® enema)	15 to 30 mL diluted 1:4

vated charcoal has been demonstrated to be more effective in producing a stool in a shorter period of time compared to saline cathartics.[74,78,79,90,96] After an orally administered dose it is slowly absorbed and metabolized to fructose; that which remains in the gut acts osmotically to draw free water into the lumen and cause diarrhea.[78–80,90]

The addition of sorbitol to activated charcoal imparts sweetness to the suspension, and its viscosity may mask the grittiness of the charcoal and maintains the particles in suspension for a prolonged period of time without reducing the adsorptive properties of the charcoal.[81,98] Sorbitol has also been shown to enhance the antidotal activity of charcoal when the two are combined; its use is therefore recommended by an increasing number of toxicologists,[62] and sorbitol is now commercially available. The dose is 1 to 2 mL/kg administered as a 70% solution (Table 2-11).[65,78,79] Toxicity from sorbitol is unlikely to occur unless there has been improper or overly aggressive use, as when it is used too frequently in patients being treated with multiple-dose activated charcoal or in excessive amounts in the pediatric patient.[80]

Contraindications

Although there are no documented reports of severe toxicity from the use of cathartics in the treatment of poisoning, a cathartic should be avoided with patients who have adynamic ileus because they may not respond[95]. A patient with diarrhea does not require a cathartic. A patient who overdoses and has concomitant intestinal obstruction (a rare circumstance) should not be given a cathartic because it may worsen the patient's condition and cause a perforation of the intestine.

In a patient with potential myoglobinuria and subsequent renal failure, a saline cathartic other than the magnesium salt should be selected.[1] Sodium cathartics should be avoided in patients in whom restricted salt intake is indicated and in patients with a history of congestive heart failure.[94] Oil-base cathartics such as castor oil or mineral oil, which are advocated by some (especially after an ingestion of glutethimide), are contraindicated because they may be hazardous if aspirated.[1] Finally, a cathartic should be used cautiously in the very young and the very old.

SUMMARY

Attempts at preventing absorption of a compound may be the most important aspect of the early care of the poisoned patient. Preventing the absorption of an orally ingested material consists of ipecac or lavage followed by activated charcoal and a cathartic. Because of the importance of using activated charcoal and the prolonged vomiting that occurs secondary to administration of ipecac, gastric lavage is advocated in significant overdoses if carried out in a timely fashion. Although magnesium sulfate had previously been the cathartic of choice, sorbitol now appears to be superior. Finally, there is an increasing importance being ascribed to the administration of activated charcoal both as single therapy and, in select cases, in a multiple-dose regimen.

REFERENCES

1. Rodgers G, Matyunas N: Gastrointestinal decontamination for acute poisoning. *Pediatr Clin North Am* 1986; 33:261–285.

2. Gaudreault P, McCormick M, Lacouture P, et al: Poisoning exposures and use of ipecac in children less than 1 year old. *Ann Emerg Med* 1986;15:808–810.

3. Kulig K, Bar-Or D, Cantrill S, et al: Management of acutely poisoned patients without gastric emptying. *Ann Emerg Med* 1985;14:562–567.

4. Tenenbein M, Cohen S, Sitar D: Efficacy of ipecac-induced emesis, or gastric lavage, and activated charcoal for acute drug overdose. *Ann Emerg Med* 1987;16:838–841.

5. Lanphear W: Gastric lavage. *J Emerg Med* 1986; 4:43–47.

6. North D: Meprobamate and bezoar formation. *Ann Emerg Med* 1987;16:472–473.

7. Corby D, Decker W, Moran M, et al: Clinical comparison of pharmacologic emetics in childhood. *Pediatrics* 1968;42:361–364.

8. Dean B, Krenzelok E: Syrup of ipecac: 15 mL versus 30 mL in pediatric poisonings. *Clin Toxicol* 1985; 23:165–170.

9. Neuvonen P: Clinical pharmacokinetics of oral activated charcoal in acute intoxications. *Clin Pharmacokinet* 1982;7:465–489.

10. Wheeler-Usher D, Wanke L, Bayer M: Gastric emptying: Risk versus benefit in the treatment of acute poisoning. *Med Toxicol* 1986;1:142–153.

11. Chafee-Bahomon C, Lacouture P, Lovejoy F: Risk assessment of ipecac in the home. *Pediatrics* 1985; 75:1105–1109.

12. Manno B, Manno J: Toxicology of ipecac: A review. *Clin Toxicol* 1977;10:221–242.

13. Moran D, Crouch D, Finkle B: Absorption of ipecac alkaloids in emergency patients. *Ann Emerg Med* 1984; 13:1100–1102.

14. Weaver J, Griffith J: Induction of emesis by detergent ingredients and formulations. *Toxicol Appl Pharmacol* 1969; 14:214–220.

15. King W: Syrup of ipecac: A review. *Clin Toxicol* 1980;17:353–356.

16. Eisenga B, Meester W: Evaluation of the effect of motility on syrup of ipecac–induced emesis. *Vet Human Toxicol* 1978;20:462–465.

17. Palmer E, Guay A: Reversible myopathy secondary to abuse of ipecac in patients with major eating disorders. *N Engl J Med* 1985;313:1457–1459.

18. Uden D, Davison G, Kohen D: Effect of carbonated beverages on ipecac-induced emesis. *Ann Emerg Med* 1981; 10:79–81.

19. Easom J, Lovejoy F: Efficacy and safety of gastrointestinal decontamination in the treatment of oral poisoning. *Pediatr Clin North Am* 1979;26:827–836.

20. Manoguerra A, Krenzelok E: Rapid emesis from high-dose ipecac syrup in adults and children intoxicated with antiemetics or other drugs. *Am J Hosp Pharm* 1978; 35:1360–1362.

21. Amitai Y, Mitchell A, McGuigan M, et al: Ipecac-induced emesis and reduction of plasma concentrations of drugs following accidental overdose in children. *Pediatrics* 1987;80:364–367.

22. Grbcich P, Lacouture P, Kresel J, et al: Expired ipecac syrup efficacy. *Pediatrics* 1986;78:1085–1089.

23. Czajka P, Russell S: Nonemetic effects of ipecac syrup. *Pediatrics* 1985;75:1101–1104.

24. Krenzelok E, Dean B: Syrup of ipecac in children less than one year of age. *Clin Toxicol* 1985;23:171–176.

25. Cooney D: In vitro evidence for ipecac inactivation by activated charcoal. *J Pharm Sci* 1978;67:426–427.

26. Freedman G, Pasternak S, Krenzelok E: A clinical trial using syrup of ipecac and activated charcoal concurrently. *Ann Emerg Med* 1987;16:164–166.

27. Krenzelok E, Freedman G, Pasternak S: Preserving the emetic effect of syrup of ipecac with concurrent activated charcoal administration: A preliminary study. *Clin Toxicol* 1986;24:159–166.

28. Ordog G, Vann P, Owashi N, et al: Intravenous prochlorperazine for the rapid control of vomiting in the emergency department. *Ann Emerg Med* 1984;13:253–258.

29. Wolowodiuk O, McMicken D, O'Brien P: Pneumomediastinum and retropneumonoperitoneum: An unusual complication of syrup of ipecac–induced emesis. *Ann Emerg Med* 1984;13:1148–1151.

30. Smith R, Smith D: Acute ipecac poisoning—Report of a fatal case and review of literature. *N Engl J Med* 1961; 265:523–525.

31. Klein-Schwartz W, Gorman R, Oderda G, et al: Ipecac use in the elderly: The unanswered question. *Ann Emerg Med* 1984;13:1152–1154.

32. Brushwood D, Tietze K: Regulatory controversy surrounding ipecac use and misuse. *Am J Hosp Pharm* 1986; 43:157–161.

33. Rumack B: Ipecac use in the home. *Pediatrics* 1985; 75:1148.

34. Rumack B, Rosen P: Emesis: Safe and effective? *Ann Emerg Med* 1981;10:551.

35. Tandberg D, Liechty E, Fishbein D: Mallory-Weiss syndrome: An unusual complication of ipecac-induced emesis. *Ann Emerg Med* 1981;10:521–523.

36. Miser J, Robertson W: Ipecac poisoning. *West J Med* 1978;128:440–443.

37. Adler A, Walinsky P, Krall R, et al: Death resulting from ipecac-syrup poisoning. *JAMA* 1980;243:1927–1928.

38. Bennett H, Spiro A, Pollack M, et al: Ipecac-induced myopathy simulating dermatomyositis. *Neurology* 1982; 32:91–94.

39. Brotman M, Forbath N, Garfinkel P, et al: Myopathy due to ipecac syrup poisoning in a patient with anorexia nervosa. *Can Med Assoc J* 1981;125:453–454.

40. MacLeod J: Ipecac intoxication—Use of a cardiac pacemaker in management. *N Engl J Med* 1963;268: 146–147.

41. Dournon E, Bure A, Desplaces N, et al: Legionnaires' disease related to gastric lavage with tap water. *Lancet* 1982;1:797–798.

42. Stein R, Jenkins D, Korns M: Death after use of cupric sulfate as emetic. *JAMA* 1976;235:801.

43. Schwartz E, Schmidt E: Refractory shock secondary to copper sulfate ingestion. *Ann Emerg Med* 1986; 15:952–954.

44. Gieseker D, Troutman W: Emergency induction of emesis using liquid detergent products: A report of fifteen cases. *Clin Toxicol* 1981;18:277–282.

45. Krenzelok E: High-*p*H automatic dishwashing detergents. *Ann Emerg Med* 1987;16:470.

46. MacLean W: A comparison of ipecac syrup and apomorphine in the immediate treatment of ingestion of poisons. *J Pediatr* 1973;82:121–124.

47. Schofferman J: A clinical comparison of syrup of ipecac and apomorphine use in adults. *JACEP* 1976; 5:22–25.

48. Auerbach P, Osterloh J, Braun O, et al: Efficacy of gastric emptying: Gastric lavage versus emesis induced with ipecac. *Ann Emerg Med* 1986;15:692–698.

49. Arnold F, Hodges J, Barta R, et al: Evaluation of the efficacy of lavage and induced emesis in the treatment of salicylate poisoning. *Pediatrics* 1959;23:286–301.

50. Burke M: Gastric lavage and emesis in the treatment of ingested poisons: A review and a clinical study of lavage in ten adults. *Resuscitation* 1972;1:91–105.

51. Matthew H: Gastric aspiration and lavage. *Clin Toxicol* 1970;3:179–183.

52. McDougal C, MacLean M: Modifications in the technique of gastric lavage. *Ann Emerg Med* 1981;10:514–517.

53. Rudolph J: Automated gastric lavage and a comparison of 0.9% normal saline solution and tap water irrigant. *Ann Emerg Med* 1985;14:1156–1159.

54. Bartecchi C: A modification of gastric lavage technique. *JACEP* 1974;3:304–305.

55. Blake D, Bramble M, Grimley-Evans J: Is there excessive use of gastric lavage in the treatment of self poisoning? *Lancet* 1978;2:1362–1364.

56. Askenasi R, Abramowicz M, Jeanmart J, et al: Esophageal perforation: An unusual complication of gastric lavage. *Ann Emerg Med* 1984;13:146.

57. Boba A: Rapid whole-gut evacuation. *IMJ* 1979; 155:156–157.

58. Davis G, Santa Ana C, Morawski S, et al: Development of a lavage solution associated with minimal water and electrolyte absorption or secretion. *Gastroenterology* 1980; 78:991–995.

59. Porter R, Baker E: Drug clearance by diarrhea induction. *Am J Emerg Med* 1985;3:182–186.

60. Tenenbein M: Whole bowel irrigation for toxic ingestions. *Clin Toxicol* 1985;23:177–184.

61. Tenenbein M: Inefficacy of gastric emptying procedures. *J Emerg Med* 1985;3:133–136.

62. Cereda J, Scott J, Quigley E: Endoscopic removal of pharmacobezoar of slow-release theophylline. *Br Med J* 1986;293:1143.

63. Marstellar H, Gigler R: Endoscopic management of toxic masses in the stomach. *N Engl J Med* 1977; 296:1003–1004.

64. Czajka P, Konrad J: Saline cathartics and the adsorptive capacity of activated charcoal for aspirin. *Ann Emerg Med* 1986;15:548–551.

65. Mofenson H, Caraccio T, Greensher J, et al: Gastrointestinal dialysis with activated charcoal and cathartic in the treatment of adolescent intoxications. *Clin Pediatr* 1985; 24:678–684.

66. Curd-Sneed C, Parks K, Bordelon J, et al: In vitro adsorption of sodium pentobarbital by Superchar, USP and Darco G-60 activated charcoals. *Clin Toxicol* 1987;25:1–11.

67. Katona B, Siegel E, Cluxton R: The new black magic: Activated charcoal and new therapeutic uses. *J Emerg Med* 1987;5:9–18.

68. Neuvonen P, Vartiainen M, Tokola O: Comparison of activated charcoal and ipecac syrup in prevention of drug absorption. *Eur J Clin Pharmacol* 1983;24:557–562.

69. Harvey R, Read A: Mode of action of the saline purgatives. *Am Heart J* 1975;89:810–813.

70. Neuvonen P, Elonen E: Effect of activated charcoal on absorption and elimination of phenobarbitone, car-

bamazepine, and phenylbutazone in man. *Eur J Clin Pharmacol* 1980;17:51–55.

71. Holt L, Holz P: The black bottle. *J Pediatr* 1970; 63:306–314.

72. Hayden J, Comstock E: Use of activated charcoal in acute poisoning. *Clin Toxicol* 1975;8:515–533.

73. Kulig K: Interpreting gastric emptying studies. *J Emerg Med* 1984;1:447–448.

74. Krenzelok E, Keller R, Stewart R: Gastrointestinal transit times of cathartics combined with charcoal. *Ann Emerg Med* 1985;14:1152–1155.

75. Comstock E, Boisaubin E, Comstock B, et al: Assessment of the efficacy of activated charcoal following gastric lavage in acute drug emergencies. *J Toxicol Clin Toxicol* 1982;19:149–165.

76. Nau C, Neal J, Stembridge V: A study of the physiological effects of carbon black: II: Skin contact. *Arch Ind Health* 1958;18:511–520.

77. Nau C, Neal J, Stembridge V, et al: Physiological effects of carbon black: Inhalation. *Arch Environ Health* 1962;4:415–420.

78. Minocha A, Herold D, Bruns D, et al: Effect of activated charcoal in 70% sorbitol in healthy individuals. *J Toxicol Clin Toxicol* 1985;22:529–534.

79. Minocha A, Krenzelok E, Spyker D: Dosage recommendations for activated charcoal–sorbitol treatment. *Clin Toxicol* 1985;23:579–587,

80. Farley T: Severe hypernatremic dehydration after use of an activated charcoal–sorbitol suspension. *J Pediatr* 1986;109:719–722.

81. Mayersohn M, Perrier D, Picchioni A: Evaluation of a charcoal-sorbitol mixture as an antidote for oral aspirin overdose. *Clin Toxicol* 1977;11:561–567.

82. Olkkola K, Neuvonen P: Do gastric contents modify antidotal efficacy of oral activated charcoal? *Br J Clin Pharmacol* 1984;18:663–669.

83. Picchioni A, Chin L, Laird H: Activated charcoal preparations—Relative antidotal efficacy. *Clin Toxicol* 1974;7:97–108.

84. Tsuchiya T, Levy G: Drug adsorption efficacy of commercial activated charcoal tablets in vitro and in man. *J Pharm Sci* 1972;61:624–625.

85. Chung D, Murphy J, Taylor T: In-vivo comparison of the adsorption capacity of ''superactive charcoal'' and fructose with activated charcoal and fructose. *J Toxicol Clin Toxicol* 1982;19:219–224.

86. Curtis R, Barone J, Biacona W: Efficacy of ipecac and activated charcoal/cathartic: Prevention of salicylate absorption in a simulated overdose. *Arch Intern Med* 1984; 144:48–52.

87. Gwilt P, Perrier D: Influence of thickening agents on the antidotal efficacy of activated charcoal. *Clin Toxicol* 1976;9:89–92.

88. Levy G, Soda D, Lampman T: Inhibition by ice cream of the efficacy of activated charcoal. *Am J Hosp Pharm* 1975;32:289–291.

89. Burton B, Bayer M, Barron L, et al: Comparison of activated charcoal and gastric lavage in the prevention of aspirin absorption. *J Emerg Med* 1984;1:411–416.

90. Jones J, Heiselman D, Dougherty J, et al: Cathartic-induced magnesium toxicity during overdose management. *Ann Emerg Med* 1986;15:1214–1218.

91. Berlinger W, Spector R, Goldberg G, et al: Enhancement of theophylline clearance by oral activated charcoal. *Clin Pharmacol Ther* 1983;33:351–356.

92. True R, Berman J, Mahutte C: Treatment of theophylline toxicity with oral activated charcoal. *Crit Care Med* 1984;12:113–119.

93. Picchioni A, Chin L, Verhulst H, et al: Activated charcoal vs ''universal antidote'' as an antidote for poisons. *Toxicol Appl Pharmacol* 1966;8:447–454.

94. Shannon M, Fish S, Lovejoy F: Cathartics and laxatives: Do they still have a place in the management of the poisoned patient? *Med Toxicol* 1986;1:247–252.

95. Riegel J, Becker C: Use of cathartics in toxic ingestions. *Ann Emerg Med* 1981;10:79–81.

96. Krenzelok E: Sorbitol—A safe and effective cathartic. *Ann Emerg Med* 1987;16:729–730.

97. Martin R, Lisehora G, Braxton M, et al: Fatal poisoning from sodium phosphate enema. *JAMA* 1987;257:2190–2192.

98. Picchioni A, Chin L, Gillespie T: Evaluation of activated charcoal–sorbitol suspension as an antidote. *J Toxicol Clin Toxicol* 1982;19:433–444.

ADDITIONAL SELECTED REFERENCES

Goulding R, Volans G: Emergency treatment of common poisonings: Emptying the stomach. *Proc Royal Soc Med* 1977;70:766–770.

Morris M, Levy G: Absorption of sulfate from orally administered magnesium sulfate in man. *J Toxicol Clin Toxicol* 1983;20:107–114.

Pollack M, Dunbar B, Holbrook P, et al: Aspiration of activated charcoal and gastric contents. *Ann Emerg Med* 1981;10:528–529.

Schwartz H: Acute meprobamate poisoning with gastrostomy and removal of a drug-containing mass. *N Engl J Med* 1976;295:1177–1178.

Stewart J: Effects of emetic and cathartic agents on the gastrointestinal tract and the treatment of toxic ingestion. *J Toxicol Clin Toxicol* 1983;20:199–253.

Thoman M: The use of emetics in poison ingestion. *Clin Toxicol* 1970;3:185–188.

Vale J, Rees A, Widdop B, et al: Use of charcoal haemoperfusion in the management of severely poisoned patients. *Br Med J* 1975;1:5–9.

Varipapa R, Oderda G: Effect of milk on ipecac induced emesis. *N Engl J Med* 1977;296:112–113.

chapter 3

Methods of Enhancing Drug Excretion

The elimination of certain drugs from the body may be aided by methods that make use of pharmacokinetic parameters that effect drug excretion.[1] These include (1) forced diuresis with or without ion-trapping methods, (2) the use of multiple-dose activated charcoal, (3) dialysis, (4) hemoperfusion, and (5) plasmapheresis (Table 3-1).[2–8] Except for the use of activated charcoal, these methods have one feature in common: the vasculature must deliver the drug to the site of removal, whether this be the chamber of an extracorporeal machine, the peritoneal space, or the kidney.[9]

FORCED DIURESIS

The processes involved in the urinary excretion of drugs include glomerular filtration, active tubular secretion, and tubular reabsorption. Only the last process can be influenced so that drug elimination is significantly enhanced. If tubular reabsorption is inhibited, less drug is allowed back into the body and more is excreted by the kidney. Decreasing the concentration gradient between the urine and the blood by diluting the urine by diuresis may decrease tubular reabsorption. This process shortens the time of a drug's exposure to the reabsorptive sites in the distal tubules.[10]

Factors Involved in Diuresis

A major factor accounting for the renal elimination of a drug or metabolite is the chemical molecule's polarity. Most lipid drugs, which are nonpolar, are not readily excreted unchanged by the kidney because of their ability to be readily reabsorbed through the membrane of the kidney tubules. If the liver adds more polar groups to the molecule the drug becomes more soluble in water, and renal excretion can occur. Addition of polar groups is achieved by acetylation, conjugation (with acetate, glycine, sulfate, or glucuronic acid), reduction, oxidation, or hydroxylation. In most cases, however, an attempt to increase urine flow and output will not result in an increase in renal clearance unless a reasonable fraction of the drug is eliminated through the kidneys in comparison with other routes of

---

Table 3-1 Methods To Enhance Drug Elimination

Diuresis with or without Ion Trapping
Multiple-Dose Activated Charcoal
   Interruption of enterohepatic circulation
   "Intestinal dialysis"
Dialysis
   Hemodialysis
   Peritoneal dialysis
Hemoperfusion
Plasmapheresis

---

elimination, such as metabolism or fecal excretion. In general, for many drugs elimination by renal excretion is independent of urine flow rates. Therefore the enhancement of excretion of only a few drugs is increased solely by forced diuresis. In general, drugs with a large volume of distribution or a high degree of plasma protein binding will not be removed by forced diuresis. The few drugs whose excretion can be enhanced by a neutral diuresis (sodium chloride) are isoniazid, bromides, and lithium (Table 3-2). It is also believed that the excretion of both isoniazid and lithium are enhanced by an alkaline diuresis.

Ion-Trapping Methods

Ion trapping can be helpful in increasing the elimination of some drugs (Table 3-2). Drugs that have a dissociable group, either acidic or basic, carry a charge at a pH value that is distant from their pK_a value (at a pH equal to the pK_a, a drug is half dissociated and half undissociated). Ion-trapping methods essentially cause a solution to become more alkaline or acidic, depending on the pK_a of the substance, so that the substance is trapped in the kidney and excretion is enhanced. Low degrees of ionization and high lipid solubility favor rapid movement across membranes. Weak acids are more ionized in an alkaline medium, and weak bases are more

ionized in an acidic medium. If there is a pH difference across a membrane ion trapping will occur, and drug will accumulate in the compartment where ionization is greater because the nonionized form crosses the lipid-cell membrane much more readily than the ionized form.

Alkaline Diuresis

Both salicylate and phenobarbital are weak acids. By promoting an alkaline urine these drugs will become more ionized in the distal tubular lumen, which will slow tubular reabsorption and allow a larger fraction of drug to be excreted without being reabsorbed back into the body. This mechanism makes use of more effective renal excretion rather than saturation of the liver. This concept of ion trapping also allows phenobarbital and salicylate to move from the central nervous system into the blood compartment and then to be trapped in the tubular lumen of the kidney and excreted in the urine.

Drugs whose excretion can be enhanced by an alkaline diuresis are therefore the long-acting barbiturates, such as phenobarbital and drugs converted to phenobarbital in the body (mephobarbital and primidone), as well as salicylates, lithium (controversial), and isoniazid[11] (Table 3-2). The short- and intermediate-acting barbiturates must be metabolized before being excreted by the kidney; their excretion is not enhanced by diuresis.

An alkaline diuresis is achieved by administering one or two ampules of sodium bicarbonate dissolved in a liter of one-half normal saline. It is necessary to check the pH of the urine both before and after an effective urine flow is obtained. Potassium depletion should be carefully monitored, and the addition of potassium chloride may be necessary to ensure the adequate alkalization of the urine. Sodium bicarbonate can increase urinary pH by 2 or 3 units, which will have a pronounced effect on the renal clearance of weakly acidic drugs.

Acetazolamide (Diamox) is a carbonic anhydrase inhibitor that will cause an alkaline urine through bicarbonate loss. It will also cause a hyperchloremic metabolic acidosis (non–anion-gap metabolic acidosis), however, and should not be used for urinary alkalization.

Table 3-2 Drugs Whose Excretion Can Be Enhanced by Diuresis or Ion Trapping

Neutral Diuresis
  Bromides
  Lithium (controversial)
  Isoniazid (controversial)
Alkaline Diuresis
  Phenobarbital
  Primidone
  Mephobarbital
  Salicylates
  Isoniazid (controversial)
  Lithium (controversial)
Acid Diuresis
  Phencyclidine (not advised)
  Amphetamines (not advised)

Acid Diuresis

Drugs whose excretion can be enhanced by an acid diuresis include amphetamines and phencyclidine. Although acidifying the urine to enhance the excretion of these two drugs has been suggested and may be effective, many physicians do not recommend its use owing to the possibility of developing acute tubular necrosis secondary to rhabdomyolysis. In other words, although there is the potential for enhancing the renal excretion of these compounds, there is also the likelihood that these compounds will cause rhabdomyolysis with subsequent myoglobinemia and myoglobinuria.[12] Because the excretion of myoglobin is decreased in an acid urine, there is a greater likelihood of causing an acute tubular necrosis. It is therefore held that the risks of the procedure outweigh the potential benefit.[12]

It has been suggested that 500 mg to 1 g of ascorbic acid should be added to each liter of normal saline to acidify the urine. There have been some questions raised regarding the efficacy of intravenous and oral preparations of ascorbic acid in producing an acid urine.[1,12,13] Ammonium chloride, 75 mg/kg intravenously or orally per day, has also been suggested, but caution is advised for patients with kidney or liver disease.

MULTIPLE-DOSE ACTIVATED CHARCOAL

In the past, the applicability of charcoal was thought to be limited to its ability to bind whatever drug remained in the gastrointestinal tract after emesis or gastric lavage was performed. It is now widely accepted that the clearance of some drugs and poisons is increased when activated charcoal is administered in multiple oral doses; for this reason, activated charcoal has recently emerged as a valuable new modality to increase the elimination of certain agents.[14]

There are three ways in which activated charcoal can be effective. One involves prevention of absorption of a toxin, and the other two involve enhancing excretion of the toxin. The first makes use of a single dose of activated charcoal, which is effective because it prevents primary absorption of the toxin. Multiple-dose activated charcoal may aid excretion of drugs by two different mechanisms: interruption of enterohepatic recirculation of certain drugs, and adsorption of drug secreted across intestinal membranes into the bowel lumen ("intestinal dialysis").

Preventing Primary Absorption of a Drug

Activated charcoal may adsorb any remaining drug in the gastrointestinal tract. There is ample documentation that this is clinically important (see Chapter 2).

Enhancing Elimination of a Drug

Interruption of Enterohepatic Circulation

The activity of some drugs, particularly the high–molecular weight polar compounds, can be decreased if their natural cycle of enterohepatic recirculation is interrupted. Because of enterohepatic circulation, these drugs are reabsorbed into the stomach or intestine through the biliary system. Interruption of this pathway facilitates fecal elimination of the toxin.

Agents that interfere with enterohepatic recirculation include anionic exchange resins such as cholestyramine or colestipol. Activated charcoal is another agent that appears to have a useful role in binding drugs in the gastrointestinal tract that are recycled enterohepatically. At this time, such methods are promising but still in the experimental stage because no definite advantage has been shown in controlled studies. Activated charcoal can be employed in serious overdoses of the compounds listed in Table 3-3 because it offers no major adverse effects.

"Intestinal Dialysis"

Most nonionized drugs and poisons dissolved in the blood can diffuse across gastrointestinal membranes. Furthermore, many drugs can be concentrated in gastrointestinal fluids by ion trapping as predicted by the *p*H partition gradient. Therefore, there exists a persistent concentration gradient favoring the passive

Table 3-3 Drugs That Undergo Enterohepatic Recirculation or Secretion into the Stomach

Carbamazepine
Digitoxin
Glutethimide
Meprobamate
Nadolol
Phencyclidine
Phenylbutazone
Tricyclic antidepressants

diffusion of poison into the gastrointestinal lumen. Intestinal dialysis is an attempt at using the intestinal wall as a dialysis membrane. Drugs or poisons that can easily diffuse across gastrointestinal membranes and also have small volumes of distribution (less than 1L/kg) are effectively removed by multiple-dose activated charcoal. Drugs with large volumes of distribution are not effectively removed by orally administered activated charcoal.[14]

Overall, the principles that govern the ability of oral activated charcoal to increase the clearance of drugs and poisons from the body are analogous to the principles that govern the effectiveness of hemodialysis and hemoperfusion for removing drugs and poisons. It has been postulated that gastrointestinal dialysis is comparable in effect to peritoneal dialysis.[15,16] It is believed that a large amount of unbound charcoal in the intestine creates a large drug concentration gradient between the blood and intestinal contents, favoring diffusion of the drug from the circulation into the intestinal lumen and onto the charcoal. This increases the clearance of some compounds from the body. For example, substantial decreases in serum half-life have been reported for theophylline, phenobarbital, and dapsone.[15-17] In theory, multiple-dose activated charcoal may also be effective for enhancing the elimination of salicylates and phenytoin. In addition, mulitiple-dose activated charcoal may prevent desorption of drug from the charcoal as it passes down the gastrointestinal tract. For this reason, there are many toxicologists that advocate the use of multiple-dose activated charcoal as a safe alternative to extracorporeal methods of drug removal in mild to moderate poisonings with these drugs.

Considerations in the Use of Multiple-Dose Activated Charcoal

As can be seen, not many compounds undergo enhanced elimination by multiple-dose activated charcoal, and the pharmacokinetic characteristics of the compound should be considered before patients are treated in this way. A drug whose excretion may be enhanced by multiple-dose activated charcoal must have a small volume of distribution, be extensively bound to plasma proteins or other blood components, must be lipophilic (uncharged), or it must undergo enterohepatic or enteroenteric circulation.[17] Most compounds have some degree of protein binding, so that the upper limit of hepatic blood flow will only apply to the clearance of unbound drug. The administration of activated charcoal should not replace supportive care, nor should it be relied on as the sole treatment of an intoxication.[16]

Method of Administration

The optimal dose and frequency of administration of activated charcoal are not well defined. The dosage usually recommended for adults is 20 to 100 g every 2 to 8 hours until objective evidence and clinical observations indicate that serum drug concentrations have declined to a subtoxic range. A dosage of 5 to 10 g every 4 to 8 hours is recommended for children.

When using this method it is important to keep the gut continuously full of charcoal, at least as far as is practical, and it may not be necessary to administer sorbitol or other cathartics more than once. There is also the potential for fluid and electrolyte depletion if sorbitol or other cathartics are used with each dose of activated charcoal in a multiple-dose regimen. Multiple doses of saline cathartics, such as magnesium sulfate, should not be administered because this regimen has resulted in hypermagnesemia with acute neuromuscular deterioration that required dialysis.[18] Furthermore, gastrointestinal obstruction has been reported after repeated doses of activated charcoal along with a cathartic.[19] Repeated doses of activated charcoal may also adsorb orally and parenterally administered drugs necessary for the management of the overdosed patient. These medications may therefore have to be administered more frequently.

THE ROLE OF EXTRACORPOREAL MEANS FOR DRUG REMOVAL

Hemodialysis, hemoperfusion, and plasmapheresis are considered the state of the art in invasive detoxification. There are certain similarities among the three procedures. They all require an extracorporeal chamber through which blood is passed, either a membrane dialyzer (dialysis) or a bed of charcoal or other sorbent (hemoperfusion and plasmapheresis). They make use of blood anticoagulation treatments, pumps, and safety devices to detect or prevent air embolism.

Dialysis

Although dialysis can be a useful means of removing endogenous wastes in the event of poor renal function, it has a limited application in toxicology. The use of hemodialysis in the treatment of drug overdose has waned in recent years because of the good results obtained with conservative management[20] and the poor clearance of many drugs with standard dialysis procedures.[21] The overwhelming majority of overdosed patients can be treated conservatively, and procedures such as peritoneal dialysis and hemodialysis are seldom indicated in the modern treatment of drug intoxication. In many instances claims of efficacy have been based on uncontrolled observations. With very few exceptions, dialysis should be considered only a part of the supportive care of a poisoned patient and not the primary form of treatment.

In general, the rate of removal of a dialyzable substance is usually 5 to 10 times greater with hemodialysis than with peritoneal dialysis. In the presence of severe hypotension or vasoconstriction, effective hemodialysis can sometimes be performed when peritoneal dialysis is ineffective.

Criteria for Dialysis

No single criterion determines the dialyzability of any drug; often there may be a complex relationship that determines this factor. Essentially, to be dialyzed a substance should (1) be of small molecular weight, (2) have limited protein and lipid binding, (3) have a small volume of distribution, and (4) diffuse readily across a dialysis membrane (Table 3-4). Therefore, agents that are highly protein bound, have low aqueous solubility, or are poorly distributed in plasma water are poorly dialyzable.

Molecular weight. Drugs with a low molecular weight cross the dialysis membrane more readily than compounds with high molecular weight because the membrane's pores allow the smaller compounds to pass.

Water solubility. Drugs that are poorly solubilized in water are poorly diffused in the aqueous dialysate solution.

Volume of distribution. If the apparent volume of distribution is large, only a small amount of the drug will be available for elimination by dialysis because only a small amount of the drug is in the vascular compartment.

Protein binding. Albumin is not well filtered by the kidneys, so that drugs bound to proteins in the plasma are also not diffusible through the dialysis membrane. Therefore, only the free drug is available for removal.

Active metabolites. All these criteria apply as well to active metabolites of the parent compound (Table 3-5).

Contraindications for Dialysis

Dialysis is contraindicated for many of the drugs previously thought to yield an effective return from dialysis (Table 3-6).

Table 3-4 Criteria for Dialysis

Low molecular weight
Water solubility
Small volume of distribution
Small degree of protein binding
Dialyzable active metabolites

Table 3-5 Pharmacologically Active Metabolites of Drugs

Drug	Metabolite
Acetylsalicylic acid	Salicylic acid
Amitriptyline	Nortriptyline
Chloral hydrate	Trichloroethanol
Chlordiazepoxide	Desmethylchlordiazepoxide
Codeine	Morphine
Diazepam	Desmethyldiazepam
Digitoxin	Digoxin
Flurazepam	Desmethylflurazepam
Glutethimide	4-Hydroxyglutethimide
Imipramine	Desipramine
Lidocaine	Desethyllidocaine
Meperidine	Normeperidine
Methamphetamine	Amphetamine
Phenacetin	Acetaminophen
Phenylbutazone	Oxyphenbutazone
Prednisone	Prednisolone
Primidone	Phenobarbital
Procainamide	N-Acetylprocainamide
Propranolol	4-Hydroxypropranolol

Source: Adapted from *Clinical Pharmacokinetics: Concepts & Application* (p 125) by M Rowland and T Tozer with permission of Lea & Febiger, © 1980.

Table 3-7 Drugs for Which Dialysis Is Indicated on the Basis of Patient Condition

Alcohols	Phenobarbital
Amphetamines	Potassium
Bromides	Quinidine
Chloral hydrate	Salicylate
Ethylene glycol	Strychnine
Isoniazid	Theophylline
Isopropanol	Thiocyanate
Lithium	
Methanol	

Table 3-8 Conditions for Which Dialysis Is Required

Renal failure (when this is the major route of elimination)

If there is uncorrectable
  acid-base disorder
  osmolality
  hyperthermia or hypothermia
  electrolyte disorder
  respiratory problem
  hypertension or hypotension

Indications for Dialysis

Immediate dialysis. Immediate dialysis is indicated for only two drugs, ethylene glycol and methanol, which cause toxicity because of their breakdown products. If a patient presents with a history of ingestion of either of these compounds and has acidotic or visual symptoms, then dialysis should be instituted immediately.

Dialysis on the basis of patient condition. Although dialysis may be effective in the removal of certain other drugs (Table 3-7), it is usually not necessary unless certain conditions exist (Table 3-8). Even then, dialysis is usually reserved for salicylates, theophylline, long-acting barbiturates, and lithium.

Table 3-6 Drugs for Which Dialysis Is Contraindicated

Antidepressants	Glutethimide
Antihistamines	Methaqualone
Benzodiazepines	Methyprylon
Digitalis	Opiates
Ethchlorvynol	Phenothiazines

Hemoperfusion

Hemoperfusion, first described approximately 40 years ago,[22] is a procedure in which blood is passed through various adsorbent materials, such as activated charcoal or amberlite (a polymeric resin that has an affinity for lipid-soluble organic molecules).[22,23] These adsorbent materials contain granules of either activated charcoal or resins coated with a semipermeable membrane through which blood may pass.[23,24] The cartridges are disposable, and conventional hemodialysis tubing, pumps, and monitoring devices are used. Hemoperfusion is essentially dialysis against an adsorbent.[22,25–27]

Advantages and Disadvantages of Hemoperfusion

The advantage of hemoperfusion is that it circumvents some of the physical drug characteristics, such as molecular weight, water solubility, and protein binding, that limit dialysis.[28] Agents that are highly protein bound, have a low aqueous solubility, or are poorly distributed in plasma water are poorly dialyzable. With these agents, the technique of hemoperfusion may be appropriate. In general, drugs are removed from the blood at a more rapid rate by hemoperfusion than by dialysis. For example, a 2- or 3-hour hemoperfusion may remove as much drug as an 8-hour hemodialysis.[9]

Pharmacokinetic parameters such as volume of distribution limit the applicability of hemoperfusion, however. In addition, the affinity of the drug for the adsorbent material and the binding capacity of the adsorbent material must be considered as well as the hazards involved in the procedure.[25] Because direct contact of blood with activated charcoal results in significant damage to blood-forming elements, embolization of adsorbent particles, destruction of red and white blood cells, and, more commonly, destruction of platelets and the removal of certain normal body fluids such as plasma proteins and solutes are frequent consequences of the procedure.[29] Other methods for hemoperfusion that have been developed recently involve microencapsulation of charcoal solutions or polymers; these methods have largely overcome some of the problems.

Since the 1960s most clinical investigators have used encapsulated filters,[30] which embed the charcoal on a column,[23,31] but complications such as platelet destruction, hypotension, hypothermia, hypocalcemia,[10] and the risks associated with heparinization[32] still exist. Another important aspect of hemoperfusion is that it does not correct any acid-base or electrolyte disorders that may be secondary to the ingestion of the drug.[20]

Indications for Hemoperfusion

Hemoperfusion is indicated for a massive intoxication when the extracellular distribution of the drug is significant and when the plasma level of the drug is at its maximum.[21,22,28,30,33,34] Typically, hemoperfusion is successful with the same compounds that can be dialyzed (barbiturates, salicylates, and theophylline) and has been found to be ineffective for drugs with weak extracellular distribution (digoxin, tricyclic antidepressants, heavy metals, and glutethimide).[33–36] Some investigators seriously question the efficacy of hemoperfusion in comparison to supportive and conservative care.[37] Others hold that hemoperfusion should

never be employed for drug overdose, especially in view of its drawbacks.[36,37]

Plasmapheresis

Plasmapheresis uses the technique of phlebotomy and modifies it so that the cellular components of the blood are returned to the patient. The plasma and plasma proteins are then replaced with fresh plasma or a suitable colloid.[38] Although modifications of this procedure were used for centuries, it was successfully utilized for clinical manifestations of hyperviscosity in the 1960s.[38] Since that time it has been suggested for many disorders but only in anecdotal reports, not in controlled studies.

Plasmapheresis can be considered a modification of exchange transfusion.[9] Many of the same requirements for hemodialysis or hemoperfusion also apply to plasmapheresis, especially that the drug have a small volume of distribution so that it will be present in sufficient quantity in the plasma for there to be an effective extraction. If the drug has a large volume of distribution, even an efficient system of plasmapheresis will remove only a small amount. In addition, both hemoperfusion and hemodialysis are generally able to clear much larger volumes of plasma than plasmapheresis.[38] Plasmapheresis is most useful with drugs that are strongly protein bound, have a long half-life, and are not well dialyzed or hemoperfused.

Many of the side effects associated with other extracorporeal methods are noted with plasmapheresis, including bleeding from anticoagulation, extracorporeal blood clotting, thrombotic complications, hypocalcemia, fluid overload, citrate toxicity, infection, and problems associated with vascular access. In addition, plasmapheresis can be a very expensive procedure.

SUMMARY

Although there are methods to enhance excretion of various compounds, they are effective for very few compounds. Forced diuresis, dialysis, and hemoperfusion are all limited in the number of compounds for which they are effective. Many of the advantages and disadvantages of extracorporeal means of drug removal are not likely to change markedly as a result of improved technology because it is the chemical charac-teristics of toxic substances that limits the role of these procedures. Multiple-dose activated char-coal appears to offer the advantage of not having dangerous side effects but still being an effective means for removing certain compounds.

REFERENCES

1. Arena J: The clinical diagnosis of poisoning. *Pediatr Clin North Am* 1970;17:477–494.

2. Cashman T, Shirkey H: Emergency management of poisoning. *Pediatr Clin North Am* 1970;17:525–534.

3. Gilles C, Ford P, Lovejoy F, et al: Management of pediatric poisoning. *Pediatr Nurs* 1980;6:33–44.

4. Gossel T, Wuest J: The right first aid for poisoning. *RN* 1981;44:73–75.

5. Kaufman R, Levy S: Overdose treatment. *JAMA* 1974;227:411–416.

6. Keller E: Poisoning in children. *Postgrad Med* 1979;65:177–186.

7. Sullivan J, Rumack B, Peterson R: Management of the poisoned patient in the emergency department: Poison-ings and overdose. *Top Emerg Med* 1979;1:1–12.

8. Sunshine I: Basic toxicology. *Pediatr Clin North Am* 1970;17:509–513.

9. Peterson R, Peterson L: Cleansing the blood: Hemo-dialysis, peritoneal dialysis, exchange transfusion, charcoal hemoperfusion, forced diuresis. *Pediatr Clin North Am* 1986;33:675–689.

10. Watanabe A, Rumack B, Peterson R: Enhancement of elimination in poisonings. *Top Emerg Med* 1979;1:19–26.

11. Matthew H: Acute poisoning: Some myths and mis-conceptions. *Br Med J* 1971;1:519–522.

12. Barton C, Sterling M, Thomas R, et al: Ineffec-tiveness of intravenous ascorbic acid as an acidifying agent in man. *Arch Intern Med* 1981;141:211–212.

13. Nahata M, Shimp L, Lampman T, et al: Effect of ascorbic acid on urine pH in man. *Am J Hosp Pharm* 1977;34:1234–1237.

14. Park G, Spector R, Goldberg M, et al: Expanded role of charcoal therapy in the poisoned and overdosed patient. *Arch Intern Med* 1986;146:969–973.

15. Katona B, Siegel E, Cluxton R: The new black magic: Activated charcoal and new therapeutic uses. *J Emerg Med* 1987;5:9–18.

16. Levy G: Gastrointestinal clearance of drugs with acti-vated charcoal. *N Engl J Med* 1982;307:676–678.

17. Pond S: Role of repeated oral doses of activated charcoal in clinical toxicology. *Med Toxicol* 1986;1:3–11.

18. Jones J, Herselman D, Dougherty J, et al: Cathartic-induced magnesium toxicity during overdose management. *Ann Emerg Med* 1986;15:1214–1218.

19. Watson W, Cremer K, Chapman J: Gastrointestinal obstruction associated with multiple-dose activated char-coal. *J Emerg Med* 1986;4:401–407.

20. Koffler A, Bernstein M, LaSette A, et al: Fixed-bed charcoal hemoperfusion. *Arch Intern Med* 1978;138:1691–1694.

21. Vale J, Rees A, Widdop B, et al: Use of charcoal hemoperfusion in the management of severely poisoned patients. *Br Med J* 1975;1:5–9.

22. Rosenbaum J, Kramer M, Raja R: Resin hemoperfu-sion for acute drug intoxication. *Arch Intern Med* 1976;136:263–265.

23. Rosenbaum J, Kramer M, Raja R, et al: Current status of hemoperfusion in toxicology. *Clin Toxicol* 1980;17:493–500.

24. Pond S, Rosenberg J, Benowitz N, et al: Phar-macokinetics of hemoperfusion for drug overdose. *Clin Pharmacokinet* 1979;4:329–354.

25. Lorch J, Garella S: Hemoperfusion to treat intoxica-tions. *Ann Intern Med* 1979;91:301–304.

26. Muirhead E, Reid A: A resin artificial kidney. *J Lab Clin Med* 1948;33:841–844.

27. Okonek S: Hemoperfusion in toxicology: Basic con-siderations of its effectiveness. *Clin Toxicol* 1981;18:1185–1198.

28. Bismuth C, Fournier P, Galliot M: Biological evalua-tion of hemoperfusion in acute poisoning. *Clin Toxicol* 1981;18:1213–1223.

29. Mamdani B, Dunea G: Long-term hemoperfusion with coated activated charcoal. *Clin Toxicol* 1980;17:543–546.

30. Trafford A, Horn C, Sharpstone P, et al: Hemoperfu-sion in acute drug toxicity. *Clin Toxicol* 1980;17:547–556.

31. Chang T: Clinical experience with ACAC-coated charcoal hemoperfusion in acute intoxication. *Clin Toxicol* 1980;17:529–542.

32. De Groot G, Maes R, Van Heijst A: A toxicological evaluation of different adsorbents in hemoperfusion. *Clin Toxicol* 1981;18:1199–1211.

33. Gelfand M, Winchester J: Hemoperfusion in drug overdosage: Conservative management is not sufficient. *Clin Toxicol* 1980;17:583–602.

34. Gelfand M: Hemoperfusion in drug overdose. *JAMA* 1978;240:2761–2762.

35. Gibson T: Hemoperfusion of digoxin intoxication. *Clin Toxicol* 1980;17:501–513.

36. Garella S, Lorch J: Hemoperfusion for acute intoxications. *Clin Toxicol* 1980;17:515–527.

37. Dumont C, Rangno R: Argument against hemoperfusion in drug overdose. *JAMA* 1979;242:1611.

38. Jones J, Dougherty J: Current status of plasmapheresis in toxicology. *Ann Emerg Med* 1986; 15:474–482.

ADDITIONAL SELECTED REFERENCES

Krenzelok E, Keller R, Stewart R: Gastrointestinal transit times of cathartics combined with charcoal. *Ann Emerg Med* 1985;14:1152–1155.

Mofenson H, Caraccio T, Greensher J, et al: Gastrointestinal dialysis with activated charcoal and cathartic in the treatment of adolescent intoxications. *Clin Pediatr* 1985;24:678–684.

Oderda G, Klein-Schwartz W: General management of the poisoned patient. *Crit Care Q* 1982;4:1–18.

Ordog G, Vann P, Owashi N, et al: Intravenous prochlorperazine for the rapid control of vomiting in the emergency department. *Ann Emerg Med* 1984;13:253–258.

Watanabe A: Pharmacokinetic aspects of the dialysis of drugs. *Drug Intell Clin Pharm* 1977;11:407–416.

chapter *4*

The Role of the Laboratory

The laboratory can provide a great deal of information to the emergency department physician and can aid in the diagnosis and care given to the overdosed patient.[1] Some physicians, however, have unrealistic expectations of how the laboratory can be of help. In the toxicologic setting the laboratory can aid the physician diagnostically in a qualitative manner through a toxicologic screen for the presence of one or more suspected toxins or prognostically through a quantitative analysis of a particular toxin. The laboratory can also aid in the therapeutic monitoring of drugs and in testing for drugs of abuse.[2]

Certain specific intoxicants require specific antidotal therapies; in these cases expedient laboratory investigation is warranted. For most other substances, little change in supportive therapy may be needed, and, if the patient is stable and properly monitored, laboratory work may not be urgently required.[3]

Because relatively few classes of drugs are responsible for the great majority of drug intoxications, most laboratories can routinely identify prototypical members of these drug classes.[4] Yet screens do not identify all toxins, and the limited scope of such a test must be understood by the practitioner.[3,5]

Methods such as spectrophotometry and spectrophotofluorometry can measure serum drug concentrations of milligrams per liter, which is the typical concentration when drugs are given in doses of several hundred milligrams. Some of the new techniques such as gas chromatography, mass spectrometry, and the immunoassays can determine fractions of nanograms or less. This is an important advance in toxicology as well as in the area of therapeutic monitoring of drugs.[6–8]

Although it may be important to know whether a patient's altered mental status is caused by ingestion or exposure to a drug or toxin, often it is not mandatory to know the concentration of the toxin to initiate treatment.[3] For instance, it is useful to know from a toxicologic screen whether a barbiturate is causing the picture of CNS depression in a particular patient, but knowing the exact concentration is not as important as following the patient clinically and determining the necessary treatment.

Qualitative drug screening continues to be a prevalent practice despite its limitations. A toxicologic screen may be referred to as an "overdose panel," "comprehensive screen," "tox screen," "coma panel," or "drug screen." The name given might imply that a toxicologic screen is truly comprehensive, but a negative screen is not conclusive evidence that no drug that can account for a patient's symptoms has been ingested because most laboratories observe an abridged procedure limited to a few sequential analyses.[9] A screen is performed for only certain classes of compounds, and each laboratory uses a different type of screen. Because there is no one accepted screen that is uniformly performed, and because the protocol for a toxicologic screen is typically determined by the historic needs of the institution, it is of the utmost importance to know exactly what is *not* included in a toxicologic screen for a particular laboratory.[4,5] It is extremely important to have good ongoing communication between emergency department personnel and laboratory technicians so that the most efficient job can be performed by both parties.[4,10]

Appropriate use of the laboratory entails knowing which specific tests to order, whether the presence of a substance (qualitative results) or the concentration of the substance in the blood (quantitative results) is most important, what the "turn-around time" for the results will be, and the type of specimen that should be obtained (eg, urine or blood).[4] (For therapeutic and toxic laboratory values, see Appendix A.)

URINE COMPARED TO BLOOD SCREENING

Generally, quantitative analysis is performed on blood or plasma samples, whereas urine is required to perform the qualitative drug screen. The importance of a urine sample in facilitating the toxicology analyses cannot be understated[10] because, as a general rule, urine has a much higher drug concentration than blood. The belief lingers, however, that blood is the preferred sample for a general evaluation.[10]

There are many different methods for drug analysis, and the laboratory must decide on the appropriate degree of sophistication. Laboratories can choose spot tests; thin-layer, gas, liquid, or high-performance liquid chromatography; spectrophotometry; immunoassays, including radioimmunoassay and enzyme-modified immunoassay; gas chromatography with mass spectroscopy; and, recently, nuclear magnetic resonance spectroscopy.[10] Methods that are normally used in measuring serum drug concentrations usually do not differentiate between drugs bound to serum proteins (which are therefore inactive) and those that are free. In most situations, however, free drug concentration is a fairly constant percentage of the total, which

makes total serum drug levels indicative of the active drug concentration.

Typically, laboratory methodology is an area of relative ignorance for the emergency department physician. The following discussion is not meant to be an in-depth analysis of each laboratory test but is an attempt to familiarize the physician with the various laboratory procedures available (Table 4-1).

SPOT TESTS

Spot tests are simple colorimetric tests that rely on a change in the sample color after addition of certain reagents.[4] Spot tests are among the simplest and quickest initial screening processes. Although this method is inexpensive, it is characterized by both poor sensitivity and specificity and also requires subjective interpretation (Table 4-2).

There are also some basic "bedside" qualitative spot tests that are available for many compounds, but these are also characterized by poor sensitivity and specificity. Their chief advantage is that they are inexpensive.

Table 4-1 Toxicologic Laboratory Analyses

Spot Tests
Chromatography
   Thin-layer chromatography (TLC)
   Gas chromatography (GC)
   Liquid chromatography (LC)
   High-performance liquid chromatography (HPLC)
Electrophoresis
Immunoassay
   Radioimmunoassay (RIA)
   Enzyme-modified immunoassay
   Fluorescence polarization immunoassay
   Latex particle immunoassay
Enzymatic methods
Spectroscopy
   Visible
   Ultraviolet
   Infrared
   Fluorometry
   Nuclear magnetic resonance (NMR)
Gas Chromatography with Mass Spectroscopy (GC-MS)

Table 4-2 Spot Tests and Their Sensitivity and Specificity

Drug	Sensitivity	Specificity
Acetaminophen	+	+
Carbamates	+	−
Carbon monoxide	−	−
Ethanol	+	−
Ethchlorvynol	+	+
Iron	−	−
Imipramine	−	−
Phenothiazines	−	−
Salicylate	+	+

CHROMATOGRAPHY

Chromatography refers to a group of separation processes of closely related compounds by adsorption from a solution to an adsorbent medium. These methods are classified according to the physical state of the solute or mobile phase. Thin-layer, gas, liquid, and high-performance liquid chromatography are all based on the flow of a liquid or gas over a solid or liquid stationary phase that contains the unknown compound. Characteristic patterns of drug distribution between the stationary and mobile phases occur.

Thin-Layer Chromatography

The earliest technical approaches to drug screening were primarily based on thin-layer chromatography (TLC).[11] TLC is one of the most widely used screening procedures; it is inexpensive and requires no automation.[12] It is an excellent method for screening or for the confirmation of drugs.[11,13] The results from TLC are qualitative in nature, and positive results cannot be quantified.[11]

In TLC, a liquid solvent containing the sample diffuses through a solid adsorbent, which may be glass plates coated with silica.[11] Different compounds migrate by capillary action across this uniform thin layer at different rates, resulting in a separation of the sample constituents. The constituents are then identified by their rate of migration, their response to chemical treatment when the plate is sprayed with a color-complex-ing reagent, and their morphologic appearance in the adsorbent. The fractional distance that each constituent travels is called the migration distance, or R_f value. Visualization of the spots on the thin layer can be achieved through illumination with ultraviolet or fluorescent light. An experienced technician is of utmost importance because of the subjectivity of data interpretation.[4]

Thin-layer chromatography is one of the least sensitive screening methods; a negative result from TLC may be positive from some other, more sensitive method. With TLC most drugs are detected only when their concentration in urine is 1000 to 2000 ng/mL.[11] Although this is usually adequate for drug overdoses, there is a lack of specificity associated with TLC, so that its results must always be compared to those of a confirmatory test. The confirmatory test should always be based on a different principle of analysis and should be more specific than the screening test.[11] Another disadvantage of TLC is the relatively long turn-around time required.

The advent of high-performance or high-efficiency TLC has greatly reduced its disadvantages,[3,13] and many modern techniques are highly specific. In some cases the specificity is beyond that of gas chromatography.

Gas Chromatography

Gas chromatography (GC) is a rigorous and complicated technique that allows a multitude of compounds within a single sample to be separated and measured simultaneously.[14] In GC, molecules in a vaporized sample are separated by means of a glass or metal tube that is packed with material of a particular polarity.[11] The stationary phase may be either liquid or solid; the gas is the mobile phase.

When a mixture of substances is injected at the inlet of the column and vaporized, each component is swept through the column and toward a detector. If the substance in question has no affinity for the solvent, then it is deposited on the solid packing material of the column. The column therefore permits graded retardation of the components of the mixture to establish a relatively clean separation among groups of similar molecules.

Once these groups are separated, they leave the column and enter the detection system. When a particular molecule reaches the detector, a signal is produced. The time between injection of the sample and appearance of the signal is referred to as the retention time and is characteristic of each substance.

Separation of drugs by GC, then, is based on the characteristic vapor pressures that different compounds establish above the liquid phase of a stationary separation medium. Theoretically, any compound that can be vaporized or converted to a volatile derivative can be analyzed by GC. The technique is usually limited to organic molecules because inorganic compounds lack sufficient volatility. For screening purposes, samples can be chromatographed on a single column or injected into various compound-selective columns to enhance specificity and sensitivity.

Although GC is an excellent tool for analysis, it requires several steps to prepare the samples for analysis. Relatively large volumes of blood or urine are required for the extraction process, although recent advances have made microsampling possible on a more routine basis. One of the major disadvantages of GC is the complexity of instrumentation, which necessitates a highly trained and skilled analyst.

High-Performance Liquid Chromatography

High-performance (pressure) liquid chromatography (HPLC) is similar to GC except that liquid pressurization rather than evaporation is used to force the sample through the adsorbent.[11] HPLC can analyze complex mixtures from microsamples and is rapid and specific, but it is also expensive. The advantage of HPLC is the high resolution of similar compounds, which is made possible by the separating power of the system. HPLC is therefore most useful in situations where more than one substance is being measured. The power of HPLC also lies in its ability to separate structurally similar drugs, such as tricyclics and benzodiazepines. Most commonly, theophylline and related compounds, antiepileptic drugs, tricyclics, procainamide, disopyramide, the aminoglycosides, and a host of other drugs can be measured by HPLC systems. HPLC and other chromatographic methods are similar in many respects, so that HPLC complements rather than supplants these other methods. The greatest limitation of HPLC is the success of competing immunoassay systems.

ELECTROPHORESIS

Electrophoresis is a separation technique based on the movement of charged particles under the influence of an external electric field. Different molecules can be separated in an electric field if they carry different charges. The electric field is applied to a solution through oppositely charged electrodes placed in the solution and a particular ion then travels through the solution toward the electrode of opposite charge. Electrophoresis is not used very often in toxicology.

IMMUNOASSAYS

Immunoassays are widely employed in drug assays because they provide a high degree of sensitivity and specificity. Immunoassays measure substances by exploiting the immunochemical reaction between antigen and antibody. Antigens are substances that induce an immune response. The most potent antigens are macromolecules with molecular sizes greater than 100,000 daltons. Drugs usually have molecular sizes that are too small for them to act as antigens, so that it is necessary to couple the drug to a larger molecule, which is usually a protein. The most commonly used protein is albumin, which is taken from a species other than that in which the antibody is to be raised.

The general theory concerning the immunoassay is that a labeled drug is competitively displaced from an antibody complex by an unlabeled drug in a sample. The amount of labeled drug that is displaced from the antibody is proportional to the amount of unlabeled drug in the sample.[15]

Immunoassays for toxic substances use radioisotopic labels,[16] fluorescent labels,[17,18] latex particles, red cells, and enzymes. These techniques differ according to how the drug is labeled and in the method of detection of the displaced labeled drug. Because clinical laboratories frequently have sensitive spectrophotometers and technologists who are experienced in the handling of enzyme-based systems, emphasis has recently shifted to the use of enzyme markers.[4]

Radioimmunoassay

In radioimmunoassay (RIA), known quantities of drug-specific antibody and known amounts of isotopically labeled drug are mixed with a sample. The mixture is then scanned for the emission of gamma radiation after the displacement of the labeled antigen by the drug in the sample.[4,19] Labeled and unlabeled drug molecules compete for a limited number of binding sites on a specific drug antibody. The amount of displaced label correlates directly with the concentration of drug in the added sample. The sensitivity of this procedure can be at the picogram or nanogram level.[19]

The sensitivity of RIA results primarily from the binding affinity between antigen and antibody. The specificity of RIA is a reflection of the uniqueness of fit between an antigen and its corresponding antibody. The affinity of the unknown drug for the antibody is plotted as a curve, which is compared to standard curves so that the unknown drug can be identified.[19] Because there is no difference between the bound and free labeled drug, it is necessary to separate the two before measurement; therefore these assays are referred to as heterogeneous immunoassays.

The major advantages of RIA are its microcapability, accuracy, relative rapidity, and ease of operation. The disadvantages are that it is limited to those drugs for which antibodies are available and that its specificity is limited to classes of compounds rather than to individual drugs.[20]

Fluorescence Polarization Immunoassay

Fluorescence polarization immunoassay makes use of competitive binding principles and directly measures the binding of labeled drug without the need for a separation process. With fluorescence polarization immunoassay the unknown sample and a known labeled substance compete for a limited and known number of antibody sites specific for the drug. The more drug present, the lower the measured fluorescence polarization of the labeled drug. As with other immunoassays standard curves are prepared from calibrated drug concentrations, and the unknown is determined from the standard curve.[18,21] Although this procedure has great potential, it has seen little clinical utility primarily because of a lack of a simple, low-cost, high-performance instrumentation.

Enzyme-Modified Immunoassay

Assays in which the antibody or hapten is bound to an enzyme are called enzyme-modified immunoassays.[22] Enzyme-multiplied immunoassay technique (EMIT) has been found to be accurate, specific, and easier to use than RIA.[23] This technique generally requires only the addition of one, two, or three reagents in an orderly, timed sequence. The sample size rarely exceeds 100 μL. In addition, EMIT is applicable to many classes of compounds.[24] This system makes use of a nonisotopic label and is usually less sensitive than RIA; nevertheless, it has become the prevailing means of toxicologic analysis in hospital laboratories during the past few years because it can be performed directly and expeditiously on a given sample.

In EMIT, the inhibition of an enzyme-substrate reaction is proportional to the amount of drug in the sample. A labeled hapten is added to an unlabeled sample to be assayed; that is, the drug is labeled by chemical attachment to an enzyme, which is then allowed to equilibrate with a specific antibody. When the enzyme-labeled drug becomes bound to an antibody to the drug, the activity of the enzyme is reduced. The remaining enzyme activity is then measured by adding a known amount of substrate; the amount of added substrate needed to neutralize the remaining enzyme equals the concentration of the hapten being measured.

Because there is a difference between the free and bound labeled drug, no separation step is necessary.[25,26] These immunoassays are therefore referred to as homogeneous immunoassays.

A wide variety of homogeneous immunoassays are available as commercial kits that identify many common poisons (Table 4-3). In contrast to RIA, the shelf-life of EMIT reagents is usually long.[25] This system is adaptable to many automated and semiautomated instruments, so that with enzyme immunoassay technology hundreds of specimens can be run per day with a turn-around time of approximately 20 minutes. The use of automation has significantly reduced reagent costs because a small volume of material can be used.

Enzyme-modified immunoassay is designed to achieve accurate measurement in the therapeutic range of the drug being assayed. Biochemically accurate measurement of higher concentrations requires dilution of samples with drug-free serum. Concentrations below the therapeutic range are also less accurately measured.

Enzyme-modified immunoassay measures total drug concentration and does not separate free from protein-bound drug. To this effect, it does not give an estimate of the pharmacologically active drug but only of the total, potentially available drug circulating in the serum. In addition, it does not measure metabolic products in a single system that may or may not contribute to pharmacologic action or toxicity.

Although this procedure gives the highest percentage of positive results, by itself it does not provide the necessary comprehensive result. Therefore, confirmation of a presumptive positive finding carried out by a second analytically distinct method is prudent because it ensures the quality of the data reported.

SPECTROSCOPY

Spectroscopy measures the ability of a substance to absorb electromagnetic radiation. The wavelengths of maximum absorbance and the shape and pattern of the spectrum identify the compound. There are many types of spectrophotometry, although many have drawbacks for practical use in an emergency setting. The three types of spectrophotometry most often used in toxicology are ultraviolet spectroscopy, fluorescence spectroscopy, and nuclear magnetic resonance spectroscopy.

Ultraviolet Spectroscopy

Ultraviolet spectroscopy identifies a substance by measuring its pattern of peak absorbance of light of monochromatic wavelength.

Table 4-3 Drugs That Can Be Assayed by EMIT

Urine	Serum	Therapeutic Monitoring
Amphetamines	Acetaminophen	Amikacin
Barbiturates	Barbiturates	Disopyramide
Benzodiazepines	Benzodiazepines	Ethosuximide
Cannabinoids	Ethyl alcohol	Gentamicin
Cocaine metabolites	Phencyclidine	Lidocaine
Ethyl alcohol	Tricyclic antidepressants	Methotrexate
Methadone	Carbamazepine	Netilmicin
Methaqualone	Digoxin	Phenobarbital
Opiates	Phenytoin	Primidone
Phencyclidine		Procainamide
Propoxyphene		Quinidine
		Theophylline
		Tobramycin
		Valproic acid

Source: Adapted with permission from *Emergency Medicine Clinics of North America* (1986;4:367–376), Copyright © 1986, WB Saunders Company.

Ultraviolet spectroscopy has a relatively poor specificity unless the unknown drug is isolated by other procedures. This is because many compounds have overlapping or similar ultraviolet spectra. This method is useful as a confirming test or in conjunction with immunoassay techniques.[4]

Fluorescence Spectroscopy

Fluorescence spectroscopy is one of the most widely used luminescence techniques primarily because of its intrinsic sensitivity and selectivity. This technique measures the intensity of emitted energy of a compound after it is exposed to an exciting light source. Some drugs have natural fluorescence, such as quinine and imipramine, and some have derivatives that fluoresce.

Nuclear Magnetic Resonance Spectroscopy

Nuclear magnetic resonance (NMR) spectroscopy measures a molecule's absorption of energy in an externally applied magnetic field. As the frequency of incident radio waves changes, the molecules undergo characteristic atomic resonances that are recorded as a spectrum, which identify the chemical structure of the drug. Although NMR spectroscopy is used in many institutions to detect disease states and can be adapted for use in toxicology, it is rarely used for this purpose at present primarily because of its high cost.

GAS CHROMATOGRAPHY WITH MASS SPECTROSCOPY

Computer-assisted gas chromatography with mass spectroscopy (GC-MS) is a sophisticated but not readily available method of testing. It has long been recognized as the most definitive technique for positive identification of compounds. The drug must generally be extracted from the sample before GC can be performed, and the drug must either be volatile or derivatized to make it volatile.

Mass spectroscopy measures the masses of fragments of a molecule produced by bombardment of the molecule with electrons. The mass-to-charge ratio as well as the relative abundance of the ions produced are recorded as a characteristic spectrum. GC-MS can be used both qualitatively and quantitatively and has a sensitivity of nanograms to picograms. It is applicable to a wide range of samples, there being more than 30,000 known standards.[27] These standards are listed in computer libraries by the mass of the parent compound and its characteristic fragments. Not surprisingly, GC-MS requires a high level of sophistication to operate the equipment and is therefore usually reserved for certain reference laboratories.[11]

DRUG TESTING IN THE EMERGENCY SETTING

Qualitative Compared to Quantitative Testing

When attempting to rule out a drug as a cause of coma, qualitative drug screening is often adequate.[3,9,28] Nevertheless, for certain drugs or toxins the early clinical symptoms correlate poorly with the patient's eventual outcome.[29] A quantitative screening for these drugs may be important in determining treatment. Also, some toxins must be identified quickly so that proper treatment can be promptly administered.[30] A laboratory should therefore be prepared to perform the tests listed in Table 4-4 on an immediate (stat) basis, or it should have easy access to a reference laboratory that can perform these analyses.

When "Stat" Quantitation Is Desirable

There may be substances whose levels would be helpful to know, but in actuality such information would not change the treatment offered to the patient and so would just be obtained for scientific interest. These levels could be obtained, if possible, but it is not necessary to have them available on a stat basis. The following levels should be available on a stat basis

Table 4-4 Substances and Parameters That Require Stat Quantitative Analysis

---

Iron and iron binding capacity
Methanol
Ethylene glycol
Acetaminophen
Salicylates
Carbon monoxide (carboxyhemoglobin)
Ethanol
Digoxin
Lithium
Methemoglobin
Serum osmolality
Theophylline

---

because they will change or determine the treatment provided.

Iron and Total Iron Binding Capacity

Although iron and iron binding capacity are relatively specialized tests and are typically not available on a stat basis, their usefulness in toxicology cannot be overstated in a suspected case of iron overdose. If the iron exceeds the iron binding capacity, then specific chelation therapy is immediately required. The results of iron overload tests are unreliable, and such tests should not be attempted.

Methanol and Ethylene Glycol

The metabolites of methanol and ethylene glycol are extremely toxic, and immediate laboratory confirmation is necessary so that specific therapy can be instituted rapidly. Methanol concentration is relatively simple to measure. Most laboratories, however, are not able to measure ethylene glycol concentrations; for this reason, the diagnosis of ethylene glycol toxicity may be based on other findings, such as history, anion gap, metabolic acidosis, osmolal gap, and crystalluria.

Acetaminophen

Plotting the acetaminophen concentration on the acetaminophen nomogram is absolutely necessary because without this measurement there may be no accurate way to foresee which patient may go on to have hepatic necrosis and which

patient may be discharged from the emergency department.

Salicylates

As with acetaminophen, it is important to measure the salicylate concentration and to plot it on the salicylate nomogram so as to have a prognostic indicator that will determine the extent of treatment necessary.

Carbon Monoxide

Carbon monoxide (carboxyhemoglobin) concentrations are important to know because the history may be spurious, and the diagnosis may be missed without an immediate test.

Ethanol

Ethanol concentrations are measured for comparison with the patient's condition. For example, a low ethanol concentration in the face of an advanced stage of coma would alert the physician that the coma is due to another cause. A high concentration, on the other hand, may not be the sole cause of coma. The patient's condition should continue to be monitored and will improve as the ethanol is metabolized.

Digoxin

A serum digoxin concentration may be diagnostic in the chronically overdosed patient, but it should not determine treatment. The condition of the patient determines the course of treatment because a serum digoxin concentration may not adequately reflect the clinical course in the acute overdose.

Lithium

Blood lithium concentrations should be measured because a toxic level may require diuresis and dialysis. Early in an acute intoxication, however, blood lithium concentration may not adequately reflect the future clinical outcome.

Methemoglobin

Because methemoglobinemia is a potentially fatal condition that can be treated with an antidote, tests for the measurement of methemoglobin should be readily available. A co-oximeter can measure both carboxyhemoglobin and methemoglobin concentrations in the same sample.

Serum Osmolality

A serum osmolality test by freezing point depression should be available to detect some of the more toxic alcohols such as methanol and ethylene glycol. This measurement is compared with the calculated serum osmolality for evidence of an osmolal gap.

Theophylline

Measurement of the serum theophylline concentration may be helpful as an adjunct in deciding whether a patient requires extracorporeal means of drug removal.

REFERENCES

1. Arena J: The clinical diagnosis of poisoning. *Pediatr Clin North Am* 1970;17:477–494.

2. Hansen H, Caudill S, Boone J: Crisis in drug testing: Results of CDC blind study. *JAMA* 1985;253:2382–2387.

3. Kellermann A, Fihn S, LoGergo J, et al: Impact of drug screening in suspected overdose. *Ann Emerg Med* 1987;16:1206–1216.

4. Epstein F, Hassan M: Therapeutic drug levels and toxicology screen. *Emerg Med Clin North Am* 1986; 4:367–376.

5. Kulig K: Utilization of emergency toxicology screens, editorial. *Am J Emerg Med* 1985;6:573–574.

6. Baselt R, Wright J, Cravey R: Therapeutic and toxic concentrations of more than one hundred toxicologically significant drugs in blood, plasma, or serum: A tabulation. *Clin Chem* 1975;21:44–62.

7. Jellett L: Plasma concentrations in the control of drug therapy. *Drugs* 1976;11:412–422.

8. Koch-Weser J: Serum drug concentrations as therapeutic guides. *N Engl J Med* 1972;287:227–231.

9. Bailey D: The role of the laboratory in treatment of the poisoned patient: Laboratory perspective. *J Anal Toxicol* 1983;7:136–141.

10. Helper B, Sutheimer C, Sunshine I: Role of the toxicology laboratory in suspected ingestions. *Pediatr Clin North Am* 1986;33:245–260.

11. Gold M, Dackis C: Role of the laboratory in the evaluation of suspected drug abuse. *J Clin Psychiatr* 1986;47:17–23.

12. Michaud J: Thin-layer chromatography for broad spectrum drug detection. *Am Lab* 1980;12:104–108.

13. Martel P, Lones D, Rousseau R: Application of Toxi-Lab: A broad spectrum drug detection system in emergency toxicology. *Am Assoc Clin Chem* 1983;2:1–4.

14. Finke B: A GLC-based system for the detection of poisons, drugs and human metabolites encountered in forensic toxicology. *J Chromatogr Sci* 1971;9:393–396.

15. Brattin W, Sunshine I: Immunological assays for drugs in biological samples. *Am J Med Tech* 1973; 39:223–230.

16. Skelley D, Brown L, Besch P: Radioimmunoassay. *Clin Chem* 1973;19:146–186.

17. Bakerman S: Substrate-labeled fluorescence immunoassay. *Lab Manage* 1983;21:13–16.

18. Jolley M, Stroupe S, Schwenzer K, et al: Fluorescence polarization immunoassay: Part III: An automated system for therapeutic drug determination. *Clin Chem* 1981;27:1575–1579.

19. Castro A, Mittleman R: Determination of drugs of abuse in body fluids by radioimmunoassay. *Clin Biochem* 1978;11:103–105.

20. Spector S: Application of radioimmunoassay to pharmacology. *Clin Pharmacol Ther* 1974;16:149–154.

21. Lu-Steffes M, Pittluck G, Jolley M, et al: Fluorescence polarization immunoassay: Part IV: Determination of phenytoin and phenobarbital in human serum and plasma. *Clin Chem* 1982;28:2278–2281.

22. Rubenstein K, Schneider R, Ullman E: Homogenous enzyme immunoassay: A new immunochemical technique. *Biochem Biophys Res Commun* 1972;47:846–854.

23. Bastiani R: Homogenous immunochemical drug assays. *Am J Med Technol* 1983;39:211–223.

24. Drost R: EMIT-st drug detection system for screening of barbiturates and benzodiazepines in serum. *J Toxicol Clin Toxicol* 1982;19:303–312.

25. Helper B, Sutheimer C, Sunshine I: The role of the toxicology laboratory in emergency medicine. *J Toxicol Clin Toxicol* 1982;19:353–365.

26. Helper B, Sutheimer C, Sunshine I: The role of the toxicology laboratory in the treatment of acute poisoning. *Med Toxicol* 1986;1:61–75.

27. Ullucci P: A comprehensive GC/MS drug screening procedure. *J Anal Toxicol* 1978;2:33–38.

28. Baker S, Davey D: The predictive value for man of toxicological tests of drugs in laboratory animals. *Br Med Bull* 1976;26:208–211.

29. Green V: Use of the toxicology laboratory. *Crit Care Q* 1982;19–23.

30. Weisman R, Howland M: The toxicology laboratory. *Top Emerg Med* 1983;5:9–15.

ADDITIONAL SELECTED REFERENCES

Opheim K, Raisys V: Therapeutic drug monitoring in pediatric acute drug intoxications. *Ther Drug Monit* 1985;7:148–158.

Pippenger C: Rationale and clinical application of therapeutic drug monitoring. *Pediatr Clin North Am* 1980;27:891–925.

Teitelbaum D, Morgan J, Gray G: Nonconcordance between clinical impression and laboratory findings in clinical toxicology. *Clin Toxicol* 1977;10:417–422.

Vere D: The significance of blood levels of drugs. *Sci Basis Med* 1972;363–384.

chapter 5

Pharmacokinetics and Toxicokinetics

Pharmacokinetics and toxicokinetics are relatively new areas of pharmacology and toxicology, respectively. An understanding of pharmacokinetics can greatly aid in the treatment of medical conditions and in therapy for substance overdose. Pharmacokinetics is the study of the changes in a drug or its metabolites in the body from the time it enters the body until it is fully eliminated.[1-3] It encompasses many factors, such as absorption, distribution, extent of body storage, amount of protein binding, metabolites of the parent compound and the toxicity associated with those metabolites, as well as the method and mode of excretion of the compound and metabolites.[4,5] Pharmacologic principles are also important in predicting whether the various methods of enhancing elimination will be effective (these methods are discussed in Chapter 3).

Toxicokinetics is a mathematical conceptualization of clinical pharmacology in an overdosed patient. By using toxicokinetic principles, numbers (such as the volume of distribution) and rates are assigned to the biologic processes. An understanding of toxicokinetics is important in predicting how a drug acts in the body and why it acts in that manner. It may also explain why compounds are more easily removed from the body by extracorporeal methods or with multiple doses of activated charcoal. This chapter presents some of the terminology and concepts in pharmacokinetics and toxicokinetics.

GENERAL CONSIDERATIONS

For a drug to exert the desired biologic effect, it must reach and interact with the receptors regulating that specific effect. The site of action of a drug is the location at which a given drug acts; this is also called the receptor site. The mechanism of action of a drug is the means by which, at a specific site, the drug initiates its biologic effect.[3] The mechanism of action of most drugs depends on a chemical interaction with a functionally viable component of the physiologic system.

After a drug is administered, the pharmacologic effect achieved is a direct consequence of the reversible formation of bonds between the drug and tissue receptors controlling a particular response.[6] For most drugs, the intensity of a pharmacologic effect tends to be proportional to the drug concentration in extracellular fluid. A drug present in extracellular fluid can enter tissues and interact with specific receptors.[7] For a drug to be therapeutically effective, it must reach the site of its intended pharmacologic activity within the body at a sufficient rate and in sufficient amount to yield an effective concentration. Factors important in determining the serum drug concentrations attained and eventually reflected at receptor sites include (1) disease, (2) drug pharmacokinetics, (3) bioavailability, (4) physiological factors, (5) patient compliance, and (6) drug interactions.

The most commonly employed approach to the pharmacokinetic characterization of a drug is to represent the body as a system of compartments, even though these compartments usually have no physiologic or anatomic reality.[4,8] The one-compartment model, the simplest one, depicts the body as a single, kinetically homogeneous unit. This model is particularly useful for drugs that distribute relatively rapidly throughout the body. Therefore, models should only serve as a general guideline unless specific patient data are obtained.

PHARMACOKINETICS AND PATIENT AGE

Much of the important work in the last decade in the area of pharmacokinetics has been performed with young adults. Because of this, estimates of drug disposition in children and the elderly have been made with the use of pharmacokinetic parameters derived from the study of young adults. Neonates and the elderly, however, generally have a lower metabolic capacity compared with subjects between these extremes of age.[8] There are many other reasons why these parameters may be incorrect, owing to the continuous and rapid physiologic changes associated with the basic stages of human development.

In the first 2 weeks of life the microsomal enzymes responsible for metabolism are immature and not fully active. In the newborn, there is also an impaired glomerular filtration rate as well as impaired tubular secretory and reabsorbing capacities. Furthermore, very young children do not have the necessary plasma-binding proteins. Shortly after 2 weeks until approximately 10 years of age the activity of these systems increases, and drug elimination usually occurs at a significantly higher rate than in adults because maturing organ function contributes to a greater drug effect per unit body weight than in the adult.[3] At puberty (10 to 14 years of age), the child's physiologic pattern for metabolizing drugs rapidly approaches that of an adult. Children older than 15 years of age typically exhibit adult patterns of drug utilization. These changes are directly associated with the initial onset of puberty and are observed earlier in females than in males. In elderly subjects, there appears to be a decreasing capacity for drug metabolism as a consequence of a gradual decline in overall physiological efficiency. These differences should be kept in mind when interpreting pharmacologic data.

BIOAVAILABILITY

Bioavailability, in simple terms, refers to the rate and extent of drug absorption in the general circulation.[8] In other words, it is the fraction of a drug dose that is absorbed intact by any given route compared with intravenous administration.[9] Bioavailability depends on a number of factors, some of which relate to how a drug product is designed and manufactured and others to its physiochemical properties. Bioavailability is directly proportional to the total amount of unchanged drug in the blood.

An important concept that describes bioavailability is the 'area under the plasma concentration curve' (AUC). This term is frequently used in discussing pharmacokinetics and is an indicator of total drug absorption. Because it reflects bioavailability the AUC is more appropriate than peak serum level, which is dependent on the rate of drug absorption. The AUC, then, is the most important measurement of bioavailability and is based on serum concentration plotted against time (Fig. 5-1). The AUC repre-

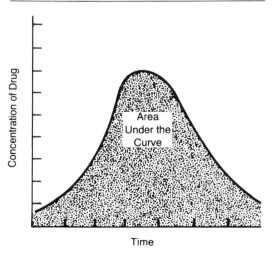

Figure 5-1 Serum Concentration Plotted against Time for Hypothetical Drug.

sents the amount of drug that enters the systemic circulation during the distribution phase, early after administration. The distribution phase, or alpha phase, lasts approximately 30 minutes to 2 hours for most drugs. During this phase concentrations in the plasma decrease more rapidly than during the second phase, or elimination phase (beta phase).

VOLUME OF DISTRIBUTION

The apparent volume of distribution is a useful pharmacokinetic parameter that relates the plasma or serum concentration of a drug to the total amount of drug in the body.[1,2] After a drug is absorbed it is distributed within the body; the measure of the compartment into which the drug distributes is termed the apparent volume of distribution. The volume of distribution is defined as that volume of fluid into which a drug *appears* to distribute to a concentration equal to that in plasma. It is calculated from the dose of a drug administered and the resulting plasma concentration. A drug concentration in body fluids other than plasma may be used, but different values for the volume of distribution are obtained for each fluid. It is therefore important to note which fluid is being used. In this text, the volumes of distribution are based on plasma concentrations.

The concept of volume of distribution is relatively simplistic because it assumes that the body acts as a single compartment with respect to the drug. In reality, this volume is a hypothetical value that does not refer to any actual physiologic space in the body.[10] The real distribution volume of a drug is related to body water and cannot exceed total body water, which is about 60% of body weight in the normal adult. In an individual of average weight (150 lb) this corresponds to approximately 40 L of fluid. Total body water may be divided into three separate compartments: the plasma water, interstitial water, and intracellular water. Extracellular water is a combination of plasma water and the interstitial water. Intracellular fluid also includes the fluid in the erythrocytes and other formed elements. Most drugs, however, are significantly bound in either the vascular or extravascular space (or both). This is divided into

approximately 25 L of intracellular water, 12 L of interstitial water, and 3 L of plasma water.

The term volume of distribution gives some idea of the extent to which a drug is taken up by tissues in the body or whether a drug is found to a greater extent in the plasma. When the volume of distribution is large, the tissue concentration is large and plasma concentration is small. When the volume of distribution is small, most of the drug remains in the plasma.[11]

The volume of distribution, then, is a measure of the compartment into which a drug distributes. The equation for the volume of distribution defines the relation between the amount of drug in the body and the amount of drug in the bloodstream. If a drug is highly concentrated in tissues, its apparent volume of distribution may be many times the total body water.[10] Because the volume of distribution does not represent a real body space, it may be as small as the plasma volume or as large as several hundred liters. Often the volume of distribution is characteristic of a drug and constant over a wide dose range.[12] The formula for the apparent volume of distribution is

$$V_d = A/(C_p)(M)$$

where V_d is the volume of distribution (in liters per kilogram), A is the amount of drug in the body (in milligrams), C_p is the concentration of drug in plasma (in milligrams per liter or micrograms per milliliter), and M is body weight (in kilograms).

The volume of distribution may also be affected by a number of different factors.[10] These include the amount of body fat (because certain drugs distribute to fat to a greater or lesser extent), renal function, age (because both the very young and the elderly metabolize drugs differently and have different volumes of distribution), cardiac output (because all drugs are distributed by the bloodstream throughout the body), and the degree of protein binding for a drug (Table 5-1).[1,13] Drugs that are highly bound to albumin and other proteins, although they may have a small volume of distribution and are found to a great extent in the plasma, are inactive[15] and therefore do not account for any drug activity.[19,20] Binding to serum albumin thus decreases the maximum intensity of action

Table 5-1 Factors Affecting the Volume of Distribution

Surface area
Degree of obesity
Sex
Physical stress
Thyroid condition
Renal function
Age
Cardiac output
Protein binding

of most drugs because it lowers the peak drug concentration achieved at the sites of action.[14]

Basic drugs are quickly taken up by tissues and fat and thus have a large volume of distribution (greater than 1 L/kg). The volume of distribution then exceeds the volume of total body fluids. Acidic drugs are not taken up by fat and thus have a small volume of distribution (less than 1 L/kg) (see Appendix B). In terms of body compartments, a drug with a volume of distribution of 3 L in a person weighing 70 kg can be thought of as being contained in the plasma volume. A volume of distribution of approximately 15 L in the same person is contained in the extravascular interstitial fluid and plasma. A drug such as alcohol has a volume of distribution of approximately 40 L and is thought of as being contained in total body water.

In toxicology, the volume of distribution can be useful (1) in calculating the amount of substance in the body to help verify the history of the quantity ingested, (2) in determining the amount of antidote needed if the serum level of the ingested substance is known, or (3) in deciding whether to attempt to enhance elimination of the toxic substance. Knowledge of the volume of distribution may also provide a reasonable basis for the design of typical dosage regimens and may indicate whether dosage adjustments will be necessary in the event of renal impairment.[16]

To verify the history of the quantity of an ingested substance after the plasma concentration is determined, the equation given above for the volume of distribution is rearranged as

$$A = V_d \times C_p \times M$$

For example, a patient weighing 70 kg states that she ingested approximately 30 100-mg phenobarbital tablets (phenobarbital has a volume of distribution of 0.75 L/kg). Blood is drawn and sent to the laboratory, and the peak plasma concentration is determined to be 60 mg/L. The history is verified as follows.

$$\begin{aligned} A &= V_d \times C_p \times M \\ &= 0.75 \text{ L/kg} \times 60 \text{ mg/L} \times 70 \text{ kg} \\ &= 3150 \text{ mg} \end{aligned}$$

The amount calculated from the equation is essentially equal to that from the patient's history, and the history is therefore verified.

As another example, involving therapeutic dosing in an emergency situation, a 110 pound patient with a history of taking xanthine bronchodilators enters the emergency department with bronchoconstriction. If the plasma theophylline concentration is 5 µg/mL (therapeutic concentration, 10 to 20 µg/mL), the amount of aminophylline it would take to raise the patient's level to the mid-therapeutic range (15 µg/mL) is calculated as follows. The necessary change in plasma concentration is 10 µg/mL. The change in the dose is then the volume of distribution (0.46 L/kg) multiplied by the patient's weight and the change in concentration.

$$\begin{aligned} A &= V_d \times (\text{change in } C_p) \times M \\ &= 0.46 \text{ L/kg} \times 10 \text{ µg/mL} \times 50 \text{ kg} \\ &= 230 \text{ mg} \end{aligned}$$

The dose required is 230 mg and can be given as a loading dosage over a 20-minute period (in actuality, this may be an underestimate because aminophylline is only 80% to 85% theophylline).

If the equation is rearranged, then the plasma concentration after a given quantity of drug has been ingested can also be estimated. For example, if a 60-kg patient ingests approximately 20 tablets of phenytoin (100 mg each; volume of distribution, 0.75 L/kg), the peak plasma concentration is calculated as follows:

$$\begin{aligned} C_p &= A/(V_d)(M) \\ &= 2000 \text{ mg}/0.75 \text{ L/kg} \times 60 \text{ kg} = 44.4 \text{ µg/mL} \end{aligned}$$

Knowing this level before receiving the laboratory report may aid in determining the extent of toxicity and treatment required.

As another example, an 8-month-old child weighing 10 kg is given 2 tablespoons of 80-proof bourbon to soothe teething pain. The peak plasma concentration of ethanol is calculated as follows. Two tablespoons (30 mL) of 80-proof whiskey (40% ethanol) is approximately 9.5 g of ethanol (40% of 30 mL, or 12 mL, times the density of ethanol, 0.79 g/mL). This is then divided by the volume of distribution (0.60 L/kg) times the child's weight to yield more than 150 mg/dL. This value means that the infant requires immediate attention, and appropriate measures must be taken to prevent complications (eg, seizures, hypoglycemia, hypothermia, apnea, and hypotension). If a person weighing 70 kg ingests the same 2 tablespoons of bourbon, the plasma concentration is only about 23 mg/dL because this person has a markedly larger space into which the ethanol is distributed (70 kg × 0.6 L/kg), making the peak plasma level only 23 mg/dL.

$$12,500 \text{ mg}/42 \text{ L} \times 0.79 = 22.7 \text{ mg/dL}$$

These examples show that the volume of distribution is not simply a concept but a number that can aid in certain predictions of outcome and the extent of toxicity in various therapeutic and overdose situations.

Drugs with a relatively small volume of distribution (less than 1 L/kg) are present in substantial amounts in the circulation at any given time and may be removed with some success by extracorporeal methods. This is by no means always true because there are many other variables that determine whether the excretion of a substance may be enhanced by extracorporeal means.[17] The degree of protein binding and the volume of distribution of the compound are only two factors. Substances with a large volume of distribution (greater than 1 L/kg) are not present in the blood in high concentrations, and generally a significant fraction of the total drug in the body is not recovered by extracorporeal means.

PROTEIN BINDING

Often, drugs are transported in the blood in two forms: attached to carrier proteins, or unbound in solution. Interaction between binding proteins in the serum and drugs is a reversible event.[3] Albumin and α_1-acid glycoprotein are the most important carrier proteins for many therapeutic agents. In general, acidic drugs bind to albumin and basic drugs to α_1-acid glycoprotein.

The drug concentration in extracellular fluid is in equilibrium with the drug concentration in plasma water.[18–21] The latter, known as the free drug concentration, is an indirect measure of drug concentration at the site of action. On entering the systemic circulation any drug that is characteristically protein bound binds to the plasma proteins. Bound drug is unable to cross cell membranes and consequently exerts no biologic effect. This is because the drug-protein complex is usually a large molecule that cannot leave the blood to reach the cell membranes. Only the unbound or free drug is able to cross the various lipoprotein membranes and is dissolved in plasma water. It is then transported across cell membranes and interacts with specific receptors to elicit a desired pharmacologic response. A drug that is highly protein bound has a small volume of distribution.

Each drug has its own characteristic protein binding pattern that is dependent on the physical and chemical properties of that drug. Drugs are either tightly or loosely bound, depending on their affinity for the plasma proteins. A drug with a greater affinity for plasma proteins can displace a weakly bound drug from its plasma protein binding site. Those drugs that are tightly bound are not displaced rapidly. Heredity, sex, age, disease, and other physiologic conditions may also affect the extent of drug binding to proteins. Displacement of a drug from its plasma protein binding site can, under certain circumstances, elevate free drug concentrations at the tissue receptor sites with resultant clinical toxicity, even though the total plasma drug concentration remains unchanged.[3]

As plasma protein-binding sites become saturated in overdose the unbound fraction of the drug increases, resulting in an increased volume of distribution for the drug. Increases in the amount of free drug may then lead to a greater clinical or toxic effect than would be expected from the drug's total concentration because free concentrations generally correlate more closely with clinical effect.

ROUTES OF EXCRETION AND ELIMINATION

Clearance

The elimination of drugs from the body can also be described quantitatively by the term clearance. Clearance is a measure of the amount of drug that is eliminated per unit time. This elimination may be accomplished through major routes, such as excretion by the kidneys or metabolism by the liver as well as through minor routes, such as the lungs, sweat, and feces. How a drug is cleared and by what mechanism is important in deciding on a method for detoxification. For most drugs, clearance by glomerular filtration by the kidney and metabolism by the liver is directly proportional to the amount of free drug in the serum. Consequently, an increase in free drug concentration makes more drug available for elimination.

The elimination rate, or clearance, does not necessarily refer to the actual elimination of the drug from the body because drug metabolism converts drugs from pharmacologically active to inactive compounds. Thus the pharmacologically active portion of the drug may be eliminated even though the metabolite is still present in the body. This type of elimination is dependent only on plasma concentration.

First-Pass Effect

Drugs that are administered intravenously enter the systemic circulation as soon as they are injected. They then may be redistributed into various tissues or remain in the blood compartment. Drugs that are ingested orally first traverse the hepatic portal system before reaching the systemic circulation. Thus if a drug is extensively cleared by the liver only a small fraction of it will reach the systemic circulation. This is called the first-pass effect and occurs with a number of therapeutic agents. It is also called the extraction ratio, the proportion of a drug that enters the liver and is then eliminated from the plasma in a single passage.

Drugs that have a significant first-pass effect can be administered as sublingual tablets or by rectal suppositories, which avoids the first pass through the portal circulation. For example, naloxone is absorbed by almost all routes with significant serum concentrations being achieved. This is not true for the oral route because of the significant first-pass effect; by this route the drug is 2% as potent as when it is parenterally administered. Other drugs that have a significant first-pass effect are listed in Table 5-2.

The liver transforms a drug into one or more metabolites, and the kidneys excrete variable amounts of a drug and its metabolites. That is why the liver is the most important organ to remove drugs by metabolism and the kidneys are the second in importance. In general, there are two types of metabolic processes in the liver: one in which more polar groups are introduced into the drug molecule by processes such as oxidation, reduction, or hydrolysis; and the other in which the drug is conjugated with glucuronic acid, sulfate, glycine, or other groups.

First-Order, Zero-Order, and Michaelis-Menten Elimination

Drugs are eliminated in one of three ways: first-order elimination, zero-order elimination, or a combination of the two. Drugs that are charged or highly polar are either not metabolized or, what is more likely, the metabolism is

Table 5-2 Drugs That Exhibit Significant First-Pass Effect

Alprenolol
Hydralazine (Apresoline®)
Isoproterenol (Isuprel®)
Labetalol (Normodyne®, Trandate®)
Lidocaine (Xylocaine®)
Meperidine (Demerol®)
Metoprolol (Lopressor®)
Morphine
Naloxone (Narcan®)
Naltrexone (Trexan®)
N-Acetylcysteine (Mucomyst®)
Nitroglycerin
Pentazocine (Talwin®)
Propoxyphene (Darvon®)
Propranolol (Inderal®)
Salicylamide (Codalan®, Korigesic®)
Verapamil (Calan®, Isoptin®)

rapid enough that the highly polar metabolites are excreted directly by the kidneys. This is referred to as first-order elimination. Drugs that are highly lipid soluble are first metabolized by the liver to introduce a charge or highly polar group and are then excreted by the kidneys. When elimination depends in this way on metabolism and when the enzymes responsible for the breakdown of the compound are saturated, it is referred to as zero-order elimination. A combination of the two types of elimination, in which a drug changes its elimination pattern from first order to zero order, is called Michaelis-Menten elimination.

First-order elimination (renal elimination) means that the higher the plasma concentration of a drug, the greater the amount of drug excreted in a given time interval. This also means that, regardless of how much drug is in the body, one-half the total amount will be excreted in one drug half-life. Doubling the plasma concentration will thus result in a doubling of the rate at which the drug is eliminated. In other words, the rate of clearance is directly proportional to the concentration of the drug in the system.[3] Because of this there is a linear relation between plasma concentration of the drug and the total amount of drug. Renal elimination therefore is linear when plotted on semilogarithmic graph paper and is called first order because a constant fraction of the drug is eliminated per unit of time.

Urinary excretion is the major pathway for the elimination of drugs and drug metabolites. Any change in renal function will alter plasma concentrations of drugs that are not metabolized extensively. If renal function is impaired, plasma drug concentrations may be elevated.

The half-life for first-order elimination is a constant. It can be a useful kinetic parameter as long as renal function is normal. For example, in a drug excreted by first-order elimination a plasma concentration of 200 μg/mL will fall to 100 μg/mL after one half-life, to 50 μg/mL after two half-lives, and so on. A rule of thumb is that after five to six half-lives, there will be no significant drug effect (Table 5-3).[3]

The half-life of a drug has practical implications. Drugs with short half-lives accumulate in the body minimally and with multiple doses reach steady-state concentrations shortly after

Table 5-3 Percentage of Steady-State Plasma Concentrations Achieved at Each Half-Life Interval

Number of Half-Lives	Percentage of Steady-State Concentration
1	50
2	75
3	88
4	94
5	97
6	98
7	99

Source: Reprinted with permission from *Pediatric Clinics of North America* (1980;27:906), Copyright © 1980, WB Saunders Company.

initiation of therapy. They also leave the body rapidly once therapy has been discontinued. For drugs with long half-lives the converse is true; that is, they accumulate extensively in the body with multiple doses, reach steady-state concentration slowly, and leave the body slowly on termination of therapy.

Zero-order elimination (hepatic metabolism) occurs with compounds that require degradation in the liver before excretion. This type of elimination involves enzymes that are easily saturable, and the rate at which a drug is metabolized can only be increased to a certain point, which is the maximal rate at which the particular enzyme can act. Since the enzyme system generally has a slow rate of metabolism, the rate of elimination is fixed and depends on the activity of the saturated enzymes irrespective of the drug concentration. Therefore, unlike the renal mechanism in which the greater the plasma level the larger the amount of drug excreted, hepatic metabolism has an upper limit for metabolism that cannot go higher regardless of the plasma level. Once the hepatic enzymes are saturated, the plasma level increases abruptly. This rate of elimination can be predicted by simply plotting it on linear graph paper, with concentration on the *y* axis and time on the *x* axis. An example of a drug that undergoes this type of elimination is ethanol, which is broken down at 15 to 25 mg%/ hour regardless of the concentration.

At a certain concentration point, drug absorption, excretion, and biotransformation become independent of concentration. It is thought that all drugs convert from first-order to zero-order kinetics because a point is reached at which enzyme or transport mechanisms become saturated.

Most drugs never achieve concentrations in the body that approach the transition point from first-order to zero-order kinetics. In most cases, the serum concentrations of a drug achieved at therapeutic doses is low relative to the drug concentration necessary to saturate the particular system involved, and therefore most drugs follow first-order elimination. For most drugs, then, first-order kinetics is usually observed throughout the therapeutic range. When the drug elimination system is saturated, linear kinetics then switch to zero order, in which a constant amount of the drug that is present is eliminated per unit of time. This is typically seen when patients ingest toxic amounts of a drug.

There are some drugs, however, that switch their kinetics in therapeutic amounts, which has important clinical ramifications. Salicylates, phenytoin, theophylline, and ethyl alcohol are examples of drugs that undergo dose-dependent or Michaelis-Menten elimination in the therapeutic range (Table 5-4). As concentration increases, the half-life of the drug increases as well because there is an early saturation of the various enzymes in the liver. Further administration of these drugs may result in accumulation of the drug, and a small change in dose may, over several days, result in anywhere from a modest to large change in plasma concentration. In other words, once the plasma level approaches the saturation concentration a very small change in dose will, over several days, result in a very large change in plasma concentration.[1,2]

The proportion of drug elimination falls as the drug concentration rises, resulting in a longer elimination half-life. As an example, an overdose of phenytoin may change the drug's elimination half-life from 22 hours to 4 days because first-order elimination is changed to zero-order when the enzyme system is saturated. A 50% increase in the maintenance dose of aspirin has resulted in a 300% increase in steady-state salicylate concentrations in the plasma. Therefore, the half-life for drugs such as phenytoin and salicylates may not be constant, even in therapeutic doses, but can change as a result of the amount of drug in the body.

Summary of Elimination

The difference between first-order and zero-order elimination is a matter of degree. Although first-order elimination is "equivalent" to renal elimination, almost all drugs require some degree of metabolism before excretion. That is why the liver is the most important organ for removing drugs by metabolism and the kidneys are the second in importance. When the metabolic processes are not saturated, then the drug does not accumulate and is said to be excreted by first-order elimination. When the metabolic processes are saturated early, then zero-order kinetics prevail. In most nonoverdose situations, first-order kinetics prevail. In certain nonpurposeful overdose situations, kinetics switch from first order to zero order as a result of enzyme saturation (Michaelis-Menten kinetics). In most large overdoses, in which hepatic metabolism of the substance is required, the enzymes are overwhelmed and zero-order kinetics prevails.

SUMMARY

The principles of pharmacokinetics and toxicokinetics can be used by emergency department personnel in many different ways. Knowledge of the volume of distribution of a substance can help in determining approximate plasma concentrations or aid in deciding whether elimination will be facilitated by diuresis, dialysis, or hemoperfusion. Drugs with a large volume of distribution are concentrated in the tissues and fat of the body and so are not found to a great extent in the serum. For that reason,

Table 5-4 Drugs That Undergo Michaelis-Menten Elimination at Therapeutic Concentrations

Dicumarol
Ethanol
Phenylbutazone
Phenytoin
Probenecid
Salicylates
Theophylline

diuresis, dialysis, and hemoperfusion are effective. In addition, although many drugs undergo first-order kinetics in therapeutic situations, they may change their kinetics in the overdose situation and thereby accumulate and change their half-life.

REFERENCES

1. Gibaldi M, Levy G: Pharmacokinetics in clinical practice: Concepts. *JAMA* 1976;235:1864–1867.

2. Gibaldi M, Levy G: Pharmacokinetics in clinical practice: Applications. *JAMA* 1976;235:1987–1992.

3. Pippenger C: Rationale and clinical application of therapeutic drug monitoring. *Pediatr Clin North Am* 1980;27:891–925.

4. Greenblatt D. Koch-Weser J: Clinical pharmacokinetics. *N Engl J Med* 1975;293:702–708.

5. Watanabe A: Pharmacokinetic aspects of the dialysis of drugs. *Drug Intell Clin Pharmacol* 1977;11:407–416.

6. Gilette J: The importance of tissue distribution in pharmacokinetics. *J Pharmacokinet Biopharmacol* 1973;1:497–520.

7. Ariens E: Drug levels in the target tissue and effect. *Clin Pharmacol Ther* 1974;16:155–175.

8. Greenblatt D, Sellers E, Shader R: Drug disposition in old age. *N Engl J Med* 1982;306:1081–1088.

9. Levy G: Pharmacokinetic control and clinical interpretation of steady-state blood levels of drugs. *Clin Pharmacol Ther* 1975;16:120–134.

10. Chiou W, Peng G, Nation R: Rapid estimation of volume of distribution after a short intravenous infusion and its application to dosing adjustments. *J Clin Pharmacol* 1978;18:266–271.

11. Pagliaro L, Benet L: Pharmacokinetic data: Critical compilation of terminal half-lives, percent excreted unchanged, and changes of half-life in renal and hepatic dysfunction for studies in humans with references. *J Pharmacokinet Biopharmacol* 1975;3:333–383.

12. Kowarski C, Kowarski A: Simplified method for estimating volume of distribution at steady state. *J Pharm Sci* 1980;69:1222–1223.

13. Gilman AG, Goodman L, Gilman A: *Pharmacological Basis of Therapeutics*, ed 6. New York, MacMillan, 1980.

14. Klotz U: Pathophysiological and disease-induced changes in drug distribution volume: Pharmacokinetic implications. *Clin Pharmacokinet* 1976;1:204–218.

15. Wagner J: A modern view of pharmacokinetics. *J Pharmacokinet Biopharmacol* 1973;1:363–401.

16. Graham G, Chinwah P, Kennedy M, et al: Monitoring plasma concentrations of drugs. *Med J Aust* 1980;2:124–130.

17. Knoben J, Anderson P, Watanabe A: *Handbook of Clinical Drug Data*, ed 4. Hamilton, Ill, Drug Intelligence Publications, 1979.

18. Koch-Weser J: Bioavailability of drugs. *N Engl J Med* 1974;291:233–237.

19. Koch-Weser J, Sellers E: Binding of drugs to serum albumin, part 1. *N Engl J Med* 1976;294:311–316.

20. Koch-Weser J, Sellers E: Binding of drugs to serum albumin, part 2. *N Engl J Med* 1976;294:526–531.

21. Vesell E: Factors causing interindividual variations of drug concentrations in blood. *Clin Pharmacol Ther* 1974;16:135–148.

part II

THE AUTONOMIC NERVOUS SYSTEM, NEUROTRANSMITTERS, AND DRUGS

The Autonomic Nervous System: An Overview of Receptors, Neurotransmitters, and Drugs

The autonomic nervous system is involved with the functions of almost all organs and tissues of the body.[1,2] The toxicologist must therefore have a working knowledge of this system to understand the effects seen with many overdoses. This chapter reviews the autonomic nervous system, and subsequent chapters focus on the drugs that affect it.

The autonomic nervous system is also called the visceral, vegetative, or involuntary nervous system. It provides the innervation to the heart, blood vessels, glands, visceral organs, and smooth muscles of the body.[3-5] The nerves of this system are widely distributed throughout the body and regulate functions that are not under conscious control.

The autonomic nervous system is divided into two major branches—the sympathetic (adrenergic), and parasympathetic (cholinergic) branches[6]—on the basis of anatomy, neurotransmitters, receptors, and physiologic effects. A characteristic feature of the sympathetic and parasympathetic modulation is the reciprocal activities of the two nervous systems. Both systems consist of a preganglionic fiber, a ganglion, a postganglionic fiber, and a neuroeffector organ.

The peripheral sympathetic and parasympathetic nerve endings secrete two synaptic transmitter substances, norepinephrine and acetylcholine, respectively. In general those fibers that secrete norepinephrine are adrenergic, and those that secrete acetylcholine are cholinergic. Epinephrine is a circulating hormone; that is, it is not released from postganglionic fibers but from the adrenal medulla.[1,7,8] All preganglionic neurons are cholinergic in both the sympathetic and parasympathetic nervous system. Therefore, acetylcholine excites both sympathetic and parasympathetic preganglionic neurons. The postganglionic neurons of the parasympathetic system are also cholinergic. Most postganglionic sympathetic neurons are adrenergic except for sympathetic fibers to sweat glands and a few blood vessels (Table 6-1).

Table 6-1 Division and Actions of the Autonomic Nervous System

Organ or Tissue	Action	
	Parasympathetic	*Sympathetic*
Eye	Constriction	Dilation
Blood vessels	Dilation	Constriction
Heart rate	Decrease	Increase
Intestine motility	Increase	Decrease
Salivation	Thin	Thick
Skin (pilomotor)	No effect	Contraction
Stomach acid secretion	Stimulation	Inhibition
Stomach motility	Increase	Decrease
Urinary bladder	Relaxation	Constriction

THE ROLE OF RECEPTORS

Virtually all hormones, drugs, and neurotransmitters released from postganglionic fibers initiate their biologic actions by binding to specific cellular recognition sites that are termed receptors.[1,2,6,9,10] A receptor is a distinct molecule, usually a large protein or glycoprotein on the membrane of the receiving neuron synapse, into which the neurotransmitter chemical molecule fits.[3–5] Receptors may be enzymes, ion channels, macromolecules coupled to enzymes or ion channels, or structural macromolecules.[1,2] They may be located intracellularly or at the cell surface. The binding of the receptor is then followed by alterations of cellular metabolic events, such as enzyme activities or ion fluxes, that are ultimately expressed as characteristic physiologic or pharmacologic effects.

The impulse from one neuron is transferred to the next by means of neurotransmitters, which comprise the catecholamines, norepinephrine, epinephrine, and dopamine[11] as well as acetylcholine, serotonin, γ-aminobutyric acid, glycine, glutamate, histamine, and substance P.[1,2,12]

NEUROTRANSMISSION: GENERAL CONSIDERATIONS

Normal neuromuscular transmission begins with a nerve impulse that is conducted along the prejunctional neuron and reaches the motor nerve terminal.[11] The axon terminal of the prejunctional neuron makes a close approximation with the dendrite of the motor nerve terminal through a narrow space called the synaptic cleft.[11] This cleft separates the presynaptic membrane (the axon and axon terminal) from the postsynaptic membrane of the dendrite.[12] The presynaptic terminal consists of mitochondria and numerous synaptic vesicles. Transmitter chemical is stored in these vesicles before it is released and is capable of altering the permeability of the dendritic membrane of the next neuron, resulting in either a depolarization or hyperpolarization of the dentrites of that neuron.[12]

The impulse that reaches the prejunctional neuron then depolarizes the membrane, and calcium ions enter the prejunctional axoplasm and facilitate release of the excitatory or inhibitory chemical transmitter from storage vesicles into the junctional space.[1,2,12] The neurotransmitter then diffuses across the junctional space and combines with receptors at the prejunctional membrane surface, resulting in permeability changes to small ions such as sodium and potassium. Depolarization (excitation) or hyperpolarization (inhibition) of the membrane then occurs[12] and is followed by the effector response.

CHOLINERGIC RECEPTORS

Acetylcholine and choline are synthesized from enzymes within the nerve terminal, the former from acetylcoenzyme A and the latter from choline acetyltransferase.[13] Acetylcholine is stored in synaptic vesicles at the axon terminal.[14] When a nerve is stimulated, acetylcholine is released from the presynaptic terminal, traverses the synaptic cleft, and binds reversibly to the cholinergic receptor on the motor endplate (see Figure 6-1).[14] Once the acetylcholine has been secreted by the cholinergic nerve ending, most of it is hydrolyzed within 2 to 3 msec into acetic acid and choline by the enzyme acetylcholinesterase, which is present in the terminal nerve ending itself and on the surface of the receptor organ.[13,14] The choline that is formed is in turn transported back into the terminal nerve ending, where it is used again for synthesis of new acetylcholine. Pseudocholinesterase, a nonspecific enzyme, also hydrolyzes acetylcholine should any of it be transported into the plasma.

Location of Cholinergic Receptors

Cholinergic neurons are found in certain synapses in the central nervous system, all autonomic ganglia, postganglionic parasympathetic fibers, a few sympathetic neuroeffectors (sweat glands), the neuromuscular junction or motor endplate of skeletal muscle innervated by the somatic or voluntary nervous system, and the adrenal medulla.[6]

Cholinergic receptors are categorized as muscarinic and nicotinic, depending on their response to the receptor agonists muscarine or nicotine.[6] Muscarine mimics the acetylcholine effects at the end organ of visceral smooth muscle of the gastrointestinal tract, urinary tract, uterus, bronchi, heart, vascular tissue, some secretory glands, and the central nervous system. Nicotine acts as an agonist at the neuromuscular junction of skeletal muscle, preganglionic portions of the autonomic nervous system, portions of the central nervous system, and the chromaffin cells of the adrenal medulla[6] (Table 6-2).

As an example of receptor function, at the cellular level the nicotinic cholinergic receptor forms a chemically regulated channel for sodium ions. The subunits of this receptor-channel complex carry a recognition and binding site for acetylcholine, and on binding with acetylcholine the subunits change their configuration. This transducer function results in the opening of the previously closed channel, and the sodium ions flow into the cell, initiating depolarization. This is measured as an intercellular decrease (ie, a shift toward zero) in the membrane's resting potential (-90 mV).

Although acetylcholine is the transmitter at both the nicotinic and muscarinic receptor sites, some agents display a degree of selectivity in blocking acetylcholine from nicotinic receptors at neuromuscular junctions or from those at autonomic ganglia. In addition, transmission in cholinergic neuroeffector junctions of skeletal muscle, viscera, autonomic ganglia, and heart differs with respect to the time limits of acetylcholine inactivation, which vary from milliseconds (motor endplate) to several seconds (heart).

Table 6-2 Types of Cholinergic Receptors

Muscarinic	Nicotinic
Postganglionic	Preganglionic
Visceral smooth muscle	Autonomic NS
Gastrointestinal tract	Voluntary NS
Urinary tract	Postganglionic
Uterus	Voluntary NS
Bronchi	Central NS
Heart	Adrenal Medulla
Vascular tissue	

Antimuscarinic Drugs

Antimuscarinic drugs compete with acetylcholine on smooth muscle receptors and only inhibit acetylcholine on nicotinic receptors at high concentrations. Atropine, for example, is a competitive antagonist to the muscarinic actions because it occupies the cholinergic receptor sites on autonomic effector cells and on the secondary muscarinic receptors of autonomic ganglion cells. *d*-Tubocurarine blocks transmission at both motor endplates and autonomic ganglia.

Botulinum Toxin

Botulinum toxin prevents the release of acetylcholine by all types of cholinergic fibers and thereby blocks transmission at the skeletal neuromuscular junction as well as at the autonomic cholinergic synapses.[15] Only a minuscule amount of this toxin is necessary to bind irreversibly to their sites of action, producing an essentially irreversible blockade of all cholinergic junctions and resulting in anticholinergic symptoms.

Acetylcholinesterase Inhibitors

Drugs that inhibit the enzyme acetylcholinesterase are called anticholinesterase agents or acetylcholinesterase inhibitors. They cause acetylcholine to accumulate at cholinergic receptor sites and thus produce effects equivalent to excessive stimulation of cholinergic receptors. On inhibition of acetylcholinesterase, the transmitter is removed principally by diffusion. Under these circumstances, the effects of released acetylcholine are potentiated and prolonged. Carbamates such as physostigmine, neostigmine, pyridostigmine, edrophonium, and the carbamate insecticides act in this manner. The organophosphate insecticides parathion, malathion, and others also act in this manner but at some point in time become irreversible.

Black Widow Spider Venom

Black widow spider venom causes a transient release of acetylcholine and a subsequent permanent block. This results in transient cho-linomimetic effects that are followed by anticholinergic effects.

Muscarinic Receptors at Sympathetic Sites

In recent years it has been shown that sympathetic nerve terminals contain muscarinic receptors that can be activated by acetylcholine released from nerve fibers.[16] This muscarinic activation inhibits the release of norepinephrine. Activation of muscarinic receptors can therefore powerfully modulate the positive inotropic, electrophysiologic, and metabolic effects of catecholamines acting on adrenergic receptors.[16] These antagonistic effects of acetylcholine are directed at cyclic adenosine monophosphate actions within the cell and not specifically at the β-adrenergic receptor.[13]

ADRENERGIC RECEPTORS

In the early 1900s, it was shown that preparations of ergot abolished the motor effects of sympathetic stimulation.[17] In 1948, Ahlquist concluded that there were two distinct types of adrenergic receptors, α and β.[1,2,17,18] α receptors referred to those adrenergic receptors most sensitive to norepinephrine and least sensitive to isoproterenol, and β receptors referred to those showing the reverse pattern.[1,2,19]

The adrenergic neuroeffector junction consists of the sympathetic neuron, which synthesizes, stores, and releases norepinephrine, and the effector cell.[6,11] Sympathetic effector cells in different organs generally have a preponderance of one type of receptor. α refers to the receptors associated with most of the excitatory functions of the sympathetic nervous system, and β refers to receptors associated with most of the inhibitory functions.[19] The myocardium is an important exception to this rule.

α receptors are most abundant in the resistance vessels of the skin, mucosa, intestine, and kidney, and they cause vasoconstriction in these vascular beds. α-Adrenergic receptors classically mediate catecholamine effects, such as smooth muscle contraction. In contrast, smooth muscle relaxation and other β-adren-

ergic receptor–mediated responses to catecholamines are those for which isoproterenol is more potent than either epinephrine or norepinephrine.[3–5] β receptors are predominant in the heart, the arteries and arterioles of skeletal muscle, and the bronchi, where they cause cardiac excitation, vasodilatation, and bronchial relaxation, respectively (Table 6-3).

Sympathetic Agonists

Sympathetic agonists vary in their action on the receptors. Among the catecholamines, norepinephrine acts mainly on α receptor sites and has little β stimulating activity, except in the heart; epinephrine acts on β receptors in the heart and bronchial tree and on both α and β receptors in the blood vessels; isoproterenol is almost a pure β receptor agonist.[3–5] Norepinephrine, its immediate precursor dopamine, and epinephrine are also neurotransmitters in the central nervous system (Table 6-4). Dopamine serves two functions: it is a precurser of norepinephrine, and it is a neurotransmitter in the area of the brain involved in coordinating motor activity.

Norepinephrine

Norepinephrine is an endogenous catecholamine synthesized from tyrosine and stored in vesicles in adrenergic nerve endings.[11] When sympathetic nerves are activated, norepinephrine is released from its stores and stimulates α-adrenergic receptors.[1,2] As mentioned earlier, norepinephrine is a neurotransmitter in the central nervous system and in sympathetic postganglionic nerves of the peripheral nervous system. Norepinephrine is also released from the adrenal medulla.

Table 6-3 Adrenergic Receptors (Not Absolute)

Alpha	Beta
Resistance vessels of:	Heart
Skin	Skeletal muscle
Mucosa	Bronchi
Intestine	Metabolic effects
Kidney	Uterus

Table 6-4 Differences between α and β Adrenoceptor Action

Organ	Action	
	Alpha Receptor	*Beta Receptor*
Heart		Increases heart rate Increases contractility Increases conduction velocity
Blood vessels	Constriction	Dilation
Bronchi		Dilation
Stomach	Contracts sphincter	Decreases motility
Intestine	Relaxation	Relaxation
Uterus	Contraction	Relaxation
Urinary bladder	Contraction	Relaxation
Eye	Pupil dilation	

Source: Reprinted with permission from *Medical Clinics of North America* (1968;52:1009–1016), Copyright © 1968, WB Saunders Company.

Dopamine

Dopamine is principally a centrally acting neurotransmitter. In the brain there are at least two types of dopamine receptors: the D_1 receptor (which is linked to adenyl cyclase) and the D_2 receptor. Dopamine is linked to fine motor coordination, emotion, memory, and neurohormonal balance. Peripherally, dopamine receptors are found in the renal and mesenteric vasculature and cause vasodilatation.

Epinephrine

Epinephrine is a hormone manufactured in and released from the adrenal medulla. In contrast to norepinephrine, it acts at a distant site from where it is released. Many of the actions of epinephrine and norepinephrine are similar.

Termination of Neurotransmission

The actions of norepinephrine, epinephrine, and dopamine are terminated by various methods, including (1) reuptake of the agonist into

nerve terminals, (2) dilution of the agonist by diffusion out of the junctional cleft and uptake at extraneuronal sites, (3) metabolic transformation of the agonist, and (4) actions on α inhibitory receptors (α_2 receptors).[20,21]

Although catecholamines can be inactivated by the enzymes monoamine oxidase and catechol *o*-methyltransferase, this is not usually how an action is terminated.[22] Termination primarily occurs through the active process of catecholamine reuptake across the presynaptic nerve membrane back into the presynaptic nerve ending. The catecholamines are then stored again in the synaptic vesicles for reuse.[11] This process differs from the hydrolysis that occurs with acetylcholine.

The principle of agonist reuptake into the nerve terminal and then into the storage vesicles is of crucial importance because there are drugs that may block either the active reuptake process into the nerve terminal, thus potentiating the synaptic action of the transmitter, or the reuptake of the transmitter from the intracellular fluid in the presynaptic nerve terminal back into the storage granule (synaptic vesicles), where it is stored and protected from monoamine oxidase.[11] An example of the latter type of drug is reserpine. As a result of blockage by reserpine, norepinephrine may be metabolized by monoamine oxidase and the nervous system depleted of the transmitter, with the result of sedation and emotional depression. Cocaine and the tricyclic antidepressants are examples of the former type of drug; they block reuptake of norepinephrine from the synaptic cleft back into the nerve terminal, thus increasing its action at the synapse.[11]

Some drugs are capable of blocking the enzyme monoamine oxidase, thereby increasing the norepinephrine concentration in the nerve terminal. Tranylcypromine (Parnate®) is one such monoamine oxidase inhibitor. Some compounds (ephedrine) are capable of stimulating the postsynaptic norepinephrine receptor; others (such as phenoxybenzamine) are capable of blocking the receptor.

The Role of Cyclic Adenosine Monophosphate

A key compound that is involved in the mediation of sympathetic effects is cyclic adenosine monophosphate (AMP).[23–26] The sympathetics enhance the accumulation of cyclic AMP by activating adenyl cyclase, an enzyme located on the internal surface of the plasma membrane.[27] Adenyl cyclase converts adenosine triphosphate into cyclic AMP. Cyclic AMP appears to activate a class of enzymes known as protein kinases, which phosphorylate a wide variety of important substrates.[1,2] This action in turn creates an open pore through which sodium and potassium ions may flow to cause depolarization. Cyclic AMP is involved with β-adrenergic receptors, serotonin receptors, histamine receptors, and dopamine receptors.

Classification of Adrenergic Receptors

Although the use of the terms α and β adrenoceptors for describing catecholamine receptors is now generally accepted, adrenoceptors are much more complicated than what was first described.[9,10,18,28] The current concept is that there are subtypes of adrenergic receptors—α_1, α_2, β_1, and β_2—that are distinguished by the relative potencies of particular agonists and antagonists.[18] Receptors are also subdivided morphologically as pre- and postsynaptic adrenoceptors.[18] Morphologically, presynaptic receptors are located before the synapse, at the nerve terminal or nerve ending; a synonymous term is prejunctional.[29] Postsynaptic or postjunctional receptors are located at the muscle cell. Another classification is based on pharmacologic or functional characteristics: α_1 receptors are located postsynaptically and cause stimulation, and α_2 receptors are located presynaptically and cause sympathetic inhibition.[30]

Three of the four subtypes of adrenergic receptors are linked to the same biochemical effector, the adenyl cyclase system. This system generates cyclic AMP, which acts as a messenger provoking a series of reactions that leads to a physiologic response within the effector cell.[9] The β receptors are thought to activate adenyl cyclase by a coupling protein that binds guanosine triphosphate. The β_1 and β_2 receptors stimulate adenyl cyclase, whereas the α_2 receptors inhibit it.[3–6] The α_1 receptors appear not to be coupled to adenyl cyclase but rather to processes that regulate cellular calcium ion fluxes

possibly mediated by increased phosphatidylinositol hydrolysis.[1,2,6]

α Adrenoceptors

α_1 adrenoceptors. Peripheral α receptors located postsynaptically on the vascular smooth muscle cell are termed α_1.[19] These receptors are under the influence of the neurotransmitter norepinephrine, which is liberated from postganglionic adrenergic fibers by the nerve impulse. Stimulation of these receptors results in typical adrenergic effects.

α_2 adrenoceptors. Receptors located presynaptically on the sympathetic nerve ending that inhibit peripheral neuronal neurotransmitter release are termed α_2.[18] These presynaptic autoregulatory α receptors are located peripherally and differ in their pharmacologic properties from postsynaptic α receptors mediating typical α-adrenergic effects.[19] The peripheral α_2 receptors located at presynaptic sites on the nerve ending itself reduce the amount of norepinephrine released by nerve impulses when stimulated by norepinephrine in the synaptic cleft.[12] When high concentrations of norepinephrine are present, subsequent nerve impulses release less norepinephrine.[31,32] Thus the presynaptic α_2 receptor forms part of a feedback loop that maintains the local level of sympathetic activity.[19] Stimulation of the α_2 receptors therefore inhibits adenyl cyclase activity and in turn decreases cellular concentrations of cyclic AMP (Table 6-5, Fig. 6-1).[33]

Although the exact function, distribution, and location of central α_2 receptors is currently under investigation, it is clear that they modulate autonomic nerve outflux from medullary brain structures.[34] The α_2 adrenoceptors in the brain that mediate the central hypotensive action of clonidine are probably located at postsynaptic sites.[3–5] Stimulation of these receptors causes decreased sympathetic and increased parasympathetic nerve outflux from the central nervous system. This is a result of a decrease in cyclic AMP by inhibition of adenyl cyclase. Drugs that inhibit α_2 receptors increase central epinephrine and norepinephrine turnover, resulting in increased sympathetic and decreased vagal nerve outflux from the central nervous system.[19] Originally it was thought that α_2 adrenoceptors were located exclusively presynaptically,

Table 6-5 Characteristics of α Adrenoceptors

Receptor Type	Location	Function	Distribution
α_1	Postsynaptic	Raises intracellular calcium concentration	Myocardium, vascular smooth muscle
α_2	Presynaptic (peripheral)	Inhibits norepinephrine release	Peripheral nervous system, cholinergic nerve endings
	Postsynaptic (central)	Inhibits adenyl cyclase	Central nervous system
	Nonsynaptic (platelets)		

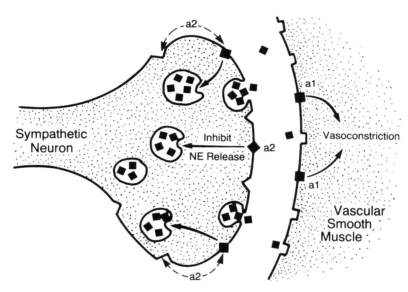

Figure 6-1 Configuration of receptors. Schematic illustrating the suggested neuronal location of α_2 and vascular smooth muscle location of α_1 receptor prototypes. However, there is evidence for postsynaptic location in other organs for this α_2 receptor. Thus, the classification is functional rather than anatomic. *Source:* Reprinted with permission from *Life Sciences* (1977;21:595–606), Copyright © 1977, Pergamon Press, Inc.

but at present there is ample evidence for the existence of α_2 adrenoceptors outside noradrenergic terminal axons, on some organelles lacking synapses, and at postsynaptic sites.[19–21,35–37] The important point is that the designation α_2 is based on pharmacologic studies and specific drugs and does not necessarily imply a presynaptic location (Table 6-6).[3–5,34,38]

Substances that decrease noradrenergic neurotransmission include purines (such as adenosine triphosphate and adenosine), prostaglandins of the E series, acetylcholine (by way of muscarinic receptors), dopamine, histamine, serotonin, morphine, and opioid peptides.[35] Substances that facilitate noradrenergic neurotransmission include β adrenoceptor agonists, acetylcholine (by way of nicotinic receptors), angiotensin, possibly prostaglandins of the F series, and thromboxane.[32]

β Adrenoceptors

Since 1967 it has been generally accepted that the β receptors are divided functionally into β_1

Table 6-6 Location and Action of α Receptors

Location	Action
α₁ Receptors	
Smooth muscle	Contraction
Liver	Glycogenolysis
CNS	Increase in locomotor activity
α₂ Receptors	
Terminal noradrenergic axons	Inhibition of norepinephrine release
Cholinergic neurons	Inhibition
CNS	Sedation
Smooth muscle	Contraction
Platelets	Aggregation
Fat cells	Inhibition of lipolysis
Pancreatic islets	Inhibition of insulin release

and β_2 (Table 6-7).[39] The receptors are located in the heart and mediate the positive inotropic effects[6]; they are also located in the kidneys. The β_2 receptors mediate smooth muscle relaxation and are located in the vasculature, bronchi, and uterus.[18] Actually, both receptor types appear to be present in these areas; for example, a small number of β_2 receptors appear to exist in the heart, and β_1 receptors are also present in the lung.[6]

In physiologic terms, the β_1 receptors generally mediate the effects of the neuronally released neurotransmitter norepinephrine,[6] whereas β_2 receptors that mediate vasodilation are not under neuronal control and generally respond to the hormone epinephrine, which is released from the adrenal medulla.[3–5] Stimulation of β_1 receptors causes tachycardia and accentuation of cardiac contraction and atrioventricular conduction. The results of β_2 stimulation are bronchodilation, vasodilation, glycogenolysis, and fibrinolysis. Both β_1 and β_2 adrenoceptors activate adenyl cyclase.[1,2,24–26]

Agonists and Antagonists

Receptor agonists have an affinity for a receptor and, when combined with the receptor, transform it in such a way that a cellular response is initiated. A full agonist causes a maximal response, whereas a partial agonist causes a response that is qualitatively similar but always less in magnitude than that of a full agonist.[3] A receptor antagonist interacts with the receptor but elicits no response on its own. By occupying the receptor, however, an antagonist may reduce the effect of an agonist.[9] Through structural modifications, an agonist may become an antag-

Table 6-7 Characteristics of β Adrenoceptors

Receptor Type	Location	Effect	Function	Distribution
β_1	Heart	Cardiac stimulation	Increases cyclic AMP	Peripheral nerve endings
	Kidney	Renin release		
	Fat	Lipolysis		
	Eye	Decreased aqueous humor production		
β_2	Bronchi	Bronchodilation	Increases cyclic AMP	Peripheral nerve endings
	Blood vessels	Vasodilation		
	Endocrine glands	Glycolysis, insulin release, lactic acid production		
	Uterus	Uterine relaxation		

onist by retaining its affinity for a receptor and losing its ability to initiate the reactions necessary for a response.

Methoxamine and phenylephrine are directly acting sympathomimetic amine agonists that selectively stimulate α_1 receptors.[40] Clonidine is an α_2-selective agonist.[29,41] Epinephrine and norepinephrine, having approximately equal potency at α_1 and α_2 receptors, are nonselective agonists (Table 6-8).

Among α-adrenergic antagonists, prazosin, terazosin, and corynanthine are considered α_1 selective. Prazosin is probably the most potent α_1-blocking agent currently available.[3–5] Yohimbine and Rauwolscine, both plant alkaloids, are specific α_2 antagonists.[41] Phentolamine is generally equipotent at α_1 and α_2 receptors.[42] It is therefore nonselective, so that both the postsynaptic receptor on the vascular smooth muscle cell and the presynaptic receptor on the peripheral nerve ending are blocked.[40]

Among the β agonists, isoproterenol is nonselective and dobutamine is selective for β_1 receptors.[4] Propranolol is a nonselective β-adrenergic blocking agent, and metoprolol is a selective β_1-blocking agent.

Table 6-8 Partial List of α and β Adrenoceptor Agonists and Antagonists

Receptor Type	Agonists	Antagonists
α (nonselective)	Norepinephrine	Phentolamine
	Epinephrine	Tolazoline
α_1	Methoxamine	Prazosin
	Phenylephrine	Corynanthine
		Terazosin
α_2	Clonidine	Yohimbine
	Guanabenz	Rauwolscine
	Guanefesine	Piperoxan
	Methyldopa	
	Naphazoline	
	Oxymetazoline	
β (nonselective)	Isoproterenol	Nadolol
		Propranolol
		Timolol
β_1	Dobutamine	Acebutolol
	Tazolol	Alprenolol
	Prenalterol	Atenolol
		Metoprolol
		Practolol
β_2	Terbutaline	Butoxamine
	Salbutamol	
	Isoetharine	
	Fenoterol	
	Rimiterol	

REFERENCES

1. Abboud F: The sympathetic nervous system and α-adrenergic blocking agents in shock. *Med Clin North Am* 1968;52:1049–1060.

2. Abboud F: Concepts of adrenergic receptors. *Med Clin North Am* 1968;52:1009–1016.

3. Hoffman B: Regulation of α- and β-adrenergic receptors in man. *Clin Endocrinol Metab* 1983;12:1–13.

4. Hoffman B, Lefkowitz R: α-Adrenergic receptor subtypes. *N Engl J Med* 1980;302:1390–1396.

5. Hoffman B, De Lean A, Wood C, et al: α-Adrenergic receptor subtypes. *Life Sci* 1979;24:1739–1746.

6. Casale T: The role of the autonomic nervous system in allergic diseases. *Ann Allergy* 1983;51:423–429.

7. Motulsky H, Insel P: Adrenergic receptors in man. *N Engl J Med* 1982;307:18–29.

8. Nadel J, Barnes P: Autonomic regulation of the airways. *Annu Rev Med* 1984;35:451–467.

9. Lefkowitz R, Caron M, Stiles G: Mechanisms of membrane receptor regulation. *N Engl J Med* 1984; 310:1570–1579.

10. Lefkowitz R: β-Adrenergic receptors: Recognition and regulation. *N Engl J Med* 1976;295:323–328.

11. Axelrod J, Weinshilboum R: Catecholamines. *N Engl J Med* 1972;287:237–242.

12. Brown R, Mann J: A clinical perspective on the role of neurotransmitters in mental disorders. *Hosp Community Psychiatr* 1985;36:141–150.

13. Loeffelholz K, Pappano A: The parasympathetic neuroeffector junction of the heart. *Pharmacol Rev* 1985; 37:1–24.

14. DeGramo B, Dronen S: Pharmacology and clinical use of neuromuscular blocking agents. *Ann Emerg Med* 1983;12:48–55.

15. Mellanby J: Comparative activities of tetanus and botulinum toxins. *Neuroscience* 1984;11:29–34.

16. Burnstock G: Autonomic neurotransmitters and trophic factors. *J Auton Nerv Syst* 1983;7:213–217.

17. Ahlquist R: A study of the adrenotropic receptors. *Am J Physiol* 1948;153:586–600.

18. Berthelsen S, Pettinger W: A functional basis for classification of α-adrenergic receptors. *Life Sci* 1977; 21:595–606.

19. Colucci W: New developments in α-adrenergic receptor pharmacology: Implications for the initial treatment of hypertension. *Am J Cardiol* 1983;51:639–643.

20. Langer S: Presynaptic regulation of catecholamine release. *Biochem Pharmacol* 1974;23:1793–1800.

21. Langer S: Presynaptic receptors and their role in the regulation of transmitter release. *Br J Pharmacol* 1977; 60:481–497.

22. Eckstein J, Abboud F: Circulatory effects of sympathomimetic amines. *Am Heart J* 1962;63:119–135.

23. Sutherland E, Robison G: Metabolic effects of catecholamines. *Pharmacol Rev* 1966;18:145–161.

24. Wit A, Hoffman B, Rosen M: Electrophysiology and pharmacology of cardiac arrhythmias: Part IX: Cardiac electrophysiologic effects of β-adrenergic receptor stimulation and blockade: Part A. *Am Heart J* 1975;90:521–533.

25. Wit A, Hoffman B, Rosen M: Electrophysiology and pharmacology of cardiac arrhythmias: Part IX: Cardiac electrophysiologic effects of β-adrenergic receptor stimulation and blockade: Part B. *Am Heart J* 1975;90:665–675.

26. Wit A, Hoffman B, Rosen M: Electrophysiology and pharmacology of cardiac arrhythmias: Part IX: Cardiac electrophysiologic effects of β-adrenergic receptor stimulation and blockade: Part C. *Am Heart J* 1975;90:795–803.

27. Epstein S, Levey G, Skelton C: Adenyl cyclase and cyclic AMP. *Circulation* 1977;43:437–450.

28. Williams J: New developments and therapeutic applications of cardiac stimulating agents. *Am J Cardiol* 1973;32:491–496.

29. Doxey J, Smith C, Walker J: Selectivity of blocking agents for pre- and postsynaptic α adrenoceptors. *Br J Pharmacol* 1977;60:91–96.

30. Kobinger W: Central blood pressure regulation. *Chest* 1983;83(suppl):296–299.

31. Weiss R, Tobes M, Wertz C, et al: Platelet α_2 adrenoceptors in chronic congestive heart failure. *Am J Cardiol* 1983;52:101–105.

32. Westfall T: Evidence that noradrenergic transmitter release is regulated by presynaptic receptors. *Fed Proc* 1984; 43:1352–1357.

33. Fitzgerald G, Watkins J, Dollery C: Regulation of norepinephrine release by peripheral α_2 receptor stimulation. *Clin Pharmacol Ther* 1981;29:160–167.

34. Starke K, Docherty J: α_1 and α_2 Adrenoceptors: Pharmacology and clinical implications. *J Cardiovasc Pharmacol* 1981;3:S14–S23.

35. Bannister R: Clinical studies of autonomic function and dysfunction. *J Auton Nerv Syst* 1983;7:233–237.

36. Docherty J, Hyland L: Evidence for neuroeffector transmission through postjunctional α_2 adrenoceptors in human saphenous vein. *Br J Pharmacol* 1985;84:573–576.

37. Gross F: Central α adrenoceptors in cardiovascular regulation. *Chest* 1983;83(suppl):293–296.

38. DiJoseph J, Taylor J, Mir G, et al: α_2 Receptors in the gastrointestinal system: A new therapeutic approach. *Life Sci* 1984;35:1031–1042.

39. Lands A, Arnold A, McAuliff J, et al: Differentiation of receptor systems activated by sympathomimetic amines. *Nature (London)* 1967;214:597–598.

40. Goldberg M, Robertson D: Evidence for the existence of vascular α_2 adrenergic receptors in humans. *Hypertension* 1984;6:551–556.

41. Drew G: What do antagonists tell us about α adrenoceptors? *Clin Sci* 1985;68(suppl 10):15s–19s.

42. Jie K, Brummelen P, Vermey P: Identification of vascular postsynaptic α_1 and α_2 adrenoceptors in man. *Circ Res* 1984;54:447–452.

chapter **7**

Anticholinergic Drugs and Plant Alkaloids

More than 600 pharmaceutical preparations, including the tricyclic antidepressants, major tranquilizers, antipsychotics, antiparkinsonism agents, belladonna alkaloids, ophthalmic solutions, and antihistamines, contain some form of natural or synthetic anticholinergic agent (Table 7-1). Anticholinergic toxicity is therefore widespread and can be easily recognized.[1] The anticholinergic agents are also called antimuscarinics because they competitively inhibit the muscarinic effects of acetylcholine.

MECHANISM OF ACTION OF ANTICHOLINERGIC AGENTS

Acetylcholine is the neurotransmitter found at the sympathetic and parasympathetic ganglia, parasympathetic nerve endings, voluntary muscle (myoneural) junctions, and certain synapses

within the central nervous system. Anticholinergics or antimuscarinic agents act by competitively blocking acetylcholine at its parasympathetic effector site (the muscarinic site or postganglionic cholinergic nerve ending).[2] Because most organs receive both sympathetic and parasympathetic nerves and because these tend to oppose each other, parasympathetic blockade in most organs results in sympathetic dominance and sympathomimetic effects. At therapeutic doses, anticholinergics have little or no effect on cholinergic stimuli at skeletal muscle or ganglionic (nicotinic) receptors.

TYPES OF ANTICHOLINERGIC AGENTS

Antihistamines

The term antihistamine has been taken to indicate a compound that competitively antagonizes the H_1 receptors in areas such as the bronchi, gastrointestinal tract, blood vessels, and uterus. These H_1 blockers neither block the release of nor chemically inactivate histamine but rather prevent the action of histamine on the cell. Antihistamines are not blockers of H_2 receptors, which are located in the parietal cells of the stomach.

Antihistamines are the major components of most over-the-counter sedatives and sleeping

---

Table 7-1 Types of Anticholinergic Compounds

Antihistamines
Antiparkinsonian agents
Antipsychotic agents
Belladonna alkaloids
Ophthalmic solutions
Plants
Tricyclic antidepressants

---

aids (Table 7-2).[3] The antihistamines have a number of other actions besides anticholinergic; for example, they are used as local anesthetics and antispasmodics and to treat motion sickness. Some antihistamines also demonstrate a quinidine-like effect on myocardial conduction, and some enhance the pressor action of norepinephrine. Part of the antiemetic and anti–motion-sickness actions of some antihistamines are a result of their central anticholinergic and central nervous system depressant properties.

In general, the ethylenediamine derivatives have relatively weak central nervous system effects, but drowsiness may occur in some patients. Ethanolamine derivatives commonly cause central nervous system depression. Propylamine derivatives cause less drowsiness and more central nervous system stimulation than the other antihistamines. These effects are frequently present when these drugs are used therapeutically, and they predominate when overdosage occurs.

Although antihistamines have relatively high therapeutic indexes, overdosage may result in death, especially in infants and children. Absorption of transdermal antihistamines as well as aerosol antihistamines has resulted in intoxication and organic psychosis in children.[4]

Most of the clinical features of antihistamine poisoning are due to anticholinergic toxicity, and the patient with this toxicity may present with a central or peripheral anticholinergic syndrome.[2,5] Cardiogenic shock refractory to pharmacologic intervention has been reported secondary to ingestion of a massive amount of pyrilamine. Delayed-release preparations are available and should be considered when estimating the onset of drug effect.[6]

Antipsychotic Agents

Antipsychotic agents are discussed in Chapter 12.

Antiparkinsonism Agents

The antiparkinsonism agents (Table 7-3) are used mainly in the prophylactic management of the side effects secondary to the major tranquilizers.

Table 7-2 Antihistamines with Selected Trade Names

Parent Compound	Derivatives
Ethylenediamine	Antazoline (Arithmin®)
	Methapyrilene (Histadyl®)
	Pyrilamine (Histalon®, Neo-Pyramine®)
	Tripelennamine (Pyribenzamine®, PBZ®)
Ethanolamine	Bromodiphenhydramine (Ambenyl®)
	Carbinoxamine (Clistin®, Rondec®)
	Clemastine (Tavist®)
	Dimenhydrinate (Dramamine®, Dimate®, Dimetabs®, Dramocen®, Eladryl®, Hydrate®, Marmine®, Vertiban®)
	Diphenhydramine (Benadryl®, Benahist®, Benylin®, Dihydrex®, Fenylhist®, Noradryl®)
	Diphenylpyraline (Hispril®)
	Doxylamine (Decapryn®)
	Phenyltoloxamine (Atrohist®, Histaminic®, Naldecon®, Percogesic®)
Propylamine	Brompheniramine (Bromamine®, Bromphen®, Dimetane®, Spentane®, Veltane®)
	Chlorpheniramine (AL-R®, Allerchlor®, Chlor-Trimeton®, Phenetron®, Chloramate®, Alermine®, Ornade®, Teldrin®, Chloro-Amine®, Chlorspan®, Histrex®, Trymegen®)
	Dexbrompheniramine
	Dexchlorpheniramine (Polaramine®)
	Dimethindene
	Pheniramine (Ru-Tuss®, Citra Forte®)
	Pyrobutamine
	Triprolidine (Actidil®)
Phenothiazine	Methdilazine (Tacaryl®)
	Promethazine (Phenergan®)
	Trimeprazine (Temaril®)
Piperazine	Buclizine (Bucladin-S®)
	Chlorcyclizine (Mantadil®)
	Cyclizine (Marezine®)
	Hydroxyzine (Vistaril®)
	Meclizine (Antivert®, Bonine®)
Miscellaneous	Azatadine (Optimine®)
	Cyproheptadine (Periactin®)
	Orphenadrine (Disipal®)
	Phenindamine (Nolahist®)

Table 7-3 Antiparkinsonism Agents with Selected Trade Names

Benztropine (Cogentin®)
Biperiden (Akineton®)
Ethopropazine (Parsidol®)
Orphenadrine (Norflex®, Flexon®, Norgesic®)
Procyclidine (Kemadrin®)
Trihexyphenidyl (Artane®, Tremin®, Trihexane®)

Benztropine resembles atropine in chemical structure, and its anticholinergic effect is about equal to that of atropine. Benztropine also exhibits antihistaminic and local anesthetic properties.[7–11] Although benztropine is successfully used to treat dystonia secondary to the major tranquilizers, it has also caused dyskinesia and dystonia in some individuals.[12] This may result from a dopamine excess secondary to inhibition of dopamine reuptake.

Orphenadrine is a tertiary amine antimuscarinic agent that may also have skeletal muscle relaxant properties, possibly through an atropine-like central action on cerebral motor centers or on the medulla. It is also widely used in Parkinson's disease and in drug-induced parkinsonism. Some overdoses of this product have resulted in death.

Ethopropazine is an antiparkinsonism agent derived from phenothiazine that has a strong atropine-like blocking agent. In addition to antimuscarinic action, the drug exhibits antihistaminic, local anesthetic, ganglionic blocking, and weak adrenolytic activity. Adverse reactions to ethopropazine are mainly extensions of its anticholinergic effects.

Trihexyphenidyl is a synthetic tertiary amine antimuscarinic antiparkinsonism agent that has atropine-like blocking action on parasympathetic innervated peripheral structures.

Plant Alkaloids

The tropane alkaloids, often called belladonna alkaloids, include atropine (hyoscyamine), scopolamine (hyoscine), and ecgonine (cocaine). This group contains the large and commercially important family Solanaceae, which includes the medicinal belladonna, the poisonous jimson weed, and the food staples potato, tomato, eggplant, and pepper (Table 7-4).

Hyoscyamine

The genus *Datura* belongs to the family Solanaceae, which includes a great number of plants with hypnotic properties, among them the mandrake, deadly nightshade, and henbane.[13] Tropane alkaloids, including scopolamine, hyoscyamine, norhyoscyamine, and atropine, have been isolated from these plants. There is great variation in the amounts and percentages of these alkaloids present, depending on the portion of the plant analyzed and the stage of maturation. Those plants of the genus *Datura* produce most cases of anticholinergic plant poisoning in the United States.

Jimson weed. In the United States, poisoning with jimson weed (*Datura stramonium*) has shifted from accidental childhood poisonings to inadvertent overdoses in persons experimenting with mind-altering drugs. Recreational users usually ingest the seeds whole or make a tea with the leaves, but all parts of the plant are toxic. *Datura stramonium* has also been marketed as

---

Table 7-4 Plant Alkaloids That Have Anticholinergic Activity

Alkaloid	*Plant (Common Name)*
Hyoscyamine	*Datura sarvolens* (angel's trumpet)
	Datura stramonium (jimson weed)
	Hyoscyamus niger (henbane)
	Atropa belladonna (deadly nightshade)
	Lycium halimifolium (matrimony vine)
Solanine	*Solanum dulcamara* (European bittersweet)
	Solanum nigrum (black nightshade)
	Solanum tuberosum (common potato)
	Solanum pseudocapsicum (jerusalem cherry)
	Solanum melongena (eggplant)
	Solanum gracile (wild tomato)
Lycopersicon	(tomato)
Amanitin	*Amanita muscaria* (mushroom)

Asthmador, a preparation sold in health food stores as an asthma medication. The plant is also smoked in cigarettes and prepared as a powder.

Datura stramonium is found throughout the United States. The plant has large white or purple trumpet-shaped flowers that in autumn become thorny capsules filled with many blackish seeds. These are common annuals, and more than a dozen species occur across the country. Other common names include Jamestown weed, loco weed, devil's weed, and thornapple. Most cases of poisoning relate to ingestion or inhalation of extracts of *Datura stramonium*.

Belladonna. Belladonna is a term applied to the various preparations of the naturally occurring solanaceous alkaloids. Belladonna leaf is derived from the dried leaf and flowering or fruiting top of *Atropa belladonna*. Belladonna leaf contains several alkaloids, principally *l*-hyoscyamine and scopolamine. The pharmacologic activity of belladonna derives principally from its atropine (*d,l*-hyoscyamine) content.[14] *Atropa belladonna* is native to Europe and rare in the United States. Preparations of belladonna are marketed as Donnatal®, Hyosophen®, Bellalphen®, Barbidonna®, and Kinesed®.

Atropine

Atropine, a naturally occurring tertiary amine muscarinic agent is the prototype of the antimuscarinic drugs and, in adequate doses, provides all the effects described for the group as a whole. The drug may be prepared synthetically but is usually obtained by extraction from various members of the Solanaceae family of plants. It has a volume of distribution of 2 to 4 L/kg.

The pharmacologic activity of atropine results almost completely from *l*-hyoscyamine; *d*-hyoscyamine has essentially no antimuscarinic activity. In general, atropine is more potent than scopolamine in its antimuscarinic action on the heart, bronchi, and intestinal smooth muscle.

Poisoning with atropine is uncommon but has been reported in children given atropine eye drops, in individuals who have ingested plants containing belladonna alkaloids, in errors in prescribing and dispensing, and in cases of deliberate self-poisoning.

Scopolamine

Scopolamine (*l*-hyoscine) is a belladonna alkaloid and is among the oldest drugs in medicine.[15] The drug may be prepared synthetically but is usually obtained by extraction from various members of the Solanaceae family of plants. The peripheral cholinergic blocking actions of scopolamine and atropine are similar; the two drugs differ mainly in their central nervous system effects. Unlike atropine and most other anticholinergic agents, scopolamine, at usual dosages, produces central nervous system depression manifested as drowsiness, euphoria, amnesia, fatigue, and dreamless sleep. Higher doses of scopolamine produce central nervous system effects similar to those produced by toxic doses of other anticholinergics.[9] A transdermal preparation is now available for treatment of motion sickness. This route allows for a controlled release of medication with fewer side effects.[16] Pure scopolamine intoxications are extremely rare.

Tricyclic Antidepressants

The tricyclic antidepressants are described in Chapter 11.

Miscellaneous Compounds

Other anticholinergic agents include the synthetic relatives of the belladonna alkaloids,[17] ophthalmic solutions, and antispasmodic agents (Table 7-5).

CLINICAL MANIFESTATIONS OF INTOXICATION

The blocking of the action of acetylcholine on the muscarinic receptors results in the anticholinergic syndrome:

> "Hot as a hare,
> Blind as a bat,
> Dry as a bone,
> Red as a beet,
> Mad as a hatter."

Table 7-5 Miscellaneous Anticholinergic Agents with Selected Trade Names

Agent Class	Drugs
Antispasmodic	Adiphenine (Trasentine®)
	Clidinium bromide (Quarzan®, Librax®, Clindex®)
	Dicyclomine (Bentyl®)
	Methantheline bromide (Banthine®)
	Methixene (Trest®)
	Oxyphencyclimine (Daricon®)
	Propantheline bromide (Pro-Banthine®)
	Mepenzolate bromide (Cantil®)
Synthetic belladonna alkaloids	Glycopyrrolate (Robinul®)
	Homatropine (Dia-Quel®, Homapin®)
	Methscopolamine bromide (Pamine®)
	Hexocyclium (Tral®)
Ophthalmic solutions	Cyclopentolate (Cyclogyl®)
	Eucatropine (Euphthalmine®)
	Tropicamide (Mydriacyl®)

The signs and symptoms of anticholinergic poisoning can be divided into peripheral and central effects (Table 7-6).

Table 7-6 Signs and Symptoms of Anticholinergic Poisoning

Peripheral Effects
Tachycardia
Mydriasis
Blurred vision
Vasodilation
Dry skin
Hyperpyrexia
Hypertension
Decreased secretions
  Bronchi
  Pharynx
  Nasal
  Salivary
Urinary retention
Decreased bowel motility
Central
Delirium
Anxiety
Hyperactivity
Hallucinations
Disorientation
Incoherence
Confusion
Paranoia
Restlessness
Seizure
Impairment of recent memory
Clonus
Hyperreflexia
Coma

Peripheral Manifestations of Toxicity

Peripheral toxicity may be manifested by sinus tachycardia; dilated and unreactive pupils; blurred vision; vasodilation and flushing; dry skin; hyperpyrexia; hypertension; decreased bronchial, pharyngeal, nasal, and salivary secretions; urinary retention; and decreased bowel motility.

Central Nervous System Manifestations of Toxicity

Acute overdosage generally produces CNS stimulation with subsequent depression. These manifestations may resemble acute psychosis characterized by various neuropsychiatric signs and symptoms, including disorientation, incoherence, confusion, hallucinations (which are usually visual but may also be auditory or tactile), delusions, and paranoia. Disturbed speech and abnormal motor behavior such as ataxia, incoordination, agitation, and restlessness may also occur. In children anticholinergic toxicity is commonly manifested as hyperpyrexia.[18] Severe impairment of recent memory is a prominent symptom. Comatose patients may display clonic movements, hyperreflexia, and extensor plantar reflexes. Grand mal seizures are also a result of central anticholinergic activity.

Typically, adults manifest CNS depression as somnolence, weakness, and coma after overdose; seizures are uncommon. Children manifest CNS stimulation as agitation, hallucinations, and ataxia; seizures are more common than in adults.

Cardiac Manifestations of Toxicity

In addition to sinus tachycardia, cardiac manifestations may also include electrocardiographic abnormalities similar to those produced by quinidine toxicity.[19,20] This includes widening of the QRS complex, prolongation of the QT interval, and ST segment depression. These abnormalities result from enhanced reentrant excitation secondary to reduced conduction velocity.

Systemic Manifestations after Ophthalmic Administration

Anticholinergic eye drops have caused systemic effects. After instillation of the compound into the conjunctival sac, systemic absorption may occur through the conjunctival capillaries by simple diffusion[21] as well as through the nasal mucosa, oral pharynx, and gastrointestinal tract after passage through the lacrimal drainage system.[22] Reactions to ophthalmic ointments are less frequent than reactions to eye drops because of reduced absorption of ointments by the conjunctiva and lack of lacrimal duct passage. In some cases, atropine may produce an initial transitory central vagal stimulant action before the blocking effect is manifested. This is especially true when it is taken in large amounts.[14] Symptoms noted after ophthalmic administration consist of restlessness, insomnia, ataxia, hallucinations, confusion (which at times progresses to supraventricular tachycardia), seizures, coma, and death.[21,22] Agents that have caused these symptoms include atropine, scopolamine, homatropine, and cyclopentolate.

Manifestations of Severe Overdosage

In severe overdosage, CNS depression, circulatory collapse, and hypotension may occur. Coma and skeletal muscle paralysis may also occur and may be followed by death from respiratory failure. Death has also reportedly resulted from hyperpyrexia, especially in children: Additive adverse effects resulting from cholinergic blockade may occur when anticholinergics are administered concomitantly with pheno-

thiazines, amantadines, antiparkinsonism drugs, glutethimide, meperidine, tricyclic antidepressants, quinidine, disopyramide, antihistamines, or any other drug with prominent anticholinergic effects.

LABORATORY ANALYSIS

In all cases of acutely altered mental status, blood should be obtained and analyzed for glucose, blood urea nitrogen, serum electrolytes, complete blood count, toxicologic screen, and arterial blood gas. Specific testing for anticholinergics is usually of no value.

TREATMENT

The treatment of an acute overdose of an anticholinergic agent consists of symptomatic and supportive therapy (Table 7-7). Removal of the material from the gastrointestinal tract should be attempted in the acute overdose and should be followed by administration of activated charcoal and a cathartic. Fluid therapy and other standard treatments of shock should be administered as needed.

Patients with any evidence of cardiac dysrhythmias must be monitored. Ventricular ectopy in the absence of atrioventricular block may be treated with lidocaine. Because many of the anticholinergic agents have a quinidine-like action, the use of procainamide, quinidine, or disopyramide should be avoided. Precautions against seizure must be undertaken. Hyperther-

Table 7-7 Treatment of Anticholinergic Toxicity

Condition	Treatment
Acute overdose	Monitor, prevent absorption
Ventricular ectopy	Lidocaine (1 mg/kg IV)
Seizure	Diazepam (5 to 10 mg IV)
Hyperthermia	Active cooling
Acute psychosis	Diazepam (5 to 10 mg IV)
	?Physostigmine (1 to 2 mg IV)
Urinary retention	Urinary catheterization

mia is usually treated with cold packs, mechanical cooling devices, or sponging with tepid water. Diazepam may be administered to control excitement, delirium, or other symptoms of acute psychosis. Phenothiazines should not be used because they may contribute to anticholinergic effects. If the patient is comatose, urinary catheterization should be performed to avoid urinary retention.

Because most of the anticholinergic agents are rapidly distributed to the tissues and have large volumes of distribution, little free drug is present in the plasma. Thus treatment modalities such as hemodialysis, hemoperfusion, and forced diuresis are of little benefit.[23] In addition to supportive care, the intravenous use of physostigmine may be efficacious under certain circumstances.

Antidotal Therapy with Acetylcholinesterase Inhibitors

Anticholinesterase agents are antidotal agents that inhibit acetylcholinesterase, the enzyme that breaks down acetylcholine and allows acetylcholine to accumulate and to overcome the competitive inhibition of anticholinergic agents.[24] Some of these agents include physostigmine (Antilirium), neostigmine (Prostigmin®), pyridostigmine (Mestinon®), and edrophonium (Tensilon®).

Physostigmine

Physostigmine belongs to a class of drugs known as acetylcholinesterase inhibitors.[25] These anticholinesterases allow for the buildup of naturally generated acetylcholine, thereby reversing the effects of anticholinergic overdose.[26] Physostigmine differs from other anticholinergic compounds in that it is a tertiary amine, a nonionized lipophilic compound that can cross the blood-brain barrier and reverse both the peripheral and central effects of an anticholinergic overdose.[27] The other compounds are quaternary ammonium compounds, and, because they are charged molecules, they are not able to cross the blood-brain barrier and therefore will reverse only the peripheral anticholinergic effects.[26,28]

Indications for Use of Physostigmine

Treatment with physostigmine must be based on the presence of the anticholinergic syndrome and not merely on a history of ingestion because the use of physostigmine is not without complications (Table 7-8).[29] Because of the potential for producing severe adverse effects, its use should be reserved for treatment of patients with extreme delirium or agitation who have the potential for inflicting injuries on themselves; for patients with severe, hemodynamically significant sinus tachycardia or supraventricular tachycardia; for patients with repetitive or long-lasting seizures; or for patients with extreme hyperthermia unresponsive to mechanical cooling.[1] In other words, physostigmine should be used only in situations where a potential life-threatening emergency exists.[30] Coma is not an indication for the use of physostigmine, other than to confirm a diagnosis.

Table 7-8 Use of Physostigmine for Anticholinergic Overdose

Indications
  Diagnostic
  Therapeutic
    Supraventricular dysrhythmias
    Seizures
    Myclonus
    Hallucinations
    Hypertension
Dosage
  Adult: 1 to 2 mg IV, slowly
  Child: 0.5 mg or 0.02 mg/kg IV, slowly
Cholinergic Side Effects
  Bradycardia
  Miosis
  Increased secretions
  —Salivation
  —Lacrimation
  —Rhinorrhea
  —Pulmonary
  Urination
  Defecation
  Seizures
Cardiac Side Effects
  Shift of pacemaker from sinoatrial node to another site
  Slowing of conduction through atrioventricular node
  Prolonging of refractory period
  Production of atrioventricular block
  Asystole

Dosage

In adults, 1 to 2 mg of physostigmine may be administered intravenously. In children, a dose of 0.5 mg[31] or 0.02 mg/kg[14] may be administered intravenously. Physostigmine is available in 2-mL sterile vials containing 1 mg/mL. It should be diluted to 10 mL in dextrose in water or normal saline and given over two to five minutes.[15] The half-life of physostigmine is 90 minutes, which may necessitate repeated doses for long-acting anticholinergic compounds.[32]

Contraindications to the Use of Physostigmine

Relative contraindications to the use of physostigmine are diabetes, glaucoma, asthma, heart block, coronary artery disease, gangrene, peptic ulcer disease, and ulcerative colitis. The absolute contraindications are mechanical obstruction of the gastrointestinal and genitourinary tracts.[2]

Complications from Physostigmine

The most common complications from the use of physostigmine are nausea and vomiting.[27] Seizures have also been reported after the use of physostigmine and may be attributable to the rapidity of administration.[31] If physostigmine is used in the absence of anticholinergic overdose, patients may manifest the signs of cholinergic toxicity, including salivation, lacrimation, urination, defecation, gastrointestinal upset, and emesis. If cholinergic crisis occurs, an anticholinergic agent may be necessary.

REFERENCES

1. Goldfrank L, Flomenbaum N, Lewin N, et al: Anticholinergic poisoning. *J Toxicol Clin Toxicol* 1982; 19:17–25.

2. Richmond M, Seger D: Central anticholinergic syndrome in a child: A case report. *J Emerg Med* 1985;3: 453–456.

3. Feldman M, Behar M: A case of massive diphenhydramine abuse and withdrawal from use of the drug. *JAMA* 1986;255:3119–3120.

4. Filoux F: Toxic encephalopathy caused by topically applied diphenhydramine. *J Pediatr* 1986;108:1018–1020.

5. Sankey R, Nunn A, Sills J: Visual hallucinations in children receiving decongestants. *Br Med J* 1984;288:1369.

6. Meadow S, Leeson G: Poisoning with delayed-release tablets. *Arch Dis Child* 1974;49:310–312.

7. Koppel C, Ibe K, Tenczer J: Clinical symptomatology of diphenhydramine overdose: An evaluation of 136 cases in 1982 to 1985. *Clin Toxicol* 1987;25:53–70.

8. Bratt K, Zagerman A: Dyskinesias after antihistamine use. *N Engl J Med* 1977;196:111–114.

9. Crowell E, Ketchum J: The treatment of scopolamine-induced delirium with physostigmine. *Clin Pharmacol Ther* 1978;8:409–414.

10. Hestand H, Teske D: Diphenhydramine hydrochloride intoxication. *J Pediatr* 1977;90:1017–1018.

11. Lavenstein B, Cantor F: Acute dystonia: An unusual reaction to diphenhydramine. *JAMA* 1976;236:291–292.

12. Howrie D, Rowley A, Krenzelok E: Benztropine-induced acute dystonic reaction. *Ann Emerg Med* 1986; 15:594–596.

13. Hayman J: *Datura* poisoning—The angel's trumpet. *Pathology* 1985;17:465–466.

14. Spoerke D, Hall A, Dodson C, et al: Mystery root ingestion. *J Emerg Med* 1987;5:385–388.

15. Thornton W: Sleep aids and sedatives. *JACEP* 1977;6:408–412.

16. Wilkinson J: Side effects of transdermal scopolamine. *J Emerg Med* 1987;5:389–392.

17. Slovis C, Daniels G, Wharton D: Intravenous use of glycopyrrolate in acute respiratory distress due to bronchospastic pulmonary disease. *Ann Emerg Med* 1987;16:898–900.

18. Magera B, Betlach C, Sweatt A, et al: Hydroxyzine intoxication in a 13-month-old child. *Pediatrics* 1981; 67:280–283.

19. Burton B, Rice M, Schmertzier L: Atrioventricular block following overdose of decongestant cold medication. *J Emerg Med* 1985;2:415–419.

20. Freedberg R, Friedman G, Palu R, et al: Cardiogenic shock due to antihistamine overdose. *JAMA* 1987; 257:660–661.

21. Merli G, Weitz H, Martin J, et al: Cardiac dysrhythmias associated with ophthalmic atropine. *Arch Intern Med* 1986;146:45–47.

22. Adler A, McElwain G, Merli G, et al: Systemic effects of eye drops. *Arch Intern Med* 1982;142:2293–2294.

23. Worth D, Davison A, Roberts T, et al: Ineffectiveness of hemodialysis in atropine poisoning. *Br Med J* 1983;286:2023–2024.

24. Ullman K, Groh R: Identification and treatment of acute psychotic states secondary to the usage of over-the-counter sleeping preparations. *Am J Psychiatry* 1972;128:64–68.

25. Brashares Z, Conley W: Physostigmine in drug overdose. *JACEP* 1975;4:46–48.

26. Nattel S, Bayne L, Ruedy J: Physostigmine in coma due to drug overdose. *Clin Pharmacol Ther* 1979; 25:96–102.

27. Granacher R, Baldessarini R: Physostigmine: Its use in acute anticholinergic syndrome with antidepressant and antiparkinson drugs. *Arch Gen Psychiatry* 1975; 32:375–379.

28. Janowsky D, Risch S, Heuy L: Central cardiovascular effects of physostigmine in humans. *Hypertension* 1985;7:140–145.

29. Levy R: Arrhythmias following physostigmine administration in jimson weed poisoning. *JACEP* 1977;6:107–108.

30. Hussey H: Physostigmine: Value in treatment of central toxic effects of anticholinergic drugs. *JAMA* 1975;231:1066.

31. Rumack B: Anticholinergic poisoning: Treatment with physostigmine. *Pediatrics* 1973;52:449–451.

32. Lauwers L, Daelemans R, Baute L, et al: Scopolamine intoxications. *Intensive Care Med* 1983;9:283–285.

ADDITIONAL SELECTED REFERENCES

Bailie G, Nelson M, Krenzelok E, et al: Unusual treatment response of a severe dystonia to diphenhydramine. *Ann Emerg Med* 1987;16:705–715.

Cockrell J: Acute hallucinogenic reaction to carbinoxamine maleate. *Clin Toxicol* 1987;25:161–167.

Furlanut M, Bettio I, Bertin G, et al: Orphenadrine serum levels in a poisoned patient. *Human Toxicol* 1985; 4:331–333.

Hooper R, Conner C, Rumack B: Acute poisoning from over-the-counter sleep preparations. *JACEP* 1979; 8:98–100.

Kaplan M, Register D, Bierman A, et al: A nonfatal case of intentional scopolamine poisoning. *Clin Toxicol* 1974; 7:509–512.

Krenzelok E, Anderson G, Mirick M: Massive diphenhydramine overdose resulting in death. *Ann Emerg Med* 1982;11:212–213.

Lacouture P, Lovejoy F, Mitchell A: Acute hypothermia associated with atropine. *Am J Dis Child* 1983; 137:291–292.

Pentel P, Peterson C: Asystole complicating physostigmine treatment of tricyclic antidepressant overdose. *Ann Emerg Med* 1980;9:588–590.

Schuster P, Gabriel E, Kufferle B, et al: Reversal by physostigmine of clozapine-induced delirium. *Clin Toxicol* 1977;10:437–441.

Spaulding B, Choi S, Gross J, et al: The effect of physostigmine on diazepam-induced ventilatory depression: A double-blind study. *Anesthesiology* 1984;61:551–554.

chapter 8

The α-Adrenergic Agents

The α-adrenergic agents are adrenoceptor agonists or antagonists, and there are clinical uses for both. Although there are many α-adrenergic agents used in medicine, this chapter concentrates on those agents that may be taken as a purposeful or accidental overdose outside the hospital situation: (1) clonidine, guanabenz, and methyldopa, which are antihypertensive α₂ receptor agonists; (2) yohimbine, which is an α₂ receptor antagonist and a drug of abuse; and (3) prazosin, an antihypertensive α₁ receptor antagonist.

α₂-ADRENERGIC AGONISTS

Clonidine

Clonidine (Catapres®) is an imidazoline derivative[1] originally synthesized as a sympathomimetic agent for use as a nasal decongestant.[2] Clonidine is structurally similar to the α receptor blockers phentolamine and tolazoline and was one of the first drugs for which a central mechanism was recognized to be the most important factor in its hypotensive activity.[3,4]

Clinical Use

Clonidine is primarily used as an antihypertensive agent.[3,4] In this regard, it is frequently used for the management of hypertensive urgen-cies.[5] In addition, it is used in the prophylaxis of migraine or recurrent vascular headaches[6] and in the treatment of menopausal flushing (Table 8-1).[7,8] Clonidine has also been used for detoxification of opiate-dependent individuals because it blocks the symptoms of narcotic withdrawal.[9,10] The mechanism of action is thought to be an inhibition in the locus coeruleus through α₂ adrenergic receptors.[11] Because of this, clonidine has become a street drug used by opiate addicts during withdrawal or during periods of opiate scarcity. Lofexidine, a clonidine analog, is being investigated as a safe alternative in clinical settings.

Recently clonidine was made available as a transdermal patch, which allows for a constant delivery of the drug over a 7-day period. Usually, a steady state is reached approximately 48 hours after the patch is applied. Toxicity has been noted in cases of irregular delivery or in children coming in contact with used patches.[12]

Table 8-1 Medical Uses of Clonidine

Antihypertensive agent
Migraine prophylaxis
Vascular headache prophylaxis
Menopause
Narcotic withdrawal

Pharmacokinetics

Clonidine is absorbed from the gastrointestinal tract and widely distributed into body tissues. After oral administration the onset of action is usually within 30 to 60 minutes, and blood concentrations reach a peak 3 to 5 hours after ingestion.[3,4] The plasma half-life is 12 to 16 hours in patients with normal renal functions.[13,14]

Mechanism of Action

Clonidine appears to stimulate postsynaptic α_2-adrenergic receptors in the central nervous system, mainly in the medulla oblongata, and cause inhibition but not blockade of sympathetic vasomotor centers.[15,16] This results in decreased sympathetic outflux to the heart, kidneys, and peripheral vasculature.[3] Cardiovascular reflexes remain intact, and normal homeostatic mechanisms and hemodynamic responses to exercise are maintained.[17]

Clonidine also acts peripherally, especially in high doses, partly by inhibiting neuronal uptake of norepinephrine and by stimulating α-adrenergic receptors.[8,14] Because clonidine does not display absolute selectivity for α_2 adrenoceptors, high blood concentrations of clonidine as in an overdose may cause a pressor response. In the therapeutic dose range, the peripheral α-adrenergic agonist effect of clonidine is not important. In a massive overdose, however, the vasoconstrictor effect may compete with or overcome the drug's central hypotensive mechanism.

Side Effects

Intimately connected with the desired circulatory effect are α_2-adrenergic side effects such as sedation and dryness of the mouth,[2] the latter being at least partly due to α_2-adrenergic inhibition of cholinergic transmission to the salivary glands. Dizziness, lethargy, insomnia, hallucinations, depression, and delirium have also been reported[18,19] (Table 8-2).

Withdrawal Symptoms

The abrupt cessation of clonidine may precipitate withdrawal symptoms related to the drug's sympatholytic mechanism of action.[4,20] The

Table 8-2 Side Effects of Clonidine

Delirium
Depression
Dizziness
Dryness of mouth
Insomnia
Hallucinations
Lethargy
Sedation

frequency and severity of symptoms appear to be greater in patients treated with high doses for long periods and in those with severe hypertension before treatment.[21] This syndrome of adrenergic overactivity is mediated by a sudden increase in circulating catecholamines and is manifested by rebound hypertension, tachycardia, tremor, flushing, insomnia, nausea, vomiting, palpitations, and cardiac dysrhythmias (Table 8-3).[22] Withdrawal from clonidine can begin as soon as 8 hours or up to 36 hours after the last dose and can last for 72 to 96 hours.[23] The blood pressure may rise to values greater than those recorded before therapy is initiated. Death due to hypertensive encephalopathy has been reported.[14] Concomitant β-blocker therapy may predispose the patient to overshoot hypertension.

Because of the rather severe withdrawal symptoms, clonidine therapy should be terminated gradually, especially in a high-risk population.[20] Nevertheless, withdrawal reactions have been reported even when the drug was slowly and gradually withdrawn.[24] Symptoms secondary to withdrawal are treated by readministering clonidine orally.[25,26]

Table 8-3 Symptoms of Clonidine Withdrawal

Sinus tachycardia
Rebound hypertension
Flushing
Insomnia
Tremor
Nausea
Vomiting
Palpitations
Cardiac dysrhythmias

Toxicity

Accidental or intentional overdose with clonidine can result in severe toxicity with variable clinical presentation and may mimic the clinical picture of an overdose of narcotics (Table 8-4).[4,27] Signs and symptoms of clonidine overdosage usually occur within 30 to 60 minutes after ingestion.

The most common features of overdose are CNS depression, hypotension, miosis, and bradycardia[16]; prolonged coma has also been reported.[28] Central and presumably peripheral presynaptic cardiac α_2 adrenoceptors are involved in the bradycardic action of clonidine.[29] Other symptoms include weakness, respiratory depression sometimes leading to apnea, cardiac conduction defects, cardiac dysrhythmias, hypothermia, and hypertension.[14,30,31] Hypertension may be transient and may lead to hypotension even without therapy.[32] The mechanism proposed for the paradoxic hypertension observed in some overdose patients is stimulation of peripheral receptors for α_1 receptor agonists.[14,31] Other symptoms occurring less frequently include irritability, agitation, seizures, or paralytic ileus. Atrioventricular conduction delays of all degrees have also been noted.[31]

Laboratory Analysis

Methods for measuring clonidine concentration in body fluids are not widely available, and at present the usual toxicology screening tests will not detect clonidine. Although serum concentrations appear to correlate with the sedative effects of the drug, the correlation with blood pressure is poorly defined. An electrocardiogram should be obtained to evaluate cardiac rhythm and atrioventricular conduction.

Treatment

Treatment must include the basics of overdose resuscitation and careful cardiovascular monitoring. Seizures can be managed with intravenous diazepam. If the patient has an altered mental status, 50% dextrose in water, thiamine, and naloxone should be administered (Table 8-5). In acute clonidine overdose an attempt should be made to empty the stomach by inducing emesis or by gastric lavage followed by administration of activated charcoal and a cathartic. Naloxone has been used with and without success.[16,27,33,34] Although naloxone has been advocated in the treatment of clonidine overdose due to an adrenergic-opioid interaction,[35] its effectiveness has not been demonstrated. Because naloxone is relatively innocuous, and clonidine overdose closely resembles narcotic overdose, it should be administered.

Blood pressure should be closely monitored after overdose because hypotension, if it occurs, will be detected within the first several hours after ingestion.[32] Hypotension can initially be managed with intravenous fluids and by placing the patient in Trendelenburg's position. In most cases, hypotension associated with clonidine overdose responds to intravenous fluids.[3,32]

Table 8-4 Symptoms of Clonidine Overdose

Central Nervous System
 Sedation
 Weakness
 Impaired consciousness
 Irritability
 Agitation
 Apnea
 Miosis
 Seizures
 Coma
Cardiovascular
 Hypertension (transient)
 Hypotension
 Conduction defects
 Cardiac dysrhythmia
 Bradycardia

Table 8-5 Treatment of Clonidine Overdose

Indication	Treatment
Altered mental status	Dextrose and thiamine
Decreased respiration	Naloxone
Acute overdose	Ipecac or lavage
Acute overdose	Charcoal and cathartic
Bradycardia with hypotension	Fluids
	Atropine
	Tolazoline
	Dopamine
Seizures	Diazepam

Dopamine may be useful for severe hypotension.

When bradycardia with hypotension is present and unresponsive to intravenous fluids, atropine may be effective. Tolazoline may be effective in reversing the hypotensive, bradycardic, and hypertensive effects of clonidine.[8,14] Tolazoline, an imidazoline compound with a structure similar to that of clonidine, has both central and peripheral nonspecific α-adrenergic inhibitory effects.[13] Tolazoline penetrates into the brain and thereby reverses part of clonidine's central nervous system effects. It may be administered intravenously (0.5 to 1 mg/kg, up to 25 mg, in children and 25 mg per dose in adults) every 5 to 10 minutes to a maximum of four doses. Tolazoline may be tried if fluids, atropine, and dopamine do not reverse hypotension and bradycardia.[3,4] It may cause dysrhythmias, angina, and hypertension, however.[36]

Although forced diuresis has been suggested to enhance the elimination of clonidine, there is no strong evidence that it increases urinary excretion and therefore should not be attempted. Dialysis and hemoperfusion are also not effective.[3,4]

Guanabenz and Guanfacine

Guanabenz (Wytensin®) and guanfacine (Tenex®) are guanidine derivatives that are centrally acting α₂-adrenergic agonists with pharmacological properties and side effects that are similar to those of clonidine.[36–38] The mode of action is stimulation of central α₂ receptors that cause suppression of the vasomotor center.

Guanabenz and guanfacine are rapidly absorbed after oral administration. Guanabenz undergoes substantial first-pass hepatic metabolism. Its onset of action is 1 to 2 hours, and peak plasma concentrations are achieved within 4 hours. Guanabenz has a duration of effect of 8 to 12 hours and a volume of distribution of 4 to 17 L/kg.[36] It is 90% bound to human plasma protein.[37] Guanfacine has a half-life of 15 to 20 hours, which is significantly longer than that of clonidine.[38] Development of tolerance to the drug as well as withdrawal reactions may be seen.[37] Symptoms associated with withdrawal include headache, dizziness, hypertension, nau-

sea, vomiting, palpitations, agitation, anxiety, and abdominal pain. Symptoms of overdose and treatment are identical to those of clonidine.

Methyldopa

The mode of action of methyldopa (Aldomet®) is also interference with central α adrenoceptors, although in a more complicated manner than is the case with clonidine. After oral ingestion of methyldopa, plasma concentrations reach a peak in approximately 3 to 6 hours. Methyldopa is a drug precursor in the sense that it needs to be converted to an active product. This occurs when it penetrates into the brain stem, where it is decarboxylated enzymatically to yield α-methyldopamine, which is in turn converted by enzymatic hydroxylation into α-methylnorepinephrine. α-Methylnorepinephrine, an α-adrenoceptor agonist, then stimulates central inhibitory α adrenoceptors in a manner similar to that of clonidine, causing a fall in arterial pressure.

Methyldopa does not appear to cause withdrawal reactions with any measurable frequency. This may be due to the active metabolite, which persists in nerve endings for some time and thus permits a gradual offset of effect.

Overdosage with methyldopa may produce acute hypotension, sedation, weakness, bradycardia, dizziness, lightheadedness, constipation, diarrhea, nausea and vomiting (Table 8-6).[39] Treatment is similar to that for clonidine overdosage.

α-ADRENERGIC BLOCKING AGENTS

Although there are many α-adrenergic blocking agents, very few are encountered as an overdose. Two of these are prazosin[40] and yohimbine.

Prazosin

Prazosin (Minipress®) is a quinozoline derivative used in the treatment of hypertension by reducing peripheral vascular resistance. The major mechanism of action of prazosin is com-

Table 8-6 Signs and Symptoms of Methyldopa Overdose

Central Nervous System
Dizziness
Lightheadedness
Sedation
Weakness
Cardiovascular
Hypotension
Bradycardia
Gastrointestinal
Constipation
Diarrhea
Nausea
Vomiting

---

petitive blockade of the vascular postsynaptic α_1-adrenergic receptor.[40–42] It is thought that, by leaving the inhibitory prejunctional α_2 receptors unblocked, prazosin does not alter the negative feedback loop through which norepinephrine regulates its own release.[43] This is in contrast with vasodilators that directly relax arteriolar vascular muscle; these include hydralazine, diazoxide, and phentolamine (which blocks both pre- and postsynaptic receptors). As a result of its vasodilating effects, prazosin produces both arterial and venous dilation. Unlike hydralazine, the antihypertensive effect of prazosin is accompanied by little or no increase in heart rate.[42] This lack of reflex tachycardia is probably attributable to a number of reasons, one of which is that prazosin does not interrupt the α_2-adrenergic autoinhibition of norepinephrine release.[44]

Prazosin is the most potent α_1 blocking drug currently available and has no α_2- or β-adrenergic activity. Also, unlike methyldopa and clonidine, prazosin appears to have no central action on blood pressure.

Pharmacokinetics

After oral administration of prazosin, plasma concentrations of the drug reach a peak in 2 to 3 hours. Plasma concentrations generally do not correlate with therapeutic effects. The plasma half-life of prazosin is 2 to 4 hours. Prazosin is 97% bound to human plasma proteins and has an apparent volume of distribution of approximately 0.6 to 1 L/kg.

Side Effects

Commonly reported side effects from prazosin include headache, lassitude, dryness of the mouth, nausea, and urinary frequency with urgency (Table 8-7). The major side effect of prazosin therapy in patients with hypertension is postural hypotension, which is usually most pronounced after the initial drug administration. This postural hypotension is accompanied by tachycardia and palpitations and occasionally proceeds to bradycardia and syncope.[41] This "first dose phenomenon" may occur 30 to 90 minutes after the initial dose.[42] It may be due to a combination of prazosin's failure to cause tachycardia and the effect of venous dilatation. Occasionally, bradycardia may be noted. Postural hypotension is not usually a problem during continued treatment.

Toxicity

Overdosage of prazosin has caused drowsiness but no severe hypotension (Table 8-8). Priapism has also been noted with prazosin overdose and is thought to be related to the sympatholytic effects from blockade of postsynaptic α-adrenergic receptors.[45] This blockade appears to favor erection, which is parasympathetically mediated, and to inhibit ejaculation and detumescence, which are sympathetically mediated.

Table 8-7 Side Effects of Prazosin

Bradycardia
Dryness of mouth
Headache
Lassitude
Nausea
Postural hypotension
Urinary frequency

Table 8-8 Signs and Symptoms of Prazosin Overdose

Hypotension (rare)
Drowsiness
Priapism

Treatment

If overdosage of prazosin causes hypotension, supportive therapy should be initiated. The patient should be kept in the supine position; if necessary, shock may be treated with plasma volume expanders and vasopressor drugs. Prazosin is not dialyzable because of its high degree of protein binding.

Yohimbine

Yohimbine is an indole alkylamine alkaloid that is chemically similar to reserpine and is the prototype of the α_2 blocking agents. It is a plant alkaloid derived from the bark of *Corynanthe johimbe* and has prominent CNS effects.[46,47] Yohimbine acts by selectively blocking the central α_2 receptors that cause the release of norepinephrine. Thus yohimbine antagonizes α-adrenergic inhibition of adrenergic actions and reverses the effects of many centrally acting antihypertensive agents such as clonidine. Non-α_2 effects of yohimbine include local anesthetic actions and inhibition of monoamine oxidase.[46,47]

Although yohimbine hydrochloride is available under the brand names Yohimex® and Yocon® and is suggested as a sympatholytic and mydriatic and for erectile dysfunction, its medical use is questionable. Yohimbine has no FDA sanctioned indications and is a drug of abuse (its street name is "yo-yo"). Although it has been promoted as an aphrodisiac for many years, in actuality it stimulates erectile tissue without increasing sexual desire and thus is not a true aphrodisiac.

Ingestion of yohimbine may result in hypertension, tachycardia, mydriasis, lacrimation, salivation, diaphoresis, priapism, and tremors.[48] Central nervous system excitation is also a characteristic response to yohimbine, with anxiety, increased motor activity, and irritability noted. Mild hallucinations have also been noted (Table 8-9).

Treatment of yohimbine intoxication consists mainly of supportive care. Attempts to empty the stomach are usually of no benefit. Clonidine is the agent of choice for treating anxiety, hypertension, and other autonomic symptoms.[49] Clonidine should be administered in an initial oral loading dose of 0.1 to 0.2 mg followed by several additional hourly doses of 0.1 mg.[50]

Table 8-9 Signs and Symptoms of Yohimbine Overdose

Hypertension
Tachycardia
Anxiety
Increased motor activity
Irritability
Mydriasis
Lacrimation
Salivation
Penile erection
Tremors
Mild hallucinations

REFERENCES

1. Gallanosa A, Spyker D, Shipe J, et al: Human xylazine overdose: A comparative review with clonidine, phenothiazines, and tricyclic antidepressants. *Clin Toxicol* 1981; 18:663–678.

2. Lowenstein J: Clonidine. *Ann Intern Med* 1980; 92:74–77.

3. Anderson R, Hart G, Crumler C, et al: Clonidine overdose: Report of six cases and review of the literature. *Ann Emerg Med* 1981;10:107–112.

4. Anderson R, Hart G, Crumler C, et al: Oral clonidine loading in hypertensive urgencies. *JAMA* 1981;246: 848–850.

5. Houston M: Oral clonidine loading in the treatment of hypertensive urgencies and emergencies. *Cardiovasc Rev Rep* 1985;6:1249–1252.

6. Shafer I, Tallett E, Knowlson P: Evaluation of clonidine in prophylaxis of migraine—Double-blind trial and follow-up. *Lancet* 1972;1:403–407.

7. Clayden J, Bell J, Pellard P: Menopausal flushing: Double-blind trial of a nonhormonal medication. *Br Med J* 1974;9:490.

8. Mathew P, Addy D, Wright N: Clonidine overdose in children. *Clin Toxicol* 1981;18:169–173.

9. Hughes P, Morse R: Use of clonidine in a mixed drug detoxification regimen: Possibility of masking of clinical

signs of sedative withdrawal. *Mayo Clin Proc* 1985; 60:47–49.

10. Johnson D, Bohan M: Propoxyphene withdrawal with clonidine. *Am J Psychiatr* 1983;140:1217–1218.

11. Javel A: Mixed substance abuse withdrawal treated by clonidine. *J Med Soc N J* 1983;80:1035–1036.

12. Hamblin J: Transdermal patch poisoning. *Pediatrics* 1987;79:161.

13. Mendoza J, Medalle M: Clonidine poisoning with marked hypotension in a 2½ year old child. *Clin Pediatr* 1979;18:123–127.

14. Mofenson H, Greensher J, Weiss T: Clonidine poisoning: Is there a single antidote? *Clin Toxicol* 1979;14: 271–275.

15. Augustine S, Tachikawa S, Lokhandwala M, et al: Central α adrenergic control of blood pressure. *Chest* 1983; 83(suppl):328–331.

16. Gremse D, Artman M, Boerth R: Hypertension associated with naloxone treatment for clonidine poisoning. *J Pediatr* 1986;108:776–778.

17. Korner P, Angus J, Lew M, et al: Characterization of the clonidine receptor site. *Chest* 1983;83:345–349.

18. MacFaul R, Miller G: Clonidine poisoning in children. *Lancet* 1977;1:1266–1267.

19. Brown M, Salmon D, Rendell M: Clonidine hallucinations. *Ann Intern Med* 1980;93:456–457.

20. Peters R, Hamilton B, Hamilton J, et al: Cardiac arrhythmias after abrupt clonidine withdrawal. *Clin Pharmacol Ther* 1983;34:435–439.

21. Collis M, Shepherd J: Antidepressant drug action and presynaptic α receptors. *Mayo Clin Proc* 1980;55:567–572.

22. Hamilton B, Mersey J, Hamilton J, et al: Withdrawal phenomena in subjects with essential hypertension on clonidine or tiamenidine. *Clin Pharmacol Ther* 1984; 36:628–633.

23. Stiff J, Harris D: Clonidine withdrawal complicated by amitriptyline therapy. *Anesthesiology* 1983;59:73–74.

24. Reid J, Campbell B, Hamilton C: Withdrawal reactions following cessation of central α-adrenergic receptor agonists. *Hypertension* 1984;6(suppl II):71–75.

25. Ferguson R, Alvino E: Rebound hypertension after low-dose clonidine withdrawal. *South Med J* 1983;76:98.

26. Catapano M, Marx J: Management of urgent hypertensive: A comparison of oral treatment regimens in the emergency department. *J Emerg Med* 1986;4:361–368.

27. Banner W, Lund M, Clawson L: Failure of naloxone to reverse clonidine toxic effect. *Am J Dis Child* 1983;137: 1170–1171.

28. Patnode R, Brouhard B, Travis L: Prolonged clonidine overdosage in a child. *J Pediatr* 1977;90:848–849.

29. Van Zwieten P, Timmermans P: Pharmacology and characterization of central α adrenoceptors involved in the effect of centrally acting antihypertensive drugs. *Chest* 1983; 83(suppl):340–343.

30. Williams P, Krafeik J, Potter B, et al: Cardiac toxicity of clonidine. *Chest* 1977;72:784–785.

31. Neuvonen P, Vilska J, Keranen A: Severe poisoning in a child caused by a small dose of clonidine. *Clin Toxicol* 1979;14:369–374.

32. Artman M, Boerth R: Clonidine poisoning. *Am J Dis Child* 1983;137:171–174.

33. Kulig K, Duffy J, Rumack B: Naloxone for treatment of clonidine overdose. *JAMA* 1982;247:1697.

34. Olsson J, Pruitt A: Management of clonidine ingestion in children. *J Pediatr* 1983;103:646–649.

35. Niemann J, Getzug T, Murphy W: Reversal of clonidine toxicity by naloxone. *Ann Emerg Med* 1986;15: 1229–1231.

36. Hall A, Smolinske S, Kulig K, et al: Guanabenz overdose. *Ann Intern Med* 1985;102:787–788.

37. Holmes B, Brogden R, Heel R, et al: Guanabenz: A review of its pharmacodynamic properties and therapeutic efficacy in hypertension. *Drugs* 1983;26:212–229.

38. Malini P, Strocchi E, Ambrosioni E, et al: Comparison of antihypertensive activity and tolerability of guanfacine and methyldopa. *Int J Clin Pharmacol Res* 1983; 1:35–39.

39. Shnaps Y, Almog S, Halkin H, et al: Methyldopa poisoning. *J Toxicol Clin Toxicol* 1982;19:501–513.

40. Von Bahr C, Lindstrom B, Seideman P: α-Receptor function changes after the first dose of prazosin. *Clin Pharmacol Ther* 1982;32:41–47.

41. Brogden R, Hell R, Speight T, et al: Prazosin: A review of its pharmacological properties and therapeutic efficacy in hypertension. *Drugs* 1977;14:163–197.

42. Colucci W: α-adrenergic receptor blockade with prazosin. *Ann Intern Med* 1982;97:67–77.

43. Cambridge D, Davey M, Massingham R: Prazosin, a selective antagonist of postsynaptic α adrenoceptors. *Br J Pharmacol* 1977;59:514–515.

44. Kobrin I, Stessman J, Yagil Y, et al: Prazosin-induced bradycardia in acute treatment of hypertension. *Arch Intern Med* 1983;143:2019–2020.

45. Robbins D, Crawford D, Lackner L: Priapism secondary to prazosine overdose. *J Urol* 1983;130:975.

46. Goldberg M, Hollister A, Robertson D: Influence of yohimbine on blood pressure, autonomic reflexes, and plasma catecholamines in humans. *Hypertension* 1983; 5:772–778.

47. Goldberg M, Robertson D: Yohimbine: A pharmacological probe for study of the α2 adrenoreceptor. *Pharmacol Rev* 1983;35:143–180.

48. Holmberg G, Gershon S: Autonomic and psychic effects of yohimbine hydrochloride. *Psychopharmacologia* 1961;2:93–106.

49. Charney D, Heninger G, Redmond D: Yohimbine-induced anxiety and increased noradrenergic function in humans: Effects of diazepam and clonidine. *Life Sci* 1983; 33:19–29.

50. Linden C, Vellman W, Rumack B: Yohimbine: A new street drug. *Ann Emerg Med* 1985;14:1002–1004.

ADDITIONAL SELECTED REFERENCES

Buffum J: Pharmacosexology update: Yohimbine and sexual function. *J Psychoactive Drugs* 1985;17:131–132.

Dunn F, Messerli F, Dreslinski G: Clonidine in hypertensive urgencies. *JAMA* 1982;247:1274–1275.

Houston M: Treatment of hypertensive emergencies and urgencies with oral clonidine loading and titration. *Arch Intern Med* 1986;146:586–589.

Louis W, Taylor H, McNeil J, et al: Clinical pharmacology of adrenergic adrenoreceptor blocking drugs. *Am Heart J* 1982;104:407–412.

Quart B, Guglielmo B: Prolonged diarrhea secondary to methyldopa therapy. *Drug Intell Clin Pharmacol* 1983; 17:462.

Schaut J, Schnoll S: Four cases of clonidine abuse. *Am J Psychiatry* 1983;140:1625–1627.

Schieber R, Kaufman N: Use of tolazoline in massive clonidine poisoning. *Am J Dis Child* 1981;135:77–78.

Siegel G, Bonfiglo J, Ritschel W, et al: Investigation of clonidine and lofexidine for the treatment of barbiturate withdrawal in mice. *Vet Hum Toxicol* 1985;27:503–505.

β-Adrenergic Blocking Agents

The β-adrenergic blocking agents have come into increasing use in recent years, and their medical indications continue to expand. They have become the most commonly used drugs for a number of cardiovascular diseases. Because of this extensive use, inadvertent self-poisoning as well as deliberate overdosing with β-adrenergic blocking drugs is becoming an increasingly frequent and important problem.

The β receptors are divided into β_1 and β_2. The β_1 receptors are located primarily in cardiac tissue and the kidneys. The β_2 receptors mediate smooth muscle relaxation and are located in the vasculature, bronchi, and uterus. This is not absolute; β_1 receptors are present in the lung, and a small number of β_2 receptors are present in the heart.[1,2] The β_1 receptors are under the control of the neurotransmitter norepinephrine, which is released from the sympathetic neuron. The β_2 receptors are not innervated and are under the control of circulating epinephrine.

THERAPEUTIC INDICATIONS FOR USE

Therapeutic indications for β-adrenergic blocking agents (Table 9-1) include exertion-induced angina pectoris; hypertension; atrial, nodal, or ventricular tachydysrhythmias[3]; prophylaxis against reinfarction and sudden death after an acute myocardial infarction[4–6]; alcohol and narcotic withdrawal; thyrotoxicosis; prophylaxis against migraine; obstructive cardiomyopathy; pheochromocytoma; essential tremor; anxiety; and dissecting aortic aneurysm.[7] The β-adrenergic blocking agents share some indications with the centrally active α_2 agonist clonidine.

MECHANISM OF ACTION

All the β-adrenergic blocking agents competitively antagonize the action of catecholamines and other sympathomimetic agents at the β-adrenergic receptor.[8] Nearly all the β-

Table 9-1 Therapeutic Indications for β-Adrenergic Blocking Agents

Angina pectoris
Anxiety
Dissecting aortic aneurysm
Essential tremor
Glaucoma
Hypertension
Infarction prophylaxis
Migraine prophylaxis
Obstructive cardiomyopathy
Pheochromocytoma
Substance withdrawal
Thyrotoxicosis
Ventricular tachydysrhythmias

adrenergic blocking agents used clinically share with isoproterenol, the prototypical β receptor agonist, an isopropyl-substituted amine group thought to produce a high affinity for the β receptor.[1]

When an adrenergic agonist combines with a receptor site, a response is elicited and the drug-receptor complex rapidly dissociates, leaving the receptor ready for further stimulation. The β receptor blocking agents are competitive antagonists, which means that the blocking agent occupies the same β receptor site as does the agonist isoproterenol but that the attachment results in little or no activation of adenyl cyclase or transmission of response to the tissue. This prolonged occupation of the receptor results in a reversible blockade.[9] The result of β blockade is that higher concentrations of endogenous agonists or higher doses of exogenously administered agonists are required to induce the same β receptor–mediated response.[10] This is important to remember when treating overdoses with β-adrenergic blocking agents.[11]

Although all the β-adrenergic blocking agents competitively interact with β adrenoceptors, some are lipophilic, β_1 cardioselective, possess intrinsic sympathomimetic (partial agonist) activity, and have membrane-stabilizing properties.[5,6,12,13] Differences in potency, route of elimination, half-life, and protein binding are also recognized.[14] In equivalent doses, β-adrenergic blocking drugs are equally effective in the treatment of hypertension, angina, and dysrhythmias, but they may differ in other respects.[12,13]

There are many β-adrenergic blocking drugs approved for use in the United States. The major differences among the available β-adrenergic blocking drugs are summarized in Table 9-2. Trade names for some of these drugs are listed in Table 9-3.

Route of Elimination

Broadly speaking, the β receptor blockers are divided into two groups: those that are largely metabolized by the liver, such as propranolol, practolol, and timolol; and those that are excreted predominantly unchanged by the kidneys, such as atenolol and nadolol (Table 9-4).

Table 9-2 Differences among β-Adrenergic Blocking Agents

Route of elimination
Lipophilicity
Cardioselectivity
Membrane-stabilizing activity
Intrinsic sympathomimetic activity
Potency
Half-life
Protein binding

Table 9-3 Partial Listing of β-Adrenergic Blocking Agents and Their Trade Names

Generic Name	Trade Name
Acebutolol	Sectral®
Atenolol	Tenormin®
Betaxolol	Betoptic®
Esmolol	Brevibloc®
Labetalol	Trandate®, Normodyne®
Levobunolol	Betagan®
Metoprolol	Lopressor®
Nadolol	Corgard®
Pindolol	Visken®
Propranolol	Inderal®
Timolol	Timoptic®

Table 9-4 Metabolized and Renally Excreted β-Adrenergic Blocking Agents

Metabolized	Renally Excreted
Propranolol	Atenolol
Practolol	Nadolol
Timolol	

Lipid Solubility

Drugs such as propranolol and metoprolol are highly lipid soluble and cross the blood-brain barrier easily. These drugs may therefore have more of an effect on the CNS than drugs such as nadolol and atenolol, which are water soluble and penetrate tissues less readily (Table 9-5).

Cardioselectivity

Certain β-adrenergic receptor blocking agents exhibit a higher affinity for β_1 than β_2 adre-

Table 9-5 Solubility of β-Adrenergic Blocking Agents

Lipid Soluble	Water Soluble
Alprenolol	Atenolol
Labetalol	Nadolol
Metoprolol	Practolol
Oxprenolol	Sotalol
Propranolol	

noceptors. This property is called cardioselectivity[15] and is a beneficial attribute of β receptor blocking agents in treating patients with bronchospastic disorders.

The nonselective cardiac β-adrenergic receptor blocking agents (Table 9-6) have both negative chronotropic and inotropic effects, may cause bronchospasm, and impair glycogenolysis and the hyperglycemic response to epinephrine, thus predisposing the patient to hypoglycemia. They may also exert an adverse effect on the peripheral circulation: cold hands and feet as well as more severe forms of vasospasm have been described with these drugs. The cardioselective β-adrenergic blocking drugs (Table 9-6) antagonize β receptors in the heart at lower doses than those required for other tissue and therefore do not produce bronchospasm or inhibit glycogenolysis at therapeutic doses.

Cardioselectivity of the β-adrenergic blocking drugs is not an "all or none" phenomenon. Pharmacologically, it is the relative ability of a blocking drug to block the effects of a marked sympathetic stimulus on the β_1 receptors while not affecting the influence of the stimulus on β_2 receptors. These agents begin to lose their β selectivity at high doses and exert the same effects as the nonselective agents.

Membrane-Stabilizing Activity

Membrane-stabilizing activity refers to the ability of certain drugs to interact with sodium channels, thereby impeding the depolarization of excitable tissues.[16] These drugs are considered to stabilize the cellular membrane, which results in depression of myocardial cells. Local anesthetics, quinidine, the tricyclic antidepressants, and β-adrenergic blocking agents with membrane-stabilizing activity (Table 9-7) all share this property, which is unrelated to competitive inhibition of catecholamines. This property is also described as quinidine-like and causes an effect similar to that of a local anesthetic, decreasing the reduction in the rate of rise in the cardiac action potential without affecting the overall duration of the spike or the resting potential.[2,9] The membrane-stabilizing properties of these compounds come into play at doses greater than those used in clinical practice.

Intrinsic Sympathomimetic Activity

Because almost all β blockers are chemical relatives of isoproterenol, it is not surprising that some have intrinsic sympathomimetic or partial agonist activity (Table 9-8).[13] These drugs cause a

Table 9-6 Cardioselective and Nonselective β-Adrenergic Blocking Drugs

Nonselective	Cardioselective
Alprenolol	Acebutolol
Esmolol	Atenolol
Labetalol	Betaxolol
Levobunolol	Metoprolol
Nadolol	Practolol
Oxprenolol	
Pindolol	
Propranolol	
Sotalol	
Timolol	

Table 9-7 β-Adrenergic Blocking Drugs with and without Membrane-Stabilizing Activity

With Membrane-Stabilizing Activity	Without Membrane-Stabilizing Activity
Acebutolol	Atenolol
Alprenolol	Betaxolol
Labetalol	Nadolol
Metoprolol	Practolol
Oxprenolol	Sotalol
Pindolol	Timolol
Propranolol	

Table 9-8 β-Adrenergic Blocking Drugs with and without Intrinsic Sympathomimetic Activity

With Intrinsic Sympathomimetic Activity	Without Intrinsic Sympathomimetic Activity
Acebutolol	Atenolol
Alprenolol	Betaxolol
Oxprenolol	Labetalol
Pindolol	Metoprolol
Practolol	Nadolol
	Propranolol
	Sotalol
	Timolol

Table 9-9 Summary of β-Adrenergic Blocking Drugs

Name	Lipophilic	β₁	ISA	MSA
*Acebutolol	±	+	+	+
Alprenolol	+	−	+	+
*Atenolol	−	+	−	−
*Betaxolol	0	+	−	−
*Esmolol	0	+	0	0
*Labetalol	+	−	−	+
*Levobunolol	0	−	0	0
*Metoprolol	+	+	−	±
*Nadolol	−	−	−	−
Oxprenolol	+	−	+ +	+
*Pindolol	+	−	+ + +	+
Practolol	−	+	+ +	−
*Propranolol	+ +	−	−	+ +
*Sotalol	−	−	−	−
*Timolol	+	−	−	−

* indicates FDA approval
+ = effect
− = no effect
0 = effect not known
ISA = Intrinsic sympathomimetic activity
MSA = Membrane-stabilizing activity

slight to moderate activation of the β receptors in addition to preventing the access of natural or synthetic catecholamines to the receptor site.[8,17,18] There is no strong evidence that β blocking drugs with intrinsic sympathomimetic activity are inherently safer than those without it.[9]

SELECTED β-ADRENERGIC BLOCKING AGENTS

Acebutolol (Sectral®)

Acebutolol is a β₁ selective adrenoceptor blocking agent. It also has some partial intrinsic sympathomimetic activity, as well as weak membrane-stabilizing activity (Table 9-9).[19]

Acebutolol is completely absorbed from the gastrointestinal tract and undergoes extensive first-pass hepatic metabolism, but its major metabolite is also active. The pharmacologic half-life of acebutolol is about 8 hours. Acebutolol has been associated with the development of antinuclear antibodies.

Alprenolol

Alprenolol closely resembles propranolol in its pharmacologic properties. It differs from propranolol only in that it has significant intrinsic sympathomimetic activity. The half-life of alprenolol is approximately 2 hours, and its maximum effects occur 1 to 3 hours after oral ingestion.

Atenolol (Tenormin®)

Atenolol is cardioselective but does not exhibit intrinsic sympathomimetic activity.[20] It also does not have membrane-stabilizing properties.[21] The cardioselective properties that atenolol exhibits at low doses may be lost at high doses. After oral administration, blood concentration reaches a peak between 2 and 4 hours. The elimination half-life in patients with normal renal function is approximately 6 to 7 hours, and the volume of distribution is 0.56 L/kg. Because of its low lipid solubility, atenolol penetrates poorly into the central nervous system. Because of the long half-life, in the event of overdose supportive measures may be needed for an extended period.[21]

Betaxolol (Betalol®)

Betaxolol is structurally similar to metoprolol and displays cardioselectivity. Its only approved use is to reduce elevated intraocular pressure by topical administration. It is one of the most potent and selective β-adrenergic blocking agents currently available. It does not exhibit intrinsic sympathomimetic activity and does not have substantial membrane-stabilizing activity. It also causes no change in the size of the pupils.

Esmolol (Brevibloc®)

Esmolol is a parenterally administered cardioselective β-adrenergic blocking agent. It has a half-life of approximately 10 minutes and is metabolized by cholinesterase.

Labetalol (Trandate®, Normodyne®)

Labetalol possesses neither cardioselectivity nor partial agonist activity.[22] It does possess weak membrane-stabilizing properties at high doses. In addition, labetalol exhibits α-adrenergic blocking activity and is able to inhibit the reuptake of norepinephrine into nerve terminals.[23] It is the only agent in this class that blocks both $α_1$ and β receptors, but it is 4 to 16 times more potent at β than at α receptors.[24] These properties yield a drug that hemodynamically resembles a combination of propranolol and prazosin.[24] Because it undergoes significant first-pass metabolism, its bioavailability is 30% to 40%. Labetalol is approximately 50% bound to plasma proteins and has a volume of distribution of 11 L/kg. Intravenous labetalol is available for use in patients who require rapid control of severe hypertension.

Metoprolol (Lopressor®)

Metoprolol has no intrinsic sympathomimetic activity and only weak membrane-stabilizing activity.[25] Plasma concentrations of metoprolol reach their peak between 1 and 2 hours after administration.[26–28]

Nadolol (Corgard®)

Nadolol is noncardioselective and lacks both intrinsic sympathomimetic activity and membrane-stabilizing properties.[29] It is distinguished from other β-adrenergic blocking drugs on the basis of its long plasma half-life, which is about 20 to 24 hours.[29] Plasma concentrations of nadolol reach their peak between 3 to 4 hours after administration. Unlike propranolol and metoprolol, most nadolol is not metabolized; about 75% of the amount absorbed is excreted unchanged by the kidneys. The drug is 30% bound to plasma protein and has a large volume of distribution of 2 L/kg.

Oxprenolol

Oxprenolol has approximately the same β-adrenergic blocking potency as propranolol but less local anesthetic activity and less membrane-stabilizing action. Like alprenolol, it has significant intrinsic sympathomimetic activity.[30] Oxprenolol may be used interchangeably with alprenolol.

Pindolol (Visken®)

Pindolol is noncardioselective, acts as a weak adrenergic agonist, and has weak membrane-depressant activity. It is absorbed almost completely from the gastrointestinal tract and achieves peak plasma concentrations within 1 hour of administration. Approximately 13% of a dose of pindolol undergoes first-pass metabolism, and the rest is excreted by the kidney. It has a relatively short half-life. The intrinsic sympathomimetic activity of pindolol may be blocked by other β blockers. Because of its intrinsic sympathomimetic activity, it does not decrease cardiac contractility or resting cardiac output as much as other β-adrenergic blocking drugs.

Practolol (Eraldin®)

Practolol has cardioselectivity, partial agonist activity, and no membrane-stabilizing effect. It is associated with a unique, serious, delayed adverse reaction known as oculocutaneous syndrome. This syndrome consists of a sclerosing peritonitis, psoriasiform rash, secretory otitis media, pleurisy, ocular involvement, and pericarditis. These symptoms have not been reported with other β blockers.[12] Practolol is no longer available for general use in the United States.

Propranolol (Inderal®)

Propranolol is the prototype of the β-adrenergic blocking drugs and was the first to come into wide clinical use. It remains the β-adrenergic blocking drug most commonly used in clinical medicine. Of all the β-adrenergic blocking drugs, propranolol seems consistently to produce the most severe picture with overdosage.[31] Self-induced poisoning with propranolol is increasing in frequency as the therapeutic indications for this medication continue to grow.

Propranolol is noncardioselective and has no intrinsic sympathomimetic activity, although it does induce membrane-depressant effects.[13] In the usual dose range for propanolol this membrane-depressant effect is of little importance, but with massive ingestion this effect may be clinically manifested.[32,33] Propranolol is extremely lipid soluble and crosses the blood-brain barrier rapidly, concentrating in brain tissue.[34,35]

After oral administration propranolol is completely absorbed from the gastrointestinal tract, but it undergoes substantial first-pass metabolism by the liver. The volume of distribution is 3 to 5 L/kg,[9] and the plasma half-life is 3 to 6 hours. Propranolol is metabolized to 4-hydroxypropranolol, an active metabolite that is present in almost equal amounts. Several other β-adrenergic blocking drugs, including oxprenolol and alprenolol, appear to have kinetics similar to that of propranolol.

Sotalol

Sotalol is noncardioselective and has neither partial agonist nor membrane-depressant properties. It has the properties of an antidysrhythmic agent and may induce ventricular tachy-dysrhythmias because it prolongs the duration of the action potential.[36,37] This appears as a prolonged QT interval. Because of this action, sotalol has been reported as a cause of torsades de pointes–type ventricular tachycardia.

Timolol (Timoptic®)

Timolol is noncardioselective, has no demonstrable membrane-stabilizing properties, and has no intrinsic sympathomimetic activity.[20,38–40] It is less lipid soluble than propranolol or metoprolol; thus it penetrates the brain to a low degree and causes few side effects in the central nervous system. Timolol is approved for treatment of glaucoma and reduces intraocular pressure without changing the pupil size.[39,40] Although it is used locally, because of its absorption through the nasal mucosa systemic side effects have been reported.[41–43] Orally administered timolol is completely absorbed from the gastrointestinal tract. It has a half-life of 3 to 4 hours and binds poorly to plasma proteins.

WITHDRAWAL OF β-ADRENERGIC BLOCKING DRUGS

Abrupt discontinuation of therapy with β-adrenergic blocking drugs has led to a syndrome resembling rebound adrenergic hyperactivity.[2,44] Unstable angina, myocardial infarction, or increased preponderance of dysrhythmias may ensue. Treatment for withdrawal consists of reinstituting the drug and further treatment of secondary medical problems.[45] There are no controlled studies demonstrating that slow withdrawal of the drug prevents the withdrawal syndrome. In addition, some researchers have failed to confirm the existence of β blocker withdrawal.[46]

TOXICITY

The β-adrenergic blocking drugs are relatively safe when properly administered, and there is a wide gap between therapeutic and toxic doses. In general, adverse effects of β-adrenergic blocking drugs appear to be an extension of their pharmacologic properties.[12,13] Because all the β-adrenergic blocking drugs are rapidly absorbed from the gastrointestinal tract, the first critical signs of overdosage can appear 20 minutes after ingestion but are more commonly seen within 1 to 2 hours after ingestion.

The principal manifestations of massive overdosage are bradycardia, hypotension, lowered cardiac output, left ventricular failure, respiratory depression, and cardiogenic shock (Table 9-10). Bradycardia is caused by the slowing of spontaneous diastolic depolarization in cardiac conducting tissue, an effect that is prominent in the sinoatrial node and accounts for the reduction in sinus rate. Not all seriously ill patients have a bradycardia, and sinus tachycardia and tachydysrhythmias have been reported in overdoses of practolol and sotalol. In massive overdoses, sudden rapid deterioration with cardiovascular collapse is common. Death is usually due to asystole.[30]

Changes in mental and neurologic status have been reported in patients treated with highly lipid-soluble drugs. This may be due either to direct toxicity or to reduced cerebral blood flow. Grand mal seizures may occur especially with propranolol, which is highly lipid soluble and thus gains access to the central nervous system easily. Peripheral cyanosis and coma are less frequent.

Because mobilization of liver glycogen is an α receptor function and mobilization of glycogen is a β receptor function, β-adrenergic blocking

---

Table 9-10 Symptoms of Toxicity from β-Adrenergic Blocking Drugs

---

Cardiovascular
  Sinus bradycardia
  Hypotension
  Prolonged atrioventricular conduction
  Bundle branch block
  Asystole
  Sinus tachycardia (rare)
  Cardiogenic shock
  Congestive heart failure
Central Nervous System
  Loss of consciousness
  Delirium
  Seizures
Respiratory
  Bronchospasm (rare)
  Acute pulmonary edema
  Respiratory arrest
Metabolic
  Hypoglycemia
Miscellaneous
  Peripheral cyanosis

---

drugs may retard recovery from hyperglycemia. If glycogen is reduced, they may prolong recovery from hypoglycemia because alternative glycogen stores cannot be mobilized. Hypoglycemia has been reported in diabetic patients on insulin who have taken β-adrenergic blockers, and cases of spontaneous hypoglycemia have also been reported.[47,48] Masking of hypoglycemia is more common.

Bronchospasm is a rare complication of overdosage with β-adrenergic blocking drugs, except in patients who already have bronchospastic disease.

The usual electrocardiographic manifestations of β blockade include first-degree atrioventricular heart block and sinus bradycardia.[30] With massive intoxication, disappearance of P waves, intraventricular conduction defects, and asystole may be seen. The widening of the QRS complex appears to be related to the membrane-depressant effect of some of the β-adrenergic blocking drugs. It has been estimated that, for this change to appear in humans, the plasma concentration must be 50 to 100 times that needed for β blockade. Not all seriously ill patients have a bradycardia. Sinus tachycardia and tachydysrhythmias have been reported in overdoses of practolol and sotalol, respectively.[49–51]

LABORATORY ANALYSIS

Although plasma drug concentrations can be measured, they do not always reflect the degree of β-adrenergic blocker intoxication. Moreover, certain compounds yield active metabolites that may not be easily detected in plasma assays. It is therefore important that the physician recognize the clinical manifestations of overdose and not rely on plasma drug concentrations. In addition, because the effects of β-adrenergic blocking drugs on the body last longer than their chemical half-life in plasma, intensive care may have to be continued for several days.

TREATMENT

All patients should be carefully observed by cardiac monitoring and venous access should be readily available, even if they are clinically stable on presentation (Table 9-11). All overdoses with β-adrenergic blocking drugs can be treated in a similar fashion. The major goals of treatment are to remove quickly any ingested tablets, to counteract life-threatening cardiovascular and pulmonary effects, and to treat central nervous system disturbances.

If the ingestion is recent, emesis or lavage should be initiated and followed by administration of activated charcoal and a cathartic. Intravenous diazepam should be used to treat seizure activity. Hemodialysis and hemoperfusion have not been shown to enhance excretion of β-adrenergic blocking drugs. In the pharmacologic therapy for overdoses with β-adrenergic blocking drugs, patients are symptomatic as a result of a competitive antagonism of the drug with the receptor. To be effective, large doses of selected agents are usually necessary.[52]

Sympathomimetics

Epinephrine may be given intravenously as needed for bradycardia or hypotension (or both). Epinephrine is a good choice in that it has maximal β effect on the myocardium as well as peripheral vasoconstrictor effects. The dose of epinephrine administered may be inadequate, however, because the β-receptors are being competitively blocked. It is for this reason that larger doses than what might be normally recommended are necessary.[52] This is similar to the use of larger doses of atropine than usually required to overcome the competitive block seen with the organophosphates and other acetylcholinesterase inhibitors.

Other sympathomimetic agents such as dopamine, isoproterenol, dobutamine, and norepinephrine are usually administered as intravenous infusions and are not effective if a bolus of epinephrine is not effective. Bradycardia may be resistant to the traditional drugs such as epinephrine, atropine, isoproterenol, dopamine, and dobutamine, even in large doses. In addition, although isoproterenol is often thought of as the agent of choice, a great disadvantage to its use is that it has vasodilator properties and may reduce diastolic blood pressure.

Other Methods

Intravenous atropine may be given to reduce unopposed vagal activity. A temporary transvenous pacemaker may be inserted if heart block or severe bradycardia cannot be readily controlled by pharmacologic means. The rarely reported occurrence of significant bronchospasm after overdose with β-adrenergic blocking drugs may be treated with epinephrine and aerosol β receptor agonists. Aminophylline, which acts independently of β-adrenergic receptors and produces an accumulation of cyclic AMP, may also be used.

Table 9-11 Treatment of Overdoses of β-Adrenergic Blocking Drugs

Indication	Treatment
Acute ingestion	Ipecac or lavage
	Charcoal and cathartic
Hypotension or bradycardia, asystole	Sympathomimetics (epinephrine, dopamine)
Bradycardia or hypotension, asystole	Atropine
Bradycardia or hypotension, asystole	Glucagon
Hypotension	Fluids
Bradycardia or hypotension, asystole	Pacemaker

Glucagon

Glucagon is considered the agent of choice for overdoses of β-adrenergic blocking drugs by many clinicians. Glucagon is a naturally occurring polypeptide hormone produced by the α cells of the pancreatic islets.[30,53–56] This hormone has been known to have inotropic and chronotropic effects on the heart.[57–59] Its action stems from its ability to increase cyclic AMP by stimulation of adenyl cyclase. Its effects are not blocked by β-adrenergic blocking drugs,[12,13,58] and unlike other positive inotropic agents it has the advantage of not increasing cardiac irritability.[50,51,53,60]

Glucagon is the drug of choice for initial treatment of myocardial depression and hypotension in overdoses with β-adrenergic blockers because the inotropic response is not affected by even high degrees of β receptor blockage.[53] Like digitalis, glucagon augments the movement of calcium ions into myocardial cells. Glucagon receptors have been demonstrated in fat and liver cells, and it is postulated that direct stimulation of glucagon-specific receptors in the myocardium may contribute to its efficacy.[61,62] These receptors, which produce cyclic AMP, are probably not blocked by β-adrenergic blockers.[50,63]

Glucagon is considered superior to the sympathomimetic agents in that it has no dysrhythmia-producing properties and its effects are sustained over a long period of time. The recommended dosage of glucagon is 50 μg/kg as an initial intravenous dose or 3 to 10 mg infused over 1 to 2 minutes with subsequent continuous infusion of 2 to 5 mg/hour or 0.07 mg/kg/hour.[50,53] The onset of glucagon's effects is within 1 to 3 minutes, with peak activity occurring within 5 to 7 minutes and persisting for 15 to 20 minutes.[53]

When given parenterally, glucagon has few side effects; the most important side effects are hyperglycemia and nausea. The nausea is usually transient, lasting only 1 to 2 minutes in most cases. Vomiting may also occasionally occur.[51] Hyperglycemia rarely requires the administration of insulin. Lesser effects are hypokalemia and hypocalcemia. Potassium concentrations should be monitored frequently during glucagon therapy because of the possible intracellular shifts of potassium that may occur.[53]

Glucagon has successfully reversed hypotension and dysrhythmias in patients unresponsive to other pharmacologic therapies.[61,62,64] It should be administered early in the management of severe overdose. It is postulated that glucagon, by increasing myocardial cyclic AMP, increases the inotropic and chronotropic activity of the heart and circumvents the β blockade effect on the heart.

The diluent provided with glucagon is 0.2% phenol. Phenol, which is chemically related to benzene, denatures proteins and is considered a general protoplasmic poison. Venous thrombosis has also resulted from some phenol injections.[65] If large doses of glucagon are necessary, the glucagon should be reconstituted with 5% dextrose instead of the diluent provided.[66] Glucagon is stable in dextrose solutions but will precipitate if mixed with solutions containing sodium, potassium, or calcium chloride.[50]

REFERENCES

1. Louis W, McNeill J, Jarrott B, et al: β-Adrenoreceptor blocking drugs: Current status and the significance of partial agonist activity. *Am J Cardiol* 1983;52:104A–107A.

2. Black C, Mann H: Intrinsic sympathomimetic activity: Physiological reality or marketing phenomenon. *Drug Intell Clin Pharmacol* 1984;18:554–559.

3. Singh B, Jewitt D: β-Adrenergic receptor blocking drugs in cardic arrhythmias. *Drugs* 1974;7:426–461.

4. Mueller H, Ayres S: The role of propranolol in the treatment of acute myocardial infarction. *Prog Cardiovasc Dis* 1977;19:405–412.

5. Shand D: Clinical pharmacology of the β blocking drugs: Implications for the postinfarction patient. *Circulation* 1983;67(suppl I):2–5.

6. Shand D: Pharmacokinetic properties of the β-adrenergic receptor blocking drugs. *Drugs* 1974;7:39–47.

7. Tinker J: β-Adrenergic agonists and antagonists. *Contemp Anesthesiol Pract* 1983;7:97–112.

8. McDevitt D, Shanks R, Prichard B: The clinical pharmacology of β-adrenergic blocking drugs. *J R Coll Physicians* 1976;11:21–34.

9. Conolly M, Kersting F, Dollery, C: The clinical pharmacology of β-adrenergic blocking drugs. *Prog Cardiovasc Dis* 1976;19:203–234.

10. Gerber J, Nies A: β-Adrenergic blocking drugs. *Annu Rev Med* 1985;36:145–164.

11. Shanks R: The properties of β adrenoceptor antagonists. *Postgrad Med J* 1976;52(suppl 4):14–20.

12. Ahlquist R: Adrenergic β blocking agents. *Prog Drug Res* 1976;20:27–43.

13. Ahlquist R: Present state of α and β adrenergic drugs: Part III: β-Blocking agents. *Am Heart J* 1977;93:117–120.

14. Crowe D: The β and calcium channel blockers. *Top Emerg Med* 1986;8:26–33.

15. McDevitt D: Clinical significance of cardioselectivity. *Drugs* 1983;25(suppl 2):219–226.

16. McDevitt D: β-Adrenoceptor blocking drugs and partial agonist activity: Is it clinically relevant. *Drugs* 1983;25:331–338.

17. Wood A: Pharmacologic differences between β blockers. *Am Heart J* 1984;108:1070–1077.

18. Dollery C, Paterson J, Conolly M: Clinical pharmacology of β receptor blocking drugs. *Clin Pharmacol Therap* 1969;10:765–798.

19. Sangster B, Wildt D, Dijk A: A case of acebutolol intoxication. *Clin Toxicol* 1983;20:69–77.

20. Frishman W: Atenolol and timolol: Two new systemic β-adrenoceptor antagonists. *N Engl J Med* 1982;306:1456–1462.

21. Brown H, Carruthers G, Johnston G, et al: Clinical pharmacologic observations on atenolol, a β-adrenoceptor blocker. *Clin Pharmacol Therap* 1976;20:524–534.

22. MacCarthy E, Bloomfield S: Labetalol: A review of its pharmacology, pharmacokinetics, clinical uses and adverse effects. *Pharmacotherapy* 1983;3:193–219.

23. Brogden R, Heel R, Speight T, et al: Labetalol: A review of its pharmacology and therapeutic use in hypertension. *Drugs* 1978;15:251–270.

24. Carter B: Labetalol. *Drug Intell Clin Pharmacol* 1983;17:704–712.

25. Anthony T, Jastremski M, Elliott W, et al: Charcoal hemoperfusion for the treatment of a combined diltiazem and metoprolol overdose. *Ann Emerg Med* 1986;15:1344–1348.

26. Wallin C, Hylting J: Massive metoprolol poisoning treated with prenalterol. *Acta Med Scand* 1983; 214:253–255.

27. Shore E, Cepin D, Davidson M: Metoprolol overdose. *Ann Emerg Med* 1981;10:524–527.

28. Smit A, Mulder P, Jong P, et al: Acute renal failure after overdose of labetalol. *Br Med J* 1986;293:1142–1143.

29. Frishman W: Nadolol: A new β adrenoceptor antagonist. *N Engl J Med* 1981;305:678–682.

30. Khan M, Miller M: β-Blocker toxicity—The role of glucagon. *South Afr Med J* 1985;67:1062–1063.

31. Langerfelt J, Matell G: Attempted suicide with 5.1 g of propranolol. *Acta Med Scand* 1976;199:517–518.

32. Shand D: Propranolol. *N Engl J Med* 1975; 293:280–285.

33. Shand D: Pharmacokinetics of propranolol: A review. *Postgrad Med J* 1976;52(suppl 4):22–25.

34. Seides S, Josephson M, Batsford W: The electrophysiology of propranolol in man. *Am Heart J* 1974; 88:733–741.

35. Voltolina E, Thompson S, Tisue J: Acute organic brain syndrome with propranolol. *Clin Toxicol* 1971; 4:357–359.

36. Kontopoulos A, Manoudis F, Filindris A, et al: Sotalol-induced torsade de pointes. *Postgrad Med J* 1981;57:321–323.

37. Totterman K, Turto H, Pellinen T: Overdrive pacing as treatment of sotalol-induced ventricular tachyarrhythmias (torsade de pointes). *Acta Med Scand* 1982;668:28–33.

38. Aronow W, Ferlinz J, Del Vicaro M, et al: Effect of timolol versus propranolol on hypertension and hemodynamics. *Circulation* 1976;54:47–51.

39. Boger W, Puliafito C, Steinert R, et al: Long-term experience with timolol ophthalmic solution in patients with open-angle glaucoma. *Am J Ophthalmol* 1978;85:259–267.

40. Boger W, Steinert R, Puliafito C, et al: Clinical trial comparing timolol ophthalmic solution to pilocarpine in open-angle glaucoma. *Am J Ophthalmol* 1978;86:8–18.

41. Fraunfelder F: Ocular β-blockers and systemic effects. *Arch Intern Med* 1986;146:1073–1074.

42. Munroe W, Rindone J, Kershner R: Systemic side effects associated with the ophthalmic administration of timolol. *Drug Intell Clin Pharmacol* 1985;19:85–89.

43. Swenson E: Severe hyperkalemia as a complication of timolol, a topically applied β-adrenergic antagonist. *Arch Intern Med* 1986;146:1220–1221.

44. Myers J, Horwitz L: Hemodynamic and metabolic response after abrupt withdrawal of long-term propranolol. *Circulation* 1978;58:196–203.

45. Alderman E, Coltart J, Wettach G, et al: Coronary artery syndromes after sudden propranolol withdrawal. *Ann Intern Med* 1974;81:625–627.

46. Lindenfeld R, Levine S, Pontiel M, et al: Adrenergic responsiveness after abrupt propranolol withdrawal in normal subjects and in patients with angina pectoris. *Circulation* 1980;62:704–710.

47. Kotler M, Berman J, Rubenstein A: Hypoglycemia precipitated by propranolol. *Lancet* 1966;2:1389–1390.

48. Mackintosh T: Propranolol and hypoglycemia. *Lancet* 1967;1:104–105.

49. Montagna M, Groppi A: Fatal sotalol poisoning. *Arch Toxicol* 1980;43:221–226.

50. Frishman W, Jacob H, Eisenberg E, et al: Clinical pharmacology of the new β-adrenergic blocking drugs: Part 8: Self-poisoning with β-adrenoceptor blocking agents: Recognition and management. *Am Heart J* 1979; 98:798–811.

51. Frishman W: β Adrenoceptor antagonists: New drugs and new indications. *N Engl J Med* 1981;305:500–505.

52. Kosinski E, Malindzak G: Glucagon and isoproterenol in reversing propranolol toxicity. *Arch Intern Med* 1973;132:840–843.

53. Parmley W, Glick G, Sonnenblick E: Cardiovascular effects of glucagon in man. *N Engl J Med* 1968;279:12–17.

54. Prasad K: Effect of glucagon on the transmembrane potential, contraction, and ATPase activity of the failing human heart. *Cardiovasc Res* 1972;6:684–695.

55. Smitherman T, Osborn R, Atkins J: Cardiac dose-response relationship for intravenously infused glucagon in normal intact dogs and men. *Am Heart J* 1978;96:363–371.

56. Wilkinson J: β Blocker overdoses. *Ann Emerg Med* 1986;15:982.

57. Nord H, Fontanes A, Williams J: Treatment of congestive heart failure with glucagon. *Ann Intern Med* 1970;72:649–653.

58. Peterson C, Leeder S, Sterner S: Glucagon therapy for β blocker overdose. *Drug Intell Clin Pharmacol* 1984;18:394–398.

59. Lucchesi B: Cardiac actions of glucagon. *Circ Res* 1968;22:777–787.

60. Timmis G, Ramos R, Parikh J, et al: The unique cardiotonic properties of glucagon. *Mich Med* 1973; 21:353–357.

61. Weinstein R: Recognition and management of poisoning with β-adrenergic blocking agents. *Ann Emerg Med* 1984;13:1123–1131.

62. Weinstein R, Cole S, Knaster H, et al: β Blocker overdose with propranolol and with atenolol. *Ann Emerg Med* 1984;14:161–163.

63. Salzberg M, Gallagher E: Propranolol overdose. *Ann Emerg Med* 1980;9:26–27.

64. Ward D, Jones B: Glucagon and β toxicity. *Br Med J* 1976;2:151.

65. Macek G: Venous thrombosis results from some phenol injections. *JAMA* 1983;249:1807.

66. Illingworth R: Glucagon for β blocker poisoning. *Practitioner* 1979;223:683–685.

ADDITIONAL SELECTED REFERENCES

Diamond G, Forrester J, Danzig R, et al: Acute myocardial infarction in man: Comparative hemodynamic effects of norepinephrine and glucagon. *Am J Cardiol* 1971; 27:612–616.

Dymowski J, Turnbull T: Glucagon and β blocker poisoning. *Ann Emerg Med* 1986;15:1118.

Frishman W: Pindolol: A new β adrenoceptor antagonist with partial agonist activity. *N Engl J Med* 1983; 306:940–944.

Gibson D: Pharmacodynamic properties of β-adrenergic receptor blocking drugs in man. *Drugs* 1974;7:8–38.

Gibson D, Sowton E: The use of β-adrenergic receptor blocking drugs in dysrhythmias. *Prog Cardiovasc Dis* 1969;12:16–39.

Haddad L, Dimond K, Schweistris J: Phenol poisoning. *JACEP* 1979;8:267–269.

Harrison D: The pharmacology and therapeutic use of β-adrenergic receptor blocking drugs in cardiovascular disease. *Drugs* 1974;7:1–7.

Heel R, Brogden R, Speight T, et al: Atenolol: A review of its pharmacological properties and therapeutic efficacy in angina pectoris and hypertension. *Drugs* 1979; 17:425–460.

Hiatt W, Fradl D, Zerbe G, et al: Selective and nonselective β blockade of the peripheral circulation. *Clin Pharmacol Ther* 1984;35:12–17.

Hong C, Yang W, Chiang B: Importance of membrane stabilizing effect in massive overdose of propranolol: Plasma level study in a fatal case. *Hum Toxicol* 1983;3:511–517.

Kaplan N: The present and future use of β blockers. *Drugs* 1983;25(suppl 2):1–4.

Kelly H: Controversies in asthma therapy with theophylline and the $β_2$-adrenergic agonists. *Clin Pharmacol* 1984;3:386–395.

Kristinsson J, Johannesson T: A case of fatal propranolol intoxication. *Acta Pharmacol Toxicol* 1977;41:190–192.

Mills G, Horn J: β Blockers and glucose control. *Drug Intell Clin Pharm* 1985;19:246–251.

Morelli H: Propranolol. *Ann Intern Med* 1973;78:913–917.

Theilen E, Wilson W: β-Adrenergic receptor blocking drugs in the treatment of cardiac arrhythmias. *Med Clin North Am* 1968;52:1017–1029.

Williams J: Glucagon and the cardiovascular system. *Ann Intern Med* 1969;71:419–423.

chapter 10

Theophylline

Theophylline (1,3-dimethylxanthine) is a naturally occurring alkaloid closely related to caffeine. Like caffeine and theobromine, theophylline is structurally classified as a xanthine derivative.[1-4] The most popular nonalcoholic stimulant beverages of the world are prepared from plants containing derivatives of xanthine. For example, tea contains theophylline and coffee contains caffeine.

Theophylline has been used for more than 40 years as a mainstay in the treatment of bronchoconstriction secondary to bronchial asthma and reversible bronchospasm that may occur in association with chronic bronchitis or emphysema.[5,6] It has also been used to relieve periodic apnea in the newborn[7] and in augmenting diaphragmatic contractility in respiratory failure.[8] Adverse effects and nonpurposeful overdose from theophylline occur relatively often because this drug has a narrow therapeutic index.[9,10] There is also a wide variability among individuals in the clearance of theophylline.[9] Cases of deliberate overdose and accidental accumulation of theophylline have been increasing in recent years.[11-13]

Although theophylline is the reference compound, certain physical mixtures and chemical combinations or double salts of xanthines with other substances have been introduced because they are more soluble than the free bases of theophylline.[1-3] Notable among these are aminophylline (theophylline ethylenediamine), theophylline sodium acetate or glycinate, and choline theophyllinate (oxtriphylline) (Table 10-1). Theophylline is the active constituent of aminophylline, and, on exposure to air, aminophylline solutions gradually liberate free theophylline.[14,15] Another parenteral theophylline preparation has been introduced (by Travenol) that contains no ethylenediamine. Diphylline (dihydroxypropyltheophylline) is a non–theophylline xanthine bronchodilator that is marketed in the United States under various trade names and is sometimes advertised as a theophylline derivative. Diphylline is not metabolized to theophylline.

SUSTAINED RELEASE FORMULATIONS

In addition to plain tablets and capsules there are also at least 30 sustained release formulations of theophylline,[16] whose pharmacokinetic properties are prolonged.[17,18] These preparations offer the potential advantages of longer dosing intervals and less fluctuation of serum concentration during long-term therapy.[5] Many clinicians prefer the sustained release formulations over the regular formulations for these reasons.[16]

Table 10-1 Selected Theophylline Xanthine Compounds by Trade Name

Compound	Trade Name
Theophylline	Accurbron
	Aquaphyllin
	Asmalix
	Elixicon
	Lanophyllin
	Liquophylline
	Physpan
	Theolixir
	Theon
	Theostat
Theophylline, Sustained Release Formulations	Aerolate
	Aminodur Dura-tab
	Bronkodyl
	Constant-T
	Elixophyllin
	Quibron-T
	Respbid
	Slo-Phyllin
	Sustaire
	Theobid
	Theo-Dur
	Theolair
	Theospan
	Theovent
	Uniphyl
Oxtriphylline	Choledyl*
Diphylline (not a theophylline preparation)	Dilin
	Dilor
	Dioxine
	Dyflex
Aminophylline	Lixaminol
	Phyllocontin*
	Somophyllin*

Note: (*) sustained release preparation available

CLINICAL USE

Four major clinical uses of theophylline are (1) bronchodilatation in patients with acute symptoms of asthma with or without an inhaled or ingested β_2-adrenergic agonist, (2) maintenance therapy for prevention of symptoms and signs of chronic asthma, (3) treatment of recurrent apnea of prematurity[7] (not FDA approved for this use), and (4) augmenting diaphragmatic contractility in respiratory failure (not FDA approved for this use).

PHARMACOKINETICS

Bioavailability

There are major differences in the bioavailability of the various theophylline preparations. Theophylline is not very water soluble, and preparations have been manufactured in an attempt to increase its solubility. Theophylline does not form stable compounds with the various strong bases such as ethylenediamine, choline, or calcium salicylate that are used to produce the so-called salts. For all practical purposes these substances are simply mixtures of theophylline and an excipient. For example, ethylenediamine (aminophylline) serves the purpose of increasing the pH sufficiently to allow theophylline to dissolve at a convenient concentration. Aminophylline is 85% theophylline, and oxtriphylline, the choline salt of theophylline and the ingredient in many theophylline preparations such as Choledyl®, contains 64% theophylline.[11] The calcium salt is approximately 50% theophylline. In recent years there has been a trend back toward the use of anhydrous theophylline in the treatment of chronic asthma (Table 10-2).

Route of Administration

Theophylline concentrations in the blood reach their peak almost immediately after intravenous and intramuscular administration of the

Table 10-2 Theophylline Preparations and Anhydrous Theophylline Content

Drug	Anhydrous Theophylline (percent)
Aminophylline (anhydrous)	85
Aminophylline (hydrous)	79
Diphylline	0
Oxtriphylline	64
Theophylline calcium salicylate	50
Theophylline monohydrate	90
Theophylline sodium glycinate	46

drug, approximately 2 to 3 hours after oral administration of tablets,[19] 5 hours after administration of enteric-coated tablets, and 3 to 5 hours after rectal administration.[12] Because rectal suppositories result in erratic absorption,[20] the drug must be in solution if this route is to be used.[11] A sustained release formulation has an increased absorption lag time or a prolonged absorption half-life, so that peak concentrations and effects may not occur until 24 to 36 hours after ingestion.[21]

Theophylline and Age

The pharmacokinetics of theophylline changes with age. Maximal clearance is thought to be achieved in patients 1 to 9 years of age. Clearance decreases in adolescence and tends to stabilize in the mid-teen years.[22] The average half-life for theophylline is approximately 5 hours in adults, but this varies widely. In young children the half-life is slightly shorter (3.5 hours), and in the newborn it is approximately 30 hours.[23,24] Prolonged half-life in neonates and premature infants may be due to incomplete neonatal development of the cytochrome P-450 monoxygenase system, which is responsible for the *N*-demethylation of this compound.[25] In addition the neonate metabolizes 20% to 30% of theophylline to caffeine, which does not occur in adults. There is also reduced protein binding of theophylline in full-term infants, which may result in increased free or pharmacologically active drug in any given serum concentration.[26] This increased free drug–to–serum concentration ratio may produce toxic manifestations at serum concentrations generally considered nontoxic.

Metabolism

Most of an administered dose of theophylline is biotransformed by the hepatic microsomal mixed-function oxygenase system, with less than 10% being eliminated unchanged in the urine.[27,28] In the liver, theophylline is demethylated and oxidized to methylxanthine, dimethyluric acid, and methyl uric acid.[11,12,14,15] These metabolites are inactive and are excreted in the urine. Hepatic cellular dysfunction is the most important cause of delayed theophylline elimination.

Theophylline and Michaelis-Menten Elimination

The metabolic pathways of degradation, especially the *N*-demethylation processes, are capacity limited; that is, the rate of elimination cannot increase proportionately to increases in drug concentration.[2,3,29–31] As a result, the biologic half-life increases with increasing dose or plasma concentration.[24,27] Theophylline follows Michaelis-Menten kinetics where at low serum levels, theophylline exhibits first-order kinetics and at high serum levels theophylline switches to zero-order kinetics.[32] Therefore, in the therapeutic range a small increase in the amount of drug administered may result in a disproportionately large increase in the serum level. This is an important aspect of pharmacological dosing because the elimination pattern changes in the therapeutic range, which can lead to inadvertent toxicity with long-term administration.

Theophylline Clearance

Factors Increasing Serum Theophylline Concentration

Factors increasing the plasma half-life of theophylline and therefore the serum theophylline concentration include upper respiratory infections,[33] sustained high fever, obesity, and administration of cimetidine (Table 10-3).[17,34] Other drugs that increase the half-life include the macrolide antibiotics erythromycin and troleandomycin.[35] Troleandomycin has been shown to slow elimination of theophylline sufficiently to double its serum concentration. Elderly patients and those with congestive heart failure or severe liver disease[14,15] have a markedly reduced capacity to eliminate or metabolize theophylline.[11] This may therefore result in chronic accumulation of the drug. Elderly patients and neonates may also have reduced theophylline clearance as a result of decreased protein binding.[6]

Table 10-3 Factors Affecting Theophylline Half-Life

Factor	Effect on Half-Life
Smoking	Decrease
Upper respiratory infection	Increase
Sustained high fever	Increase
Old age	Increase
Liver disease	Increase
Congestive heart failure	Increase
Cor pulmonale	Increase
Use of oral contraceptive	Increase
Obesity	Increase
Infections	Increase
Drug interactions	
Allopurinol	Increase
Caffeine	Increase
Cimetidine	Increase
Erythromycin	Increase
Propranolol	Increase
Troleandomycin	Increase
Isoproterenol	Decrease
Phenobarbital	Decrease
Phenytoin	Decrease

Factors Decreasing Serum Theophylline Concentration

Smokers of cigarettes and marijuana metabolize theophylline rapidly; therefore in these individuals the drug has a shorter half-life.[11] This occurs through an induction of hepatic enzymes. In addition, simultaneous administration of phenytoin, phenobarbital, and intravenous isoproterenol decreases the half-life of theophylline (Table 10-3).[6]

Volume of Distribution and Protein Binding

The apparent volume of distribution of theophylline in adults and children is relatively constant, averaging 0.5 L/kg.[11,12] It is elevated in premature neonates to 0.69 L/kg and decreased in obese patients, but otherwise it is not significantly affected by age, sex, smoking, heart failure, or airway obstruction.

Approximately 60% of theophylline is bound to plasma proteins. Because serum theophylline reflects both the bound and unbound drug, a patient with hypoalbuminemia may have toxic symptoms at normal serum levels.[36]

Actions

Theophylline has actions resembling those of the other xanthine derivatives, such as caffeine and theobromine (Table 10-4). These actions are CNS stimulation, cardiac muscle stimulation, relaxation of smooth muscle, and diuresis.[2,8,29] Theophylline has greater potency as a dilator of bronchial smooth muscle and as a relaxant of involuntary muscle than the other two derivatives. Its diuretic action, although stronger than that of caffeine, is of shorter duration. The pharmacologic actions of theophylline also include stimulation of respiration, cerebral vascular constriction, and gastric acid secretion; augmentation of cardiac inotropy and chronotropy; and relaxation of uterine smooth muscle.[12]

Because it is a methylxanthine, theophylline increases plasma and urinary catecholamine concentrations.[8,37] Theophylline also increases the release of catecholamines from the sympathoadrenal medullary system, increases cyclic adenosine monophosphate concentration, and inhibits nonneuronal uptake and metabolism of catecholamines.[38] In addition, theophylline is a potent glycogenolytic, gluconeogenic, and lipolytic agent and is synergistic in these respects with the catecholamines.[37,39]

Mechanism of Action

The methylxanthines inhibit the enzyme phosphodiesterase, which is responsible for the degradation of cyclic AMP. Thus the actions of theophylline are due to an inhibition of an

Table 10-4 Actions of Theophylline

Diuresis
Relaxes involuntary smooth muscle, bronchi (blood vessels, uterus)
Increases plasma catecholamines
Increases cyclic AMP
Stimulates respiration
Stimulates cerebrovascular constriction
Stimulates gastric acid secretion
Increases glycogenolysis
Increases lipolysis
Increases cardiac inotropy and chronotropy

enzyme that normally breaks down the mediator of adrenergic activity.[24,40] This results in bronchial smooth muscle relaxation and the inhibition of the release of histamine by mast cells.

Although the elevated concentration of cyclic AMP has been cited to explain how theophylline produces bronchodilation, the concentrations obtained do not appear to be sufficient to produce this effect, nor does this theory explain why other phosphodiesterase inhibitors do not result in bronchodilation.[2,3,5,40,41] Other proposed mechanisms of action of theophylline include inhibition of prostaglandin activity with consequent decreased contraction of bronchial smooth muscle, stimulation of catecholamine release, β-adrenergic receptor agonism, and adenosine receptor antagonism.[2,5,41]

Serum Theophylline Concentration

Serum theophylline concentrations are among the most clinically useful of all the serum drug concentrations that can be measured. Assays to measure the serum concentration of theophylline have improved the ability to diagnose theophylline intoxication and assess its prognosis.[42] It has been shown that theophylline concentrations of 8 to 20 μg/mL are needed to produce maximal bronchodilation; some patients with mild pulmonary disease experience relief of bronchospasm with serum theophylline concentrations of 5 μg/mL.[6] Because of the low therapeutic index for theophylline, serum concentrations only slightly higher than the therapeutic range may be toxic.[18,27,43]

Each increase of 1 μg/mL in serum concentration requires a loading dose of approximately 0.5 mg/kg. Stated another way, each milligram per kilogram of theophylline administered will result in an average increase of 2 μg/mL in serum theophylline concentration. Plasma concentrations of theophylline may change as a result of a change in dosage interval of the drug, the rate of biotransformation, the rate of clearance from the body, or the volume of distribution.[44,45] Because of the many factors that may account for different clearance rates of theophylline (see Table 10-3), it is difficult to design a safe and effective dosage regimen without monitoring plasma concentrations.[9]

There is an important difference between chronic and acute theophylline intoxication because of the lag between the serum concentration and toxic effect.[16] Therefore, at a given serum concentration, patients with chronic theophylline intoxication may experience more severe symptoms than patients with acute theophylline intoxication.

TOXICITY

As stated earlier, theophylline intoxication is a common problem that occurs in two distinct settings: chronic and acute intoxication.[8,38,46] Patients who have been repeatedly administered standard doses of the drug may develop subacute or chronic intoxication that is often attributable to excessive dosage or decreased clearance due to heart failure, liver disease, or drug interactions. Such patients may have serious complications at blood concentrations that are just above the therapeutic range. Chronic theophylline intoxication may occur when the dose of theophylline administered on a repeated basis is excessive compared to the patients' capacity to metabolize and excrete it. Acute accidental or suicidal overdoses of theophylline may result in high blood concentrations that may be somewhat better tolerated initially than in the chronically intoxicated patient.

Sustained Release Preparations

Ingestion of an overdose of a sustained release theophylline preparation may cause dramatic late increases in serum theophylline concentration. The delay before the onset of symptoms may be as much as 10 hours, and there may be a prolonging of toxic manifestations as well.[17,18]

Clinical Manifestations of Toxicity

The clinical manifestations of theophylline intoxication (Table 10-5) result from an accentuation of the drug's pharmacologic effects. The systems mainly affected are the gastrointestinal system, the cardiovascular system, and the central nervous system.[8,11,46] Because theophylline

Table 10-5 Clinical Manifestations of Theophylline Intoxication

---

Mild
  Anorexia
  Abdominal pain
  Vomiting

Moderate
  Cardiac
    Sinus tachycardia
    Hypertension
    Hypotension

  Neurologic
    Increased wakefulness
    Restlessness
    Irritability
    Tremor
    Hallucinations

Severe
  Cardiac dysrhythmia

  Neurologic
    Seizures
    Coma

  Metabolic
    Hyperthermia
    Hypokalemia
    Hyperkalemia
    Hyperglycemia
    Hypophosphatemia
    Metabolic acidosis

---

has been shown to stimulate catecholamine release, acute theophylline poisoning may produce a state of increased β-adrenergic stimulation that accounts for many of the toxic effects, including cardiac dysrhythmias, hypotension, tremor, agitation, and metabolic disturbances.[8]

Gastrointestinal manifestations include nausea and vomiting.[11] Cardiovascular manifestations affect both the heart and the vasculature. In the heart, theophylline toxicity can produce both supraventricular and ventricular dysrhythmias. Among supraventricular dysrhythmias encountered are sinus tachycardia, multifocal atrial tachycardia, and atrial flutter and fibrillation.

Hemodynamic changes are dose dependent. At low doses, theophylline induces a transitory hypertension secondary to an increase in cardiac output and total peripheral resistance. At high doses the direct effect of theophylline on the blood vessels predominates. This β_2-adrenergic

effect reduces the total peripheral resistance, resulting in a decrease in blood pressure.

Mild Intoxication

Theophylline toxicity increases in parallel with serum theophylline concentration and increases notably at serum concentrations exceeding 20 μg/mL.[18,27] Adverse effects observed with serum theophylline concentrations greater than 20 μg/mL include gastrointestinal reactions, an early sign of toxicity that may be misdiagnosed as evidence of a gastrointestinal abnormality not attributable to drug toxicity.[35] Vomiting is a common early sign of toxicity from all routes of administration and reflects stimulation of the medulla oblongata.[11,12] Vomiting may also be partly due to an irritation of the gastric mucosa and an increase in the volume of gastric secretions.[29] Diarrhea may also be noted as a result of increased secretion of fluid by the intestinal mucosa.[11,12] Vomiting is generally violent and persistent but may be slight or absent in poisonings from sustained release preparations.

Other early signs of toxicity are restlessness and irritability, which are attributable to the stimulatory actions of theophylline on all parts of the central nervous system. These actions may progress to extreme agitation, tremors, delirium, seizures, and coma.

Moderate Intoxication

A moderate overdose of theophylline may produce symptoms of increased wakefulness, mild sinus tachycardia, tachydysrhythmias, and hypertension or hypotension.[12] Hypotension is a common but poorly understood complication of massive theophylline ingestion. It is frequently refractory to conventional vasopressors and contributes significantly to mortality. Hyperthermia, albuminuria, and dehydration may also be noted. As toxicity increases vomiting becomes more frequent, and hematemesis may ensue. Manic behavior as well as hallucinations may be noted.

Severe Intoxication

Life-threatening theophylline toxicity includes cardiac dysrhythmias, seizures, dehydration, severe metabolic abnormalities, extreme hyperthermia, coma, and death. Although seizures have been associated with theophylline concentrations as low as 25 μg/mL, they are usually associated with concentrations of 40 to 50 μg/mL.[8] Seizures are usually preceded by other signs of drug toxicity, although they have occurred without any prodromal signs.[47] When seizures do occur in the low toxic range in chronically intoxicated patients, these patients often have cirrhosis, cor pulmonale, viral illnesses, prior history of seizures, congestive heart failure, or focal central nervous system lesions as well. Acutely intoxicated patients may not have seizures until a serum concentration of approximately 90 μg/mL is attained.[37] The actual mechanism of action by which theophylline causes seizures is unknown. Once seizures have occurred, the outcome in cases of both acute and chronic theophylline poisoning is often poor regardless of the therapy used.[7,38,48] For this reason there has been considerable interest in using hemodialysis or hemoperfusion to remove the drug before seizures occur.

Metabolic Abnormalities

Metabolic abnormalities are an aspect of theophylline toxicity that has not been previously well recognized.[49] Metabolic abnormalities include hypokalemia, hyperglycemia, hypophosphatemia, leukocytosis, and, less commonly, hyperkalemia.[11,12,38,49,50] Metabolic acidosis has also been reported and is probably due to accumulation of lactic acid secondary to increased glycolysis in muscles.[38] These abnormalities are characteristic features of acute but not of chronic theophylline overdose and may be related to the adrenergic overdrive. Hypokalemia and hyperglycemia appear to result from hyperinsulinemia and glycogenolysis.[12] Elevated serum concentration of insulin and glucose promotes an intracellular shift of glucose and potassium that results in relative hypokalemia.[37] This does not represent a total body depletion of potassium but results from various cellular shifts of fluid and electrolyte.[11] Hypokalemia may also be a result of vomiting and diarrhea. These abnormalities are not usually associated with clinical or electrocardiographic changes. Many times their severity correlates with the serum theophylline measurements.[49]

The risk of life-threatening theophylline toxicity depends on the chronicity of the overdose. Patients with acute single theophylline ingestion typically tolerate levels of up to 80 to 100 μg/mL without seizures or other serious complications. Older patients with a higher prevalence of underlying cardiopulmonary disease are also more susceptible to life-threatening complications. Acute overdose is therefore suggested by a history of suicidal or accidental single ingestion and the presence of hypotension, hypokalemia, and metabolic acidosis. With acute overdose, seizures and severe cardiovascular manifestations are unlikely to occur unless peak serum concentrations are high (greater than 80 μg/mL).

LABORATORY DETERMINATIONS

The concentration of theophylline is important to measure, and a toxicologic screen may be necessary to rule out co-ingestants (Table 10-6). In the severely intoxicated patient, theophylline concentration should be measured at frequent intervals to ensure that clearance is not prolonged. In cases of a potentially toxic overdose with a sustained release formulation, early plasma theophylline concentrations will not reflect accurately the degree of intoxication; concentrations should be measured every 2 hours until a peak is reached, and then every 4 hours when the concentration is declining, until a therapeutic level is attained.[16]

Because of the various electrolyte abnormalities that may ensue, serum electrolytes are also important to monitor.[8] A determination of arterial blood gas may also be necessary. In addition to continuous cardiac monitoring, an electrocardiogram should also be obtained.

Table 10-6 Laboratory Determinations in Theophylline Overdose

Toxicologic screen
Serum theophylline concentration
Serum electrolytes
Arterial blood gas
Electrocardiogram

Examination of the gastric contents and stool for blood may be necessary as well.[8]

After an acute intoxication, serum theophylline concentrations correlate with the development of toxic manifestations. When patients are chronically intoxicated, the correlation between theophylline serum concentrations and the appearance of serious toxic manifestations is less obvious. Relatively low concentrations over a long period may result in more neurotoxicity and poorer outcome than high concentrations in acute intoxication.

Age is also an important factor to consider when interpreting theophylline serum concentrations. Older patients seem to experience serious toxic manifestations such as seizures and dysrhythmias at lower concentrations than those that induce such symptoms in children.

TREATMENT

Every theophylline overdose should be regarded as potentially fatal, and all patients should be closely observed (Table 10-7).[13,37] Most patients with acute theophylline intoxication can be managed in a traditional manner that includes careful attention to serum electrolytes, acid-base balance, glucose, and neurologic complications. Cardiovascular monitoring should also be performed until theophylline concentration and the patient's clinical course have excluded the possibility of toxicity.

Table 10-7 Treatment of Theophylline Overdose

Indication	Treatment
Acute overdose	Emesis or lavage
	Charcoal and cathartic
	Pulse charcoal
Hypotension	Fluids
Hypotension	Pressor agents
Supraventricular tachycardia	Verapamil
Ventricular ectopy	Lidocaine
Ventricular ectopy	β_1 Blocking agent
Seizures	Diazepam
Refractory seizures, refractory dysrhythmias, deterioration	Hemoperfusion or dialysis

Because of the differences in pharmacokinetic characteristics of sustained formulations, the approach to a patient who has overdosed with these preparations must be modified. In the absence of toxicity, observation on the basis of history alone may be necessary for a much longer period than for conventional formulations.[18]

Standard techniques to reduce drug absorption such as emptying the stomach via emesis or gastric lavage should be performed in the acute overdose.[12] This should be followed by the administration of activated charcoal and a cathartic.[51–55] This may be useful even late after an acute overdose, especially if a sustained release preparation has been ingested.[38] Most theophylline overdoses respond to supportive measures.[13]

Treatment of Metabolic Abnormalities

Biochemical abnormalities respond to conservative management and resolve rapidly with fluid replacement and modest potassium supplementation. Administration of phenothiazines for intractable hyperthermia may be warranted in life-threatening situations. Conventional antiemetics do not appear to relieve vomiting,[37] but the administration of H_2 antagonists such as ranitidine (50 mg every 6 hours) or droperidol (5 mg intravenously) has been successful in controlling vomiting.[29] Ranitidine is a good choice because, unlike cimetidine, it does not interfere with the clearance of theophylline.

Treatment of Cardiac Abnormalities

Tachycardia rarely requires treatment. Although verapamil has been used effectively for the supraventricular tachycardia associated with theophylline overdose, there are reports of increased mortality with the use of this drug. Therefore, verapamil should not be used until further studies are performed.[11,12] Lidocaine may be of benefit for ventricular ectopy. A cardiospecific β-adrenergic blocking agent may be useful in the treatment of serious tachydysrhythmias because catecholamine release has been implicated in their genesis.

Propranolol may prevent or reverse the metabolic and cardiovascular consequences of theophylline toxicity. The risk of precipitating bronchospasm with its administration to patients with asthma is uncertain, however, and caution should be exercised in this patient population. An ultra-short–acting parenteral β blocking agent such as esmolol may be useful since it is easily titratable and disappears rapidly from the circulation.

Hypotension should be initially treated with intravenous crystalloid. Hypotension that does not respond to intravenous fluids can be treated with the cautious administration of pressor agents.[51–53]

Treatment of Seizures

Seizures may be treated with diazepam. As an alternative, the prophylactic administration of phenobarbital to prevent seizures and associated complications should be considered for patients with severe theophylline intoxication.[11,12,51–53] Seizures secondary to theophylline toxicity are frequently refractory to diazepam, phenobarbital, and phenytoin; nevertheless these agents should be tried.[10–12,51–53] Status seizures that are unresponsive to those drugs may merit treatment with paralyzing drugs and general anesthesia.

Attempts To Enhance Elimination

Diuresis

Although theophylline is a weak base, there is probably little to be gained by acidification of the urine to enhance excretion. In addition, because theophylline is mainly metabolized by the liver with only a fraction excreted unchanged in the urine, it is unlikely that forced diuresis would significantly increase elimination.

Multiple-Dose Activated Charcoal

Multiple-dose activated charcoal can be administered in an attempt to increase elimination of theophylline by the gastrointestinal tract.[29,56] This has been successful in the removal of other drugs, such as phenobarbital, carbamazepine, and phenylbutazone.[42,48,57] Some studies have shown a twofold increase in the systemic elimination of theophylline when multiple-dose activated charcoal is administered.

Oral activated charcoal is therefore useful in the acute overdose because it adsorbs the drug and also because it may promote drug elimination, thereby shortening the duration of toxic symptoms.[38,58] This latter action is due to gastrointestinal dialysis,[12,59] whereby the charcoal absorbs the drug entering the intestine, which acts as a dialysis membrane[16,42,60,61] (see Chapter 3). Although biliary excretion of theophylline has not been demonstrated,[56] activated charcoal appears to enhance the rate of diffusion into the intestines by absorbing theophylline in gastrointestinal fluids, thereby maintaining a constant diffusion gradient into the intestine.[59] This method has been shown to reduce the serum half-life of theophylline that is administered both intravenously and orally.[60]

Activated charcoal should be administered in dosages of 0.5 to 1 g/kg every 2 to 4 hours until serum theophylline concentrations are within normal limits.[61] Unless there are specific indications, a cathartic should be administered only once.

Early treatment with orally administered activated charcoal, although it may enhance theophylline elimination, may not avert a large delayed elevation in serum theophylline concentrations in patients who have ingested sustained release preparations.[18]

Extracorporeal Removal

The efficacy of extracorporeal means of removal of theophylline is controversial. Hemodialysis[62] and hemoperfusion[63,64] have been shown to increase plasma clearance of theophylline, yet no controlled studies of the use of these methods have been performed.[17,37] Although there seems to be the potential for theophylline-intoxicated patients to benefit significantly from hemodialysis or hemoperfusion, these procedures are expensive and not without risks, including hypotension, bleeding, hemolysis,[65] hypocalcemia, thrombocytopenia, and sepsis.[11,12,38] In addition, both hemodialysis and hemoperfusion are invasive and require time and specialized facilities before they can be instituted.[66]

Hemodialysis[67] or charcoal or resin hemoperfusion in the acute overdose should only be used for the severely intoxicated patient.[68] These methods may be considered if the patient manifests intractable seizures, dysrhythmias, or clinical deterioration.[69] Hemoperfusion with a resin column or an activated charcoal column appears to be more effective than hemodialysis in removing theophylline.[11,12,17,64,70,71] Also, a rebound effect is possible when hemoperfusion is completed.[5,63,72]

Although hemoperfusion is the most efficient method for removing theophylline, multiple-dose activated charcoal is less expensive, more widely accessible, and probably safer.[56,57] Because hemoperfusion is an extracorporeal system of removal, it should only be performed in a hemodialysis area or an intensive care unit by a physician and technical team familiar with the procedure. If hemoperfusion is performed because of signs of neurotoxicity such as seizures, it should be done as early as possible.[73]

In the acute overdose with serum concentrations less than 80 μg/mL, patients have been managed with supportive care alone. In the chronic overdose, in patients with underlying cardiovascular disease, in clinically unstable patients, or in patients with a high serum concentration that is still increasing, extracorporeal means may be attempted early in the course.

Conservative Management

The vast majority of theophylline overdoses can be managed in a traditional manner with careful monitoring, intensive supportive measures, and thorough evacuation of remaining drug from the gastrointestinal tract. Repeated doses of activated charcoal should be administered at least until charcoal is visible in the stool. Patients may recover completely from a substantial overdose with conservative management.[74-77]

REFERENCES

1. Weinberger M, Riegelman S: Rational use of theophylline for bronchodilatation. N Engl J Med 1974;291:151–153.

2. Weinberger M: Theophylline for treatment of asthma. J Pediatr 1978;92:1–7.

3. Weinberger M: The pharmacology and therapeutic use of theophylline. J Allergy Clin Immunol 1984;73:525–541.

4. Labovita E, Spector S: Placental theophylline transfer in pregnant asthmatics. JAMA 1982;247:786–788.

5. Heath A, Knudsen K: Role of extracorporeal drug removal in acute theophylline poisoning: A review. Med Toxicol 1987;2:294–308.

6. Mountain R, Neff T: Oral theophylline intoxication. Arch Intern Med 1984;144:724–727.

7. Gal P, Roop C, Robinson H, et al: Theophylline-induced seizures in accidentally overdosed neonates. Pediatrics 1980;65:547–549.

8. Albert S: Aminophylline toxicity. Pediatr Clin North Am 1987;34:61–73.

9. Elenbaas R, Payne V: Prediction of serum theophylline levels. Ann Intern Med 1984;13:92–96.

10. Greenberg A, Piraino B, Kroboth P, et al: Severe theophylline toxicity. Am J Med 1984;76:854–860.

11. Gaudreault P, Guay J: Theophylline poisoning. Med Toxicol 1986;1:169–191.

12. Gaudreault P, Wason S, Lovejoy F: Acute pediatric theophylline overdose: A summary of 28 cases. J Pediatr 1983;102:474–476.

13. Mant T, Cochrane M, Henry J: ABCs of poisoning: Respiratory drugs. Br Med J 1984;289:1133–1135.

14. Piafsky K, Sitar D, Rangno R, et al: Theophylline disposition in patients with hepatic cirrhosis. N Engl J Med 1977;296:1495–1497.

15. Piafsky K, Ogilvie R: Dosage of theophylline in bronchial asthma. N Engl J Med 1973;292:1218–1222.

16. Minocha A, Spyker D: Acute overdose with sustained release drug formulations. Med Toxicol 1986;1:300–307.

17. Ahlemen C, Heath A, Herlitz H, et al: Treatment of oral theophylline poisoning. Acta Med Scand 1984;216:423–426.

18. Corser B, Youngs C, Baughman R: Prolonged toxicity following massive ingestion of sustained release theophylline preparation. Chest 1985;88:749–750.

19. Carrier J, Shaw R, Porter R, et al: Comparison of intravenous and oral routes of theophylline loading in acute asthma. Ann Emerg Med 1985;14:1145–1151.

20. Nolke A: Severe toxic effects from aminophylline and theophylline suppositories in children. JAMA 1956;161:693–697.

21. Hendeles L, Weinberger M, Milavetz G, et al: Food-induced "dose dumping" from a once a day theophylline product as a cause of theophylline toxicity. Chest 1985;87:758–765.

22. Rangsithienchai R, Newcomb R: Aminophylline therapy in children: Guidelines for dosage. J Pediatr 1977;91:325–330.

23. Rosen J, Danish M, Ragni M, et al: Theophylline pharmacokinetics in the young infant. *Pediatrics* 1979;64:248–251.

24. Rothstein R: Intravenous theophylline therapy in asthma: A clinical update. *Ann Emerg Med* 1980;9:327–330.

25. Simons F, Friesen F, Simons K: Theophylline toxicity in term infants. *Am J Dis Child* 1980;134:39–41.

26. Arwood L, Dasta J, Friedman C: Placental transfer of theophylline: Two case reports. *Pediatrics* 1979; 63:844–846.

27. Davis R, Ellsworth A, Justus R, et al: Reversal of theophylline toxicity using oral activated charcoal. *J Fam Prac* 1985;20:73–75.

28. Mangione A, Imhoff T, Lee R, et al: Pharmacokinetics of theophylline in hepatic disease. *Chest* 1978;73:616–622.

29. Amitai Y, Yeung A, Moye J, et al: Repetitive oral activated charcoal and control of emesis in severe theophylline toxicity. *Ann Intern Med* 1986;105: 386–387.

30. Weinberger M, Matthay R, Ginchansky E, et al: Intravenous aminophylline dosage. *JAMA* 1976; 235:2110–2113.

31. Weinberger M, Bronsky E, Bensch G, et al: Interaction of ephedrine and theophylline. *Clin Pharmacol Ther* 1975;17:585–592.

32. Kadlec G, Jarboe C, Pollard S, et al: Acute theophylline intoxication: Biphasic first-order elimination kinetics in a child. *Ann Allergy* 1978;41:337–339.

33. Vozeh S, Powell R, Riegelman S, et al: Changes in theophylline clearance during acute illness. *JAMA* 1978;240:1882–1884.

34. Jackson J, Powell J, Wandell M, et al: Cimetidine decreases theophylline clearance. *Am Rev Respir Dis* 1981;123:615–617.

35. Anderson J, Poklis A, Slavin R: A fatal case of theophylline intoxication. *Arch Intern Med* 1983; 143:559–560.

36. McGuigan M, Tenenbein M: Planning an effective strategy for theophylline poisoning in adults. *Emerg Med Rep* 1987;8:41–48.

37. Kearney T, Manoguerra A, Curtis G, et al: Theophylline toxicity and the β-adrenergic system. *Ann Intern Med* 1985;102:766–769.

38. Biberstein M, Ziegler M, Ward D: Use of β blockade and hemoperfusion for acute theophylline poisoning. *West J Med* 1984;141:485–490.

39. Vaucher Y, Lightner E, Watxon P: Theophylline poisoning. *J Pediatr* 1977;90:827–830.

40. Marney S: Asthma: Recent developments in treatment. *South Med J* 1985;78:1084–1096.

41. Weinberger M, Hendeles L, Wong L, et al: Relationship of formulation and dosing interval to fluctuation of serum theophylline concentration in children with chronic asthma. *J Pediatr* 1981;99:145–152.

42. Brashear R, Aronoff G, Brier R: Activated charcoal in theophylline intoxication. *J Lab Clin Med* 1985;106: 242–245.

43. Olson K, Benowitz N, Woo O, et al: Theophylline overdose: Acute single ingestion versus chronic repeated overmedication. *J Emerg Med* 1985;3:386–394.

44. Jacobs M, Senior R, Kessler G: Clinical experience with theophylline. *JAMA* 1976;235:1983–1986.

45. Jenne J, Wyze E, Rood F, et al: Pharmacokinetics of theophylline. *Clin Pharmacol Ther* 1972;13:349–360.

46. Bertino J, Walker J: Reassessment of theophylline toxicity. *Arch Intern Med* 1987;147:757–760.

47. Zwillich C, Sutton R, Neff T, et al: Theophylline-induced seizures in adults. *Ann Intern Med* 1975; 82:784–787.

48. Gal P, Miller A, McCue J: Oral activated charcoal to enhance theophylline elimination in an acute overdose. *JAMA* 1984;251:3130–3131.

49. Hall K, Dobson K, Dalton J, et al: Metabolic abnormalities associated with intentional theophylline overdose. *Ann Intern Med* 1984;101:457–462.

50. Sawyer W, Caravati M, Ellison M, et al: Hypokalemia, hyperglycemia, and acidosis after intentional theophylline overdose. *J Emerg Med* 1985;3:408–410.

51. Goldberg M, Park G, Berlinger W: Treatment of theophylline intoxication. *J Allergy Clin Immunol* 1986;78:811–817.

52. Goldberg M, Spector R, Miller G: Phenobarbital improves survival in theophylline-intoxicated rabbits. *Clin Toxicol* 1986;24:203–211.

53. Goldberg M, Spector R, Park G, et al: The effect of sorbitol and activated charcoal on serum theophylline concentrations after slow-release theophylline. *Clin Pharmacol Ther* 1987;41:108–111.

54. Lim D, Sing P, Nourtsis S, et al: Absorption inhibition and enhancement of elimination of sustained-release theophylline tablets by oral activated charcoal. *Ann Emerg Med* 1986;15:1303–1307.

55. True R, Berman J, Mahutte K: Treatment of theophylline toxicity with oral activated charcoal. *Crit Care Med* 1984;12:113–114.

56. Kulig K, Bar-Or D, Rumack B: Intravenous theophylline poisoning and multiple dose charcoal in an animal model. *Ann Emerg Med* 1987;16:842–846.

57. Berlinger W, Spector R, Goldberg M, et al: Enhancement of theophylline clearance by oral activated charcoal. *Clin Pharmacol Ther* 1982;33:351–354.

58. Park G, Spector R, Roberts R, et al: Use of hemoperfusion for treatment of theophylline intoxication. *Am J Med* 1983;74:961–966.

59. Levy G: Gastrointestinal clearance of drugs with activated charcoal. *N Engl J Med* 1982;307:676–678.

60. Ginoza G, Strauss A, Iskra M, et al: Potential treatment of theophylline toxicity by high surface area activated charcoal. *J Pediatr* 1987;1:140–143.

61. Shannon M, Amitai Y, Lovejoy F: Multiple-dose activated charcoal for theophylline poisoning in young infants. *Pediatrics* 1987;80:368–370.

62. Levy G, Gibson T, Whitman W, et al: Hemodialysis clearance of theophylline. *JAMA* 1977;237:1466–1467.

63. Lawyer C, Aitchison J, Sutton J, et al: Treatment of theophylline neurotoxicity with resin hemoperfusion. *Ann Intern Med* 1978;88:516–517.

64. Laggner A, Kaik G, Lenz K, et al: Treatment of severe poisoning with slow release theophylline. *Br Med J* 1984;288:1497.

65. Gallagher E, Howland M, Greenblatt H: Hemolysis following treatment of theophylline overdose with coated charcoal hemoperfusion. *J Emerg Med* 1987;5:19–22.

66. Ohning B, Reed M, Blumer J: Continuous nasogastric administration of activated charcoal for the treatment of theophylline intoxication. *Pediatr Pharmacol* 1986;5:241–245.

67. Weinberger M, Hendeles L: Role of dialysis in the management and prevention of theophylline toxicity. *Dev Pharmacol Ther* 1980;1:26–30.

68. Russo M: Management of theophylline intoxication with charcoal-column hemoperfusion. *N Engl J Med* 1979;300:24–26.

69. Sahney S, Abarzua J, Sessums L: Hemoperfusion in theophylline neurotoxicity. *Pediatrics* 1983;71:615–619.

70. Chang T, Espinosa-Melendez E, Francoeur T, et al: Albumin-Collodion activated charcoal hemoperfusion in the treatment of severe theophylline intoxication in a 3-year old patient. *Pediatrics* 1980;65:811–814.

71. Woo O, Pond S, Benowitz N, et al: Benefit of hemoperfusion in acute theophylline intoxication. *Clin Toxicol* 1984;22:411–424.

72. Connell J, McGeachie J, Knepil J, et al: Self-poisoning with sustained-release aminophylline: Secondary rise in serum theophylline concentration after charcoal hemoperfusion. *Br Med J* 1982;284:943.

73. Kelly W, Parkin W: Charcoal hemoperfusion treatment of severe theophylline toxicity. *Aust N Z J Med* 1985;15:75–77.

74. Kossoy A, Weir M: Potentially toxic theophylline ingestions: Are heroic measures indicated? *South Med J* 1985;78:1000–1002.

75. Hendeles L, Bighley L, Richardson R: Frequent toxicity from IV aminophylline infusions in critically ill patients. *Drug Intell Clin Pharmacol* 1977;11:12–18.

76. Weibert R: Theophylline. *Clin Toxicol* 1979;14:157–160.

77. Whyte K, Addis G: Treatment of theophylline poisoning. *Br Med J* 1984;288:1835–1838.

ADDITIONAL SELECTED REFERENCES

Baker M: Theophylline toxicity in children. *J Pediatr* 1986;109:538.

Cereda J, Scott J, Quigley E: Endoscopic removal of pharmacobezoar of slow release theophylline. *Br Med J* 1986;293:1143.

Jusko W, Koup J, Vance J, et al: Intravenous theophylline therapy: Nomogram guidelines. *Ann Intern Med* 1977;86:400–404.

Kordash T, Van dellen R, McCall J: Theophylline concentrations in asthmatic patients. *JAMA* 1977;238:139–141.

Miceli J, Bidani A, Aronow R, et al: Peritoneal dialysis of theophylline. *Clin Toxicol* 1979;14:539–544.

Mitenko P, Ogilvie R: Bioavailability and efficacy of a sustained-release theophylline tablet. *Clin Pharmacol Ther* 1974;16:720–726.

Mitenko P, Ogilvie R: Rational intravenous doses of theophylline. *N Engl J Med* 1973;289:600–603.

Scott P, Tabachnik E, MacLeod S, et al: Sustained-release theophylline for childhood asthma: Evidence for circadian variation of theophylline pharmacokinetics. *J Pediatr* 1981;99:476–479.

Stine R, Marcus R, Parvin C: Clinical predictors of theophylline blood levels in asthmatic patients. *Ann Emerg Med* 1987;16:18–24.

Tattersfield A: Bronchodilator drugs. *Pharmacol Ther* 1982;17:299–313.

Wyatt R, Weinberger M, Hendeles L: Oral theophylline dosage for the management of chronic asthma. *J Pediatr* 1977;92:125–130.

Yarnell P, Chu N: Focal seizures and aminophylline. *Neurology* 1975;25:819–822.

part III

DRUGS USED IN PSYCHIATRY

chapter 11

Cyclic Antidepressants

One of the most serious types of poisoning, and one that appears to be increasing in frequency in both adults and children, is that due to cyclic antidepressants.[1-3] This group of drugs comprises the monocyclic, bicyclic, tricyclic, and the newer tetracyclic compounds. Most of the newer antidepressants are difficult to categorize according to structure and activity, and there are now numerous types of chemical structures as well as functional differences among many of the antidepressants. In this chapter the term tricyclic refers to any of the cyclic compounds as well as the noncyclic triazobipyridine derivative trazodone unless otherwise stated.[4-6]

The true tricyclics are the most well known of the cyclic compounds; this group comprises imipramine,[7,8] amitriptyline, doxepin,[6,9] trimipramine, nortriptyline,[10] protriptyline, desipramine, and others. These compounds are structurally similar to the phenothiazines and were first noted during the clinical investigation of phenothiazines in the early 1960s.[11,12] The antidepressant properties of these compounds were discovered at that time.[13] The rationale for the treatment of depression with tricyclics was a fortuitous discovery.[11,12] Imipramine was originally developed as an antipsychotic medicine, but it was noted that patients taking imipramine experienced significant relief of their depression.

The tricyclics have a relatively narrow therapeutic margin, and toxic doses are only 3 to 4 times greater than therapeutic doses. These compounds are therefore particularly dangerous in the context of overdose. Tricyclic overdoses commonly result in hospitalizations because of their potential for causing severe cardiovascular complications. As a result, they account not only for many lives lost but also for untold millions of dollars spent on hospitalizations and intensive care monitoring.[11,12]

The tricyclics have been involved in 10% to 25% of suicidal ingestions[14-16] and account for 20% to 25% of all drug-related deaths,[17-23] although some recent reports indicate that mortality has decreased. It is ironic that the individuals for whom these medications are prescribed are also at greatest risk for overdosage because they are either suicide prone and depressed[24] or young children being treated for nocturnal enuresis.[25-27] Because of the complex central and peripheral toxic effects of these drugs, the clinician who treats the overdosed patient may have to manage a number of complex problems, such as hypotension, coma with respiratory arrest, convulsions, complex dysrhythmias, and myocardial depression.[14,28,29] Because of these potential complications, a thorough understanding of the action of these drugs is important.[30-35]

The true tricyclic antidepressant drugs have a three-ring nucleus consisting of a seven-membered central ring bound by two benzene rings.[15] They may be categorized as follows: (1) dibenzocycloheptadiene derivatives (nortriptyline and amitriptyline); (2) dihydrodibenzepine derivatives (imipramine, desipramine, and chlorimipramine); (3) dibenzoxepine derivatives (doxepin); and (4) dibenzocycloheptatrine derivatives (protriptyline). Chemical alterations of the basic three-ring molecule have led to the development of similar drugs. Although there are numerous preparations on the market, there is actually little difference in the acute toxicity of these products (Table 11-1). The older "second generation" tricyclics, such as doxepin, were developed as an attempt to produce a less toxic alternative, but there were no real advantages to these agents. Recently, however, antidepressants have been developed that are radically different in structure and function. These appear to have pharmacodynamic characteristics that offer significant advantages.

MECHANISM OF ACTION

The major hypothesis of the biogenic amine theory of affective illness is that major depressive disorders arise from a functional decrease of certain biogenic amines, such as norepinephrine, dopamine, or serotonin, at functionally important synapses in the brain.[36,37] Even where neurotransmitter levels may be high, the sensitivity of the postsynaptic receptor is thought to be abnormally low as a result of agonist-induced receptor desensitization. Thus decreased central neuronal activity may arise from either an actual decrease in synaptic transmitter or a decrease in sensitivity of the postsynaptic receptor for the transmitter.

The apparent mode of action of the antidepressants is thought to be through an increase in the activity of central neurotransmitter systems (Table 11-2). This in turn is thought to be related to their abilities to block the reuptake of norepinephrine and serotonin from within the synaptic cleft into the presynaptic terminal.[13] Blockade of amine reuptake leads to increasing synaptic transmitter levels with secondary effects.

The tricyclics therefore appear to reduce depression by inhibiting the reuptake of norepinephrine, serotonin, and other amines.[15] This prolongs the action of these amine neurotransmitters by allowing them to remain at the

Table 11-1 Commonly Used Cyclic Compounds and Their Trade Names

Compound	Trade Name(s)
Amitriptyline	Amitid
	Amitril
	Elavil
	Endep
	Antipress
	Etrafon
	Limbitrol
	Perphenyline
	Triavil
Imipramine	Imavate
	Janimine
	Presamine
	SK-Pramine
	Tofranil
Doxepin	Adapin
	Sinequan
Nortriptyline	Aventyl
	Pamelor
Desipramine	Norpramin
	Pertofrane
Amoxapine	Asendin
Protriptyline	Vivactil
Trimipramine	Surmontil
Trazodone	Desyrel
Maprotiline	Ludiomil

receptors, thus increasing CNS transmission. The actual antidepressant effects seem to be related to down-regulation of presynaptic receptors and enhanced neurotransmitter release.

PHARMACOKINETICS

Tricyclics may be tertiary or secondary amines. There is a significant difference between these two types of amines in that tertiary amines are metabolized by N-demethylation to the corresponding secondary amines by the hepatic microsomal enzymes.[38-40] These secondary amines are pharmacologically active and contribute to both therapeutic and toxic effects. The tertiary amines therefore show dual toxicity.[41] On the other hand, the secondary amines are metabolized in the liver by aromatic hydroxylation and glucuronidization to compounds that have neither the therapeutic nor the toxic effects of the tricyclics.[33] Tertiary amines are therefore toxic in the parent form as well as in metabolite

Table 11-2 Inhibition of Neurotransmitter Reuptake by Various Cyclic Antidepressants

Compound	Norepinephrine	Serotonin	Dopamine	Histamine
Amitriptyline	+ + +	+ + +	+	+
Amoxapine	+ + +	+ /0	0	+
Desipramine	+ + +	+	0	0
Doxepin	+ +	+ +	0	+
Imipramine	+ + +	+ + +	+	+
Maprotiline	+ + +	0	+	+
Trazodone	0	+ +	0	0

form, whereas secondary amines are only toxic in the parent form.[42]

For example, imipramine is a tertiary amine and is partially metabolized to desipramine, its active secondary amine. Amitriptyline is also a tertiary amine that is metabolized to its active secondary amine nortriptyline. Because the demethylation reaction is not reversible, patients treated with the secondary tricyclics are only exposed to these products and not to the tertiary or parent compound (Table 11-3).

In general, secondary amines such as desipramine are more potent inhibitors of norepinephrine uptake, whereas tertiary amines such as imipramine exert more potent effects on the uptake of 5-hydroxytryptamine. Because the tertiary amines are broken down to secondary amines, they have both actions.

Absorption

Tricyclics are rapidly absorbed from the gastrointestinal tract in therapeutic doses, and after oral administration their plasma concentrations reach their peak within 2 to 4 hours. Although absorption of the tricyclics is complete, the amount of tricyclic that is bioavailable is sub-stantially less than that administered because of a significant first-pass effect. Because of their high lipid solubility, tricyclics are rapidly distributed to body tissues and fat, leaving only a small amount of the drug in the blood. In an overdose, they are absorbed more slowly because, owing to their anticholinergic effects, they decrease peristalsis and delay gastric emptying. Delayed absorption of oral doses of the tricyclics, with peak serum concentrations reached up to 12 hours after ingestion, has been noted.

Protein Binding

The tricyclics are approximately 85% to 98% protein bound to α acid glycoproteins[15]; that is, free drug concentrations are 2% to 15%.[4,43] The bound tricyclic is pharmacologically inactive but equilibrates between bound and unbound states in milliseconds. There is a direct relationship between protein binding and pH in that the more alkalotic the patient, the greater the degree of protein binding, with a consequent decrease in free or active drug concentrations at drug receptor sites.[15]

Metabolism

Metabolism occurs by demethylation, oxidation, aromatic hydroxylation, and glucuronidization by the microsomal enzyme system in the liver.[13,15,38–40] There is good evidence that the tricyclics are excreted into the biliary system after hepatic degradation and that 20% to 30% of a given dose of tricyclic may be secreted into the stomach or the bile in a 24-hour period.[15,44]

Table 11-3 Tertiary and Secondary Amine Tricyclics

Tertiary Amine	Secondary Amine
Amitriptyline	Nortriptyline
Imipramine	Desipramine
Doxepin	Nordoxepin

Volume of Distribution

The volume of distribution of the tricyclics is large and varies with the particular drug; the range is from 8 L/kg (for amitriptyline) to 34 L/kg (for desipramine). This large volume of distribution reflects the vast tissue distribution of the drugs. The large volume of distribution and the high degree of protein binding make the tricyclics virtually inaccessible to hemodialysis or hemoperfusion. Because of the high lipid solubility of these drugs, concentrations in tissue may be 10 times greater than those in the plasma. Concentrations in myocardial tissue have been reported to be as much as 50 to 200 times higher than in plasma.

ACTIONS

The tricyclics have four major actions when taken in therapeutic amounts (Tables 11-4 and 11-5). In the United States, they are approved by the FDA as antidepressant agents. They have also been used in children for enuresis. Although approved in Europe for dysrhythmias and peptic

ulcer disease, the tricyclics are not approved in the United States for those indications. Other uses not approved by the FDA include treatment for migraine, panic attacks, phobias, chronic pain, and bulimia.[45]

Antidepressant Effect

As mentioned earlier, the tricyclics are antidepressants owing to their ability to block the reuptake of norepinephrine and 5-hydroxytryptamine in the central nervous system. In patients with endogenous depression, an effect can be seen in 2 to 3 weeks. The tricyclics do not appear to offer mood elevation or euphoria to nonendogenously depressed individuals; therefore these compounds have not appeared as drugs of abuse.

Antidysrhythmic Effect

Therapeutic doses of tricyclics produce electrocardiographic changes similar to those seen with quinidine, procainamide, and disopyramide; thus the tricyclics are considered antidysrhythmic agents of the class Ia type.[15,46-49] Imipramine, for example, is attractive as a potential antidysrhythmic drug because it has a long half-life that would permit twice-daily dosing.[46,50] Although effective as antidysrhythmic agents and used in Europe for this purpose, the tricyclics are not approved for such use in the United States.

Table 11-4 Actions of the Tricyclics

Antidepressant (blocks the reuptake of
  5-hydroxytryptamine and norepinephrine)
Antidysrhythmic (class Ia type)
Antihistaminic (H_1 and H_2 antagonist)
Antienuretic (anticholinergic action)

Table 11-5 Comparison of the Actions of the Tricyclics

Compound	Orthostatic Hypotension	Anticholinergic Action	Quinidine-like Action	Adrenergic Side Effects
Amitriptyline	+ + + + +	+ + + + +	+	+
Doxepin	+ + +	+ + +	±	0
Imipramine	+ + + +	+ + + +	+	+ + +
Nortriptyline	+ +	+ +	+	+ + +
Desipramine	+ +	+ +	+	+ + + + +
Maprotiline	+	+	+	+ + + + +
Trazodone	+	+	−	0

Source: Reprinted with permission from *Medical Clinics of North America* (1986;70:1185–1201), Copyright © 1986, WB Saunders Company.

Antihistaminic Effect

The tricyclics have antihistaminic effects, exhibiting potent inhibition of both H_1 and H_2 receptors.[13] Some of the tricyclics, notably doxepin, amitriptyline, and trimipramine, are the most potent histamine antagonists currently available; they are more potent than cimetidine. Trimipramine has been used in Europe for duodenal ulcers and has been shown to be effective.[51,52] Tricyclics have also been beneficial for gastric ulcers.[53] Although these drugs are effective as histamine antagonists, they have not been approved for this use in the United States.

Antienuresis Effect

The tricyclics have been used in the pediatric age group for enuresis.[54] The mechanism of action of the tricyclics in the treatment of enuresis is not known but may involve inhibition of urination as a result of anticholinergic activity. This therapy poses a problem in that children have small fat stores, which makes more free and active drug available and creates the potential for toxicity.[31,55] The indications for the tricyclics have increased in the pediatrics age group. These now include hyperkinesis, school phobia, and sleep disorders.[15]

SECOND GENERATION ANTIDEPRESSANTS

It appears that the toxicities associated with second generation tricyclics are different from those of the more generally accepted antidepressants.[36]

Amoxapine

Amoxapine (Asendin®), a dibenzoxapine,[56] resembles imipramine and other tricyclics in both structure and pharmacology. Although amoxapine has potent antidepressant properties, it is a metabolite of the antipsychotic drug loxapine[57–59] and appears to have less cardiotoxic effects than the tricyclics. There are prominent

manifestations of CNS depression and seizures associated with an overdose.

Amoxapine, like imipramine, is a potent inhibitor of neuronal norepinephrine reuptake but has little potency as an inhibitor of the neuronal uptake of serotonin.[57] Amoxapine appears to be associated with an incidence of anticholinergic side effects similar to those of imipramine. Amoxapine is unique among antidepressants in that it has neuroleptic activity.[60,61] In psychomotor systems, amoxapine treatment is associated with many of the movement disorders classically associated with neuroleptic treatment. These include dystonia, akathisia, parkinsonism, neuroleptic malignant syndrome, and chorea (see Chapter 12).[61]

Amoxapine is rapidly absorbed and reaches peak blood concentrations within 1 to 2 hours after oral administration. It has a half-life of 8 hours, and its metabolite has a half-life of 30 hours.

Overdosage with amoxapine, especially with large doses, is characterized primarily by central nervous system toxicity, including an extremely high incidence of treatment-resistant seizures, coma, hypotension, and respiratory depression.[13,56,60–62] In addition, a substantial number of cases of amoxapine overdose have been accompanied by acute renal failure,[33] and some of these patients have required dialysis. The specific pathophysiologic cause of the acute renal failure is unclear, although the hypotension, rhabdomyolysis, and direct nephrotoxicity appear to be the most likely explanations. Because of conflicting reports concerning the cardiotoxic nature of amoxapine, no firm statement can be made regarding its cardiac toxicity.

Maprotiline

Maprotiline (Ludiomil®) was the first tetracyclic approved for clinical use in the United States and belongs to the class of anthracenes. The pharmacology of maprotiline is similar to that of the tricyclics in that it blocks the reuptake of norepinephrine at the neuronal membrane and has anticholinergic activity.[58] Maprotiline differs from the first generation tricyclics in that it has little or no effect on the reuptake of serotonin or dopamine. Maprotiline does not inhibit monoamine oxidase.

Maprotiline is slowly absorbed and has a half-life of approximately 2 days.[36] It is largely metabolized into its demethylated derivatives, which are later excreted into the urine and bile. Its extremely long half-life is of significance because toxic effects may be prolonged in overdosage and in elderly patients who may be slower to metabolize drugs.

Although there appear to be fewer cardiotoxic effects noted with overdosage of maprotiline, high doses comparable to those commonly prescribed are likely to be associated with a cardiac risk similar to that of the first generation tricyclics.[60,61] More prominent CNS effects, including a greater incidence of seizures, have been associated with maprotiline.[56,58,63] In addition, metabolic acidosis and hypokalemia have also been noted. Maprotiline-induced seizures may occur without previous history of seizure disorder, anticholinergic symptoms, or cardiac conduction or rhythm disturbances.[64] There have also been reports of seizures occurring during therapeutic use.[63] The drug's relatively long half-life has been implicated as the possible cause of the increased incidence of seizures.

Trazodone

Trazodone (Desyrel®) is chemically and structurally unrelated to the tricyclic, tetracyclic, or other known antidepressant agents. It is the first triazolopyridine derivative, a new class of antidepressant.[15,56]

Trazodone is rapidly and completely absorbed within the digestive tract after oral administration. Plasma concentrations reach their peak within 2 hours, and the half-life is 6 to 11 hours.[36] It is extensively metabolized, and less than 1% of an oral dose is excreted unchanged.

Trazodone does not appear to influence the reuptake of dopamine or norepinephrine within the central nervous system; at the same time it has been shown to block selectively the reuptake of serotonin at the presynaptic neuronal membrane.[58,60,61] It also has little clinical anticholinergic activity. Desirable central therapeutic effects may therefore be obtained with doses too small to produce any cardiovascular effects. The efficacy of trazodone appears to be equal to that of the tricyclics, and there also appears to be a lower incidence of cardiotoxic effects, anticholinergic effects, and lethal overdoses. However, CNS manifestations such as delirium and seizures have been reported.[60,61,65] Priapism is a troublesome adverse reaction and may have an onset between 6 and 14 days after treatment at therapeutic doses. Surgery has been required in some of these cases.

Compared to other agents, overdosage with trazodone alone has been reported to be relatively benign.[13,36,56,66] In an overdose its effects are comparable to those of the benzodiazepines.[18] The primary manifestations are hypotension, central nervous system effects, and gastrointestinal effects. Like the tricyclics and phenothiazines trazodone is a moderately potent α-adrenergic blocking agent, and hypotension may occur because of this action. Drowsiness, ataxia, nausea, vomiting, and dryness of the mouth may also be seen. CNS depression has been noted to progress to coma in some cases. Seizures, death, and the type of cardiovascular toxicity described for the other tricyclic agents are extremely rare.[36,66]

SIDE EFFECTS OF THERAPEUTIC AMOUNTS

It is estimated that 5% to 10% of patients placed on long-term therapy with tricyclic agents experience significant side effects, including anticholinergic effects such as dryness of the mouth, tachycardia,[58,67] and urinary retention (Table 11-6).[68,69] Although these problems can be bothersome, a tolerance develops to them.[68] Sweating, a paradoxical response, occurs by an unknown mechanism. Weakness, fatigue, and sedation have also been noted; these are possibly due to the anticholinergic actions causing drowsiness. Muscle tremors may occur in 10% to 20% of patients receiving the drug. On occasion, periods of confusion may be noted while the dosage is being increased; this abates when the medication is withheld for 1 day. Orthostatic hypotension is a significant side effect of tricyclic therapy that is unrelated to the age of the patient or to

Table 11-6 Side Effects of Therapeutic Amounts of Tricyclics

Anticholinergic
  Sweating
  Headache
  Weakness
  Fatigue
  Muscle tremors
  Cardiac toxicity
  Seizures
  Obstructive jaundice
Extrapyramidal
  Muscular rigidity
  Akathisia
  Dystonia
  Oculogyric crisis
  Opisthotonus
  Chorea
  Dysphagia
Parkinsonism
Postural Hypotension
Inappropriate Secretion of Antidiuretic Hormone

---

the duration of use of the drug. This action is due to α receptor blockade. Obstructive jaundice, when seen, is an idiosyncratic reaction (also noted with phenothiazines) that improves after discontinuance of the medication.

As with the phenothiazines, extrapyramidal symptoms may occur in patients receiving tricyclics (Table 11-6). In addition, a persistent fine tremor may develop in any age group, and parkinsonism is most commonly seen in geriatric patients receiving high doses. Other extrapyramidal side effects include rigidity, akathisia, dystonia, oculogyric crisis, opisthotonus, dysphagia, and chorea. Another relatively rare idiosyncratic reaction is the syndrome of inappropriate antidiuretic hormone secretion with resultant hyponatremia, lethargy, and seizures.[15,70]

In the healthy adult the tricyclics do not cause clinically important adverse cardiovascular effects except for postural hypotension, which can occur at therapeutic levels. Postural hypotension may result from the α blocking action of the tricyclics and is more likely to occur in the presence of existing cardiovascular disease.[71,72] Some patients with ventricular dysrhythmias have even shown improvement during treatment for their psychiatric disorder.[46,47] The patients at greatest risk for cardiac problems are those

with pre-existing bundle branch block, who have an increased risk for developing high grades of atrioventricular block.

TRICYCLIC WITHDRAWAL

A withdrawal syndrome has been described that is associated with abrupt discontinuance of tricyclics.[73] The syndrome is considered mild and consists of akathisia[74] (which may be related to a sudden decrease in dopamine concentration at the receptor site), nausea, vomiting, diarrhea, chills, headache, and malaise. No treatment is necessary for this condition except to replace the discontinued medicine if warranted.

TOXICITY

Most patients who have overdosed with tricyclics have no more than transient minor toxic effects, although serious toxic effects can certainly occur. After a significant overdose the patient may progress from a state of alertness and lucidity to unconsciousness, usually within a short period of time. Typically a patient intoxicated with tricyclics becomes symptomatic within a 3- to 4-hour period, but symptoms may begin as early as 20 to 30 minutes after ingestion.[20,21] Most patients who develop a dysrhythmia or conduction abnormality do so within 1 to 2 hours after ingestion. Myoclonus and grand mal seizures may also be noted shortly after ingestion.

Toxicity of the tricyclics is caused by a number of different mechanisms: (1) the anticholinergic actions, (2) the blocking of the reuptake of norepinephrine, (3) the membrane-stabilizing or quinidine-like action on the myocardium, and (4) miscellaneous actions (Table 11-7).[75,76] The signs and symptoms of tricyclic intoxication can also be placed in three categories: atropine-like, neurologic, and cardiovascular.

Anticholinergic Action

Because of an atropine-like action, the tricyclics bind to the cholinergic receptor in a com-

Table 11-7 Major Toxicity of the Tricyclics

Action	Manifestations
Anticholinergic	Atropine-like effects
Blocking of reuptake of norepinephrine	Sympathomimetic effects
Membrane stabilization	Quinidine-like effects
α-Adrenergic blocking action	Hypotension
Miscellaneous	Coma, bradycardia

Table 11-8 Peripheral and Central Anticholinergic Effects of Tricyclics

Peripheral
  Tachycardia
  Hypertension
  Hyperpyrexia
  Mydriasis
  Vasodilation
  Supraventricular dysrhythmias
  Urinary retention
  Decreased secretions
Central
  Anxiety
  Confusion
  Disorientation
  Myoclonus
  Choreoathetosis
  Hallucinations
  Seizures
  Medullary paralysis
  Death

petitive fashion. When acetylcholine is released it cannot bind to the receptor and is destroyed by the enzyme acetylcholinesterase, resulting in parasympathetic paralysis. This is the mechanism of action for any of the anticholinergic compounds (see Chapter 7).

Cardiac and smooth muscle, exocrine gland, and brain tissue are the most markedly affected by the tricyclics; there is little effect on autonomic ganglia or motor endplates. The competitive antagonism to acetylcholine is manifested in peripheral and central anticholinergic effects.[77]

Peripheral Effects

Peripheral effects include supraventricular tachycardia, hyperpyrexia, mydriasis, vasodilation, urinary retention, decreased gastrointestinal motility, and decreased secretions (Table 11-8).[78]

Central Effects

The central anticholinergic effects include anxiety, delirium, disorientation, hallucinations, hyperactivity, seizures, myoclonus, choreoathetosis, coma, and, possibly, death (Table 11-8).[79] Coma usually occurs within 6 hours of the ingestion and may last for 24 hours, in some cases simulating brain death with complete loss of brainstem and cerebral function.[80,81] CNS depression may cause ventilatory failure and contribute to aspiration pneumonia, and seizures, agitation, and marked muscle activity can lead to rhabdomyolysis and acute renal failure.[82] Many of these symptoms result from an imbalance of acetylcholine and dopamine, with a resultant decrease in acetylcholine relative to dopamine in the basal ganglia.

Myoclonus results from the decrease in serotonin uptake and subsequent increase in serotonin at the synapse.

Many of the movement disorders associated with these drugs are often inaccurately classified as seizures. Recognizing the movements as chorea, athetosis, or myoclonus may be important in helping to establish the correct diagnosis as well as initiating proper treatment.

Anticholinergic effects, although common after tricyclic overdose, are not the primary mechanism by which the tricyclics are lethal.

Blocking of the Reuptake of Norepinephrine

The second action of the tricyclics is an exaggeration of the beneficial mechanism of action—the central and peripheral blockage of the reuptake of norepinephrine.[83] In contrast to many metabolic processes in which the actions of pharmacologically active substances are terminated by enzymatic transformation of the substance into less active metabolites, reuptake of the neurotransmitter back into the vesicle, rather than metabolism, is the major mechanism by which an action is terminated at the adrenergic site for compounds such as norepinephrine, epinephrine, and dopamine. This action occurs by means of an active pump mechanism. The nor-epinephrine is again stored intraneuronally until released again by the next stimulus; this is the reuptake mechanism.

The tricyclics block this reuptake of nor-epinephrine both centrally and peripherally, resulting in increased neurotransmitter action at the receptor site. Such an action causes potentiation of transmitter action. Blocking of the reuptake of the neurotransmitter also eventually leads to local or generalized norepinephrine depletion because the neurotransmitter is metabolized once it is in the bloodstream. This eventually causes decreased myocardial contractility, hypotension, and bradycardia.

Membrane-Stabilizing Action

The most dangerous action of the tricyclics is the membrane-stabilizing action, sometimes referred to as the quinidine-like effect. Membrane stabilizers depress excitability in nerve and muscle tissue, including the heart, and depress both conduction and contractility of the myocardium.[84,85] This occurs through direct depression of the myocardium caused by interference with the sodium-potassium pump. This is believed to be due to an inhibition of the adenosine triphosphate phosphohydrolase enzyme, which is the enzyme involved in the maintenance of sodium and potassium balance across the myocardial cell membrane.[86] This slowing of sodium flux into cells results in altered repolarization and conduction.[83] Interruption of ionic balance across the cell therefore leads to myocardial depression and conduction defects. This is because slowing of phase 0 depolarization of the action potential results in slowing of conduction through the His-Purkinje system and myocardium.[48,49] Slow impulse conduction is responsible for QRS prolongation and atrioventricular block and contributes to ventricular dysrhythmias and hypotension. Cardiotoxicity is manifested by decreased myocardial contractile force, increased PR interval, and pronounced intraventricular conduction delays, all of which predispose the patient to re-entry and ventricular dysrhythmias.[17–19]

Because of slowed conduction in the ventricles a widened QRS may be noted. This is a

sensitive indicator of toxicity and toxic blood levels.[11,12,15,80,81] An increased QT interval may predispose the patient to torsades de pointes,[87] which is seen during treatment with drugs that prolong the QT interval.[48,49] The mechanism of torsades is thought to be increased temporal dispersion of ventricular depolarization. Drug-induced torsades de pointes is typically triggered by a premature ventricular beat on the terminal position of the T wave and often occurs after a sinus pause.[88,89] This rhythm is more likely to occur at slow heart rates and has been observed when therapeutic doses of tricyclics are administered. Torsades de pointes is unlikely to occur with tachycardia associated with tricyclic overdose. In addition to torsades, myocardial depression, hypotension, bradycardia, and asystole have been noted (Table 11-9).[90]

The QRS duration in the limb leads of an electrocardiogram is an important prognostic indicator of toxicity.[11,13,18,80] It has been found that patients with a QRS duration of less than 0.10 second are not likely to experience seizures or ventricular dysrhythmias.[14] Those with a QRS duration of 0.10 second or more have a greater incidence of seizures, and those with a QRS duration that exceeds 0.16 second are likely to experience ventricular dysrhythmias.[14] Other studies have shown that the QRS interval might not be a reliable indicator of toxicity.[91]

Inhibition of the sodium current slowing of phase 0 depolarization is the most important toxic effect of the tricyclics on the cardiac action potential. This effect on the depolarization rate is also rate dependent. At rapid heart rates

---

Table 11-9 Quinidine-like Cardiovascular Effects of Tricyclics

Primary
    Increased refractory period
    Decreased conduction velocity
    Decreased ventricular automaticity
Secondary
    Increased PR interval
    Increased QT interval
    Increased QRS duration
    Predisposition to re-entry
    Hypotension

depolarization is depressed, and the QRS complex becomes prolonged. Thus sinus tachycardia may aggravate the conduction abnormality.

Cardiac Effects

Cardiovascular toxic reactions account for most fatalities from tricyclic overdosage and are the most difficult to treat; they are therefore the major adverse action of the tricyclics. Owing to the anticholinergic action, there may be a sinus tachycardia and other evidence of a hyperdynamic state. Sinus tachycardia is considered one of the most sensitive early indicators of tricyclic toxicity.[13,49,92,93] Mild hypertension may also be produced. The anticholinergic effects are not thought to be responsible for ventricular conduction blocks because cholinergic innervation of the ventricle is sparse.

Because of the blockage of the reuptake of norepinephrine, there may also be a sinus tachycardia, hypertension, an associated increase in cardiac output, and ventricular dysrhythmias.[94] Hypotension may be noted and is caused by the α blocking action of the tricyclics or, over a longer period of time, by the depletion of norepinephrine with subsequent metabolism of the catecholamine. Hypotension may at times be severe and, when combined with marked bradycardia and heart block, may lead to cardiac arrest.[49] Hypotension may also aggravate tricyclic-induced dysrhythmias by impairing myocardial perfusion or causing systemic acidosis.[15]

Toxic doses of the tricyclics are capable of producing various rate and rhythm disturbances, including sinus tachycardia, sinus bradycardia, supraventricular and ventricular tachycardia, wandering atrial pacemaker, atrial and ventricular flutter and fibrillation, partial or complete atrioventricular block, bundle branch blocks, intraventricular blocks, ectopic beats, and asystole.[49] The most frequent dysrhythmias noted are supraventricular tachycardia, conduction defects, ventricular ectopic beats, and ventricular tachycardia or fibrillation.[95] Sometimes differentiating supraventricular dysrhythmias with aberrant conduction from ventricular dysrhythmias may be difficult, as recent studies suggest.[96]

Continuous infusion of imipramine in animals has resulted in a progression of electrocardiographic changes similar to that seen in humans.[17] These changes are typically seen in order and consist of sinus tachycardia, intraventricular conduction defects (with right bundle branch block occurring more frequently than left bundle branch block), ventricular dysrhythmias including ventricular tachycardia and ventricular fibrillation, and atrioventricular conduction defects that eventually lead to bradycardia and cardiac arrest.[97,98] First-degree atrioventricular block and intraventricular conduction delay in tricyclic antidepressant poisoning do not cause hemodynamic abnormalities and are not life threatening.[99,100] The importance of these conduction abnormalities lies in their being the most reliable premonitory signs of severe tricyclic antidepressant poisoning, heralding the increased probability of subsequent dysrhythmias, heart block, cardiac arrest, and sudden death.[12,22]

Owing to the complex pharmacokinetics of the tricyclics, many instances of delayed complications including dysrhythmias, conduction blocks, coma, and death have been reported. The recurrence of symptoms and rebound of plasma concentrations may be due to the release of the tissue-bound supply of the tricyclic.

Children may be at an increased risk of tricyclic cardiotoxicity because they have smaller lipid compartments than adults and tend to have less tricyclic stored in the fat and more available free drug. In addition, children appear to have a low capacity for drug binding to albumin, which also increases the amount of available free drug.[101]

Other Effects

Seizures

Generalized seizures may be noted after a serious tricyclic overdose. Grand mal seizures have been associated with increased mortality from tricyclic antidepressants. Seizures are more likely to occur in comatose patients.[15] Many times these seizures are noted immediately before the appearance of cardiac dysrhythmias.

This may be due to the acidemia after a seizure, which then limits protein binding and consequently allows more free drug to enter the circulation. Hypoxia, hypoglycemia, and other metabolic and structural causes of seizures must first be ruled out.[15]

Acidemia

The patient overdosed on tricyclics may experience hypotension, hypoventilation, or seizures that may lead to acidemia.[48] Vigorous management is required to treat the acidemia because it could lead to cardiac arrest.

Hyperthermia and Hypothermia

Both hypothermia and hyperthermia in tricyclic overdose have been reported.[31-33] Hyperthermia is a result of the blocking of the reuptake of norepinephrine, increased muscular generation of heat from seizures, myoclonus, or agitation combined with impaired heat loss from decreased sweating due to cholinergic blockade.[48] Hypothermia may be seen in patients with severe poisoning and is thought to be due to a combination of low cardiac output, peripheral vasodilation, and low external temperature.

Coma

Coma resulting from tricyclic overdose is generally of short duration. Although coma may be accompanied by other signs of tricyclic poisoning, this is not always the case, and coma may be the sole symptom. Respiratory failure in tricyclic overdose can occur from CNS depression, seizures, upper airway obstruction, aspiration, and pulmonary edema.

Pseudoseizures

Pseudoseizures such as myoclonus, tremor, chorea, and choreoathetosis may occur in many of the serious overdoses.[15] Myoclonus may be related to tricyclic blockade of amine neurotransmitter uptake, which then increases serotonin at peripheral synapses. Coarse myoclonic jerking may precede seizure activity and may be difficult to differentiate, but patients experiencing myoclonus usually remain awake.[13] An imbalance of dopamine and acetylcholine in the central nervous system may produce tremor and chorea.

LABORATORY ANALYSIS FOR TRICYCLIC OVERDOSE

A 12-lead electrocardiogram should be immediately obtained looking for evidence of cardiovascular effects, including sinus tachycardia and bundle branch block. Although there appears to be a positive correlation between the QRS duration and the development of significant symptoms,[11,12,14,17-19,80,81] a QRS interval of less than 0.10 second cannot be used as the sole indicator of safety.[102] This finding alone therefore does not exclude the risk of significant toxic events, including seizures and ventricular dysrhythmias.

Plasma assays of tricyclics are not a routine procedure in most hospitals, but they can be performed in larger institutions.[103,104] The tricyclics are among the most difficult drugs to analyze, and unpredictable losses of the compound can occur if scrupulous care is not taken with the specimen. It is only recently that methods have become available to measure the tricyclics at the low concentrations that occur in serum. In addition, to measure tricyclic concentrations accurately a laboratory must also assay the pharmacologically active metabolites, which may also contribute to toxicity and in some cases are more toxic than the parent compound.[105]

Although thin-layer chromatography can detect the tricyclics, it is not a quantitative method. The most widely used methods are gas chromatography with a nitrogen detector, high-performance liquid chromatography with an ultraviolet absorbance detector, and gas chromatography combined with mass spectrometry.[4,5,57] Radioimmunoassays are also available but have certain drawbacks that limit their usefulness.[106]

In general, tests for serum tricyclic concentrations are not helpful in the acute ingestion because they are relatively time consuming and because the plasma concentrations may be small (in the nanogram range) while tissue levels may be toxic.[39] In addition, the results of laboratory tests are not as helpful in determining treatment as is the interpretation of the patient's signs and symptoms. Laboratory studies can be useful, however, in confirming a diagnosis or in following the hospital course of a tricyclic-intoxicated patient.

Under therapeutic conditions the concentration of a tricyclic drug in plasma is low, usually between 20 to 500 ng/mL depending on the specific tricyclic.[4–6,28,103] In acute intoxications, tricyclic concentrations greater than 1000 ng/mL (for imipramine) are associated with severe toxicity, including electrocardiographic widening of the QRS of more than 100 msec, development of serious dysrhythmias, and coma.[12,28,80,81] High concentrations may remain high for several days, particularly if the patient overdosed with a tertiary tricyclic antidepressant. Marked differences in steady-state plasma concentrations of the tricyclics occur even in patients treated therapeutically with equal oral doses. This variation has been shown to be the result of individual differences in the rate of drug metabolism and the apparent volume of distribution.[106] Therefore, wide variations in toxic plasma concentrations may also occur. Some investigators have reported that falsely low laboratory values have been obtained if Vacutainer tubes are used for blood drawing because of the chemical in the rubber stopper.[42]

In addition to the previously mentioned laboratory analyses, serum electrolyte and arterial blood gas determinations should be performed to judge the acid-base status of the patient. A limb lead QRS duration of more than 0.10 second identifies patients at greatest risk for seizures, and a QRS duration of less than 0.16 second identifies patients at greatest risk for developing ventricular dysrhythmias or hypotension.[14]

TREATMENT

It is difficult to predict the severity of an acute intoxication on the basis of the amount of ingested drug. Therefore, as stated earlier, it is prudent to consider the ingestion of any quantity of these drugs potentially toxic and to treat it as such (Table 11-10).[78,107] Good supportive care is essential. Several studies have shown that the toxicity of the tricyclics is exaggerated by factors

Table 11-10 Summary of Treatment for Tricyclic Overdose

1. Ipecac or lavage
2. Multiple-dose activated charcoal
3. Cathartic
4. Intermittent nasogastric suction
5. Physostigmine (diagnostic or therapeutic)
   Adult: 1 to 2 mg IV slowly
   Child: 0.5 mg IV slowly
6. Alkalinization
   Sodium bicarbonate, 0.5 to 2.0 mEq/kg
   Respiratory alkalosis to pH 7.50 to 7.55
7. Phenytoin, 15-20 mg/kg IV (for ventricular dysrhythmias, conduction disturbances, or seizures)
8. Lidocaine, 1 mg/kg (for ventricular dysrhythmias)
9. β-Adrenergic blocking drugs (not recommended)
10. Bretylium (not recommended)
11. Calcium (not recommended)
12. Diazepam (for seizures)
13. Fluids (for hypotension)
14. Norepinephrine (for refractory hypotension)
15. Pacemaker (for refractory bradycardia or hypotension)

that increase cardiac work; thus efforts should be made to minimize conditions such as fluid overload, seizures, agitation, and extremes of blood pressure.

Patients are most at risk before or soon after admission to the hospital, when plasma concentrations of the drug are maximal. Most patients brought to the emergency department after tricyclic overdose who subsequently die do so within the first few hours.[13,61] The rapid decline in plasma concentration indicates that, within 2 to 3 hours of the overdose, redistribution from plasma to tissues is exceeding absorption. Toxicity also diminishes during this time. Life-threatening complications in serious tricyclic overdose almost always develop within 2 hours of the patient's presentation to the emergency department.

Prevention of Absorption

Any patient with a history of tricyclic overdose should be placed on a cardiac monitor with a patent intravenous line in place. Lavage should also be performed even late after an ingestion because of the decreased peristalsis and delayed absorption associated with anticholinergics.[18] If the patient is alert with an intact gag reflex and appears to be in no immediate danger of losing consciousness, gastric lavage can be performed.[13] Emesis may be too risky in a patient whose mental status may change rapidly.

Activated charcoal effectively binds tricyclics, and therefore 50 to 100 g of activated charcoal should be administered after adequate gastric emptying has been obtained.[13] Because of the enterohepatic recirculation and gastric resecretion, the use of multiple-dose activated charcoal every 2 to 4 hours may be effective in adsorbing the material that is recirculated.[15,20,108]

Continuous nasogastric suction has been advocated to remove any additional drug that is resecreted into the stomach; some studies have shown a removal of 5% to 15% of an ingested dose because of such resecretion. The clinical effectiveness of this method has still not been shown, however. It may be wise to administer multiple-dose activated charcoal and to apply intermittent nasogastric suction after the charcoal has been left in the gastrointestinal tract for a period of 30 to 45 minutes.

As mentioned earlier, respiratory depression or failure should be vigorously treated with intubation and mechanical ventilation because acidosis of any kind may precipitate fatal cardiac dysrhythmias.[15]

Physostigmine

Considerable controversy has arisen over the years as to the use of physostigmine (Antilirium®).[109] Although physostigmine is not considered a first-line drug for any of the problems associated with the tricyclics, it has a theoretical role in the treatment of some of the tricyclic-associated disorders.[46,47,110]

Physostigmine is a cholinergic drug that hydrolyzes the enzyme acetylcholinesterase, which is responsible for the metabolism of acetylcholine. It is considered a reversible carbamate acetylcholinesterase inhibitor. After an overdose of a tricyclic the receptor is bound by the drug, so that when acetylcholine is released it cannot bind with the receptor. Physostigmine inhibits the acetylcholinesterase, thereby allowing more acetylcholine to be available and to displace competitively the anticholinergic drug.[111,112]

Other acetylcholinesterase inhibitors are available, including neostigmine (Prostigmin®), pyridostigmine (Mestinon®), and edrophonium (Tensilon®). Although these compounds are successful in reversing the peripheral anticholinergic effects of the tricyclics, because they are all quaternary ammonium-charged compounds they do not cross the blood-brain barrier. Physostigmine is a tertiary amine and can cross the blood-brain barrier to reverse both the peripheral and the central anticholinergic effects.[15]

Clinical Indications for Use

Physostigmine may be indicated in the diagnosis of anticholinergic overdose and may be effective in reversing dysrhythmias that are the result of vagal blockade.[113] Dysrhythmias that develop from the direct effect of the antidepressant action on the myocardium are probably not affected. Supraventricular dysrhythmias that are hemodynamically significant—seizures, myoclonus (especially when violent), hallucinations (when severe), and hypertension (when marked)—are all considered indications for the use of physostigmine (Table 11-11). Because the ventricles do not have significant cholinergic innervation, beneficial effects in treating ventricular dysrhythmias with physostigmine are not expected.

Dosage

The dosage of physostigmine is 1 to 2 mg intravenously, administered slowly. In children, a dose of 0.5 mg[92] or 0.02 mg/kg[114] may be administered intravenously. Physostigmine has a short half-life; consequently it may reverse symptoms of tricyclic overdose for only 30 to 45 minutes.[15] Because physostigmine is rapidly metabolized, the dose may need to be repeated.

Contraindications to Use

Relative contraindications to the use of physostigmine include asthma, gangrene, and mechanical obstruction of the gastrointestinal tract or genitourinary tract. Caution should be

Table 11-11 The Use of Physostigmine for Tricyclic Overdose

Indications
  Diagnostic
  Therapeutic
    Supraventricular dysrhythmias
    Seizures
    Myoclonus
    Hallucinations
    Hypertension
Dosage
  Adult: 1 to 2 mg IV slowly
  Child: 0.5 mg or 0.02 mg/kg IV slowly
Cholinergic Side Effects
  Bradycardia
  Miosis
  Increased secretions
  Urination
  Defecation
  Seizures
Cardiac Side Effects
  Shift of pacemaker from sinoatrial node to another site
  Slowing of conduction through atrioventricular node
  Prolonged refractory period
  Atrioventricular block
  Asystole

exercised because physostigmine can precipitate seizures when administered too rapidly or cause a cholinergic crisis consisting of bradycardia, miosis, increased secretions, urination, and defecation if given to a patient who has not ingested an anticholinergic compound (see Table 11-11).[115] Physostigmine may also have undesirable effects in a quinidine-like overdose because it can shift the pacemaker from the sinoatrial node to another atrial site, slow conduction through the atrioventricular node, prolong the refractory period, produce atrioventricular blocks, and cause asystole (see Table 11-11).[115] Its use has therefore greatly diminished over the last few years, and it should not be considered a first-line drug. It has been suggested that physostigmine be administered to patients to make them alert enough that steps can be taken to induce vomiting.[13] This is a potentially dangerous procedure because the duration of action of physostigmine is short and the patient may lose consciousness before or during vomiting. In addition, coma is not a life-threatening condition and often may be preferable in violent, uncontrollable patients who may harm themselves. Hence, coma alone should not be an indication for the use of physostigmine.[92,93,116]

Alkalinization

Alkalinization of the patient has long been advocated in Europe and Australia, and recently it has been advocated in the United States.[117] The effectiveness of this therapy has been confirmed in both animals and humans.[83,118–120] Similar therapy has been used to treat quinidine toxicity.

Clinical Indications

Administration of sodium bicarbonate parenterally to cause metabolic alkalosis, or induction of hyperventilation[117,118] to cause respiratory alkalosis have been shown to be effective for treating ventricular dysrhythmias, specifically ventricular tachycardia and fibrillation, as well as conduction disturbances and bundle branch blocks, seizures, and hypotension due to decreased cardiac contractility (Table 11-12).[13,83,121–123] Alkalinization may be useful regardless of whether blood pH is low or normal.[83]

Dosage of Sodium Bicarbonate

Alkalinization of the patient to a blood pH of 7.50 to 7.55 is suggested as a first-line approach to treatment.[123] The optimal dose of sodium bicarbonate has not been established, but roughly 0.5 to 2 mEq/kg intravenously is effective. If the patient is experiencing controlled respirations, hyperventilation may be induced instead.[118–121,123] If sodium bicarbonate is used, the addition of potassium chloride (20 to 40 mEq/L) is useful in compensating for the potential fall in serum potassium that occurs with acute alkalinization.

Table 11-12 Indications for Alkalinization Procedures

Widened QRS interval
Ventricular dysrhythmias
Seizures
Hypotension

Mechanism of Action

The mechanism by which alkalinization is effective for the tricyclics is still unclear, but some investigators postulate that it is due to the increased protein binding that occurs in an alkaline environment, which reduces the amount of free or active drug.[118–122] Other investigators hold that the mechanism of action is due to the positive effect of the sodium ion (rather than of the bicarbonate) on the refractory period of the cardiac action potential.[83,123] It may be that the effects of increasing the extracellular sodium concentration and of increasing the blood *p*H are distinct and additive actions and that both mechanisms operate.

Although the rationale for the use of sodium bicarbonate is still unclear, that alkalinization is effective is beyond question and its use is encouraged. Sodium bicarbonate appears to be more commonly used than hyperventilation for the production of alkalemia, but hyperventilation has an advantage in that it does not predispose the patient to the hazards of sodium overload, which may then make the patient more vulnerable to pulmonary edema.[118]

Sodium bicarbonate reverses the cardiac manifestations regardless of heart rate or blood *p*H.[83,123] It is usually effective immediately after administration, and, although its effects are not long lasting, repeated administration is usually effective. If the patient is intubated, ventilatory prophylaxis ensuring a slight respiratory alkalosis and hypocapnia may be sufficient. Nevertheless, the prophylactic efficacy of alkalosis in patients who have ingested tricyclics but have no QRS prolongation or other signs of toxicity has not been well studied.[18]

Treatment of Rhythm Disturbances

There is much debate concerning whether lidocaine or phenytoin is the best drug for the ventricular dysrhythmias associated with an overdose of tricyclics.[124,125] *Lidocaine* can be useful in low to moderate doses because it has little effect on atrioventricular conduction.[13,123] Care should be exercised when high doses are administered because lidocaine also has the ability to decrease atrioventricular conduction, cause sinoatrial nodal arrest, and, at times, sei-

zures. Lidocaine can be administered relatively rapidly and can therefore control the dysrhythmias in a shorter period of time than phenytoin, which makes it highly recommended for quick control.

The use of *phenytoin* is another reasonable form of therapy for tricyclic overdose because this drug has both antidysrhythmic and anticonvulsant activity, enhances atrioventricular and intraventricular conduction, and decreases ventricular automaticity.[123,126,127] It is contraindicated in patients with severe bradycardia, second- and third-degree blocks, asystole, and ventricular fibrillation. The recommended dosage of phenytoin in an adult is 15 to 20 mg/kg (usually 1 g) intravenously, not exceeding 25 to 50 mg/min. This is the main drawback to the use of phenytoin: it may take 20 to 40 minutes to administer (Table 11-13). Phenytoin is not approved by the FDA for use as an antidysrhythmic agent, although such use is generally accepted.

The use of β-*adrenergic blockers*, although initially thought to be of benefit for the tachydysrhythmias, is not appropriate because these drugs decrease atrioventricular conduction and have some quinidine-like membrane effects.[124] In animals, the β-adrenergic blockers have also been shown not to counteract the cardiac effects and electrocardiographic changes associated with the tricyclics. In addition, it is not wise to administer a drug that may precipitate or aggravate hypotension and cardiac failure induced by the ingested drug.[124] Furthermore, using β-adrenergic blockers for treatment of tricyclic antidepressant toxicity may be hazardous

---

Table 11-13 Use of Phenytoin for Tricyclic Overdose

Actions
  Enhances atrioventricular conduction
  Enhances intraventricular conduction
  Decreases ventricular automaticity
Contraindications
  Severe bradycardia
  Second- and third-degree blocks
  Asystole
  Ventricular fibrillation
Dosage
  Adult: 1 g, not more than 25 to 50 mg/min
  Child: 15 to 20 mg/kg over 20 to 30 minutes

because increased catecholamines may be necessary to counteract the depressant actions of tricyclics on the heart rate and contractility.[123]

Bretylium causes an initial release of norepinephrine from peripheral adrenergic nerve terminals, resulting in eventual adrenergic blockade and hypotension. This initial action is similar to the effects of the tricyclics, and because of this bretylium should not be used routinely. It should only be used for refractory ventricular fibrillation or tachycardia.

Calcium, although generally not used for tricyclic overdose, has the theoretical benefit of increasing atrioventricular conduction, increasing intraventricular conduction, shortening the QT interval, and increasing contractility. Although calcium administration is not suggested, its usefulness should be kept in mind if all other agents have been tried without success.

Treatment of Seizures

Seizures secondary to the tricyclics should be first treated with bicarbonate. This is not so much an attempt to stop the seizure as to reverse the metabolic acidosis that will ensue.[13] Diazepam should be administered to control the seizure. Intractable seizures are more often seen with amoxapine and maprotiline overdoses and may require the use of anticonvulsants other than diazepam. Inducing neuromuscular paralysis with curare-like agents has also been required for overdoses of some tricyclic agents. If seizure prevention is necessary, phenytoin can be given in a loading dose. Physostigmine has also been reported to be effective for seizures secondary to anticholinergic drugs, although as stated earlier this is not considered a first-line drug.

Seizures should be treated promptly to prevent acidemia because this condition may increase the amount of free drug. Therefore, concomitant with the use of diazepam seizures due to tricyclic antidepressants should be vigorously treated with bicarbonate to correct the metabolic component of the acidosis.

Treatment of Hypotension

Blood pressure support may be required in view of the hypotensive effect of the tricyclics. Hypotension is a serious manifestation of tricyclic overdose and may be the harbinger of cardiac arrest.[119] Fluids and bicarbonate should be administered.[83] If there is no response to Trendelenburg's position or to bicarbonate and saline challenge of 10 to 20 mL/kg, pressor agents should be used. If this is ineffective, Swan-Ganz catheterization is desirable to differentiate between vasodilation and myocardial depression.

Norepinephrine or phenylephrine—direct-acting sympathetic agents—rather than an indirectly acting agent (which may first have to be taken up by the cells before it will function) should be administered.[15] Drugs such as metaraminol, ephedrine, and dopamine may have attenuated effectiveness as pressor agents because the tricyclics block their reuptake into the adrenergic neuron. An exaggerated response may occur with norepinephrine; vasopressors should therefore be reserved for refractory hypotension, and low doses should be used initially because the effect of further sensitizing the myocardium may induce or worsen dysrhythmias.

A *pacemaker* may be necessary for those patients with refractory bradydysrhythmias or refractory hypotension. In addition, a pacemaker may be effective in suppressing ventricular tachycardia associated with bradycardia or for torsades de pointes.[15,123]

Therapeutic Agents To Avoid

Class Ia antidysrhythmics should be avoided; therefore quinidine, procainamide, and disopyramide are contraindicated.[15] Forced diuresis is also contraindicated because excretion of the tricyclics is not enhanced with diuresis and because of the possibility of worsening the patient's condition through fluid overload.[127,128] Although it is theoretically possible that acidification of the urine will enhance the excretion of the tricyclics, the increase in urine output is minimal and there is a possibility of increasing the risk from systemic tricyclic toxicity. Although dialysis and hemoperfusion have been reported to be effective,[127,129-132] they should not be attempted because the volume of distribution is so large that there is no significant retrieval of material.[15,30,129,133] Charcoal hemoperfusion binds almost all the drug passing through the device but is limited in usefulness because most of the ingested drug is located in the body tissue pool, not in the blood.[30] The degree of protein binding also precludes a satisfactory removal of the drug (Table 11-14).[127]

DELAYED TOXICITY

Tricyclic overdose is widely believed to be associated with late sudden cardiac dysrhythmias. Deaths from cardiac dysrhythmia have been reported to occur as long as 5 days after ingestion.[124,134] Most patients who developed these late cardiac complications have had severe overdoses that previously required treatment. In addition, these cases did not occur after a 24-hour period of electrocardiographic normalization. Recent reports concerning delayed complications after tricyclic overdose do not support the development of delayed complications after a symptom-free period of 24 hours.[1,2,14,49,135]

In the patient who is awake and alert after an acute overdose and who does not develop any clinical signs of tricyclic overdose after 6 hours, delayed dysrhythmias are unlikely.[14] In the previously symptomatic patient, an observation period of 12 to 24 hours after recovery appears to be adequate.[136]

SUMMARY OF EFFECTS, TREATMENT, AND RECOMMENDATIONS

Sinus tachycardia is a sensitive indicator of tricyclic anticholinergic effect but an insensitive marker of the development of serious toxicity. These dysrhythmias are due to the anticholinergic effects of the tricyclics in conjunction with the blocking of the reuptake of norepinephrine. Unless they cause severe hemodynamic changes, they need not be treated. If necessary, physostigmine may be effective. It should be kept in mind that sinus tachycardia with QRS prolongation may be difficult to distinguish from ventricular tachycardia.

Table 11-14 Drugs and Procedures Contraindicated for Tricyclic Overdose

---

Class Ia Antidysrhythmics
  Quinidine
  Procainamide
  Disopyramide
Forced Diuresis
Dialysis
  Hemodialysis
  Peritoneal dialysis
Hemoperfusion

Supraventricular tachydysrhythmias, in contrast to sinus tachycardia, is relatively uncommon with tricylic intoxication.

Ventricular tachydysrhythmias are caused by increased sympathetic activity in conjunction with the direct depressant quinidine-like action of the tricyclics. Sodium bicarbonate (0.5 to 2 mEq/kg) is suggested as a first-line drug to raise the arterial *p*H to 7.50 to 7.55.[123] Antidysrhythmic therapy should then be instituted with either lidocaine or phenytoin. Propranolol, quinidine, procainamide, disopyramide, and physostigmine should be avoided. What may appear to be ectopy may actually be intermittent aberrance due to depressed conduction.

Torsades de pointes can be treated with temporary overdrive pacing. It is not clear whether bicarbonate is effective for this condition. *Bundle branch blocks* are one of the more serious disturbances and occur because of the quinidine-like action of the tricyclics.[18] Sodium bicarbonate (0.5 to 2 mEq/kg) or hyperventilation is suggested. Phenytoin may also be effective. Although QRS prolongation alone is not compromising, it is a marker for patients at highest risk of developing seizures, dysrhythmias, or hypotension.

Bradydysrhythmias are a result of the direct myocardial depressant quinidine-like effect of the tricyclics in conjunction with depletion of neurotransmitter at the myocardium and are difficult to treat. Sodium bicarbonate may be effective for this condition, but a temporary transvenous pacemaker may be lifesaving. Although therapy with atropine can be attempted, it may be ineffective. The finding of bradycardia, rather than tachycardia, usually indicates a later course or a massive overdose, unless the patient is taking a pharmacologic β-adrenergic blocking agent.

Hypotension occurs as a result of the direct depressant quinidine-like effect of tricyclics in conjunction with a depletion of neurotransmitter and the α-adrenergic blocking action of the tricyclics. Sodium bicarbonate (0.5 to 2 mEq/kg) or hyperventilation are recommended treatments in conjunction with fluid therapy. Care must be taken not to administer excessive amounts of fluids in these patients because depressed myocardial contractility makes them particularly susceptible to fluid overload and the development of heart failure and pulmonary edema.

Norepinephrine, a direct-acting sympathomimetic, is reserved for the refractory cases because an exaggerated response may ensue. An indirectly acting agent must enter the adrenergic neuron by the same uptake mechanism as the neurotransmitter, and consequently its uptake will be blocked by the tricyclic.

Generalized *seizures* have been associated with increased mortality in tricyclic overdose and have been noted immediately before cardiac arrest. Seizure may cause significant metabolic acidemia, thereby increasing unbound tricyclic in the circulation and contributing to the development of fatal dysrhythmias.

Asymptomatic Patients

In the asymptomatic individual, methods for prevention of absorption should be attempted. The patient should be placed on a cardiac monitor and observed for a period of at least 6 to 8 hours.[14] If the patient remains completely asymptomatic, has no electrocardiographic changes, has a normal 12 lead electrocardiogram, and has been given psychiatric clearance, then he or she may be discharged. Patients demonstrating an isolated sinus tachycardia that resolves with volume repletion or time, and in whom no further signs of toxicity develop, can be medically cleared for psychiatric disposition.[19] If an isolated sinus tachycardia does not resolve, the patient should be admitted.

Symptomatic Patients

For the symptomatic individual or in one with a widened QRS interval (indicating bundle branch block), admittance to the intensive care unit is recommended so that monitoring can be continued. After the patient is awake and alert and shows no evidence of cardiovascular symptoms, monitoring should be continued for 12 to 24 hours after apparent recovery.[1,2,19,48,135]

REFERENCES

1. Goldberg R, Capone R: Cardiac complications following tricyclic antidepressant overdose. *JAMA* 1985; 254:1772–1775.

2. Goldberg M, Park G, Spector R, et al: Lack of effect of oral activated charcoal on imipramine clearance. *Clin Pharmacol Ther* 1985;38:350–353.

3. Sullivan J, Rumack B, Peterson R: Management of tricyclic antidepressant toxicity, *Top Emerg Med* 1979; 1:65–71.

4. Hollister L: Tricyclic antidepressants. *N Engl J Med* 1978;299:1106–1109.

5. Hollister L: Monitoring tricyclic antidepressant concentration. *JAMA* 1979;241:2530–2533.

6. Hollister L: Doxepin hydrochloride. *Ann Intern Med* 1974;81:360–363.

7. Hong W, Mauer P, Hochman R, et al: Amitriptyline cardiotoxicity. *Chest* 1974;66:304–306.

8. Moir D, Cornwell W, Dingwall-Fordyce I, et al: Cardiotoxicity of amitriptyline. *Lancet* 1972;2:561–564.

9. Janson P, Watt J, Hermos J: Doxepin overdose. *JAMA* 1977;237:2632–2633.

10. Stinnett J, Valentine J, Abrutyn E: Nortriptyline hydrochloride overdosage. *JAMA* 1968;204:69–71.

11. Biggs J: Clinical pharmacology and toxicology of antidepressants. *Hosp Pract* 1978;13:79–84.

12. Biggs J, Spiker D, Petit J, et al: Tricyclic antidepressant overdose. *JAMA* 1977;238:135–138.

13. Fromer D, Kulig K, Rumack B: Tricyclic antidepressant overdose: A review. *JAMA* 1987;257:521–526.

14. Boehnert M, Lovejoy F: Value of the QRS duration versus the serum drug level in predicting seizures and ventricular arrhythmias after an acute overdose of tricyclic antidepressants. *N Engl J Med* 1985;313:474–479.

15. Braden N, Jackson J, Watson P: Tricyclic antidepressant overdose. *Pediatr Clin North Am* 1986; 33:287–297.

16. Bramble M, Lishman A, Diffey B: An analysis of plasma levels and 24-hour ECG recordings in tricyclic antidepressant poisoning: Implications for management. *Q J Med* 1985;56:357–366.

17. Callaham M: Tricyclic antidepressant overdose. *JACEP* 1979;8:413–425.

18. Callaham M: Antidepressant toxicity. *Ann Emerg Med* 1986;15:1036–1038.

19. Callaham M: Admission criteria for tricyclic antidepressant ingestion. *West J Med* 1982;137:425–429.

20. Manoguerra A: Tricyclic antidepressants. *Crit Care Quart* 1982;4:43–54.

21. Manoguerra A, Weaver L: Poisoning with tricyclic antidepressant drugs. *Clin Toxicol* 1977;10:149–158.

22. Petit J, Spiker D, Ruwitch J, et al: Tricyclic antidepressant plasma levels and adverse effects after overdose. *Clin Pharmacol Ther* 1976;21:47–51.

23. Fauman M: Tricyclic antidepressant prescription by general hospital physicians. *Am J Psychiatr* 1980; 137:490–491.

24. Henn F: Suicide risk with tricyclic antidepressants. *Am Fam Physician* 1980;22:23.

25. Herson V, Schmitt B, Rumack B: Magical thinking and imipramine poisoning in two school-aged children. *JAMA* 1979;241:1926–1927.

26. Hayes T, Panitch M, Barker E: Imipramine dosage in children: A comment on "Imipramine and Electrocardiographic Abnormalities in Hyperactive Children." *Am J Psychiatr* 1975;132:546–547.

27. Saraf K, Gittelman-Klein R, Groff S: Imipramine side effects in children. *Psychopharmacologia* 1974; 37:265–274.

28. Cram L, Reisby N, Ibsen I, et al: Plasma levels and antidepressive effect of imipramine. *Clin Pharmacol Ther* 1975;19:318–324.

29. Greenblatt D, Koch-Weser J, Shader R: Multiple complications and death following protriptyline overdose. *JAMA* 1974;229:556–557.

30. Crome P, Hampel G, Vale J, et al: Hemoperfusion in treatment of drug intoxication. *Br Med J* 1978;1:174–178.

31. Crome P, Newman B: The problem of tricyclic antidepressant poisoning. *Postgrad Med J* 1979;55: 528–532.

32. Crome P, Newman B: Fatal tricyclic antidepressant poisoning. *J R Soc Med* 1979;72:649–653.

33. Crome P, Ali C: Clinical features and management of self-poisoning with newer antidepressants. *Med Toxicol* 1986;1:411–420.

34. Crome P: Poisoning due to tricyclic antidepressant overdosage: Clinical presentation and treatment. *Med Toxicol* 1986;1:261–285.

35. Burks J, Walker J, Rumack B, et al: Tricyclic antidepressant poisoning. *JAMA* 1974;230:1405–1407.

36. Coccaro E, Siever L: Second generation antidepressants: A comparative review. *J Clin Pharmacol* 1985; 25:241–260.

37. Montgomery S: Development of new treatments for depression. *J Clin Psychiatr* 1985;46:3–6.

38. Gram L: Metabolism of tricyclic antidepressants. *Dan Med Bull* 1974;21:218–231.

39. Gram L: Factors influencing the metabolism of tricyclic antidepressants. *Dan Med Bull* 1977;24:81–88.

40. Gram L, Reisby N, Ibsen I, et al: Plasma levels and antidepressive effect of imipramine. *Clin Pharmacol Ther* 1976;19:318–324.

41. Christiansen J, Gram L: Imipramine and its metabolites in human brain. *J Pharm Pharmacol* 1973; 25:604–608.

42. Amsterdam J, Brunswick D, Mednels J: The clinical application of tricyclic antidepressant pharmacokinetics and plasma levels. *Am J Psychiatr* 1980;137:653–662.

43. Moody J: Some aspects of the metabolism of tricyclic antidepressants. *Postgrad Med J* 1976;52:59–61.

44. Knapp H, Hanenson I, Walle T, et al: Studies on the disposition of amitriptyline and other tricyclic antidepressant drugs in man as it relates to the management of the overdosed patient. *Adv Biochem Psychopharmacol* 1973;7:95–105.

45. Richelson E: Tricyclic antidepressants—Drugs for other diseases. *Arch Intern Med* 1982;142:231–232.

46. Bigger J, Giardina E, Kantor S, et al: Cardiac antiarrhythmic effects of imipramine hydrochloride. *N Engl J Med* 1977;296:206–208.

47. Bigger J, Kantor S, Glassman A, et al: Is physostigmine effective for cardiac toxicity of tricyclic antidepressant drugs? *JAMA* 1977;237:1311.

48. Pentel P, Benowitz N: Tricyclic antidepressant poisoning: Management of arrhythmias. *Med Toxicol* 1986; 1:101–121.

49. Pentel P, Sioris L: Incidence of late arrhythmias following tricyclic overdose. *Clin Toxicol* 1981; 18:543–548.

50. Glassman A: Bigger J: Cardiovascular effects of therapeutic doses of tricyclic antidepressants—A review. *Arch Gen Psychiatr* 1981;38:815–820.

51. Nitter L, Haraldsson A, Holck P, et al: The effect of trimipramine on the healing of peptic ulcer: A double-blind study. *Scand J Gastroenterol* 1977;12:39–41.

52. Wetterhus S, Aubert E, Berg C, et al: The effect of trimipramine on symptoms and healing of peptic ulcer: A double-blind study. *Scand J Gastroenterol* 1977;12:33–38.

53. Mangla J, Pereira M: Tricyclic antidepressants in the treatment of peptic ulcer disease. *Arch Intern Med* 1982; 142:273–275.

54. Siomopoulos V, Seneczko L: Heterocyclic antidepressants in nonpsychiatric disorders. *Am Fam Pract* 1984;29:203–208.

55. Winsberg B, Goldstein S, Yepes L, et al: Imipramine and electrocardiographic abnormalities in hyperactive children. *Am J Psychiatr* 1975;132:542–545.

56. Wedin G, Oderda G, Klein-Schwartz W, et al: Relative toxicity of cyclic antidepressants. *Ann Emerg Med* 1986; 15:797–804.

57. Rudorfer M: Tricyclic antidepressant plasma levels in overdose. *JAMA* 1981;245:703–704.

58. Rudorfer M, Golden R, Potter W: Second-generation antidepressants. *Psychiatr Clin North Am* 1984; 7:519–534.

59. Rudorfer M: Cardiovascular changes and plasma drug levels after amitriptyline overdose. *J Toxicol Clin Toxicol* 1982;19:67–78.

60. Kulig K, Rumack B, Sullivan J, et al: Amoxapine overdose—Coma and seizures without cardiotoxic effects. *JAMA* 1982;248:1092–1094.

61. Kulig K: Management of poisoning associated with ''newer'' antidepressant agents. *Ann Emerg Med* 1986; 15:1039–1045.

62. Litovitz T, Troutman W: Amoxapine overdose—Seizures and fatalities. *JAMA* 1983;250:1069–1071.

63. Shepherd G, Kerr F: Maprotiline hydrochloride and grand mal seizures. *Br Med J* 1978;1:1523–1525.

64. Northrup L, Reed G, McAnalley B, et al: Seizures due to maprotiline overdose. *Ann Emerg Med* 1984; 13:468–470.

65. Lesar T, Kingston R, Dahms R, et al: Trazodone overdose. *Ann Emerg Med* 1983;12:221–223.

66. Ali C, Henry J: Trazodone overdosage: Experience over 5 years. *Neuropsychobiology* 1986;15:44–45.

67. Alexander C, Nino A: Cardiovascular complications in young patients taking psychotropic drugs. *Am Heart J* 1969;78:757–769.

68. Stewart R: Tricyclic antidepressant poisoning. *Am Fam Physician* 1979;19:136–144.

69. Ostrow D: The new generation antidepressants: Promising innovations or disappointments? *J Clin Psychiatr* 1985;46:25–30.

70. Abbott R: Hyponatremia due to antidepressant medications. *Ann Emerg Med* 1983;12:708–710.

71. Jefferson J: A review of the cardiovascular effects and toxicity of tricyclic antidepressants. *Psychosom Med* 1975;37:160–179.

72. Veith R, Raskind M, Caldwell J, et al: Cardiovascular effects of tricyclic antidepressants in depressed patients with chronic heart disease. *N Engl J Med* 1982;306: 954–959.

73. Stern S, Mendels J: Withdrawal symptoms during the course of imipramine therapy. *J Clin Psychiatry* 1980; 41:66–67.

74. Sathananthan G, Gershon S: Imipramine withdrawal: An akathisia-like syndrome. *Am J Psychiatr* 1973; 130:1286–1287.

75. Mayron R, Ruiz E: Phenytoin: Does it reverse tricyclic antidepressant–induced cardiac conduction abnormalities? *Ann Emerg Med* 1986;15:876–880.

76. McAlpine S, Calabro J, Robinson M, et al: Late death in tricyclic antidepressant overdose revisited. *Ann Emerg Med* 1986;15:1349–1352.

77. Henry J, Volans G: Psychoactive drugs. *Br Med J* 1984;289:1291–1294.

78. Steel C, O'Duffy J, Brown S: Clinical effects and treatment of imipramine and amitriptyline poisoning in children. *Br Med J* 1967;3:663–667.

79. Noble J, Matthew H: Acute poisoning by tricyclic antidepressants: Clinical features and management of one hundred patients. *Clin Toxicol* 1969;2:403–421.

80. Spiker D, Wiess A, Chang S, et al: Tricyclic antidepressant overdose: Clinical presentation and plasma levels. *Clin Pharmacol Ther* 1975;18:539–546.

81. Spiker D, Biggs J: Tricyclic antidepressants. *JAMA* 1976;236:1711–1712.

82. Flomenbaum N, Price D: Recognition and management of antidepressant overdoses: Tricyclics and trazodone. *Neuropsychobiology* 1986;15:46–51.

83. Sasyniuk B, Jharmandas V, Valois M: Experimental amitriptyline intoxication: Treatment of cardiac toxicity with sodium bicarbonate. *Ann Emerg Med* 1986;15:1052–1059.

84. Vohra J, Burrows G, Sloman G: Assessment of cardiovascular side effects of therapeutic doses of tricyclic antidepressant drugs. *Aust N Z J Med* 1975;5:7–11.

85. Vohra J, Burrows G, Hunt D, et al: The effect of toxic and therapeutic drugs on intracardiac conduction. *Eur J Cardiol* 1975;3:219–227.

86. Tarve V, Brechtlova M: Effect of psychopharmacological agents on brain metabolism: Part III: Effects of imipramine and ouabain on the (Na and K) activated ATPase from brain microsomes and cooperative interactions with the enzyme. *J Neurochem* 1967;14:283–290.

87. Smith W, Gallagher J: Les torsades de pointes: An unusual ventricular arrhythmia. *Ann Intern Med* 1980; 93:578–583.

88. Tobis J, Aronow W: Effect of amitriptyline antidotes on repetitive extrasystole threshold. *Clin Pharmacol Ther* 1980;27:602–606.

89. Tobis J, Das B: Cardiac complications in amitriptyline poisoning. *JAMA* 1976;235:1474–1476.

90. Kantor S, Bigger J, Glassman A, et al: Imipramine-induced heart block: A longitudinal case study. *JAMA* 1975; 231:1364–1366.

91. Emermon C, Connors A, Burma G: Level of consciousness as a predictor of complications following tricyclic overdose. *Ann Emerg Med* 1987;16:326–330.

92. Rumack B: Anticholinergic poisoning: Treatment with physostigmine. *Pediatrics* 1973;52:449–451.

93. Rumack B: Physostigmine use in drug overdose questioned. *JACEP* 1975;4:555–556.

94. Raisfeld I: Cardiovascular complications of antidepressant therapy: Interactions at the adrenergic neuron. *Am Heart J* 1972;83:129–133.

95. Ramanathan K, Davidson, C: Cardiac arrhythmia and imipramine therapy. *Br Med J* 1975;1:661–662.

96. Langou R, Van Dyke C, Tahan S, et al: Cardiovascular manifestations of tricyclic antidepressant overdose. *Am Heart J* 1980;100:458–464.

97. Dumovic P, Burrows G, Vohra J, et al: The effect of tricyclic antidepressant drugs on the heart. *Arch Toxicol* 1976;35:255–262.

98. Gaultier M, Boissier J, Barceix A, et al: The cardiotoxicity of imipramine in man. *Eur Soc Study Drug Toxicol* 1965;6:174–178.

99. Marshall A, Moore K: Pulmonary disease after amitriptyline overdosage. *Br Med J* 1973;1:716–717.

100. Marshall J, Forker A: Tricyclic antidepressant overdose: Clinical and cardiovascular features. *Nebr Med J* 1980; 65:77–80.

101. Robinson D, Barker E: Tricyclic antidepressant cardiotoxicity. *JAMA* 1976;236:2089–2090.

102. Foulke G, Albertson T: QRS interval in tricyclic antidepressant overdosage: Inaccuracy as a toxicity indicator in emergency settings. *Ann Emerg Med* 1987;16:160–163.

103. Asberg M: Plasma nortriptyline levels—Relationship to clinical effects. *Clin Pharmacol Ther* 1974; 16:215–229.

104. Hackett L, Dusci L: The use of high-performance liquid chromatography in clinical toxicology: Tricyclic antidepressants. *Clin Toxicol* 1979;15:55–61.

105. Rossi G: Pharmacology of tricyclic antidepressants. *Am J Pharmacol* 1976;148:37–45.

106. Jatlow P: Therapeutic monitoring of plasma concentrations of tricyclic antidepressants. *Arch Pathol Lab Med* 1980;104:341–344.

107. Starkey I, Lawson A: Poisoning with tricyclic and related antidepressants—A ten-year review. *Q J Med* 1980; 49:33–49.

108. Gard H, Knapp D, Walla T, et al: Qualitative and quantitative studies on the disposition of amitriptyline and other tricyclic antidepressants in man as it relates to the management of the overdosed patient. *Clin Toxicol* 1973; 6:571–584.

109. Granscher R, Baldessarini R: Physostigmine. *Arch Gen Psychiatr* 1975;32:375–379.

110. Slovis T, Ott J, Teitelbaum D, et al: Physostigmine therapy in acute tricyclic antidepressant poisoning. *Clin Toxicol* 1971;4:451–459.

111. Brashares Z, Conley W: Physostigmine in drug overdose. *JACEP* 1975;4:46–48.

112. Lum B, Follmer C, Lockwood R, et al: Experimental studies on the effects of physostigmine and of isoproterenol on toxicity produced by tricyclic antidepressant agents. *J Toxicol Clin Toxicol* 1982;19:51–65.

113. Goldberger A, Curtis G: Immediate effects of physostigmine on amitriptyline-induced QRS prolongation. *J Toxicol Clin Toxicol* 1982;19:445–454.

114. Spoerke D, Hall A, Dodson C, et al: Mystery root ingestion. *J Emerg Med* 1987;5:385–388.

115. Pentel P, Peterson C: Asystole complicating physostigmine treatment of tricyclic antidepressant overdose. *Ann Emerg Med* 1980;9:588–590.

116. Bessen H, Niemann J: Improvement of cardiac conduction after hyperventilation in tricyclic antidepressant overdose. *Clin Toxicol* 1986;23:537–546.

117. Nattel S: Physostigmine in coma due to drug overdose. *Clin Pharmacol Ther* 1979;25:96–102.

118. Kingston M: Hyperventilation in tricyclic antidepressant poisoning. *Crit Care Med* 1979;7:550–551.

119. Brown T, Leversha A: Comparison of the cardiovascular toxicity of three tricyclic antidepressant drugs: Imipramine, amitriptyline, and doxepin. *Clin Toxicol* 1979; 14:253–256.

120. Brown T, Barker G, Dunlop M, et al: The use of sodium bicarbonate in the treatment of tricyclic antidepressant-induced arrhythmias. *Anaesth Intensive Care* 1973; 1:203–210.

121. Hoffman J, McElroy C: Bicarbonate therapy for dysrhythmia and hypotension in tricyclic antidepressant overdose. *West J Med* 1981;134:60–64.

122. Hedges J, Baker P, Tasset J, et al: Bicarbonate therapy for the cardiovascular toxicity of amitriptyline in an animal model. *J Emerg Med* 1985;3:253–260.

123. Pentel P, Benowitz N: Efficacy and mechanism of action of sodium bicarbonate in the treatment of desipramine toxicity in rats. *J Pharmacol Exp Ther* 1984;230:12–19.

124. Freeman J, Loughhead M: β Blockade in the treatment of tricyclic antidepressant overdosage. *Med J Aust* 1973;1:1233–1235.

125. Freeman J, Mundy G, Beattie R, et al: Cardiac abnormalities in poisoning with tricyclic antidepressants. *Br Med J* 1969;2:610–611.

126. Uhl J: Phenytoin: The drug of choice in tricyclic antidepressant overdose? *Ann Emerg Med* 1981; 10:270–274.

127. Hagerman G, Hanashiro P: Reversal of tricyclic antidepressant–induced cardiac conduction abnormalities by phenytoin. *Ann Emerg Med* 1981;10:82–86.

128. Harthorne W, Marcus A, Kaye M: Management of massive imipramine overdosage with mannitol and artificial dialysis. *N Engl J Med* 1963;268:33–36.

129. Baake O, Iversen B, Willassen Y: Charcoal hemoperfusion in nortriptyline poisoning. *Lancet* 1978; 1:388–389.

130. Diaz-Buxo J, Farmer C, Chandler J: Hemoperfusion in the treatment of amitriptyline intoxication. *Trans Am Soc Artif Intern Organs* 1978;24:699.

131. Marbury T, Mahoney J, Fuller L, et al: Treatment of amitriptyline overdose with charcoal hemoperfusion. *Kidney Int* 1977;12:458–461.

132. Pederson R, Jorgenson K, Oelsen A, et al: Charcoal hemoperfusion and antidepressant overdose. *Lancet* 1978; 1:719–722.

133. Pentel P, Bullock M, Devane C: Hemoperfusion for imipramine overdose: Elimination of active metabolites. *J Toxicol Clin Toxicol* 1982;19:239–248.

134. Sedal L, Korman M, Williams P, et al: Overdosage of tricyclic antidepressants: A report of two deaths and a prospective study of twenty-four patients. *Med J Aust* 1972; 2:74–79.

135. Greenland P, Howe T: Cardiac monitoring in tricyclic antidepressant overdose. *Heart Lung* 1981;10: 856–859.

136. Fasoli R, Glauser F: Cardiac arrhythmias and ECG abnormalities in tricyclic antidepressant overdose. *Clin Toxicol* 1981;18:155–163.

ADDITIONAL SELECTED REFERENCES

Boakes A, Laurence D, Teoh P, et al: Interactions between sympathomimetic amines and antidepressant agents in man. *Br Med J* 1973;1:311–315.

Cain N, Cain R: A compendium of antidepressants. *Clin Toxicol* 1979;14:545–574.

Collis M, Shepherd J: Antidepressant drug action and pre-synaptic α receptors, *Mayo Clin Proc* 1980;55:567–572.

Crocker J, Morton B: Tricyclic antidepressant drug toxicity. *Clin Toxicol* 1969;2:397–402.

Desautels S, Filteau C, St Jean A: Ventricular tachycardia associated with administration of thioridazine hydrochloride. *Can Med Assoc J* 1964;99:1030–1031.

El-Hage A, Balazs T, West W: Protective effects of clonidine and verapamil in experimental amitriptyline poisoning in rabbits. *J Toxicol Clin Toxicol* 1982; 19:321–335.

Goldfrank L, Melinek M: Locoweed and other anticholinergics. *Hosp Physician* 1979;8:18–26,39.

Goldfrank L, Flomenbaum N, Lewin N: Anticholinergic poisoning. *J Toxicol Clin Toxicol* 1982;19:17–25.

Hudson C: Tricyclic antidepressants and alcoholic blackouts. *J Nerv Ment Dis* 1981;169:381–382.

Hussey H: Physostigmine: Value in treatment of central toxic effects of anticholinergic drugs. *JAMA* 1975;231:1066.

Kleber H, Weissman M, Rounsaville B, et al: Imipramine as treatment for depression in addicts. *Arch Gen Psychiatr* 1983;40:649–653.

Lepor S: Antidepressant drug overdose. *Emergency* 1983; 15:36–39.

Lindstroem F, Flodmark O, Gustafsson B: Respiratory distress syndrome and thrombotic, nonbacterial endocarditis after amitriptyline overdose. *Acta Med Scand* 1977; 202:203–212.

Lundberg G: Antidepressant drugs as a cause of death: A call for caution and data. *JAMA* 1982;248:1879.

Meador-Woodruff J, Grunhaus L: Profound behavioral toxicity due to tricyclic antidepressants. *J Nerv Ment Dis* 1986;174:628–629.

Smith R, O'Mara K: Tricyclic antidepressant overdose. *J Fam Pract* 1982;15:247–253.

Thompson T, Cardoni A: Tricyclic antidepressant overdose: Case report and review of the literature. *Poison Inf Bull* 1977;2:1–9.

Thorstrand C: Cardiovascular effects of poisoning with tricyclic antidepressants. *Acta Med Scand* 1974;195: 505–514.

Uhlenhuth E: Depressives, doctors, and antidepressants. *JAMA* 1982;248:1879–1880.

Woodhead R: Cardiac rhythm in tricyclic antidepressant poisoning. *Clin Toxicol* 1979;14:499–505.

chapter 12

The Neuroleptic-Antipsychotic Agents

Of all the psychotropic drugs, the neuroleptic agents are the most important in psychiatry. The major chemical classes of neuroleptic agents are the phenothiazines, butyrophenones, and thioxanthenes, and there are miscellaneous agents such as loxapine and molindone. The phenothiazines evolved from the aniline dyes and antihistamines, and the butyrophenones evolved from the meperidine-like analgesics. These agents are used primarily to treat psychotic disorders in adults and children. They are called neuroleptic agents because of their ability to cause a change in affect, with emotional quieting, psychomotor slowing, disinterest in surroundings, and decreased aggression and impulsivity. These drugs have a marked effect on thought disturbances associated with paranoid ideation, delusions, anxiety, and agitation.[1] These drugs do not merely sedate or calm patients; they exert a selective antischizophrenic action.

CLINICAL USES

Neuroleptic agents are widely used in various settings, including treatment of acute nausea and vomiting, as an adjunct to narcotic analgesia, for intractable hiccups, for relief of severe itching, treatment of acute intermittent porphyria, as antitussive agents, and for sedation.[1,2] In psychiatric patients, neuroleptic agents are employed in the treatment of acute and chronic schizophrenia, organic mental disorders, anxiety disorders, mixed anxiety-depressive illness, and anxiety-agitation accompanying dementia (Table 12-1). These drugs are associated with a wide variety of side effects.[2]

There are more than 20 phenothiazine derivatives available for clinical use. They have a basic three-ring structure and can be categorized in three major classes: the aliphatic derivatives, of which chlorpromazine and triflupromazine are the most widely used; the piperazine group, which includes fluphenazine, prochlorperazine, and trifluoperazine; and piperidine derivatives, which include thioridazine and mepazine (Table 12-2).[3] The thioxanthenes are derivatives of the phenothiazines. The butyrophenones are structurally unrelated to the phenothiazines, but their pharmacological actions are similar.

The physical, chemical, pharmacologic, and toxicologic properties of the various phe-

Table 12-1 Uses of Neuroleptic Agents

Antipsychotic agent
Treatment of nausea and vomiting
Preanesthetic medication
Adjunct to narcotic analgesia
Relief of itching
Antitussive agent
Sedation

Table 12-2 The Neuroleptic Agents

Compound	Derivatives (Trade Names)
Butyrophenones	Haloperidol (Haldol®)
	Droperidol (Innovar®, Inapsine®)
Phenothiazines	Aliphatic
	Chlorpromazine (Thorazine®, Chloramead®)
	Promazine (Sparine®, Prozine®)
	Promethazine (Phenergan®)
	Triflupromazine (Vesprin®)
	Piperidine
	Mesoridazine (Serentil®, Lidanar®)
	Piperacetazine (Quide®)
	Thioridazine (Mellaril®)
	Piperazine
	Acetophenazine (Tindal®)
	Butaperizine (Repoise®)
	Carphenazine (Prokethazine®)
	Fluphenazine (Prolixin®, Permitil®)
	Perphenazine (Trilafon®, Etrafon®, Triavil®)
	Prochlorperazine (Compazine®)
	Thiethylperazine (Torecan®)
	Trifluoperazine (Stelazine®)
Thioxanthenes	Chlorprothixene (Taractan®)
	Thiothixene (Navane®)
Dibenzoxepine	Loxapine (Loxitane®, Daxolin®)
Dihydroindolone	Molindone (Moban®, Lidone®)
Miscellaneous	Methoxypromazine
	Pipamazine

nothiazines are generally similar, but the relative potencies and the nature of their toxicity depend on the chemical substitutions. Piperazine derivatives, for example, are more potent as antiemetics, antipsychotics, and extrapyramidal syndrome inducers than the aliphatic and piperidine derivatives, but they have less potent hypotensive, anticholinergic, and sedative actions.[2]

ACTIONS

The pharmacology of the antipsychotic agents are complex because the drugs may affect many different sites in the body. The major pharmacologic action of the phenothiazines is on the central and autonomic nervous system, the cardiovascular system, the endocrine glands, and body metabolism.

The neuroleptic agents are antidopaminergics to varying degrees.[2] Dopamine is one of the two principal catecholamines in the brain. Receptors for dopamine occur most prominently in the reticular formation of the brainstem, the hypothalamus, the limbic system, and the basal ganglia. Blocking of the postsynaptic dopamine receptor site in the limbic system and basal ganglia is thought to account for the antipsychotic activity of the neuroleptic agents. Receptor blockade results in decreased enzyme activity with decreased cell firing and increased production rate of dopamine metabolites.

Other important physiologic properties of the neuroleptics are peripheral cholinergic blockade (anticholinergic), α-adrenergic blockade, membrane-stabilizing activity, blocking of the reuptake of norepinephrine in the peripheral synapses, serotonergenic action, and antihistaminic (H_1 receptor) action (Table 12-3).[2] Each of the neuroleptic agents differs in the degree of pharmacologic activity (Table 12-4). The effects of the neuroleptics on the autonomic nervous system are therefore complex and unpredictable because the drugs exert varying degrees of effects on many areas of the autonomic nervous system.

The phenothiazines act as potent central antiemetics by depressing the chemoreceptor trigger zone in the medulla. These drugs effectively antagonize centrally induced emesis but have no effect on emesis caused by gastrointestinal irritation or vestibular stimulation. The piperazines have a potent antiemetic effect, and thioridazine, a piperidine derivative, has no antiemetic properties.

PHARMACOKINETICS

The neuroleptics can be administered by intravenous, intramuscular, oral, and rectal routes.[1] Intramuscular absorption is variable, and some neuroleptics may cause profound hypotension when administered by this route. The neuroleptics are highly plasma protein bound (more than 90%) and lipophilic. These agents also have a large volume of distribution (more than 20 L/kg), which accounts for the large amount of

Table 12-3 Pharmacologic Actions of Neuroleptic Agents

Antidopaminergic
Anticholinergic
α-Adrenergic blockade
Antihistaminic (H_1 receptor)
Antiemetic
Membrane stabilization

---

these agents within tissues.[2] The neuroleptics are metabolized extensively in the liver by glucuronidization and sulfoxidation. There are many metabolites formed, some of which are pharmacologically active. Typically, plasma concentrations reach their peak within 2 to 4 hours of oral administration, and there is little correlation among dose, serum concentration, and antipsychotic effect.[4]

TOXIC EFFECTS

Neuroleptic agents are usually quite safe when taken in significant overdose, although abnormal electrocardiograms and sudden death of patients receiving standard therapeutic doses have been reported. Deaths have been most frequently reported in cases of overdose with thioridazine[5] and mesoridazine (a metabolite of thioridazine)[6,7] or when phenothiazines are taken in excessive amounts together with decongestants, antihistamines, or tricyclic agents. Deaths have been attributed to cardiac dysrhythmias,[8] vasodilation, hypotension, hyperpyrexia, and aspiration.

Toxicity of the neuroleptic agents can be broadly categorized into three major presentations: (1) acute or chronic overdose, (2) extrapyramidal manifestations, and (3) neuroleptic malignant syndrome.

Acute or Chronic Overdose

An acute or chronic overdose of neuroleptic agents may produce both cardiovascular and CNS toxicity. The cardiovascular effects are complex because the drugs exert both direct cardiac toxicity, described as a local anesthetic effect, as well as indirect actions on the heart and vasculature.[9] The indirect actions include peripheral vascular effects as well as a combination of autonomic changes produced by anticholinergic and antiadrenergic actions.

Cardiac Complications

The most common cardiovascular complication is orthostatic hypotension. In addition, neuroleptics are known to have a pronounced effect on the electrocardiogram, with changes includ-

Table 12-4 Comparison of Effects of Phenothiazines

Compound	Antiemetic	Antimuscarinic	Extrapyramidal	Hypotensive	Sedative
Aliphatic					
Chlorpromazine	+ + +	+ + +	+ +	+ + +	+ + +
Promazine	+ +	+ + +	+ +	+ + +	+ + +
Triflupromazine	+ + +	+ + +	+ +	+ +	+ +
Piperidine					
Mesoridazine	+	+ +	+	+ +	+ + +
Piperacetazine	+	+	+ +	+ +	+
Thioridazine	+	+ + +	+	+ +	+ + +
Piperazine					
Acetophenazine	+	+	+ +	+	+ +
Carphenazine	+	+	+ + +	+	+ +
Fluphenazine	+	+	+ + +	+	+
Perphenazine	+ + +	+ +	+ + +	+	+
Prochlorperazine	+ + +	+	+ + +	+	+ +
Trifluoperazine	+ + +	+	+ + +	+	+

ing prolongation of PR and QT intervals, slurring and notching of the T wave, and mild ST segment changes. These changes have been described as a quinidine-like effect. The hypotension seen with the neuroleptics may be due to the α-adrenergic blocking activity in combination with the quinidine-like action on the myocardium.

The incidence of serious complications or deaths resulting from neuroleptic overdose is quite low. Death from cardiac complications is of two types, both of which are considered rare. The first is death from acute overdose,[10] and the second is the sudden death of patients receiving standard doses of neuroleptic agents.[4,11] The cardiovascular manifestation of neuroleptic intoxication may include dysrhythmias such as atrioventricular dissociation, supraventricular tachycardia, ventricular tachycardia, and ventricular fibrillation.[4] The neuroleptics also have a negative inotropic effect on the myocardium. Thioridazine in particular is associated with severe electrocardiographic and adverse cardiac effects. Most reported ventricular dysrhythmias have occurred in patients taking these drugs as long-term therapy rather than after an acute overdose.

Eye Effects

Although mydriasis may be expected, miosis may also be seen. This is observed most often in the severely poisoned patient and may serve as a clinical clue to the severity of the overdose. Miosis represents an overriding of the atropine effect by the α-adrenergic blocking effect of these agents.

Seizure Threshold

The neuroleptics may also lower the seizure threshold and induce a discharge pattern associated with seizure disorders. Overt seizures may occur in patients with a history of seizure disorder.

Hyperthermia or Hypothermia

Neuroleptics have a poikilothermic effect; that is, they interfere with temperature regulation in the hypothalamus. Depending on environmental conditions, hyperthermia or hypothermia may occur. Hypothermia is most often seen with haloperidol and hyperthermia with a phenothiazine.

Treatment

The treatment of overdose with a neuroleptic agent is mostly supportive. Monitoring and support of respiratory and cardiovascular function are of primary importance. Immediate discontinuance of the agent, initiating measures to reduce the patient's fever, hydration, and vigorous monitoring of vital signs, neurologic status, fluid status, and renal function are necessary. After acute neuroleptic overdoses the potential for cardiac dysrhythmias, particularly ventricular tachydysrhythmias, should be considered, and patients should be monitored for at least 48 hours.

Syrup of ipecac has been shown to be effective in countering antiemetic effects. Lavage, even long after ingestion, may be effective because the anticholinergic effect of these agents delays gastric emptying and because neuroleptics are water soluble and therefore slowly absorbed from the gastrointestinal tract.[6] Activated charcoal and a cathartic should follow ipecac or lavage.

Phenytoin or lidocaine should be used for treatment of ventricular dysrhythmias. Drugs such as quinidine or procainamide should not be given because they will add to the quinidine effect of the neuroleptics. A pacemaker may be of value in the treatment of ventricular dysrhythmias that are unresponsive to antidysrhythmic drugs.

Because of the large volume of distribution and extensive tissue binding of these agents, hemodialysis, hemoperfusion, and forced diuresis are ineffective in enhancing elimination.[6]

Extrapyramidal Manifestations

Acute dystonic reactions, parkinsonism, and akathisia are extrapyramidal syndromes that may appear after antipsychotic drug therapy.[12] These signs occur with an acute ingestion or are side effects of long-term treatment. They may be noted within 20 minutes after ingestion of a single therapeutic dose or be delayed in onset up to 72 hours or more, or they appear intermittently.[11] These reactions often resemble symptoms of Parkinson's disease. Acute dystonic reactions, sometimes referred to as dyskinetic reactions, are involuntary tonic contractions of muscles that may occur suddenly and intermittently. Normal mentation is maintained.[13]

Pathogenesis

Extrapyramidal symptoms are the result of the disruption of the dopaminergic-cholinergic balance in the corpus striatum neurons, which results in dopamine blockade with a compensatory increase in acetylcholine activity and cholinergic dominance.[13] In the extrapyramidal system, especially the basal ganglia, acetylcholine is an excitatory transmitter and dopamine is an inhibitory transmitter.[14] Under normal conditions, the cholinergic-dopaminergic system maintains physiologic balance, which results in coordinated neuromuscular activity. When a patient takes a therapeutic dose of a neuroleptic, blockade of the dopamine receptors occurs, especially in the nitrostriatal system.[15] The acetylcholine neurotransmitters become dominant and overactive after sudden withdrawal of the dopaminergic inhibition, which leads to an acute dystonic reaction.[12]

Neuroleptics vary considerably in their ability to elicit such reactions. Neuroleptics with antidopaminergic activity far in excess of their anticholinergic potency are responsible for the greatest incidence of dystonic side effects. Piperazine phenothiazines such as trifluoperazine and fluphenazine, and butyrophenones such as haloperidol, are associated with a high incidence of such side effects. In contrast, thioridazine has a low incidence of extrapyramidal reactions. Young children tend to be prone to extrapyramidal signs and to have generalized manifestations, whereas adolescents and adults tend to have signs localized to the face and trunk. Nonneuroleptic compounds have also caused acute dystonic reactions, probably as a result of dopamine blocking effects of the compounds.[12] Nonphenothiazine antiemetics such as metoclopramide (Reglan®) and trimethobenzamide (Tigan®) have also produced dystonic reactions. Antihistamines and antipar-

kinsonism agents, although used to treat acute dystonic reactions, have also been reported to cause this reaction.[16–19]

Clinical Features

Acute dystonic reactions may be sudden in onset and consist of bizarre muscular spasms. The muscles of the head and neck are predominantly affected. Involvement of pharyngeal muscles may lead to dysarthria, dysphagia, sialorrhea, and grimacing (Table 12-5). The neck muscles are also frequently affected; thus opisthotonus and torticollis can occur and may be associated with oculogyric crisis or spasm of the external ocular muscles with painful upward gaze persisting for minutes to hours.[20] Akathisia, or the subjective desire to be in constant motion, may also be noted. Parkinsonism may also be noted as motor retardation, depression, masklike facial expression, tremor at rest, "pill-rolling" movements of the fingers, rigidity, salivation, and a shuffling gate. In most instances, spontaneous recovery occurs within 24 hours after discontinuance of the agent.

Treatment

Treatment consists of either restoring dopaminergic function by discontinuing the neuroleptic or giving the patient anticholinergic medication to alleviate the enhanced cholinergic function (or both). Dystonic reactions are reversed rapidly with several agents. Resolution of symptoms after administration of these agents is not only therapeutic but establishes the diagnosis when a clear history of recent drug ingestion is not available.[12]

Table 12-5 Extrapyramidal Signs from Neuroleptic Agents

Akathisia
Buccolingual incoordination
Dysphagia
Grimacing
Oculogyric crisis
Opisthotonus
Parkinsonism
Sialorrhea
Torticollis

The extrapyramidal symptoms in most cases respond to intravenous diphenhydramine (Benadryl®, 25 to 50 mg) or benztropine (Cogentin®, 1 to 2 mg). These agents are generally successful in 2 to 5 minutes.[21] The recommended route of administration for these agents is intravenous or intramuscular, although oral administration has shown good results. The almost immediate relief of symptoms after the initial treatment has been thought to obviate the need for continued outpatient treatment, but relapses of dyskinesia may occur. For this reason at least 48 to 72 hours of outpatient treatment is necessary.[12,13] Trihexyphenidyl (Artane®, Tremin®) is not suggested for immediate treatment because it is not available in an injectable form. Outpatient therapy of trihexyphenidyl may consist of 2-mg doses twice daily.

Neuroleptic Malignant Syndrome

An uncommon but potentially life-threatening adverse effect of antipsychotic agents, called the neuroleptic malignant syndrome,[3] has been recently recognized.[22,23] It is the rarest and least known of the complications of neuroleptic drug therapy.[24] The infrequent recognition of this disorder may be due to a lack of awareness of it on the part of many physicians.[25]

Signs and Symptoms

The clinical features of this syndrome may evolve over 24 to 72 hours and may consist of fluctuating mental status progressing to coma and extrapyramidal symptoms, especially muscle rigidity, autonomic instability, and altered level of consciousness (Table 12-6). The autonomic instability has been described as labile hypertension, profound vasoconstriction, tachycardia, and severe diaphoresis.[24] Hyperthermia appears to be caused by a disturbance of central thermal regulation in combination with the heat generated from intense central nervous system–mediated muscular contraction. Temperatures higher than 40°C may create irreversible cell damage affecting many tissues and organs, including brain, muscle, and kidney.[3] Mortality attributable to cardiac or respiratory failure may reach 20% and is related to the duration and severity of symptoms,[15,26–28] so

Table 12-6 Signs and Symptoms of Neuroleptic Malignant Syndrome

Muscle Rigidity
Extrapyramidal Effects
  Tremor
  Dysarthria
  Dysphagia
Autonomic Instability
  Hyperthermia
  Labile hypertension
  Vasoconstriction
  Pallor
  Sialorrhea
  Tachycardia
  Diaphoresis
Altered Level of Consciousness

that early recognition and prompt treatment are top priorities.

The syndrome typically begins with diffuse muscle rigidity often accompanied by extrapyramidal symptoms of tremor, dysarthria, or dysphagia.[3] Hyperpyrexia follows and is usually attended by a decreasing level of consciousness. Many of these findings are identical to those in heat stroke; temperatures higher than 42°C have been noted. Most complications of neuroleptic malignant syndrome are produced by the severe hyperthermia.

Although this syndrome resembles malignant hyperthermia,[23] the most striking difference between the two is that malignant hyperthermia occurs only minutes and rarely hours after drug administration, whereas neuroleptic malignant syndrome develops in days or longer.[24]

Neuroleptic malignant syndrome is considered a disturbance of dopamine function within the central nervous system that affects both the basal ganglia and the hypothalamus.[15] The onset of the neuroleptic malignant syndrome is not related to the duration of drug administration and can occur soon after the first dose of a drug or after prolonged treatment. Both oral and intramuscular administration of neuroleptic drugs can initiate the syndrome.

The neuroleptic malignant syndrome occurs in a small number of patients and is especially associated with haloperidol or fluphenazine.[24] These two drugs account for more than 90% of cases.[25] Although laboratory findings are abnormal, they are nonspecific. Leukocytosis and increases in lactase dehydrogenase, alanine aminotransferase, and serum creatine phosphokinase concentrations may be noted.[25] The increase in creatine phosphokinase may reflect myonecrosis after intense and sustained skeletal muscle contraction.[28] Computerized tomography reveals no acute changes, and standard cerebrospinal fluid analysis reveals no abnormalities.

Treatment

Treatment includes discontinuing the agent and immediately initiating measures to reduce the patient's fever.[3] Vigorous monitoring of the vital signs, cardiovascular function, neurologic status, fluid status, and renal function should also be attempted. Pharmacologic therapy is directed at altering the CNS dopaminergic to cholinergic ratio. Originally, anticholinergics were recommended for this purpose, but they are now considered ineffective.[3,26] Pharmacologic agents that have been suggested include bromocriptine, dantrolene, and amantadine.[29]

Bromocriptine. Bromocriptine (Parlodel®) is an ergot alkaloid and a dopamine agonist that acts postsynaptically. It has been shown to act within hours and to reverse both hyperpyrexia and muscle rigidity. It is available in tablets of 2.5 mg. Side effects are frequent and include mental changes such as confusion with occasional psychosis, nausea, vomiting, hiccups, and dyskinesias. Bromocriptine may be administered orally in a dosage of 5 to 30 mg/day.[3,29]

Dantrolene. Dantrolene (Dantrium®), a skeletal muscle relaxant, has also been reported to be successful in a few cases,[23] especially in patients with severe muscle rigidity.[24] It appears to act directly on the muscle to block heat production. This is accomplished by dissociation of the excitation-contraction coupling mechanism in peripheral muscle through inhibiting the release of calcium from the sarcoplasmic reticulum.[3] Dantrolene does not affect the rate of acetylcholine synthesis or release, nor does it have an effect on the electrical activity at the myoneural junction. It has little effect on cardiac or intestinal smooth muscle at the suggested doses.

Dantrolene may be given in divided doses of 1.0 to 2.5 mg/kg every 6 hours either orally or parenterally. Few adverse reactions are noted as long as the maximal dose of 10 mg/kg is not administered.[29] Optimal treatment consists of the concomitant use of bromocriptine and dantrolene because the effects of these drugs may be synergistic.[3,15]

Amantadine. Amantadine (Symmetrel®), a dopamine agonist that acts presynaptically, may be administered orally as 100 mg two or three times daily. If amantadine is abruptly withdrawn it may worsen or precipitate neuroleptic malignant syndrome.

Sodium nitroprusside. Sodium nitroprusside (Nipride®) has also been used to treat successfully the severe hypertension and consequently the severe hyperthermia. In patients in whom peripheral vasoconstriction rather than muscle rigidity is dominant, infusion of nitroprusside may be beneficial by lowering the patient's temperature through increasing heat loss from the skin.[3,22]

REFERENCES

1. Rivera-Calimlim L: The pharmacology and therapeutic application of the phenothiazines. *Ration Drug Ther* 1977;11:1–8.

2. Knight M, Roberts R: Phenothiazine and butyrophenone intoxication in children. *Ped Clin North Am* 1986;33:299–309.

3. Harpe C, Stoudemire A: Aetiology and treatment of neuroleptic malignant syndrome. *Med Toxicol* 1987; 2:166–176.

4. Coyle J: The clinical use of antipsychotic medications. *Med Clin North Am* 1982;66:993–1009.

5. Burgess K, Stevenson I: Fatal thioridazine cardiotoxicity. *Med J Aust* 1979;2:177–178.

6. Donlon P, Tupin J: Successful suicides with thioridazine and mesoridazine. *Arch Gen Psychiatr* 1977;34:955–957.

7. Desautels S, Filteau C, St Jean A, et al: Ventricular tachycardia associated with administration of thioridazine hydrochloride (Mellaril). *Can Med Assoc J* 1964; 90:1030–1031.

8. Alexander C, Nino A: Cardiovascular complications in young patients taking psychotropic drugs. *Am Heart J* 1969;78:757–769.

9. Ban T, St Jean A: The effect of phenothiazines on the EKG. *Can Med Assoc J* 1964;91:537–540.

10. Lumpkin J, Watanabe A, Rumack B, et al: Phenothiazine-induced ventricular tachycardia following acute overdose. *JACEP* 1979;8:476–478.

11. Tri T, Combs D: Phenothiazine-induced ventricular tachycardia. *West J Med* 1975;123:412–416.

12. Demetropoulos S, Schauben J: Acute dystonic reactions from ''street valium.'' *J Emerg Med* 1987;5:293–297.

13. Corre K, Niemann J, Bessen H, et al: Extended therapy for acute dystonic reactions. *Ann Emerg Med* 1984;13:194–197.

14. Lee A: Drug-induced dystonic reactions. *JACEP* 1977;6:351–354.

15. Granato J, Stein B, Ringel A, et al: Neuroleptic malignant syndrome: Successful treatment with dantrolene and bromocriptine. *Ann Neurol* 1983;14:89–90.

16. Baile G, Nelson M, Krenzlok E, et al: Unusual treatment response of a severe dystonia to diphenhydramine. *Ann Emerg Med* 1987;16:705–708.

17. Lavenstein B, Cantor F: Acute dystonia: An unusual reaction to diphenhydramine. *JAMA* 1976;236:216.

18. Howrie D, Rowley A, Krenzelok E: Benztropine-induced acute dystonic reaction. *Ann Emerg Med* 1986; 15:595–596.

19. Brait K, Zagerman A: Dyskinesias after antihistamine use. *N Engl J Med* 1976;296:111.

20. Lee A: Treatment of drug-induced dystonic reactions. *JACEP* 1979;8:453–457.

21. Ott D, Goeden S: Treatment of acute phenothiazine reaction. *JACEP* 1979;8:471–472.

22. Blue M, Schneider S, Noro S, et al: Successful treatment of neuroleptic malignant syndrome with sodium nitroprusside. *Ann Intern Med* 1986;104:56–57.

23. May D, Morris S, Stewart R, et al: Neuroleptic malignant syndrome: Response to dantrolene sodium. *Ann Intern Med* 1983;98:183–184.

24. Goulon M, Rohan-Chabot P, Elkharrat D, et al: Beneficial effects of dantrolene in the treatment of neuroleptic malignant syndrome: A report of two cases. *Neurology* 1983;33:516–518.

25. Henderson V, Wooten G: Neuroleptic malignant syndrome: A pathogenetic role for dopamine receptor blockade? *Neurology* 1981;31:132–137.

26. Mueller P, Vester J, Fermaglich J: Neuroleptic malignant syndrome. *JAMA* 1983;249:386–388.

27. Niemann J, Stapczynski J, Rothstein R, et al: Cardiac conduction and rhythm disturbances following suicidal ingestion of mesoridazine. *Ann Emerg Med* 1981;10:585–588.

28. Smego R, Durack K: The neuroleptic malignant syndrome. *Arch Intern Med* 1982;142:1183–1185.

29. Ellison J, Jacobs D: Emergency psychopharmacology: A review and update. *Ann Emerg Med* 1986;15: 962–968.

ADDITIONAL SELECTED REFERENCES

Ambani L, Van Woert M, Bowers M: Physostigmine: Effects on phenothiazine-induced extrapyramidal reactions. *Arch Neurol* 1973;29:444–446.

Barry D, Meyskens F, Becker C: Phenothiazines and sudden infant death syndrome. *Pediatrics* 1982;70:75–78.

Black J, Richelson E: Antipsychotic drugs: Prediction of side effect profiles based on neuroreceptor data derived from human brain tissue. *Mayo Clin Proc* 1987;62:369–372.

Craig D, Rosen P: Abuse of antiparkinsonian drugs. *Ann Emerg Med* 1981;10:98–100.

Cummingham D, Challapalli M: Hypertension in acute haloperidol poisoning. *J Pediatr* 1979;95:489–490.

Hollister L, Kosek J: Sudden death during treatment with phenothiazine derivatives. *JAMA* 1965;192:93–96.

Kahn A, Blum D: Phenothiazines and sudden infant death syndrome. *Pediatrics* 1982;70:75–78.

Klawans H: The pharmacology of tardive dyskinesias. *Am J Psychiatr* 1973;130:82–86.

Kobayashi R: Drug therapy of tardive dyskinesia. *N Engl J Med* 1977;296:257–260.

Rainey J, Nesse R: Psychobiology of anxiety and anxiety disorders. *Psychiatr Clin North Am* 1985;8:133–144.

Weisdorf D, Kramer J, Goldberg A, et al: Physostigmine for cardiac and neurologic manifestations of phenothiazine poisoning. *Clin Pharmacol Ther* 1978;24:663–668.

chapter 13

Monoamine Oxidase Inhibitors

Monoamine oxidase (MAO) is a complex flavin-containing enzyme system widely distributed throughout the body that is responsible for the metabolic decomposition of biogenic amines. The monoamine oxidase inhibitors (MAOIs) are a group of drugs that have in common the ability to block this oxidative deamination of naturally occurring monoamines. As a result, the concentration of endogenous epinephrine, norepinephrine, and serotonin increases in storage sites throughout the nervous system. It is thought that the increase in the concentration of monoamines in the CNS is the basis for the antidepressant activity of these agents, but their exact mechanism of action is unknown. The MAOIs are valuable antidepressants that have for the most part been supplanted by the tricyclic antidepressants in the treatment of endogenous depression.[1]

The MAOIs were introduced in 1957,[2] and during the 1960s they were the principal pharmacologic modality for the treatment of endogenous depression. They are now used less frequently than the tricyclic antidepressants because of their detrimental interactions with a wide variety of foods.

USE

The MAOIs are used for the treatment of neurotic and atypical depression as well as ago-raphobia, eating disorders, obsessive-compulsive disorders, and posttraumatic stress disorders. At present, the MAOIs marketed for use in depression are tranylcypromine, isocarboxazid, and phenelzine (Table 13-1). Pargyline has been used for the treatment of moderate to severe hypertension that is resistant to other pharmacologic modalities.

PHARMACOKINETICS

The MAOIs are generally classified in two main categories: hydrazines and nonhydrazines. Currently available hydrazines include isocarboxazid and phenelzine, and currently available nonhydrazines include pargyline and tranylcypromine. The MAOIs are rapidly and completely absorbed from the gastrointestinal tract. They are metabolized in the liver and excreted by the kidney.

Mechanism of Action

Monoamine oxidase is an enzyme found mainly in mitochondrial membranes in nerve tissue and in the liver, lungs, and other organs. There are at least two types of MAO isoenzymes that display different preferences for substrates

Table 13-1 The Monoamine Oxidase Inhibitors (MAOIs)

Generic Name	Trade Name(s)
Hydrazines	
Isocarboxazid	Marplan®
Phenelzine	Nardil®
Nonhydrazines	
Tranylcypromine	Parnate®
Pargyline	Eutonyl®, Eutron®

and different sensitivities to selective inhibitors.[3] The MAOIs now marketed for use are relatively nonselective. Inhibition of MAO results in an increase in the concentration of various amines throughout the body. In other words, the MAOIs exert their effects by delaying the metabolism of sympathomimetic amines and by increasing the store of releasable norepinephrine in postganglionic sympathetic neurons.

Isocarboxazid, phenelzine, and pargyline bind irreversibly to MAO. These compounds appear to attack and inactivate the flavin group after their oxidation to reactive intermediaries by MAO. This causes an irreversible inhibition of MAO.[1] Tranylcypromine binds reversibly to the enzyme. This drug bears a close resemblance to dextroamphetamine, which is a weak inhibitor of MAO. Tranylcypromine retains some of the sympathomimetic characteristics of the amphetamine, which may be due to some degree of metabolism to an amphetamine-like compound.[1,4]

The ability of these drugs to bind to MAO appears to be due to their structural similarity to the enzyme's natural substrates. Because some of them bind to MAO in an irreversible manner, despite the discontinuation of MAOI therapy enzyme inhibition may persist for several weeks until enzyme stores are repleted.[5,6]

The MAOIs also have pharmacologic properties that are unrelated to their ability to inhibit MAO. Phenelzine and tranylcypromine appear to be capable of stimulating the release of norepinephrine from sympathetic nerve endings. MAOIs also have sympatholytic activity that is due to their ability to reduce the amount of norepinephrine released from postganglionic sympathetic neurons.

Drug Interactions

The MAOIs prolong and intensify the effects of other drugs and interfere with the metabolism of various substances.[6] It is the diversity and number of substances as well as the unpredictability of the development of adverse effects that has contributed to the unpopularity of the MAOIs as therapeutic agents.[5]

The interactions fall into two categories: (1) exacerbation or prolongation of the normally occurring actions of the drug (sedation or coma caused by alcohol, anesthetics, or opiate analgesics, or atropine-like central toxicity caused by tricyclics); and (2) hypertensive crisis attributable to the release and potentiation of catecholamines. The most important reaction is the latter; hypertensive crises have sometimes led to death. These crises usually occur within several hours after the ingestion of a contraindicated substance. They are characterized by occipital headache, palpitations, neck stiffness or soreness, nausea, vomiting, mydriasis, and photophobia. The toxic effects of the MAOIs are greater when they interact with indirectly acting amines, such as amphetamine and tyramine, than with directly acting amines, such as epinephrine and phenylpropanolamine.[2] In the presence of MAOIs, exogenous sympathomimetics can cause CNS stimulation and a marked pressor response.

Certain foods containing tyramine, such as natural or aged cheese, beer, wine, pickled herring, canned figs, chocolate, large quantities of coffee, citrus fruits, chicken liver, yeast, bananas, avocados, and snails, may interact with MAOIs to cause hypertensive crisis.[2,7] MAOIs can interact with any protein food that contains decarboxylating bacteria because these produce amines by conversion of amino acids to amines such as tyramine, phenylethylamine, and histamine (Table 13-2).[5]

Hypertension with cerebrovascular accident, cardiac dysrhythmias, and pulmonary edema have been observed as an exaggerated response to sympathomimetic amines after ingestion of a MAOI.[6] Hypertension is related to varying degrees of α-adrenergic vasoconstriction and β-adrenergic cardiac stimulation. These are the most serious adverse reactions associated with MAOI therapy.[2,7] Hypotension is more com-

Table 13-2 Substances That Interact with MAOIs

Drugs
  Amphetamine
  Caffeine
  Cocaine
  Dopamine
  Ephedrine
  Epinephrine
  Levodopa
  Mephenteramine
  Metaraminol
  Methyldopa
  Methylphenidate
  Norepinephrine
  Phenylephrine
  Phenylpropranolamine
  Pseudoephedrine
  Reserpine
  Tryptophan
Foodstuffs
  Alcohol (beer, wine)
  Amine-containing foods
    Broad beans
    Canned figs
    Caviar
    Cheese
    Chicken livers
    Chocolate
    Pickled herring
    Snails
    Sour cream
    Soy sauce
    Yeast extracts
**Substances That Inhibit Hepatic Drug-
  Metabolizing Enzyme**
  Anesthetics (general and local)
  Antiparkinsonism agents
  Barbiturates
  Benzodiazepines
  Chloral hydrate
  Diuretics
  Hypoglycemia agents
  Opiate analgesics
  Thyroid extract
  Tricyclic agents

Source: Adapted with permission from *Psychiatric Clinics of North America* (1984;7:625–637), Copyright © 1984, WB Saunders Company.

mon when MAOIs are used with CNS depressant-like narcotics and anesthetics. Malignant hyperthermia is a unique feature of the toxicity of MAOIs. This syndrome has been seen especially after combined use of MAOIs and other antidepressant drugs such as imipramine, amitriptyline, and amphetamine, and mortality has been high.[8]

ACUTE TOXICITY

Acute poisoning with MAOIs is uncommon but potentially serious. In general, acute overdose produces effects that are extensions of common adverse reactions. Serious toxic symptoms rarely develop in less than 12 hours and sometimes do not develop until 24 hours after an overdose, even though the MAOIs are rapidly absorbed from the gastrointestinal tract. During the latent phase after ingestion of an acute overdose, endogenous catecholamines accumulate in the brain and elsewhere as the result of MAO enzyme inhibition.

The pharmacological basis for the delayed onset of toxic signs and symptoms after MAOI overdose is unclear. Initial reversible binding of the drugs to MAO, cumulative effects, or the time required to achieve significant enzyme inhibition with subsequent alterations of MAO substrate stores and metabolism may be responsible for delayed toxicity.

The ingestion of a MAOI can induce a complex array of hypermetabolic signs, including hyperpyrexia, tachycardia, generalized muscle rigidity, tachypnea, metabolic acidosis, hypoxemia, and hypercapnea (Table 13-3).[9] An acute overdose of MAOI does not usually produce a hypertensive crisis unless the patient deliberately provokes the interaction.

Early mild clinical features of poisoning may be consistent with neuromuscular hyperactivity and include irritability, anxiety, flushing, and sweating. Drowsiness, dizziness, and ataxia may also occur. In moderate intoxication an altered mental status as well as hyperpyrexia, hypertension, tachycardia, and tachypnea may be noted.[1] Severe intoxication may be characterized by CNS depression, coma, severe hyperpyrexia, and seizures. Although seizures may be grand mal type, myoclonus may also be noted. Decorticate or decerebrate rigidity may alternate with flaccid paralysis. Muscle rigidity may be so marked that respiration is seriously embarrassed. Dystonic-like reactions, including grimacing and writhing movements of the trunk and limbs, have also been described.

Table 13-3 Symptoms of Acute MAOI Intoxication

Mild
 Irritability
 Anxiety
 Flushing
 Diaphoresis
 Drowsiness
 Dizziness
 Ataxia
Moderate
 Altered mental status
 Hyperpyrexia
 Hypertension
 Tachycardia
 Tachypnea
Severe
 Severe hyperpyrexia
 Seizures
 Central nervous system depression
 Coma
 Cardiorespiratory depression
 Malignant hyperthermia
 Muscle rigidity

Table 13-4 Treatment of MAOI Overdose

Condition	Treatment
Acute overdose	Supportive care
	Ipecac or lavage
	Charcoal and cathartic
	Dietary precautions
Muscle irritability	Diazepam
Seizures	Diazepam
	Phenytoin
Hypertension	Phentolamine
	Sodium nitroprusside
	Labetalol
Hyperthermia	Antipyretic agents
	Cooling blankets
	Sponge baths
	Dantrolene
	Bromocriptine
Hypotension	Volume expansion
	Military antishock trousers
	Vasopressors
Cardiac dysrhythmias	Lidocaine
	Phenytoin
	Procainamide

Malignant hyperthermia is also associated with monoamine oxidase inhibitors.[6] The pathophysiologic abnormality appears to be an increase in sarcoplasmic concentrations of calcium ion, which leads to sustained contracture of the muscle, uncoupling of oxidative phosphorylation in the mitochondria, and accelerated glycolysis by activation of phosphorylase kinase.

LABORATORY ANALYSIS

Laboratory confirmation of MAOI overdose by drug assay is difficult because of the low concentrations of MAOIs in biological samples and lack of availability of assay procedures. Treatment for MAOI overdose consists mainly of supportive care as well as more specific therapy aimed at significant autonomic dysfunction (Table 13-4).

TREATMENT

Supportive Care

Good supportive care is the primary treatment for acute MAOI overdose. Because there may be delayed and severe toxicity, monitoring of the patient in the intensive care unit is necessary for a full 24 hours. Dietary precautions should be instituted, and medications should be prescribed cautiously. The rectal temperature should be monitored closely. The stomach should be emptied with either syrup of ipecac or by gastric lavage. This should be followed with activated charcoal and a cathartic.[9]

Mild to moderate CNS excitation and muscular irritability may be treated with diazepam. In addition, diazepam or phenytoin (or both) may be used if seizures develop. Sedative-hypnotic agents should be used with caution because they may potentiate the CNS depression that often develops later in the course. Narcotics also should be avoided because they may lead to exaggerated CNS and cardiorespiratory depression.[1]

Treatment of Hypertension

The recommended treatment of severe hypertension is an α-adrenergic blocking agent such as phentolamine.[6,7] Because MAOI overdose may cause a sudden rapid fall in blood pressure, α blockers should be used cautiously.[1] Sodium nitroprusside may also be used. Labetalol, an antihypertensive agent that competitively inhibits both α- and β-adrenergic receptors, has also been suggested for treatment of the acute hypertension secondary to MAOI overdose.[9] It may be administered intravenously in a dosage of 20 mg over 5 minutes.

Treatment of Hyperthermia

Antipyretic agents such as acetaminophen or salicylates, cool compresses, sponge baths, and hypothermic blankets may be effective treatment for mild to moderate hyperthermia.[1] Dantrolene relaxes skeletal muscle directly to block heat production. This drug inhibits the release of calcium ions from the sarcoplasmic reticulum by action on transverse tubular membrane-sarcoplasmic reticulum coupling or by direct action on the sarcoplasmic reticulum. Dantrolene in a dose of 2.5 mg/kg can be administered intravenously every 6 hours for 24 hours.[9] Bromocriptine, an ergot alkaloid and dopamine agonist, has also been used for hyperthermia and muscle rigidity.[1]

Treatment of Hypotension

Hypotension unresponsive to volume expansion may be treated with military antishock trousers and vasopressors. A direct-acting α-adrenergic blocking agent is preferable to an indirect pressor because the former does not require the release of intracellular amines.

Treatment of Cardiac Dysrhythmias

Cardiac dysrhythmias are usually difficult to treat. Lidocaine, phenytoin, and procainamide appear to be safe choices for the treatment of ventricular tachydysrhythmias. Bretylium should be avoided. Atropine, epinephrine, and temporary pacing may be used to treat bradydysrhythmias.

Methods To Enhance Excretion

Although MAOI excretion is enhanced by urinary acidification, there is no evidence that forced acid diuresis is effective in reducing the severity of an overdose.[1] The usefulness of extracorporeal measures such as hemodialysis or hemoperfusion in the treatment of MAOI overdose remains to be demonstrated.

REFERENCES

1. Linden C, Rumack B, Strehlke C, et al: Monoamine oxidase inhibitor overdose. *Ann Emerg Med* 1984; 13:1137–1144.

2. Smookler S, Bermudez A: Hypertensive crisis resulting from an MAO inhibitor and an over-the-counter appetite suppressant. *Ann Emerg Med* 1982;11:482–484.

3. Jones A, Pare C, Nicholson W, et al: Brain amine concentrations after monoamine oxidase inhibitor administration. *Br Med J* 1972;1:17–19.

4. Youdim M, Aronson J, Blau K, et al: Tranylcypromine (Parnate) overdose: Measurement of tranylcypromine concentrations and MAO inhibitory activity and identification of amphetamines in plasma. *Psychol Med* 1979;9:377–382.

5. Blackwell B, Schmidt G: Drug interactions in psychopharmacology. *Pyschiatr Clin North Am* 1984;7:625–637.

6. Ciocatto E, Fagiano G, Bava G: Clinical features and treatment of overdosage of monoamine oxidase inhibitors and their interaction with other psychotropic drugs. *Resuscitation* 1972;1:69–72.

7. Abrams J, Schulman P, White W: Successful treatment of a monoamine oxidase inhibitor–tyramine hypertensive emergency with intravenous labetalol. *N Engl J Med* 1985; 305:52.

8. Peebles-Brown A: Hyperpyrexia following psychotropic drug overdose. *Anaesthesia* 1985;40:1097–1099.

9. Kaplan R, Feinglass N, Webster W, et al: Phenelzine overdose treated with dantrolene sodium. *JAMA* 1986; 255:642–644.

ADDITIONAL SELECTED REFERENCES

Henry J, Volans G: Psychoactive drugs. *Br Med J* 1984; 289:1291–1294.

Pope H, Jonas J, Hudson J, et al: Toxic reactions to the combination of monoamine oxidase inhibitors and tryptophan. *Am J Psychiatr* 1985;142:491–492.

Shepherd J: β-Adrenergic blockade in the treatment of MAOI self-poisoning. *Lancet* 1974;2:1021.

chapter 14

Lithium

Lithium ion is a monovalent alkali metal cation that is chemically similar to other monovalent cations, such as sodium and potassium,[1] and that sometimes acts like a divalent cation, such as magnesium and calcium.[2,3] Lithium has no known physiological function and is present only in trace amounts in the body.[4] The term as used in this chapter refers to the non–protein-bound lithium ions or lithium salts.[5]

Lithium is one of the oldest and most effective psychotropic drugs[4,6–8] and is administered exclusively by the oral route. The most common lithium product is the salt of carbonate that is marketed as capsules or tablets. This salt is the most common because it is the most stable[9] and has the highest concentration of lithium suitable for tablets or capsules. The salt of citrate is available as a liquid but is not as frequently used. Extended-release preparations (such as Lithobid®) are also available. Other lithium salts include the chloride, sulfate, gluconate, glutamate, and acetate, although these are not used to any great extent (Table 14-1).

The actual lithium content per tablet of the 300-mg salt of carbonate is 8.1 mg. Lithium citrate solution contains 8 mEq of lithium per 5 mL.[10]

USES

In the past, lithium was used as a salt substitute but was removed from the market after deaths were attributed to its consumption.[8,11] Lithium bromide was once used as a hypnotic and sedative.[12] In 1949 it was discovered that lithium was useful as treatment for manic-depressive psychoses because it terminates the manic and hypomanic phases of this bipolar affective disorder.[12,13] It is still considered the treatment of choice for this disorder[1,14] and is also used for prophylaxis. Furthermore, there is evidence that some patients with major depressive disorders show an antidepressant response to lithium.[12,15] Lithium may also be therapeutic in a diverse group of clinical problems, including premenstrual syndrome, neutropenia, cluster headaches, and certain movement disorders.

Affective illness is divided into two subtypes: unipolar and bipolar. A bipolar psychosis is characterized by both manic and depressive epi-

---

Table 14-1 Lithium Compounds

Lithium carbonate
  Eskalith®
  Lithonate®
  Lithane®
  Lithotabs®
  Lithobid®
Lithium citrate
  Cibalith-S®

---

sodes in the same person, and unipolar psychosis is characterized by more recurrent depressions and fewer recurrent manic states. Lithium exerts a true and specific antimanic action in that euphoria, expansiveness of mood, overactivity, flight of ideas, and other symptoms of mania are suppressed.

PHARMACOKINETICS

The pharmacokinetics of lithium is of particular interest because lithium is not bound to plasma proteins, lipid, or tissue. Lithium is not metabolized but is almost entirely eliminated in urine.[3,16] Although lithium has a volume of distribution of 0.7 L/kg, which is about the same as that of total body water, it is not distributed evenly throughout the water phase.[16]

Lithium is a highly water soluble ion that is well absorbed from the gastrointestinal tract. Serum concentrations reach their peak within 2 to 3 hours after oral administration.[1] Lithium normally has a half-life of 20 to 30 hours. Because in some respects it is distributed in a fashion similar to that of sodium and potassium, it shares some of the properties of extracellular sodium and intracellular potassium with some important differences.[1]

Lithium is initially distributed into extracellular fluid and then gradually accumulates in varying amounts in tissues. Lithium crosses cell boundaries at a relatively slow rate. This slow entry into and exit from the intracellular space accounts for the delay of 6 to 10 days in achieving a full therapeutic response to lithium[3,12,17] and also accounts for the lag in onset of symptoms in the acute overdose.[14]

Because the main route of lithium excretion is through the kidneys, its elimination in the urine is of decisive importance for the safe use of this drug. Approximately 50% to 75% of a dose is eliminated by the kidneys within 24 hours. There is a prolongation of the half-life due to decreased renal excretion in patients with renal impairment.[2] In addition, the aging kidney, which has a reduced number of functioning nephrons, has an impaired ability to excrete lithium, and furthermore the drug may injure the kidney. Of equal importance is the maintenance of normal salt and fluid intake when this drug is administered.

MECHANISM OF ACTION

The mechanism of action of lithium is not fully understood. It may act by at least two nonindependent mechanisms: (1) as an imperfect substitute for other monovalent or divalent cations such as sodium, potassium, or magnesium in basic ion-transport mechanisms that affect cellular membrane properties,[18,19] or (2) by altering the cellular microenvironment by interfering with hormonal activation of adenyl cyclase, which then reduces the concentration of cyclic AMP, or by interfering with the effect of cyclic AMP.[2,20]

Lithium is also thought to inhibit the release of norepinephrine and serotonin, to increase reuptake of norepinephrine, and possibly to increase synthesis and turnover rate of serotonin.[1]

SIDE EFFECTS

Although lithium is widely acknowledged as an effective and specific therapy for bipolar affective disorders, its therapeutic index is notoriously low.[8,10] Lithium intoxication is a dose-related phenomenon that occurs when more lithium is ingested than can be excreted. Lithium intoxication is a potentially serious condition that can lead to death or permanent disability.[8]

Three main types of unwanted lithium effects can be distinguished: (1) transient effects at low serum concentrations; (2) permanent side effects at low serum concentrations; and (3) toxic effects from an acute or chronic overdose. The first type is represented by transient minor side effects occurring at the beginning of therapy at low serum concentrations. These effects take place primarily in three physiological systems: the neurological and neuromuscular, gastrointestinal, and renal systems (Table 14-2).

Neurological symptoms include cerebellar malfunctions such as incoordination, dysarthria, ataxia, and nystagmus. Gastrointestinal symptoms include gastric irritation, abdominal pain, nausea, vomiting, diarrhea, and tremor of the hands. Tremor is the most frequent adverse side effect and may fluctuate with anxiety.[10] The tremor is more severe in patients with essential tremor or in those treated with other antipsychotic medications. Renal side effects may be

Table 14-2 Side Effects from Lithium Therapy

Neurological
  Incoordination
  Dysarthria
  Ataxia
  Nystagmus
Gastrointestinal
  Irritation
  Abdominal pain
  Nausea
  Vomiting
  Diarrhea
Renal
  Nephrogenic diabetes insipidus
  Polydipsia
  Polyuria

nephrogenic diabetes insipidus with polyuria and polydipsia. This occurs because lithium reduces the effect of antidiuretic hormone on the collecting tubule cell.[2] Other renal disorders include inappropriate salt wasting, incomplete distal renal tubular acidosis, nephrotic syndrome,[13,21] and acute renal failure.[6] Many cutaneous side effects have also been associated with lithium therapy. These include folliculitis, pretibial ulcerations, psoriasis, and acne.[1] These symptoms are inconvenient rather than dangerous.[22–24]

The permanent side effects represent minor but persistent findings at low serum concentrations. The most dangerous side effects are from lithium intoxication or poisoning associated with an accumulation of lithium to serum concentrations greater than 1.5 mEq/L.

LITHIUM INTOXICATION

Lithium intoxication can result from acute overdose or from a long-term nonpurposeful accumulation.[25] This may be secondary to decreased excretion of lithium in a patient receiving optimum subtoxic therapeutic doses who is experiencing reduced sodium or water intake or concurrent illness.[26,27] Most poisonings have occurred over weeks to months of intake, not from episodes of single ingestion.[8]

The clinical course of lithium overdose is influenced by the drug's distribution kinetics. Although the volume of distribution of lithium is equal to or a little greater than the total water volume, the tissue distribution of lithium is delayed and varies with the different organs: lithium diffusion is fast for the liver and the kidneys but slow for the brain, in which equilibrium with serum concentration is reached after 8 or 10 days.[16] This slow rate of distribution explains the observation that, after an acute overdose, the severity of intoxication does not correlate well with serum concentrations: patients may be asymptomatic with relatively high serum concentrations.[3] In patients who become intoxicated during the course of long-term administration of lithium, there is a better correlation between serum lithium concentrations and the onset of neurological signs.

Acute Intoxication

In the acute overdose, slow intracellular diffusion may protect the patient from severe adverse reactions for a number of hours. Also, the lithium blood concentration may continue to rise for up to 1 week after absorption.[28] Symptoms rarely occur quickly, even when massive doses are ingested.[12]

Chronic Intoxication

The most common mode of lithium overdose results from weeks to months of ingestion or maintenance therapy. The diagnosis may therefore be difficult. In addition, various factors enter into chronic intoxication. Conditions affecting fluid and electrolyte balance, such as gastroenteritis or vomiting from any cause, diuretic treatment, dietary intake low in sodium, and decreased fluid intake, commonly precede intoxication (Table 14-3). In the presence of sodium deficiency secondary to vomiting, diarrhea, diuretics, or low-salt diet, volume contraction occurs. Under these conditions, the lithium ion is selectively reabsorbed in the renal tubules and may accumulate to toxic levels. A cycle is then set up that further exacerbates both the lithium toxicity and renal insufficiency.

Certain drugs decrease the clearance of lithium (Table 14-4). Diuretics such as hydrochlorothiazide act in this manner, as do the prosta-

Table 14-3 Conditions Affecting Lithium Toxicity

Decreased Elimination and Increased Toxicity
Fluid and Electrolyte Imbalance
    Gastroenteritis
    Diuretic therapy
    Vomiting
    Low sodium intake
    Decreased fluid intake
    Concurrent drug therapy (see Table 14-4)
Increased Elimination and Decreased Therapeutic
Concentrations
    Acute phase of therapy
    Increased sodium intake
    Concurrent drug therapy (see Table 14-4)

Table 14-4 Medications That Can Alter Lithium Elimination

Decreased Elimination and Increased Toxicity
Medications
    Diuretics
        Chlorthalidone (Hygroton®)
        Furosemide (Lasix®)
        Spironolactone (Aldactone®)
        Hydrochlorothiazide (HydroDIURIL®)
    Nonsteroidal anti-inflammatory agents
        Ibuprofen (Motrin®, Rufen®, Advil®)
        Indomethacin (Indocin®)
        Phenylbutazone (Butazolidin®)
        Salicylates
    Antihypertensives
        Methyldopa (Aldomet®)
    Antipsychotics
        Haloperidol (Haldol®)
        Thioridazine
    Miscellaneous
        Carbamazepine (Tegretol®)
        Phenytoin (Dilantin®)
        Tetracyclines
Increased Elimination and Decreased Therapeutic
Concentrations
    Xanthines
        Aminophylline
        Caffeine
        Theophylline
    Chlorpromazine (Thorazine®)
    Osmotic diuretics

glandin inhibitors such as aspirin, indomethacin, and other nonsteroidal anti-inflammatory drugs.

The prodromes of chronic intoxication are mainly gastrointestinal and cerebrovascular and precede full intoxication by several days to 1 week. Mild reactions that may be associated

with serum concentrations between 1.5 and 2 mEq/L are nausea, vomiting, diarrhea, malaise, drowsiness, muscular weakness, thirst, polyuria, polydipsia, fatigue, fine hand tremor, and mild incoordination (Table 14-5). Some of these symptoms may be confused with the spon-

Table 14-5 Signs of Lithium Intoxication

Mild (serum concentration, 1.5 to 2.0 mEq/L)
Neurologic
    Malaise
    Drowsiness
    Weakness
    Fine hand tremor
    Mild incoordination
    Sedation
    Confusion
Gastrointestinal
    Anorexia
    Nausea
    Vomiting
    Diarrhea
    Thirst
Metabolic
    Polyuria
Moderate (serum concentration, 2.0 to 2.5 mEq/L)
Neurologic
    Blurred vision
    Slurred speech
    Lethargy
    Dizziness
    Nystagmus
Gastrointestinal
    Dryness of mouth
    Abdominal pain
    Weight loss
Moderate to Severe (serum concentration, 2.5 to 3.0 mEq/L)
Neurologic
    Ataxia
    Increased deep tendon reflexes
    Choreoathetosis
    Seizures
    Confusion
    Dysarthria
    Restlessness
    Syncope
Severe (serum concentration, more than 3.0 mEq/L)
    Generalized seizures
    Oliguria
    Circulatory failure
    Coma
    Death

taneous advent of a depressive phase of a manic disorder.

When serum concentrations reach 2.0 to 2.5 mEq/L, anorexia, blurred vision, slurred speech, dryness of the mouth, abdominal pain, weight loss, lethargy, dizziness, and nystagmus may occur. Moderate to severe toxic reactions that are usually associated with serum concentrations of 2.5 mEq/L include ataxia, hyperactive deep tendon reflexes, choreathetoid movements,[14] seizures, confusion, syncope, and electrocardiographic changes.[17,28] The changes reported include T wave depression,[29] which is usually reversed with discontinuance of the drug and may be related to lithium-induced intracellular or extracellular alterations in electrolytes. First-degree atrioventricular block has also been reported.[30] Patients with moderate to severe lithium intoxication are frequently azotemic but rarely experience overt renal failure.[6] Very severe adverse reactions associated with concentrations of 3.0 mEq/L include generalized seizures,[31] oliguria, acute circulatory failure, coma, and death.

Long-Term Sequelae

Lithium intoxication can result in persistent neurological sequelae including dementia, cerebellar ataxia, polyuria, dysarthria, spasticity, nystagmus, and tremor. Permanent damage of the basal ganglia and cerebellar connections, despite effective lowering of lithium concentration by hemodialysis, has also been noted (Table 14-6).[32]

LABORATORY DETERMINATIONS

The initial laboratory examination should include a coma screen; measurements of serum lithium concentration, serum electrolytes, blood urea nitrogen, creatinine, and complete blood count; electrocardiogram; and urinalysis (Table 14-7).[17,29] It has been found that a markedly elevated serum lithium concentration is associated with a reduced anion gap.[33] This may be a helpful clue to the diagnosis in the comatose patient with no history of ingested substance. Elec-

Table 14-6 Persistent Sequelae from Lithium Intoxication

Basal Ganglia Damage
 Dysarthria
 Spasticity
 Tremor
Cerebellar Damage
 Ataxia
 Nystagmus
Dementia
Polyuria

Table 14-7 Laboratory Determinations for Lithium Overdose

Anion gap
Blood urea nitrogen
Complete blood count
Creatinine
Electrocardiogram
Serum electrolytes
Serum lithium concentration
Toxicology screen
Urinalysis

trocardiographic changes are nonspecific and may include a reversible flattening or inversion of the T waves, first-degree atrioventricular block, and sinus node dysfunction.[34]

Lithium concentrations are most frequently determined by flame photometry or atomic absorption spectrometry. A steady-state lithium concentration in the range of 0.8 to 1.2 mEq/L is considered therapeutic.[10,12,17] Somewhat lower serum concentrations, between 0.6 and 1.0 mEq/L, are necessary for prophylaxis. Clinical response to lithium, however, varies from patient to patient, and a good response may be seen at serum concentrations less than 0.5 mEq/L.[22] True toxicity seldom occurs below 1.5 mEq/L. Serum lithium concentrations of 1.5 to 2.5 mEq/L often indicate slight to moderate intoxication; concentrations of 2.5 to 3.5 mEq/L often indicate severe intoxication. Concentrations greater than 4.0 mEq/L often indicate potentially lethal intoxication (Table 14-5).

A single 300-mg dose of lithium carbonate or 600-mg dose of a sustained release preparation can be expected to raise the serum concentration by 0.2 to 0.4 mEq/L[9] in a 70-kg person. This relation does not always hold true, however, and serum concentrations may not necessarily coincide with the severity of the clinical symptoms. The concentration may be in the normal range and still be associated with clinical toxicity, especially in the acute overdose.[35] Thus the relation between serum concentration and toxicity is only an indirect one because toxicity depends on the intracellular concentration. In some cases of lithium intoxication, the patient's condition can worsen to the point of death while the lithium serum levels are diminishing.

TREATMENT

The management of lithium intoxication is still controversial (Table 14-8). Because there is no specific treatment, it is largely supportive and depends on the patient's clinical condition and the serum lithium concentration. General supportive measures consist of maintaining blood pressure and airway and correcting dehydration and electrolyte imbalance. At the same time, care must be taken to avoid iatrogenic fluid and electrolyte disorders.[17] Mere withdrawal of the drug does not always prevent serious complications or death.

Supportive Care

In the acute ingestion, induction of emesis or gastric lavage is necessary and should be followed by administration of activated charcoal

---

Table 14-8 Treatment of Lithium Intoxication

Discontinue drug
Prevent further absorption
  Ipecac or lavage
  Charcoal and cathartic
Institute supportive measures
Correct fluid and electrolyte losses
Attempt diuresis (alkaline)
Attempt dialysis (if concentration is 2.0 to 4.0 mEq/L
  with clinical signs or greater than 4.0 mEq/L without
  clinical signs)

---

and a cathartic. Activated charcoal may not be effective in adsorbing lithium, but it does no harm if used.[3] Those patients chronically intoxicated with lithium will not benefit from this procedure.

Because more than half the lithium in the body is excreted within 24 hours, merely discontinuing the drug in many instances may be the only action required. Recovery takes place gradually over 4 to 5 days in uncomplicated cases. Mild intoxication usually responds to this therapy along with correction of fluid and electrolyte abnormalities. Because more than 98% of ingested lithium is excreted in the urine, patients with serum lithium concentrations less than 2.5 mEq/L who are not stuporous and have relatively well-maintained neurological functioning can be initially treated with rapid intravenous infusion of normal saline in an attempt to rehydrate the patient and prevent hyponatremia and as a saline diuresis.[17,36] Sodium loading increases the sodium content of the glomerular filtrate. This is presumably then reabsorbed in preference to lithium in the proximal convoluted tubule.[3] Forced diuresis with furosemide appears not to be more efficacious than saline alone.[29] Alkaline diuresis in the form of added sodium bicarbonate may also enhance the elimination of lithium by decreasing lithium reabsorption in the proximal tubule, but this has not been proven.[3]

Although diuresis has been suggested for increasing the clearance of lithium, it may be that forced diuresis is not actually attained but rather that large amounts of fluid merely rehydrate the patient.[37] The glomerular filtration rate and the lithium clearance are restored through rehydration rather than through an acceleration of the usual renal clearance.[7,8]

Hemodialysis

Because lithium is located in the extracellular space, its concentrations in plasma can be lowered rapidly by dialysis.[6,25] Although hemodialysis is the treatment of choice in severe lithium intoxication,[16] patients who have taken a single acute overdose must be distinguished from those who have been taking the drug on a long-term basis.[16] In the acute overdose, hemodialysis prevents lithium diffusion into the brain and the onset of severe toxicity. In the long-term overdose, hemodialysis enhances elimination of lithium from brain but must be continued for a long period of time.

Due to lithium's location in the intracellular space though, a rebound increase in its plasma concentration may be noted after discontinuance of dialysis.[6,16] The reason is that, even though lithium is distributed throughout body water, as the extracellular concentration falls rapidly with removal the intracellular concentration is still high and takes longer to equilibrate, hence a rebound effect. A plasma lithium concentration less than 1 mEq/L 6 to 8 hours after cessation of dialysis has been considered evidence of adequate treatment.[8,38]

Indications for Dialysis

Although the usefulness of dialysis is controversial, it should be performed if the serum lithium concentration is between 2.0 and 4.0 mEq/L and the patient's clinical condition is poor or if the serum concentration is greater than 4 mEq/L regardless of the patient's condition.[3,17,39] Hemodialysis may need to be carried out for 8 to 12 hours because of the large tissue storage pool of lithium[29] and should be repeated 6 to 8 hours later if indicated. Because blood concentrations may rise for some time after an acute overdose, and because clinical symptoms may worsen during this time, some patients who do not initially appear to be ill may require dialysis after 2 to 3 days of hospitalization.

REFERENCES

1. Heng M: Lithium carbonate toxicity. *Arch Dermatol* 1982;118:246–248.

2. Myers J, Morgan T, Carney S, et al: Effects of lithium on the kidney. *Kidney Int* 1980;18:601–608.

3. Goldfrank L, Flomenbaum N, Weisman R: Management of overdose with psychoactive medications. *Emerg Med Clin North Am* 1984;2:63–76.

4. Murray J: Lithium therapy for mania and depression. *J Gen Psychol* 1984;112:5–33.

5. Sansone M, Ziegler D: Lithium toxicity: A review of neurologic complications. *Clin Neuropharmacol* 1985; 8:242–248.

6. Fenves A, Emmett M, White M: Lithium intoxication associated with acute renal failure. *South Med J* 1984; 77:1472–1473.

7. Hansen H: Renal toxicity of lithium. *Drugs* 1981;22: 461–476.

8. Hansen H, Amdisen A: Lithium intoxication. *Q J Med* 1978;47:123–144.

9. Saran B, Gaind R: Lithium. *Clin Toxicol* 1973; 6:257–269.

10. Lesar T, Tollefson G: Lithium therapy. *Postgrad Med J* 1984;75:269–286.

11. Doyal L, Morton W: The clinical usefulness of lithium as an antidepressant. *Hosp Commun Psychol* 1984; 35:685–691.

12. DePaulo J: Lithium. *Psychiatr Clin N Am* 1984; 7:587–599.

13. Bear R, Sugar L, Paul M: Nephrotic syndrome and renal failure secondary to lithium carbonate therapy. *Can Med Assoc J* 1985;132:735–736.

14. Cohen W, Cohen N: Lithium carbonate, haloperidol, and irreversible brain damage. *JAMA* 1974;230:1283–1287.

15. Campbell M, Perry R, Green W: Use of lithium in children and adolescents. *Psychosomatics* 1984;25:96–106.

16. Jaeger A, Sauder P, Kopferschmitt J, et al: Toxicokinetics of lithium intoxication treated by hemodialysis. *Clin Toxicol* 1986;23:501–517.

17. Mateer J, Clark M: Lithium toxicity with rarely reported ECG manifestations. *Ann Emerg Med* 1982; 11:208–211.

18. Singer I: Lithium and the kidney. *Kidney Int* 1981; 19:374–387.

19. Singer I, Rotenberg D: Mechanisms of lithium action. *N Engl J Med* 1973;289:254–260.

20. Fyro B, Petterson U, Sedvall G: The effect of lithium treatment on manic symptoms and levels of monoamine metabolites in cerebrospinal fluid of manic-depressive patients. *Psychopharmacologia* 1975;44:99–103.

21. Kalina K, Burnett G: Lithium and the nephrotic syndrome. *J Clin Psychopharmacol* 1984;4:148–150.

22. Hwang S, Tuason V: Long-term maintenance lithium therapy and possible irreversible renal damage. *J Clin Psychiatr* 1980;41:11–19.

23. Schou M: Lithium in psychiatric therapy and prophylaxis. *J Psychiatr Res* 1968;6:67–95.

24. Schou M, Amdisen A, Trap-Jensen J: Lithium poisoning. *Am J Psychiatr* 1968;125:112–116.

25. Jacobsen D, Aasen G, Frederichsen P, et al: Lithium intoxication: Pharmacokinetics during and after terminated hemodialysis in acute intoxications. *Clin Toxicol* 1987; 25:81–94.

26. Demers R, Heninger G: Pretibial edema and sodium retention during lithium carbonate treatment. *JAMA* 1970; 214:1845–1848.

27. Demers R, Rivenbark J: Lithium intoxication and its clinical management. *South Med J* 1982;75:738–739.

28. Kondziela J: Extreme lithium intoxication without severe symptoms. *Hosp Commun Psychol* 1984;35: 727–728.

29. Sugarman J: Management of lithium intoxication. *J Family Pract* 1984;18:237–239.

30. Martin C, Piascik M: First-degree A-V block in patients on lithium carbonate. *Can J Psychiatr* 1985;30: 114–116.

31. Massey E, Folger W: Seizures activated by therapeutic levels of lithium carbonate. *South Med J* 1984; 77:1173–1175.

32. Bejar J: Cerebellar degeneration due to acute lithium toxicity. *Clin Neuropharmacol* 1985;8:379–381.

33. Kelleher S, Raciti A, Arbert J: Reduced or absent serum anion gap as a marker of severe lithium carbonate intoxication. *Arch Intern Med* 1986;146:1839–1840.

34. Montalescot Y, Levy Y, Farge D, et al: Lithium causing a serious sinus node dysfunction at therapeutic doses. *Clin Cardiol* 1984;7:617–620.

35. Bucht C, Smigan L, Wahlin A, et al: ECG changes during lithium therapy. *Acta Med Scand* 1984;216:101–104.

36. Parfrey P, Ikeman R, Anglin D, et al: Severe lithium intoxication treated by forced diuresis. *Can Med Assoc J* 1983;29:979–980.

37. Clendennin N, Pond S, Kaysen G, et al: Potential pitfalls in the evaluation of the usefulness of hemodialysis for the removal of lithium. *J Toxicol Clin Toxicol* 1982;19: 341–352.

38. Gomolin I, Brandt J: Treatment of severe lithium intoxication. *Can Med Assoc J* 1984;130:847.

39. Goetting M: Acute lithium poisoning in a child with dystonia. *Pediatrics* 1985;76:978–980.

ADDITIONAL SELECTED REFERENCES

Bowers M, Heninger G: Lithium: Clinical effects and cerebrospinal fluid acid monamine metabolites. *Commun Psychopharmacol* 1977;1:135–145.

Danielson D, Jick H, Porter J, et al: Drug toxicity and hospitalization among lithium users. *J Clin Psychopharmacol* 1984;4:108–110.

Erwin C, Gerber C, Morrison S, et al: Lithium carbonate and convulsive disorders. *Arch Gen Psychiatr* 1973;28: 646–648.

Fava G, Molnar G, Block B, et al: The lithium loading dose method in a clinical setting. *Am J Psychiatr* 1984;141: 812–813.

Fawcett J, Clark D, Gibbons R, et al: Evaluation of lithium therapy for alcoholism. *J Clin Psychiatr* 1984;45: 494–499.

Hesketh J: Effects of potassium and lithium on sodium transport from blood to cerebrospinal fluid. *J Neurochem* 1977; 28:597–603.

Judd L, Huey L: Lithium antagonizes ethanol intoxication in alcoholics. *Am J Psychiatr* 1984;141:1517–1521.

King J, Aylard P, Hullin R: Side effects of lithium at lower therapeutic levels: The significance of thirst. *Psychol Med* 1985;15:355–361.

Lackroy G, Van Pragg H: Lithium salts as sedatives. *Acta Psychiatr Scand* 1971;47:163–173.

Louie A, Meltzer H: Lithium potentiation of antidepressant treatment. *J Clin Psychopharmacol* 1984;4:316–321.

Lyles M: Deep venous thrombophlebitis associated with lithium toxicity. *J Natl Med Assoc* 1984;76:633–634.

Prockop L, Marcus D: Cerebrospinal fluid lithium: Passive transfer kinetics. *Life Sci* 1972;11:859–868.

Rosen P, Stevens R: Action myoclonus in lithium toxicity. *Ann Neurol* 1983;13:221–222.

Spring G: Hazards of lithium prophylaxis. *Dis Nerv System* 1974;35:351–354.

Walevski A, Radwan M: Choreoathetosis as toxic effect of lithium treatment. *Eur Neurol* 1986;25:412–415.

Yassa R, Archer J, Cordoza S: The long-term effect of lithium carbonate on tardive dyskinesia. *Can J Psychiatr* 1984;29:36–37.

Yung C: A review of clinical trials of lithium in medicine. *Pharmacol Biochem Behav* 1984;21(suppl 1):51–55.

part IV

CARDIAC DRUGS

chapter 15

Cardiac Glycosides

Glycosides that have positive inotropic actions on the diseased heart occur widely in nature and can be prepared synthetically. The cardiac glycosides consist of a group of chemically and pharmacologically related substances derived from various plants (Table 15-1); each comprises a characteristic steroid molecule coupled with one or more types of sugar molecules. Cardiac glycosides of medicinal importance are obtained from *Digitalis purpurea* (purple foxglove)[1] and include digitoxin, digitalis, and gitalin. The beneficial effects of extracts of the leaves of the common foxglove were known for many years before the plant's medical usefulness was documented in 1776. *Digitalis lanata* yields digoxin, digitoxin, and deslanoside.

Table 15-1 Common Plants Containing Cardiac Glycosides

Plant	Common Name
Asclepias fruticosa	Balloon cotton
Digitalis purpurea	Foxglove
Plumeria rubra	Frangipani
Calotropis procera	King's crown
Convallaria majalis	Lily of the valley
Nerium oleander	Oleander
Cryptostegia grandiflora	Rubber vine
Cerbera manghas	Sea mango
Urginea maritima	Squill
Carissa spectabilis	Wintersweet
Thevetia peruviana	Yellow oleander

Table 15-2 Commercially Available Digitalis Preparations

Compound	Trade Names
Digoxin	Lanoxin®
	Lanoxicaps®
Digitoxin	Crystodigin®
	Purodigin®

The term digitalis is generally used to designate any of the steroid glycoside compounds that exert typical positive inotropic and electrophysiologic effects on the heart.[1] There are more than 300 compounds with this property. Powdered digitalis leaf has been superseded by purer preparations, including digoxin, digitoxin, ouabain, lanatoside C, deslanoside, and medigoxin; only the first two of these are widely prescribed. Commercially available digitalis preparations are listed in Table 15-2. Even though the frequency of digitalis intoxication appears to be decreasing, life-threatening toxicity continues to occur in patients who take overdoses by mistake or with suicidal intent.

PHARMACOKINETICS

Digoxin

Digoxin is the most commonly used cardiac glycoside primarily because it may be administered by various routes. Digoxin is 60% to 85% absorbed from the gastrointestinal tract (Table 15-3).[2–4] After oral administration the onset of action occurs in 30 minutes to 2 hours, and the drug reaches its peak plasma concentration in 3 to 8 hours. Digoxin has a volume of distribution of 7 to 10 L/kg. Approximately 23% of digoxin is bound to plasma proteins.[4] Fifteen percent undergoes hepatic transformation, and 85% is excreted unchanged by the kidney.[5] Digoxin is excreted exponentially and has an average half-life in patients with normal renal function of 36 hours, which results in a daily loss of about 37% of body stores. Renal excretion of digoxin is proportional to the glomerular filtration rate and hence to the creatinine clearance rate. The elimination half-life of digoxin is therefore greater in patients with impaired renal function. In previously undigitalized patients with normal renal function, institution of daily maintenance therapy of digoxin without a loading dose results in development of steady-state concentrations after four to five half-lives, or about 7 days.

Variation among digoxin tablets in bioavailability, and therefore in steady-state serum digoxin concentrations, was a cause of digitalis intoxication until quite recently. This was not due so much to differences in digoxin content as to differences in the dissolution rate of the tablets.[6–8] This was partly a result of differences in digoxin particularly size or in "inert" additives that had an effect on disintegration and dissolution rates within the intestinal lumen.[6–8]

Digitoxin

Oral absorption of digitoxin is considered virtually 100%.[2,4,9] This drug undergoes substantial enterohepatic circulation that is about fourfold that of digoxin.[2] It is mostly metabolized by the liver, whereas digoxin is mostly excreted by the kidney. The volume of distribution of digitoxin is approximately 0.54 L/kg. The maximum effect is attained in 4 to 12 hours. Digitoxin is 95% protein bound to serum albumin[4] and has a half-life of 5 to 7 days.[9] Administration of daily maintenance doses of digitoxin results in gradual digitalization with

Table 15-3 Differences in Pharmacokinetics between Digoxin and Digitoxin

Parameter	Digoxin	Digitoxin
Oral absorption	75% to 90%	90% to 100%
Plasma protein binding	25%	90%
Metabolism (M) compared to excretion (E)	E>M	M>E
Half-life	1.6 days	7 days
Volume of distribution	7–10 L/kg	0.5 L/kg
Enterohepatic recirculation	No	Yes

establishment of a final steady-state concentration after 3 to 4 weeks.

Digitoxin gives rise to intoxication less frequently than digoxin because its excretion is independent of renal function. Nevertheless, if intoxication does occur the signs and symptoms may persist for up to a week owing to the long half-life.[10]

Oleander

There are two common oleanders: *Thevetia peruviana* and *Nerium oleander*. The latter is more common in the United States. The plant is a flowering subtropical and tropical shrub valued for its colorful flowers, dense green foliage, and hardy nature.[11] It is common to many areas of the United States as a garden plant, and it is used widely in hedges and freeway medians.[12] Preparations of oleander containing the active ingredients have been used as rodenticides and insecticides and as remedies for fever, ringworm, leprosy, indigestion, and venereal disease.

All parts of the oleander plant are toxic, including the sap, leaves, blossoms, stems, seeds, honey, and berries. Most poisonings occur in children[13] and when the stems have been used as skewers or stirrers for outdoor picnics. Inhalation of oleander smoke has also caused toxicity. Boiling or drying the plant does not inactivate the toxins.[12]

The glycosides associated with oleander include oleandrin, digitoxigenin, and nerium from *Nerium oleander* and thevetin A and B and thevetoxin from *Thevetia peruviana*.[13] These glycosides account for the plants' cardiotoxic effects.[12] The similarities in activity and aglycone ring structure between these oleander glycosides and digoxin also allow a cross-reactivity in radioimmunoassays for digoxin.[13]

CLINICAL USES

Cardiac glycosides are used principally in the prophylactic management and treatment of heart failure and to control the ventricular rate in patients with atrial fibrillation or flutter (Table 15-4).[14] They have also been used to treat and prevent recurrent paroxysmal atrial tachycardia.[15]

ACTIONS

All cardiac glycosides produce the same qualitative therapeutic effect on the heart. This includes an increase in the force of contraction, an increase in the refractory period of the atrioventricular node, and an effect on the sinoatrial node and conduction system by way of the autonomic nervous system (Table 15-5).[1]

The main pharmacologic property of cardiac glycosides is their ability to increase the force and velocity of myocardial systolic contraction by a direct action on the myocardium.[2] Digitalis and the other cardiac glycosides can alter electrophysiological properties such as automaticity, conduction, refractoriness, and excitability of the various specialized conduction tissues, including the sinoatrial node, specialized tissues within the atrium, and atrioventricular, junctional, and Purkinje fibers.[3,4]

Table 15-4 Clinical Uses of Digitalis Preparations

Congestive heart failure
Atrial fibrillation
Atrial flutter
Paroxysmal atrial tachycardia
Atrioventricular junctional rhythm
Supraventricular tachycardia

Table 15-5 Cardiac Actions of Digitalis

Negative chronotropism
Positive inotropism
Slowing of sinus node impulse formation
Enhancement of intra-atrial conduction
Slowing of conduction velocity
Increase in rate of spontaneous depolarization

The effects of digoxin on these tissues may be to a different degree and sometimes in an opposite direction. For example, digitalis acts to cause negative chronotropic effects as well as positive inotropic effects. The negative chronotropic effect is reflected clinically as slowing of the heart rate, whereas the positive inotropic effect is reflected clinically as increased force of contraction of the cardiac muscle.[1] The negative chronotropic effect is due to an increase in vagal tone, prolongation of the refractory periods of the atrioventricular node and bundle of His, and slowing of the conduction velocity, although myocardial automaticity is increased. Digitalis can also slow sinus node impulse, hyperpolarize cells in the atrium, and enhance intra-atrial conduction.[4] The sinus slowing that accompanies digitalis therapy is therefore attributed to both a direct effect of the drug on impulse initiation by the sinus pacemaker cells and a cholinergic action mediated by the vagus nerve.[16]

Some of the pharmacologic properties of digitalis contribute to the relatively high incidence of cardiotoxic reactions.[17] This is attributable to the widespread use of cardiac glycosides coupled with the narrow margin between therapeutic and toxic doses and toxic and lethal doses.

Digitalis and the Action Potential

The transmembrane resting potential of cardiac cells is maintained by sodium and potassium gradients, which are in turn dependent on the integrity of the active sodium-potassium–activated adenosine triphosphatase (Na-K ATPase) pump. Because of the size of pores of the cells, the membrane is freely permeable to potassium and chloride ions (which are small), relatively impermeable to sodium, and essentially impermeable to organic anions (which are present as large protein molecules). The concentrations of sodium and chloride are much higher in the extracellular fluid than in the intracellular fluid, and the concentrations of potassium and organic acids are much higher in the intracellular fluid than in the extracellular fluid.[18]

As a consequence of this ionic imbalance, there is an electrical potential across the membrane. This electrical potential may reach 50 to 90 mV, with the inside of the membrane negative in relation to the outside. Such a difference in potential exists in every cell of the body and is referred to as the resting potential of the cell. When the neuron becomes less negative in relation to the extracellular fluid, the axon is said to be depolarized. When the axon is depolarized by a few millivolts, the permeability of the membrane is altered so that the membrane becomes rapidly more permeable to sodium.

Digitalis exerts a positive inotropic effect on cardiac muscle by directly binding to the membrane Na-K ATPase pump.[2,19] This enzyme is required for active transport of sodium across myocardial cell membranes.[18] By impairing active transport of these ions the increase in intracellular sodium causes a net influx of calcium, which results in an increased concentration of calcium in the sarcoplasm. The subsequent rise in intracellular calcium allows an increase in the number of actin-myosin interactions, thereby increasing the force of myocardial contraction.[19]

Because ATPase appears to be essential to couple metabolic energy to the active cation transport mechanism at the cell surface, the digitalis-poisoned myocardium cannot extrude the sodium gained or recover the potassium lost during each action potential.[2,20,21] This results in a slower rate of rise of the action potential, a slower conduction velocity with resultant conduction delays, and an increase in spontaneous depolarization.[16] This mechanism can explain the re-entrant tachydysrhythmias, the enhanced ventricular ectopic activity, and the depression of the atrioventricular conduction that are seen with toxic concentrations of digitalis.[7] In addition, toxicity results in part from loss of intracellular potassium associated with the inhibition of Na-K ATPase.[8]

Digitalis and the Autonomic Nervous System

The actions of digitalis on the autonomic nervous system are also important clinically and play a major role in determining the clinical pharmacodynamic effects of the drug.[1] At therapeutic concentrations, the predominant effect is activation of vagal tone. At toxic concentrations, there appears to be activation of sympathetic tone.[19] This may contribute to the dysrhythmogenic effects of digoxin. Therefore, digitalis causes cardiac dysrhythmias not only by mechanisms that result from its inhibition of Na-K ATPase but also by mechanisms that result from its neural effects, such as augmentation of activity on vagal and sympathetic nerves.[10]

DRUG INTERACTIONS

Calcium Antagonists

Certain calcium antagonists interact with digitalis to produce potentially undesirable electrophysiologic effects. Verapamil and diltiazem both impede conduction through the atrioventricular node. If these agents are combined with digitalis, the effect could be more marked than desirable.[4]

Quinidine

The administration of quinidine to patients taking digoxin causes a significant increase in serum digoxin concentrations, with steady-state concentrations increasing by two to three times.[22] The increase in serum digoxin concentration is due to a decrease in the apparent volume of distribution for digoxin caused by quinidine.[19,23–25] This is because quinidine displaces digoxin from tissues by decreasing the affinity of receptor sites on Na-K ATPase membranes for digoxin.[2,23,26] Thus the decrease in volume of distribution may reflect in part a decrease in the affinity of tissue receptors for digoxin.[27] Quinidine also appears to cause a decrease in the rate of digitalis elimination or the clearance of digoxin.[19,26]

PLASMA DIGITALIS CONCENTRATIONS

Radioimmunoassay uses antibodies of high affinity and specificity for cardiac glycosides and permits the rapid and accurate determination of serum digitalis concentrations.[14,20,28] A specific plasma concentration may be therapeutic or toxic in an individual patient, however, depending on factors other than dosage, such as serum electrolytes; acid-base balance; type, severity, and duration of cardiac disorder; thyroid status; autonomic nervous system tone; and concurrently administered drugs.[6,14,17] Increased serum digoxin concentrations are sometimes seen without toxicity in patients with atrial dysrhythmias or hyperkalemia (which may be protective) and in infants and children.[14] Serum digoxin concentration may also be falsely high in acute poisoning; therefore this measurement by itself lacks usefulness in the initial assessment of acute poisoning. Serum digoxin concentrations are best determined more than 6 hours after ingestion. When determined earlier than this they may give a false impression of severity.[29]

With digoxin, impairment of renal function is associated with high serum concentrations at any given dose.[14,21] Plasma digitoxin concentrations correlate poorly with renal function.

In radioimmunoassay, digoxin and oleander glycoside cross-react. This causes an increase in the digoxin concentration after ingestion of oleander. Because the degree of cross-reactivity is unknown,[11] digoxin radioimmunoassays reveal only the presence of the oleander glycoside, not the degree of toxicity.[30]

A digoxin-like immunoreactive substance that causes false-positive digoxin immunoassays has been found in adults with renal insufficiency who are not taking digoxin,[31] pregnant women,[32] and neonates, fetuses, and infants less than 2 months of age.[33] This substance may be produced by the infant before as well as after birth. This has raised concern about the reliability of the present method of digoxin measurements from the serum or plasma of neonatal patients.[31] This substance may not simply interfere in the digoxin immunoassay but may be a hormone of interest in various responses to stress or disease.[33]

TOXICITY

The molecular mechanism of digitalis intoxication is an extension of its therapeutic action. Alterations in cardiac rhythm as well as extracardiac manifestations of digitalis action, such as gastrointestinal and CNS symptoms, are dose related. Serum concentration may correlate with chronic toxicity, but there is considerable overlap between therapeutic and toxic concentrations. The single oral lethal dose of cardiac glycosides is approximately 20 to 50 times the usual daily maintenance dose.

Factors that may precipitate toxic reactions include an increasing severity of myocardial disease; electrolyte disturbance such as hypokalemia,[19] hypercalcemia, and hypomagnesemia; hypoxia; and hepatic disease (Table 15-6). A common cause of digoxin intoxication is reduced renal elimination of the drug, which may be insidious. Some patients who have certain anaerobic bacteria in the colon may require large doses of digoxin to achieve adequate serum digoxin concentrations because the organism reduces the lactone ring of the glycoside. When these patients are treated with antibiotics that abolish this organism, such as erythromycin or tetracycline, the serum digoxin concentrations can rise to toxic levels because bacterial inactivation is abruptly removed.

Two of the most significant determinants of susceptibility to digitalis poisoning are the age of the patient and the presence or absence of preexisting heart disease.[34] Except for premature infants and neonates, infants and children are

---

Table 15-6 Factors Increasing the Likelihood of Toxic Reactions to Digoxin

---

Age of patient
Degree of heart disease
Electrolyte disturbances
   —Hypokalemia
   —Hypomagnesemia
   —Hypercalcemia
Hypoxia
Hepatic disease
Renal disease
Antibiotic therapy

---

more tolerant than adults to the therapeutic and toxic actions of cardiac glycosides. Similarly, young adults are more tolerant than old adults. In addition, the clinical picture associated with acute ingestion of digitalis often is different from that seen with toxicity associated with excessive therapeutic use.[3] Young adults and children may demonstrate bradycardia with various degrees of entrance and exit blocks at the atrioventricular junction, whereas older patients with heart disease have ventricular dysrhythmias.[34] It is important, therefore, to distinguish between acute poisoning in a nondigitalized individual and the gradual development of intoxication in a patient taking the drug for heart failure. Patients without heart disease tend to tolerate high levels of serum digoxin, and the dysrhythmias encountered are most often disturbances of conduction. Patients with underlying heart disease have the greatest problems with ventricular ectopy and the worst prognosis.

Signs of intoxication do not typically occur in a regular sequence, and subjective signs of toxicity are frequently less easily recognized in infants and children than in adults. Toxicity may be manifested by gastrointestinal, CNS, psychic, visual, and cardiac symptoms.

Gastrointestinal Symptoms

Gastrointestinal symptoms are frequent in both acute and chronic digitalis intoxication.[4] Anorexia, nausea, and vomiting are common signs[3] and are usually present early in the course of an overdose and may not be recognized.[35] These symptoms are thought to be due to stimulation in the area postrema of the medulla and are seen with both intravenous and oral preparations.[4]

Central Nervous System Symptoms

Headache, fatigue, malaise, drowsiness, and generalized muscle weakness are the most common CNS signs of intoxication (Table 15-7). Irritability, vertigo, dizziness, syncope, apathy, lethargy, opisthotonus, and seizures have also occurred.

Table 15-7 CNS Disturbances Associated with Digitalis Intoxication

Dizziness
Drowsiness
Fatigue
Headache
Irritability
Lethargy
Malaise
Seizures
Syncope
Vertigo
Weakness

Table 15-8 Psychic Disturbances Associated with Digitalis Intoxication

Amnesia
Aphasia
Confusion
Disorientation
Delirium
Hallucinations
Impaired memory

Psychic Symptoms

Psychic disturbances due to digitalis intoxication may include impaired memory, amnesia, aphasia, confusion, disorientation, delusions, depression,[36] delirium, and hallucinations (Table 15-8).[37,38]

Visual Symptoms

Visual disturbances caused by toxic doses of cardiac glycosides are partly due to effects on the retina, in which the cones are affected more than the rods. Color vision is commonly affected, and objects may appear to be yellow or green and, less commonly, brown, red, blue, or white.[4,39] Blurred vision, photophobia, and perceived halos or borders on objects may also occur (Table 15-9). In addition, transient amblyopia and scotoma may occur.

Cardiac Symptoms

Cardiac manifestations are the most frequent and most dangerous sign of digitalis intoxication

Table 15-9 Visual Disturbances Associated with Digitalis Intoxication

Distorted color vision
Blurred vision
Halos around lights
Photophobia
Scotoma

Table 15-10 Cardiac Manifestations of Digitalis Intoxication

Acute intoxication
  Atrioventricular conduction disturbances
  First-degree block
  Sinus impulse formation disturbances
  Sinus bradycardia
  Sinus arrest
  Sinoatrial block
  Second-degree atrioventricular block
  Third-degree atrioventricular block
Chronic intoxication
  Paroxysmal atrial tachycardia with block
  Nonparoxysmal junctional tachycardia
  Bidirectional ventricular tachycardia
  Atrioventricular dissociation
  Second-degree atrioventricular block (Type I)
  Ventricular tachycardia
  Ventricular fibrillation

(Table 15-10).[4] Digitalis is capable of producing almost every known cardiac dysrhythmia.[19,40,41] Nevertheless, some disorders such as intraventricular block evidenced by a wide QRS interval and atrial fibrillation are rarely seen. No dysrhythmia is unique to digitalis poisoning, but cardiotonic glycosides are by far the most likely cause of nonparoxysmal nodal tachycardia, atrial tachycardia with atrioventricular dissociation, and bidirectional ventricular tachycardia. The cardiac dysrhythmias induced by digitalis are nonspecific, and electrocardiographically identical dysrhythmias may be induced by underlying heart disease,[19] drugs other than digitalis, or numerous extracardiac aberrations.[41] The cardiac manifestations of digitalis intoxication differ in the patient with underlying heart disease and chronic intoxication compared to the patient with a relatively normal myocardium and acute intoxication (Table 15-11).[3]

ACUTE INTOXICATION

In an otherwise healthy patient with acute intoxication, ventricular dysrhythmias or ectopy are uncommon. The healthy myocardium responds to an excess of digitalis by developing atrioventricular conduction disturbances with evidence of first-degree atrioventricular block.[4,40] Infants, young children, and healthy adults with digitalis intoxication therefore respond in this manner.[19] Disturbances of sinus impulse formation take the form of an inappropriate sinus bradycardia, sinus arrest, or sinoatrial block. First-degree atrioventricular block is also common. The acute overdose is further characterized by second- or third-degree atrioventricular block in the presence of normal or abnormal sinus rhythm. These effects result primarily from increased vagal activity.[19]

CHRONIC INTOXICATION

The diseased heart frequently responds with various ventricular cardiac dysrhythmias.[4] Dys-

Table 15-11 Symptoms of Acute Compared to Chronic Digoxin Overdose

Parameter	Acute Overdose (Normal Heart)	Chronic Overdose (Diseased Heart)
Serum digoxin concentration	Increased	Increased or therapeutic
Serum potassium concentration	Normal to high	Normal to low
Noncardiac manifestations	Nausea, vomiting	Anorexia, nausea, vomiting, ocular disturbances, CNS disturbances

Source: Adapted with permission from *American Journal of Hospital Pharmacy* (1978;35:268–277), Copyright © 1978, American Society of Hospital Pharmacists.

Table 15-12 Laboratory Tests in Digoxin Intoxication

Serum digoxin concentration
Serum potassium concentration
Serum magnesium concentration
Serum calcium concentration
Serum creatinine concentration
Blood urea nitrogen
Electrocardiogram

---

rhythmias that are highly suggestive of toxic reactions to long-term administration of digitalis include atrial tachycardia with block, nonparoxysmal junctional tachycardia, bidirectional ventricular tachycardia, atrioventricular dissociation usually with acceleration of the junctional focus, and other rhythms.[19,40] Second-degree block usually manifests as Wenckebach period. Mobitz type II block is also uncommon in digitalis toxicity.[4] Atrial fibrillation or atrial flutter with rapid atrioventricular conduction are not usually seen with long-term digitalis intoxication.[4]

LABORATORY TESTS

Initial laboratory studies should include serum digoxin, potassium, magnesium, calcium, and creatinine concentrations as well as blood urea nitrogen. An electrocardiogram should also be obtained (Table 15-12). Therapeutic plasma concentrations of digoxin are generally 0.5 to 2.0 ng/mL.[31] In adults, toxicity is usually but not always associated with steady-state digoxin plasma concentrations greater than 2 ng/mL (Table 15-13).[3]

Potassium and Magnesium

In general, relative hyperkalemia is protective against, and hypokalemia may exacerbate, an

Table 15-13 Therapeutic and Toxic Concentrations of Digoxin and Digitoxin

Drug	Therapeutic	Toxic
Digoxin	0.5 to 2.0 ng/mL	>2.0 ng/mL
Digitoxin	15 to 30 ng/mL	>45 ng/mL

abnormal rhythm induced by digitalis intoxication (Table 15-14). Because cardiac glycosides inhibit the Na-K ATPase pump, acute cardiac glycoside intoxication often leads to a release of intracellular potassium into the extracellular space, which results in high or even fatal elevations of serum potassium.[42,43] The hyperkalemia results from poisoning of the membrane-bound Na-K ATPase system not only in the myocardium but in all body tissues.[34,42] Hyperkalemia with serum potassium concentrations sometimes exceeding 13 mEq/L have been reported.[12,30,44] The resulting decrease in intracellular potassium concentration reduces the normal resting membrane potential.[4] The myocardial cells lose their ability to function as pacemaker cells, and asystole results. Ultimately there is a complete loss of cardiac electrical activity. Increased renal excretion of potassium may result from hyperkalemia, and thus some patients may appear to be hyperkalemic while having a total body deficit of potassium.

Hypokalemia is often a problem in chronic digitalis intoxication because of concurrent use of a diuretic, not as a direct result of the digitalis. Hypokalemia predisposes patients to ventricular ectopy and tachydysrhythmias because depletion of myocardial potassium reduces the threshold for depolarization of ectopic pacemakers. Magnesium acts in the same manner, and hypomagnesemia may potentiate digitalis toxicity.[3,4]

Calcium

Chronic digitalis intoxication may be exacerbated by rapid infusions of calcium, and intoxication may occur at low serum digoxin concentrations when hypercalcemia is present. This is probably because calcium administration

Table 15-14 Selected Electrolytes and Associated Digitalis Toxicity

Electrolyte	High Concentration	Low Concentration
Potassium	Protective	Increased toxicity
Magnesium	Protective	Increased toxicity
Calcium	Increased toxicity	Protective

decreases the serum potassium concentration. Hypocalcemia appears to be protective against dysrhythmias resulting from digitalis toxicity.[4]

TREATMENT OF DIGITALIS INTOXICATION

Treatment of acute cardiac glycoside ingestion begins with basic life support measures, including airway control and circulatory support (Table 15-15).[5] Emesis should be induced or gastric lavage performed, and activated charcoal and a cathartic should be administered.[34] In patients with heart block or sinus bradycardia, vomiting or placement of a lavage tube may lead to increased vagal tone and worsening of the rhythm or asystole.[4] If a conduction disturbance

is noted or if there is great potential for this disturbance, atropine should be administered intravenously before the administration of ipecac or performance of lavage.

Supportive Measures

There is no effective means for increasing digitalis excretion or metabolism. Because of the high degree of tissue binding of digitalis, forced diuresis, plasmapheresis, hemoperfusion, and hemodialysis do not effectively remove the drug from the body and therefore should not be attempted.[5,30,34,45–49] Hemodialysis may be of value in controlling hyperkalemia secondary to acute digitalis intoxication.[4,45]

Toxic manifestations of digoxin rapidly disappear when the drug is withdrawn, so that in the vast majority of patients digitalis cardiotoxic reactions can be handled by simply discontinuing the drug. Because digoxin is eliminated from the body by first-order kinetics, with 30% of the residual drug in the body being eliminated each day, if renal function is normal, toxic symptoms will usually disappear within 24 hours and often sooner.[50] On the basis of this first-order elimination, by obtaining a minimum of two serum digoxin concentration values the time scale for recovery can be predicted.

Dysrhythmias such as paroxysmal atrial tachycardia with atrioventricular block, atrioventricular junctional rhythm with slow rate, and atrial fibrillation or flutter with slow ventricular rate induced by digitalis can usually be treated by stopping the drug. Further management of digitalis intoxication includes close attention to the metabolic state with correction of hypoxemia, acid-base disturbances, and alterations in potassium metabolism.

Atropine

The action of atropine depends on its ability to block vagal activity and by so doing to increase impulse formation and conduction rate at the sinoatrial and atrioventricular nodes. Atropine may be administered in the hemodynamically symptomatic patient with sinus bradycardia, high-degree atrioventricular block, or sinus exit

Table 15-15 Treatment of Digitalis Intoxication

Indication	Modality
Acute ingestion	Emesis or lavage
Acute ingestion	Charcoal and cathartic
Symptomatic	Atropine
Bradycardia	
Atrioventricular block	
Sinus exit block	
Second-degree block	
Third-degree block	
Ventricular abnormalities	Phenytoin
Bigeminy	
Tachycardia	
Premature contractions	
Ventricular abnormalities	Lidocaine
Bigeminy	
Tachycardia	
Premature contractions	
Hypokalemia	Potassium
Symptomatic and unresponsive	Pacemaker
Bradycardia	
Atrioventricular block	
Second-degree block	
Third-degree block	
Severe hyperkalemia	Hemodialysis
Ventricular abnormalities	Antibody therapy
Tachycardia	
Fibrillation	
Symptomatic and unresponsive	
Bradycardia	
Second-degree block	
Third-degree block	
Severe hyperkalemia	
Significant ingestion	

block.[4,51] Atropine is likely to be more successful in reducing block in acute poisoning than in chronic poisoning. As a general rule, however, the drug is not effective,[15,46] and electrical pacing may be attempted if more aggressive treatment is indicated for a slow rate.

Phenytoin

Phenytoin is the drug of choice in treating ventricular dysrhythmias in the presence of atrioventricular blocks.[10] It depresses enhanced ventricular automaticity without affecting intraventricular conduction and also reverses digitalis-induced prolongation of atrioventricular conduction.[4] Phenytoin has been used effectively in reversing digitalis-induced ventricular dysrhythmias, including bigeminy, unifocal and multifocal premature ventricular contractions, and ventricular tachycardia.[5,52] Phenytoin increases the membrane potential toward normal and enhances atrioventricular and interventricular conduction.[52] It remains effective in the presence of acid-base imbalance and electrolyte imbalance such as hyperkalemia. Phenytoin is not approved by the FDA for use as an antidysrhythmic agent, however.

Lidocaine

Lidocaine may be useful in managing digitalis-induced ventricular tachydysrhythmias, premature contractions, and bigeminy.[10] In this respect it is similar to phenytoin but has essentially no effect on alterations of atrial activity and does not improve conduction through the atrioventricular node. Lidocaine may be given as a bolus of 1.0 mg/kg and followed by a constant infusion of 1 to 4 mg/min. Because lidocaine does not affect atrioventricular conduction, it can be used in the presence of atrioventricular block.[4]

Magnesium

In digitalis intoxication, magnesium appears either to block the transient inward current of calcium or to antagonize calcium at cellular binding sites.[30] Some investigators have shown that magnesium in adequate doses specifically counteracts the ventricular irritability caused by excessive amounts of digitalis.[53] Magnesium may also be useful in counteracting the hyperkalemia associated with digitalis by blocking the egress of potassium from the cells.[3]

The dosage of magnesium for adults is 2 g of 10% magnesium sulfate intravenously over 20 minutes.[3] Magnesium concentrations should be checked every 2 hours and a dose titrated to maintain 4 to 5 mEq/L.

Potassium

Potassium is an excellent agent for the prompt suppression of the ventricular dysrhythmias secondary to chronic digitalis intoxication associated with hypokalemia.[10] The cation may be administered intravenously in the form of potassium chloride at a rate of 0.5 mEq/min as a solution in saline or 5% dextrose containing 50 to 60 mEq of potassium per liter.

Potassium is contraindicated in the presence of renal failure or hyperkalemia. Potassium infusion in acute massive digoxin overdose is also contraindicated because massive efflux of potassium is noted after the acute overdose,[45] so that as a blind maneuver it is potentially hazardous in the face of high-normal to high serum potassium concentrations.

Treatment of Hyperkalemia

Hyperkalemia after an acute digoxin overdose may be life threatening. In addition, this serious problem may not respond to methods that are normally effective, such as calcium administration, glucose and insulin administration, or bicarbonate infusion. This is because the Na-K ATPase pump has been "poisoned" by the digoxin.[54] Potassium concentrations in hyperkalemic patients must be controlled by other measures, such as the use of resins or hemodialysis. Although such measures may lower serum potassium concentrations, they may be ineffective in re-establishing membrane potentials because of the poisoning of the Na-K ATPase pump. In stable patients, sodium polystyrene sulfonate (Kayexalate®) may help reduce serum potassium concentrations. Sodium polystyrene sulfonate (1 g per milliequivalent of excess potassium in the serum) may be administered with 70% sorbitol either orally or as a retention enema. This resin complex acts to lower serum potassium by exchange of a cation (sodium or hydrogen) for potassium, for which the resin has a high affinity. The time needed for therapeutic effect is slow. Fragment antigen-binding (Fab) antibody therapy has also been shown to lower serum potassium concentrations quickly and is the agent of choice for life-threatening hyperkalemia.

Cardiac Pacemaker

Although pacemaker insertion is relatively safe, myocardial cells poisoned by cardiac glycosides may not respond to electrical stimulation. Current indications for temporary transvenous ventricular pacing for digoxin overdose include sinus bradycardia, exit block, or high-degree atrioventricular block unresponsive to atropine and associated with signs and symptoms of inadequate organ perfusion.[55] Because cardiac glycosides lower the threshold for pacemaker-induced extrasystole, placement of a pacemaker may produce life-threatening dysrhythmias.[4]

Cardioversion

Cardioversion should be performed only when necessary because it may induce ventricular fibrillation in the digitalis intoxicated patient. When necessary, it should be done at the lowest energy setting possible.[5,30]

Bile Acid Resins

Because of the extensive enterohepatic recirculation of digitoxin, nonabsorbed substances such as cholestyramine,[56] colestipol,[57] kaolin, nonabsorbable antacids, and activated charcoal may interrupt this mechanism.[9,10,34] Although many of these agents have been used to increase the enterohepatic elimination of digitoxin, the results have often been unimpressive.[15] Cholestyramine has been administered as a 4-g dose orally every 8 hours for 3 days.[56] Nevertheless, cholestyramine has no advantages over activated charcoal, which is preferred because of its lack of side effects.

Digitalis Antibody Therapy (Digibind®)

For several decades in the past no significant advance was made in the treatment of severe digoxin intoxication and accepted treatment did not offer optimal results for the severely intoxicated patient.[58] Treatment was directed toward either inhibiting the absorption of the drug or counteracting its cardiac effects.[59] The availability of digoxin antibodies led to the development of a radioimmunoassay to measure serum digoxin concentrations; this assay is now used routinely to determine patient compliance and digoxin toxicity.[60,61] Shortly after this development it was postulated that antibodies to digoxin could be used to reverse its pharmacologic and toxic effects. Probably the most dramatic breakthrough in the treatment of severe digoxin intoxication occurred in the mid 1970s, when a report appeared describing the use of immunotherapy to reverse the signs of toxicity and hasten the elimination of the offending agent.[50,62–65]

Digitalis has a relatively low molecular weight and is therefore not immunogenic. It is rendered antigenic by coupling it to a carrier protein.

As early as 1967 it was shown that the whole antibody from the serum of animals bound digoxin, but the large size of the molecule and the lack of purity precluded its use.[66] The whole antibody to digoxin was also antigenic in its own right and had a prolonged half-life in the body because the intact antibody-digoxin complex was too large to enter the glomerular filtrate.[67] To promote more rapid excretion as well as decreased antigenicity, the antibody produced in sheep was digested with papain to yield three fragments. Two of these are called the Fab fragments, and they retain the antigen-binding properties of the molecule.[59,64–66] The other portion, which is not used, is the c fragment (F_c).[47] This is the portion involved in complement activation and other effector functions.

Each Fab segment has one combining site of the parent antigen molecule. They are smaller than the parent antigen and have intact binding affinity and specificity for digoxin when separated from nonspecific antigen fragments.[64,65] This results in more rapid distribution, a shorter elimination time, and lower immunogenicity than the parent antigen.[47]

The Fab-digoxin complex is small enough to allow rapid clearance that, coupled with the absence of c fragment, results in minimal antigenic stimulus to the patient.[66] The Fab segments, which have a molecular size of 50,000 daltons, bind free digoxin, which has a molecular size of 781 daltons, and render it inactive.[64] The affinity of digoxin-specific Fab for digoxin is greater than the affinity of digoxin for Na-K ATPase.

Because the interaction of cardiac glycosides is reversible, a concentration gradient is established that results in a progressive efflux of membrane-bound digoxin. Because the interaction of digoxin with its cellular receptors is also reversible, the reduction in free digoxin results in progressive removal of digoxin from receptor sites as the drug-receptor equilibrium is displaced in the direction of dissociation. The dissociation of the cardiac glycoside from its cellular receptor and its subsequent bonding to the high-affinity Fab antibody results in rapid reversal of the cardiac rhythm disturbances. In other words, after intravenous administration of Fab, any free digoxin is bound intravascularly. Fab antibodies then diffuse into the extracellular space and bind any free digoxin. Because of the reduction in concentration, there is an efflux of free intracellular digoxin into the extracellular fluid, where it is also immediately bound. Digoxin molecules dissociate from the membrane receptors and are removed from the site of action by binding to Fab. In patients with good renal function, the digoxin-Fab complex appears to be eliminated fairly rapidly by glomerular filtration; the elimination half-life is about 16 to 20 hours.[61,66] It is not known whether digoxin-specific Fab is removed by hemodialysis.

Fab antibodies interfere with digitalis immunoassay measurements, although serum digoxin concentrations do not decrease but rather rise dramatically.[61] These high concentrations, however, reflect the amount of digoxin bound in an inactive form to the antibody fragment that is consistent with the dissociation of digoxin from its membrane site.[66] Free digoxin decreases rapidly to undetectable concentrations after Fab administration. The antidysrhythmic effect of the antibody can be dramatic, with complete reversal of potentially lethal problems seen in as little as 30 minutes.[66,67]

The use of purified, digoxin-specific Fab antibodies therefore provides a new and exciting therapeutic approach in the management of advanced digoxin intoxication.[68] The glycosides' high potency requires that only a relatively small amount of foreign antibody protein be administered, thereby reducing the likelihood of developing serum sickness.

Indications for Fab Therapy

Fab therapy should be reserved for those cases in which there is a life-threatening situation or the potential for such.[65] Manifestations of life-threatening toxicity include severe ventricular dysrhythmias, such as ventricular tachycardia or ventricular fibrillation, or progressive bradydysrhythmias, such as severe sinus bradycardia or second- or third-degree heart block not responsive to atropine or pacemaker. Severe hyperkalemia may also be an indication for Fab therapy.[2,61,65] In addition, histories of ingestions of more than 10 mg of digoxin in previously healthy adults or 4 mg in previously healthy children, or of ingestion causing steady-state serum concentrations greater than 10 ng/mL, often result in cardiac arrest and would warrant serious consideration for Fab therapy. In patients with elevated serum digoxin concentrations but with no signs of toxicity, Fab therapy is unwarranted.[61]

Since the advent of digoxin-specific Fab antibodies, there has been a marked reduction in mortality rates. This treatment constitutes an effective and highly specific means of reversing advanced, life-threatening digitalis intoxication. The FDA recently approved digoxin-specific Fab antibodies for clinical use, and the preparation is marketed as Digibind®.

Although antibodies to a large number of drugs have been produced, their use therapeutically is likely to be limited. The immense problems in manufacturing, purifying, and administering large quantities of antibodies are such that this technique is restricted to the very few drugs that cause serious toxicity when taken in milligram amounts.[61]

Dosage

The dosage of Fab must be determined according to the severity of the poisoning and the quantity of glycoside in the body (Table 15-16).[68] Eighty milligrams of Fab bind 1 mg of glycoside. Each vial, which contains 40 mg of Fab antibody, binds approximately 0.6 mg of digoxin. In most cases, however, the quantity of glycoside is not known precisely and can therefore only be estimated. The calculated quantity of Fab is dissolved in physiologic saline to give a concentration of 2 to 4 mg/mL and is infused over 30 minutes.

Fab therapy has also been effective in cases of digitoxin poisoning. In addition, the cross-reactivity between the glycosides in oleander and in digoxin noted in radioimmunoassay may mean that treatment of oleander poisoning with digoxin-specific Fab antibody could be effective.

Table 15-16 Fab Antibody Dosage Calculation Chart

Approximate Digibind dose for reversal of single-ingestion digoxin overdose

Number of Tablets or Capsules of Digoxin Ingested				Digibind Dose	
0.05 mg capsules	0.125 mg tablets or 0.1 mg capsules	0.25 mg tablets or 0.2 mg capsules	0.5 mg tablets	mg	vials
25	12–13	6	3	85	2
50	25	12–13	6	170	4.25
100	50	25	12–13	340	8.5
200	100	50	25	680	17
300	150	75	37–38	1000	25
400	200	100	50	1360	34

Estimated adult dose in vials (v) from serum digoxin concentration (ng/mL)

Patient weight (kg)	Serum Digoxin Concentration (ng/mL)						
	1	2	4	8	12	16	20
40	0.5v	1v	2v	3v	5v	6v	8v
60	0.5v	1v	2v	5v	7v	9v	11v
70	1.0v	2v	3v	5v	8v	11v	13v
80	1.0v	2v	3v	6v	9v	12v	15v
100	1.0v	2v	4v	8v	11v	15v	19v

Estimated pediatric dose in mg from serum digoxin concentration (ng/mL)

Patient weight (kg)	Serum Digoxin Concentration (ng/mL)						
	1	2	4	8	12	16	20
1	0.5 mg*	1.0 mg*	1.5 mg*	3.0 mg	5 mg	6 mg	8 mg
3	1.0 mg*	2.0 mg*	5.0 mg	9.0 mg	13 mg	18 mg	22 mg
5	2.0 mg*	4.0 mg	8.0 mg	15.0 mg	22 mg	30 mg	40 mg
10	4.0 mg	8.0 mg	15.0 mg	30.0 mg	40 mg	60 mg	80 mg
20	8.0 mg	15.0 mg	30.0 mg	60.0 mg	80 mg	120 mg	160 mg

Source: Courtesy of Burroughs Wellcome Company, Research Triangle Park, North Carolina.

Side Effects of Fab Therapy

No serious adverse reactions have occurred from Fab therapy, yet the possibility exists. This may be especially true in patients who are subsequently exposed to antibody therapy in the future.[61]

Contraindicated Agents

Propranolol

Propranolol has been successful in terminating ventricular premature beats secondary to digitalis intoxication. Its use should be limited to controlling ectopy and tachydysrhythmias. It is contraindicated in the presence of blocks, such as atrial tachycardia with block, because its net effect is to decrease automaticity and to slow conduction velocity, thereby inducing bradycardia.[53] Propranolol cannot be thought of as a first-line drug and should not be used unless lidocaine and phenytoin have been ineffective.

Bretylium, Procainamide, and Quinidine

Bretylium should be avoided because it may worsen dysrhythmias by stimulating the release of catecholamines, which have been shown to aggravate digitalis-induced dysrhythmias.[4,5] Procainamide and quinidine should also be avoided.[53]

SUMMARY

Conventional measures such as the administration of lidocaine or phenytoin for control of ventricular dysrhythmias, the use of atropine or transvenous pacemakers for symptomatic bradycardia, restoration of potassium balance and, most important, the allowance of time for excretion of digoxin or metabolism of digitoxin are at present the best recommendations for most patients with digitalis intoxication. Fab therapy should be reserved for the severely intoxicated patient. Elderly patients with severe cardiac disease and patients with severe suicidal poisoning are at greatest risk of mortality.

REFERENCES

1. Powis D: Cardiac glycosides and autonomic neurotransmission. *J Auton Pharmacol* 1983;3:127–154.

2. Doherty J, Straub K, Murphy M, et al: Digoxin-quinidine interaction. *Am J Cardiol* 1980;45:1196–1200.

3. Reisdorff E, Clark M, Walters B: Acute digitalis poisoning: The role of intravenous magnesium sulfate. *J Emerg Med* 1986;4:463–469.

4. Sharff J, Bayer M: Acute and chronic digitalis toxicity: Presentation and treatment. *Ann Emerg Med* 1982;11:327–331.

5. Drake C: Cardiac drug overdose. *Am Fam Physician* 1982;25:181–187.

6. Smith T, Haber E: Digitalis (first of four parts), *N Engl J Med* 1973;289:945–952.

7. Smith T, Haber E: Digitalis (second of four parts), *N Engl J Med* 1973;289:1010–1015.

8. Smith T, Haber E: Digitalis (third of four parts), *N Engl J Med* 1973;289:1063–1069.

9. Baciewicz A, Isaacson M, Lipscomb G: Cholestyramine resin in the treatment of digitoxin toxicity. *Drug Intell Clin Pharmacol* 1983;17:57–59.

10. Cady W, Rehder T, Campbell J: Use of cholestyramine resin in the treatment of digitoxin toxicity. *Am J Hosp Pharmacol* 1979;36:92–94.

11. Radford D, Gillies A, Hinds J, et al: Naturally occurring cardiac glycosides. *Med J Aust* 1986;144:540–544.

12. Osterloh J, Herold S, Pond S: Oleander interference in the digoxin radioimmunoassay in a fatal ingestion. *JAMA* 1982;247:1596–1597.

13. Ansford H, Morris H: Fatal oleander poisoning. *Med J Aust* 1981;1:360–361.

14. Smith T: New advances in the assessment and treatment of digitalis toxicity. *J Clin Pharmacol* 1985;25:522–528.

15. Smith T, Willerson J: Suicidal and accidental digoxin ingestion. *Circulation* 1971;44:29–36.

16. Rosen M, Wit A, Hoffman B: Electrophysiology and pharmacology of cardiac arrhythmias: Part IV: Cardiac antiarrhythmic and toxic effects of digitalis. *Am Heart J* 1975;89:391–399.

17. Ordog G, Benaron S, Bhasin V, et al: Serum digoxin levels and mortality in 5,100 patients. *Ann Emerg Med* 1987;16:32–39.

18. Watanabe A: Digitalis and the autonomic nervous system. *J Am Coll Cardiol* 1985;5:35A–42A.

19. Bigger J: Digitalis toxicity. *J Clin Pharmacol* 1985;25:514–521.

20. Mason D, Zelis R, Lee G: Current concepts and treatment of digitalis toxicity. *Am J Cardiol* 1971;27:546–559.

21. Mason D: Digitalis pharmacology and therapeutics: Recent advances. *Ann Intern Med* 1974;80:520–530.

22. Fenster P, Hager W, Perrier D, et al: Digoxin-quinidine interaction in patients with chronic renal failure. *Circulation* 1982;66:1277–1279.

23. Ball W, Tse-eng D, Wallick E, et al: Effect of quinidine on the digoxin receptor in vitro. *J Clin Invest* 1981;68:1065–1074.

24. Chen T, Friedman H: Alteration of digoxin pharmacokinetics by a single dose of quinidine. *JAMA* 1980;244:669–762.

25. Leahey E, Bigger J, Butler V, et al: Quinidine-digoxin interaction: Time course and pharmacokinetics. *Am J Cardiol* 1981;48:1141–1146.

26. Belz G, Doering W, Aust P, et al: Quinidine-digoxin interaction: Cardiac efficacy of elevated serum digoxin concentration. *Clin Pharmacol Ther* 1982;31:548–554.

27. Hager W, Mayersohn M, Graves P: Digoxin bioavailability during quinidine administration. *Clin Pharmacol Ther* 1981;30:594–599.

28. Hobson J, Zettner A: Digoxin serum half-life following suicidal digoxin poisoning. *JAMA* 1973;223:147–150.

29. Lewander W, Gaudreault P, Einhorn A, et al: Acute pediatric digoxin ingestion. *Am J Dis Child* 1986;140:770–773.

30. Haynes B, Bessen H, Wightman W: Oleander tea: Herbal draught of death. *Ann Emerg Med* 1985;14:350–353.

31. Valdes R, Graves S, Brown B, et al: Endogenous substance in newborn infants causing false positive digoxin measurements. *J Pediatr* 1983;102:947–950.

32. Friedman H, Abramowitz I, Nguyen T, et al: Urinary digoxin-like immunoreactive substance in pregnancy. *Am J Med* 1987;83:261–264.

33. Spiehler W, Fisher W, Richards R: Digoxin-like immunoreactive substance in postmortem blood of infants and children. *J Forensic Sci* 1985;30:86–91.

34. Ekins B, Watanabe A: Acute digoxin poisonings: Review of therapy. *Am J Hosp Pharmacol* 1978;35:268–277.

35. Sonnenblick M, Abraham A, Meshulam Z, et al: Correlation between manifestations of digoxin toxicity and serum digoxin, calcium, potassium, and magnesium concentrations and arterial *p*H. *Br Med J* 1983;286:1089–1091.

36. Walker A, Cody R, Greenblatt D, et al: Drug toxicity in patients receiving digoxin and quinidine. *Am Heart J* 1983;105:1025–1028.

37. Closson R: Visual hallucinations as the earliest symptom of digoxin intoxication. *Arch Neurol* 1983;40:386.

38. Volpe B, Soave R: Formed visual hallucinations as digitalis toxicity. *Ann Intern Med* 1979;91:865–866.

39. Chuman M, LeSage J: Color vision deficiencies in two cases of digoxin toxicity. *Am J Ophthalmol* 1985;100:682–685.

40. Fisch C, Knoebel S: Recognition and therapy of digitalis toxicity. *Prog Cardiovasc Dis* 1970;13:71–95.

41. Fisch C: Digitalis intoxication. *JAMA* 1971;216:1770–1773.

42. Doherty J: Digitalis glycosides. *Ann Intern Med* 1973;79:229–238.

43. Doherty J: Digoxin antibodies and digitalis intoxication. *N Engl J Med* 1982;307:1398–1399.

44. Reza M, Kovick R, Shine K, et al: Massive intravenous digoxin overdosage. *N Engl J Med* 1974;291:777–778.

45. Warren S, Fanestil D: Digoxin overdose: Limitations of hemoperfusion-hemodialysis treatment. *JAMA* 1979;242:2100–2101.

46. Hansteen V, Jacobsen D, Knudsen K, et al: Acute, massive poisoning with digitoxin: Report of seven cases and discussion of treatment. *Clin Toxicol* 1981;18:679–692.

47. Hess T, Riesen W, Scholtysik G, et al: Digotoxin intoxication with severe thrombocytopenia: Reversal by digoxin-specific antibodies. *Eur J Clin Invest* 1983;13:159–163.

48. Lai K, Swaminathan R, Pun C, et al: Hemofiltration in digoxin overdose. *Arch Intern Med* 1986;146:1219–1220.

49. Mathieu D, Gosselin B, Nolf M, et al: Massive digitoxin intoxication: Treatment by Amberlite XAD-4 resin hemoperfusion. *J Toxicol Clin Toxicol* 1983;19:931–950.

50. Gibb J, Adams P, Parnham A: Plasma digoxin: Assay anomalies in Fab-treated patients. *Br J Clin Pharmacol* 1983;16:445–447.

51. Duke M: Atrioventricular block due to accidental digoxin ingestion treated with atropine. *Am J Dis Child* 1972;124:754–756.

52. Rumack B, Wolfe R, Gilfrich H: Phenytoin (diphenylhydantoin) treatment of massive digoxin overdose. *Br Heart J* 1974;36:405–408.

53. French J, Thomas R, Siskind A: Magnesium therapy in massive digoxin intoxication. *Ann Emerg Med* 1984;13:562–566.

54. Murphy D, Bremner F, Haber E, et al: Massive digoxin poisoning treated with Fab fragments of digoxin-specific antibodies. *Pediatrics* 1982;70:472–473.

55. Citrin D, O'Malley K, Hillis W: Cardiac standstill due to digoxin poisoning successfully treated with atrial pacing. *Br Med J* 1973;2:526–527.

56. Pieroni R, Fisher H: Use of cholestyramine resin in digitoxin toxicity. *JAMA* 1981;245:1939–1940.

57. Payne V, Secter R, Noback R: Use of colestipol in a patient with digoxin intoxication. *Drug Intell Clin Pharmacol* 1981;15:902–903.

58. Cohen S: Antibody therapy of digoxin intoxication. *Pediatrics* 1982;70:494.

59. Leikin J, Vogel S, Graff J, et al: Use of Fab fragments of digoxin-specific antibodies in the therapy of massive digoxin poisoning. *Ann Emerg Med* 1985;14:175–178.

60. Goldman R: The use of serum digoxin levels in clinical practice. *JAMA* 1974;229:331–332.

61. Rollins D, Brizgys M: Immunological approach to poisoning. *Ann Emerg Med* 1986;15:1046–1051.

62. Gibson T: Comparison of XAD-4 and charcoal hemoperfusion for removal of digoxin and digitoxin. *Kidney Int* 1980;18:S101–S105.

63. Gibson T: Hemoperfusion of digoxin intoxication. *Clin Toxicol* 1980;17:501–513.

64. Smith T, Butler V, Haber E, et al: Treatment of life-threatening digitalis intoxication with digoxin-specific Fab antibody fragments. *N Engl J Med* 1982;307:1357–1362.

65. Smith T, Haber E: Digoxin intoxication: The relationship of clinical presentation to serum digoxin concentration. *J Clin Invest* 1970;49:2377–2386.

66. Wenger T, Butler V, Haber E, et al: Treatment of 63 severely digitalis-toxic patients with digoxin-specific antibody fragments. *J Am Coll Cardiol* 1985;5:118A–123A.

67. Smolarz A, Roesch E, Lenz E, et al: Digoxin-specific antibody (Fab) fragments in 34 cases of severe digitalis intoxication. *Clin Toxicol* 1985;23:327–340.

68. Zucker A, Lacina S, DasGupta D, et al: Fab fragments of digoxin-specific antibodies used to reverse ventricular fibrillation induced by digoxin ingestion in a child. *Pediatrics* 1982;70:468–471.

ADDITIONAL SELECTED REFERENCES

Cohn J: Indications for digitalis therapy. *JAMA* 1974;229:1911–1914.

Das G: Digoxin-quinidine interaction. *Am J Cardiol* 1982;49:495.

Doering W: Is there a clinically relevant interaction between quinine and digoxin in human beings? *Am J Cardiol* 1981;48:975–976.

Gullner H, Stinson E, Harrison D, et al: Correlation of serum concentrations with heart concentrations of digoxin in human subjects. *Circulation* 1974;50:653–655.

Henry D, Lawson D, Lowe J, et al: The changing pattern of toxicity to digoxin. *Postgrad Med J* 1981;57:358–362.

Koch-Weser J, Greenblatt D: Influence of serum digoxin concentration measurements on frequency of digitoxicity. *Clin Pharmacol Ther* 1975;16:284–288.

Mooradian A, Wynn E: Pharmacokinetic prediction of serum digoxin concentration in the elderly. *Arch Intern Med* 1987;147:650–653.

Schaumann W, Kaufmann B, Neubert P, et al: Kinetics of the Fab fragments of digoxin antibodies and of bound digoxin in patients with severe digoxin intoxication. *Eur J Clin Pharmacol* 1986;30:527–533.

chapter 16

Calcium Channel Blockers

Calcium ions play a critical role in numerous essential biologic processes.[1] In particular, they catalyze enzymatic reactions that split high-energy phosphate bonds and are involved in the electrical activation of excitable cells,[2] hemostasis, and metabolism of bone (Table 16-1).[3] In terms of clinical effects that relate to calcium channel blockers, calcium ion influx is primarily involved in the genesis of the cardiac action potential,[2] facilitates the intracardiac conduction of electrical impulses,[4] promotes contraction of cardiac and smooth muscle cells, and may also cause irreversible cellular injury of anoxic tissue.[2,3]

CALCIUM ANTAGONISM

Several inorganic cations, such as cobalt and manganese, function as general calcium antagonists.[3] These agents are effective in blocking a

Table 16-1 The Role of Calcium in Biological Processes

Electrical activation of excitable cells
Enzymatic reactions
Hemostasis
Metabolism of bone
Genesis of cardiac action potential
Promotes contraction of smooth muscle

wide variety of calcium-dependent processes, but they are considered nonselective agents. This nonselectivity of action arises from the ability of these cations to substitute for calcium at various calcium-binding sites. The calcium channel blockers are different in action in that they selectively act on calcium as it relates to the "slow" channel of an action potential.

THE ROLE OF CALCIUM IN THE ACTION POTENTIAL

Calcium has important roles in the excitation-contraction coupling process of heart and vascular smooth muscle cells and in the electrical discharge of the specialized conduction cells of the heart.[3,5] The membranes of these cells contain numerous channels that carry a slow inward current and that are selective for calcium.

The calcium channel blockers are organic compounds that produce electromechanical uncoupling in heart muscle by selectively blocking the slow inward current of cardiac action potential.[2,6] By inhibiting calcium influx, the calcium channel blockers inhibit the contractile processes of cardiac and vascular smooth muscle. This in turn leads to a negative inotropic effect as well as a reduction in cardiac work and myocardial oxygen demand.[5] The effect of calcium channel blockade of the sinoatrial and atrioventricular nodes is to block or decrease impulse conduction by increasing the effective and functional refractory periods of these nodal cells. This is due to the inhibition of coupling of actin and myosin, two proteins necessary for muscular contraction of myocardial and vascular smooth muscle.[1,3,5]

In skeletal muscle, most of the calcium ion required for electromechanical coupling is derived from intracellular stores within the sarcoplasmic reticulum.[1] In cardiac and smooth muscle, most of the calcium ions reach the intracellular site from transmembrane calcium ion flow. As a result, the calcium channel blockers can only affect cardiac and smooth muscle.[3]

In the resting myocardial cell, the extracellular and intracellular calcium gradients are maintained by both cell membranes and efficient pumping systems, thereby maintaining the constancy of the environment. It is this gradient of free ionized calcium that contributes to the propagation of the action potential and determines the contractile state of the heart. The calcium channel blockers therefore exert their pharmacologic effects primarily through calcium antagonism at the cell membrane of these excitable tissues, hereby inhibiting the transmembrane influx of extracellular calcium.[2] They do not modify calcium intake, binding, or exchange by cardiac microsomes, nor do they have an effect on calcium activated ATPase or cause a change in serum calcium concentrations.[7,8]

THE ACTION POTENTIAL AND "SLOW" AND "FAST" CHANNELS

The action potential of excitable cardiac cells is the result of the movement of ions, particularly sodium and calcium.[9] It is thought that there are movable macromolecules that function as gates that allow ions to cross excitable membranes. Each ion channel has one gate that controls activation and another gate that controls inactivation. Each ion (sodium, calcium, chloride, or potassium) has a transmembrane flux that is regulated by the opening and closing of these gates.[10]

The changes in transmembrane potential that occur during the action potential of cardiac cells are divided into five phases: phase 0, rapid depolarization; phase 1, early repolarization;

phase 2, plateau; phase 3, rapid repolarization; and phase 4, diastole.[4]

When cardiac cells in normal atrial and ventricular contractile tissues are stimulated sufficiently to alter membrane permeability for sodium, a "fast" channel allows rapid sodium ionic influx during phase 0 depolarization of the action potential.[3] This is seen as a rapid upstroke of the action potential. This current is dependent on the extracellular sodium concentration and can be blocked by type I antidysrhythmics, such as quinidine and procainamide. During phase 0, when the interior of the cell becomes less negative, or depolarized, from approximately -90mV to -40mV, the membrane conductance for sodium rapidly increases.[1,10] At this point the fast sodium channel becomes inactivated, but not before it activates a second inward current.[6,11] Because the rates of activation and inactivation of this second inward current are several orders of magnitude slower than those of the fast inward current, and because these channels are approximately 100 times more selective for calcium than for sodium, this channel is termed the "slow" inward current or the calcium channel.[3,11] The plateau phase or phase 2 is largely dependent on a slow inward current through calcium-specific channels (Fig. 16-1).[4] The slow channels are not entirely calcium mediated, however.[6]

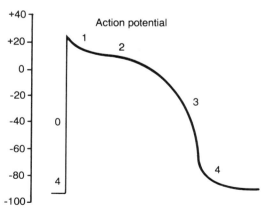

Figure 16-1 The action potential of cardiac muscle. *Source:* Adapted with permission from "Calcium Channel Blocking Agents in the Treatment of Cardiovascular Disorders" by E Antman et al in *Annals of Internal Medicine* (1980;93:875–885), Copyright © 1980, American College of Physicians.

The electrical activity of the sinoatrial and atrioventricular nodal cells has a slowly rising action potential and a reduced rate of conduction and is especially dependent on the slow current, which accounts for the effectiveness of the calcium channel blockers.[4,9] The rest of the specialized conduction system is dependent on the fast current.[2] Slow channel-dependent tissues, such as the sinoatrial and atrioventricular nodes, therefore have low diastolic potentials, slow rates of phase 0 depolarization (slow conduction velocities), spontaneous phase 4 depolarization (automaticity), and delayed recovery of excitability outlasting the duration of the action potential (long refractory periods).[12] The effects of slow-channel blocking agents are thus most evident in the sinoatrial node, atrioventricular node, and diseased fast-channel tissues.

In fast-channel tissues, such as the atrial and ventricular contractile tissues and the His-Purkinje system, electrical excitability results primarily from transmembrane sodium flux.[2] These tissues have high diastolic potentials and rapid rates of phase 0 depolarization (fast conduction velocities) and recover excitability coincident with repolarization (have short refractory periods).[9]

GENERAL OVERVIEW OF CALCIUM CHANNEL BLOCKERS

Calcium channel blockers have been found to be useful in treating a wide variety of cardiovascular disorders (Table 16-2).[3,13,14] There are three approved calcium channel blockers on the market: verapamil, nifedipine, and diltiazem. Although each drug may act as a calcium channel blocker, there are also significant differences in their clinical indications (Table 16-3) and their effects (Table 16-4). Although the calcium channel blockers share the same general mechanism of action, they are chemically unrelated.

Verapamil's most potent activity is electrophysiologic, and nifedipine's effects are hemodynamic; diltiazem acts like a less potent combination of the two.[1] All three cause an increase in coronary blood flow, with nifedipine having a greater effect than verapamil or

Table 16-2 Uses of the Calcium Channel Blockers

Stable and unstable angina
Vasospastic angina
Acute myocardial infarction
Congestive heart failure
Hypertropic cardiomyopathy
Dysrhythmias
    Paroxysmal atrial tachycardia
    Atrial fibrillation
    Atrial flutter
Systemic hypertension
Pulmonary hypertension

Table 16-3 Comparison of Indications for Use of Calcium Channel Blockers

Indication	Verapamil	Diltiazem	Nifedipine
Vasospastic angina	+	+	+
Effort angina	0	+	+
Supraventricular tachycardia	+	0	0
Left ventricular failure	0	0	+
Malignant hypertension	0	0	+
Migraine prophylaxis	+	0	0

Source: Adapted with permission from *Emergency Medicine* (1984;5:31), Copyright © 1984, Cahners Publishing Company.

Table 16-4 Comparison of Effects of Calcium Channel Blockers

Effect	Verapamil	Diltiazem	Nifedipine
Hypotension	+	+	+
Flushing	+	−	+ +
Headache	+	+	+ +
Peripheral edema	+	+	+
Palpitations	+	+	+
Chest pain	+	+	+
Conduction disturbances	+ +	+	−
Heart failure	+	−	+/−
Bradycardia	+ +	+	−

Source: Adapted with permission from "Adverse Reactions with Calcium Antagonists" by R Krebs in *Hypertension 5* (Supp 11) (pp 11-125 through 11-129), Copyright © 1983, American Heart Association.

diltiazem. All cause vasodilation of vascular smooth muscle, although diltiazem dilates coronary vessels with less potent effects on blood flow in the other vascular beds. Verapamil and nifedipine appear to be roughly equivalent in the various vascular beds.[15,16]

The bioavailability of each compound is relatively low owing to extensive first-pass metabolism in the liver.[13] Nifedipine has the shortest half-life, and verapamil has the longest half-life and partially active metabolites.[2]

Verapamil (Isoptin®, Calan®)

Verapamil, a papaverine derivative,[17] was first introduced as a smooth muscle relaxant with potent peripheral and coronary vasodilator properties.[18] It was originally thought to be an adrenergic blocking agent because its myocardial effects were opposite those resulting from catecholamine action.[15,19]

The effects of verapamil consist of negative inotropic and chronotropic actions. Of the three calcium channel blockers it has the most profound influence on the calcium current of the sinoatrial and atrioventricular nodes[1] and thus is the most useful in the treatment of supraventricular tachycardia, which is often caused by re-entry through the atrioventricular node.[2,4] Verapamil has also been shown to inhibit a second slow current carried by the sodium ion.[19]

Pharmacokinetics

After oral administration of verapamil, absorption is rapid and virtually complete.[19] The first-pass effect through the hepatic portal circulation causes 60% to 70% of the oral dose to be biotransformed; thus bioavailability of verapamil ranges from 20% to 35%.[1,20] To be effective, an oral dose must be 10 to 20 times more than the recommended intravenous dose. Plasma concentrations reach their peak within 1 to 2 hours after oral administration. The steady-state volume of distribution ranges from 4.5 to 7 L/kg, and approximately 90% of the drug is bound to plasma proteins.[10] The plasma half-life of verapamil in adults is approximately 3 to 7 hours and may be longer in children. Norverapamil, an active metabolite, achieves plasma concentrations approximately equal to those of verapamil within 4 to 6 hours after administration.[13,15]

The onset of action of intravenous verapamil is almost immediate, with the maximal effect on atrioventricular node conduction occurring in 3 to 5 minutes.[11] The slowing of atrioventricular node conduction lasts up to 6 hours because of preferential binding of the drug at atrioventricular nodal tissues.

The most prominent clinical effect of verapamil is depression of sinoatrial rate and conduction through the atrioventricular node. Although verapamil directly suppresses the sinoatrial node rate, this effect is easily overcome in most patients by reflex stimulation.[6] In contrast, the effect of delayed atrioventricular node conduction is significant and results in prolongation of the PR interval. This accounts for verapamil's efficacy in slowing or converting most supraventricular tachydysrhythmias.[13]

Adverse Effects

Reports concerning verapamil's side effects and associated acute intoxication are scarce.[13] Side effects result from the drug's action on the conducting tissue of the heart and peripheral smooth muscle (Table 16-5). Constipation, headache, dizziness, hepatic dysfunction,[18] hypotension, fatigue, prolonged atrioventricular conduction, and decreased cardiac output have been noted.[13,21]

The most significant adverse cardiovascular effects are hypotension, bradydysrhythmias, conduction disturbances, and left ventricular failure (which is normally transient and mild). Severe

---

Table 16-5 Adverse Effects of Verapamil

Noncardiac
  Constipation
  Headache
  Dizziness
  Hepatic dysfunction
  Fatigue
Cardiac
  Hypotension
  Bradydysrhythmias
  Conduction disturbances
  Left ventricular failure
  First-, second-, and third-degree block

---

hypotension has been noted most often in patients concurrently taking β blockers, so that caution must be exercised when administering calcium channel blockers to such patients.[11,15,21–23] The most frequently observed benign cardiac effects are first- or second-degree atrioventricular block (Wenckebach period) and atrioventricular junctional rhythm. Although verapamil rarely produces clinically important changes in the rate of sinoatrial node discharge or recovery time, it may reduce the resting heart rate and produce sinus arrest in patients with sinoatrial node disease.

Verapamil is contraindicated in patients who have atrioventricular node disease or block, who are concurrently taking quinidine or disopyramide, or who have congestive heart failure unless the failure is secondary to a tachycardia.[1]

Nifedipine (Procardia®)

Unlike other known cardioactive drugs, nifedipine is a dihydropyridine derivative. At the doses used clinically, it does not have a depressant effect on the sinoatrial or atrioventricular conduction in the heart.[1] This is in contrast to both verapamil and diltiazem, which produce sinoatrial and atrioventricular node depression. Nifedipine causes relaxation of blood vessels and therefore is a coronary vasodilator that increases coronary flow.[1] Because it has no important myocardial depressant actions or electrophysiologic effects in therapeutic doses, the drug has found primary clinical application in disorders associated with abnormal or inappropriate vasoconstriction.[4]

Pharmacokinetics

Approximately 90% of an oral dose of nifedipine is rapidly absorbed from the gastrointestinal tract. Of the total oral dose, 65% to 75% reaches systemic circulation unchanged because nifedipine is metabolized to some extent on first pass through the liver. In patients with normal renal and hepatic function, the plasma half-life is 2 to 5 hours.

Onset of action after oral administration is within 20 minutes, with a peak effect between 1 and 2 hours. A sublingual preparation is available and has an onset of action of 3 minutes and a peak at 20 minutes.[24]

Table 16-6 Adverse Effects of Nifedipine

Fatigue
Flushing
Headache
Hypotension
Peripheral paresthesias
Palpitations
Peripheral edema
Syncope

Adverse Effects

The adverse effects of nifedipine are related to its potent vasodilation and include flushing, headache, hypotension, fatigue, peripheral paresthesias and dysesthesia, palpitations, peripheral edema, and syncope (Table 16-6).[13,25] Caution should be used when administering nifedipine together with β blockers.[21] When administered with digoxin it may increase digoxin levels by 50%.

Diltiazem (Cardizem®)

Diltiazem is a benzothiazepine derivative. Like the other calcium channel blockers, it causes a dose-dependent inhibition of the slow inward calcium current in normal cardiac tissue. Diltiazem prolongs atrioventricular node conduction time and slows the sinoatrial node rate without the reflex changes seen with verapamil.[1] This is because diltiazem exerts only a minimal effect on blood vessels elsewhere in the body. Both verapamil and diltiazem are equivalent in their slowing of atrioventricular node conduction, but diltiazem causes less prolongation of the atrioventricular node refractory period than verapamil. Diltiazem is also a potent vasodilator of coronary vessels. It has a stronger depressant action on sinoatrial node discharge than verapamil and can cause significant bradycardia or sinus arrest in patients with sick sinus syndrome.

Pharmacokinetics

Approximately 80% of an oral dose of diltiazem is rapidly absorbed from the gastrointestinal tract. The onset of action of oral diltiazem is within 15 minutes, with peak effect within 1 to 2 hours. It has a plasma half-life of 4 to 9 hours. Diltiazem also undergoes significant first-pass metabolism by the liver, with 40% of an oral dose reaching the systemic circulation.[9] The mean volume of distribution is approximately 5 L/kg.[9]

Adverse Effects

Side effects of diltiazem are similar to those of verapamil (Table 16-7). The drug has a wide therapeutic index and is the best tolerated of the three agents. The major and potentially most serious side effects are vasodilation resulting in headache, flushing, occasional hypotension, and depression of atrioventricular nodal conduction, the last of which may result in a sinus bradycardia or various degrees of atrioventricular block[9] and asystole.[16] Hepatic dysfunction has also been reported.[16] Caution should be exercised when administering diltiazem to patients taking β blockers or with pre-existing hypotension.

OVERDOSAGE

Overdosage of the calcium channel blockers produces symptoms that are mainly extensions of common adverse reactions (Table 16-8). Acute overdose may be manifested by symptomatic hypotension due to peripheral vasodilation, bradydysrhythmias due to depression of cardiac nodal tissues, and left ventricular decompensation due to negative inotropism. Supression of the sinus node may lead to a slow ventricular escape rhythm. In addition, first-, second-, and third-degree atrioventricular block and bundle branch block have been noted.[17] Hypotension is most likely to occur in patients with poor left ventricular function in whom peripheral vasodilation and negative inotropic

Table 16-7 Adverse Effects of Diltiazem

Atrioventricular block
Flushing
Headache
Hepatic dysfunction
Hypotension
Sinus bradycardia

Table 16-8 Signs and Symptoms of Overdosage with Calcium Channel Blockers

Cardiovascular
Hypotension
Bradydysrhythmias
Congestive heart failure
First-, second-, and third-degree heart block
Bundle branch block
Neurologic
Dizziness
Syncope
Mental confusion
Miscellaneous
Anuria
Hyperglycemia
Metabolic acidosis

effects cannot be compensated. Patients with a high risk of profound bradycardia are those with prior evidence of sick sinus syndrome or atrioventricular conduction delay. Cardiac arrest and other cases of severe myocardial depression have been noted as a result of intentional or accidental overdosage.[26,27] Other clinical manifestations of overdose include mental confusion, syncope, anuria, hyperglycemia, and metabolic acidosis.[19,28]

TREATMENT OF OVERDOSAGE

Supportive and symptomatic treatment, including administration of intravenous fluids and placement of the patient in Trendelenburg's position, should be initiated in case of overdosage with calcium channel blockers (Table 16-9). Because the half-life of these drugs is short, intoxication usually responds promptly to withdrawal of the drug. Methods to prevent absorption in acute ingestion should be attempted.

Although calcium has been used empirically as the "antidote" for acute intoxication, there is limited experience to date in the proper use of either calcium or sodium.[29] The tissues most responsive to an elevated serum calcium concentration in calcium channel blocker intoxication are myocardium and vascular smooth muscle, whereas cardiac conduction tissues appear to require the addition of sodium for partial reversal of calcium channel blocker–in-

Table 16-9 Treatment of Calcium Channel Blocker Overdose

Indication	Agent
History of ingestion	Intravenous line (sodium chloride)
History of ingestion	Cardiac monitor
History of ingestion	Ipecac or lavage
History of ingestion	Charcoal and cathartic
Symptomatic bradycardia or atrioventricular blocks	Atropine
Symptomatic bradycardia, atrioventricular blocks, or hypotension	Calcium chloride Sodium chloride
Significant hypotension	Sympathomimetics
Symptomatic refractory bradycardia or atrioventricular blocks	Transvenous pacemaker

duced depression.[29] For these reasons, both calcium infusion and sodium chloride infusion may be helpful in calcium channel blocker overdose.

Both calcium chloride and calcium gluconate[28] have been used in single and infusion doses to reverse the untoward bradycardia and hypotension of the calcium channel blockers.[13,29-31] Calcium chloride (5 to 10 mL of 10% solution or 10 mg/kg[32]) or calcium gluconate (10 to 20 mL of 10% solution) may be injected over 5 minutes. If the response is temporary the dose may be repeated, or calcium mixed with 5 percent dextrose and water and titrated to the patient's response may be given by infusion.

Epinephrine has sometimes been used successfully with calcium for severe hypotension caused by the calcium channel blockers, but pressor agents probably have only an adjunctive role to other therapy.[27] A fixed high-degree atrioventricular block, symptomatic sinus bradycardia, or asystole may be indications for placement of a temporary pacemaker.[16] Although there may be only a partial response or no response to atropine, atropine should be administered for symptomatic bradycardia or a fixed second- or third-degree atrioventricular block. Cardiac failure may be treated with inotropic agents and diuretics.

The calcium channel blockers are not effectively removed by forced diuresis, hemodialysis, or hemoperfusion.

REFERENCES

1. Conti C, Mazzullo J, Meyers F: All calcium channel blockers are not created equal. *Emerg Med Rep* 1984;5:29–34.

2. Karlsberg R: Calcium channel blockers for cardiovascular disorders. *Arch Intern Med* 1982;142:452–455.

3. Braunwald E: Mechanism of action of calcium channel blocking agents. *N Engl J Med* 1982;307:1618–1627.

4. Antman E, Stone P, Muller J, et al: Calcium channel blocking agents in the treatment of cardiovascular disorders: Part 1: Basic and clinical electrophysiologic effects. *Ann Intern Med* 1980;93:875–885.

5. Donovan P, Propp D: Calcium and its role in cardiac arrest: Understanding the controversy. *J Emerg Med* 1985;3:105–116.

6. Kuhn M: Verapamil in the treatment of PSVT. *Ann Emerg Med* 1981;10:538–544.

7. Singh B, Ellrodt G, Peter T: Verapamil: A review of its pharmacological properties and therapeutic use. *Drugs* 1978;15:169–197.

8. Singh B, Hecht H, Nademanee K, et al: Electrophysiologic and hemodynamic effects of slow channel blocking drugs. *Prog Cardiovasc Dis* 1982;25:103–132.

9. Chaffman M, Brogden R: Diltiazem. *Drugs* 1985;29:387–454.

10. McGoon M, Vlietstra R, Holmes D, et al: The clinical use of verapamil. *Mayo Clin Proc* 1982;57:495–510.

11. Young G: Calcium channel blockers in emergency medicine. *Ann Emerg Med* 1984;13:712–722.

12. Mitchell L, Schroeder J, Mason J: Comparative clinical electrophysiologic effects of diltiazem, verapamil, and nifedipine: A review. *Am J Cardiol* 1982;49:629–635.

13. Crowe D: The β and calcium channel blockers. *Top Emerg Med* 1986;8:26–33.

14. Mauritson D, Winniford M, Walker S, et al: Oral verapamil for paroxysmal supraventricular tachycardia. *Ann Intern Med* 1982;96:409–412.

15. McAllister R: Clinical pharmacology of slow channel blocking agents. *Prog Cardiovasc Dis* 1982;25:83–102.

16. Snover S, Bocchino V: Massive diltiazem overdose. *Ann Emerg Med* 1986;15:1221–1224.

17. Candell J, Valle V, Soler M, et al: Acute intoxication with verapamil. *Chest* 1979;75:200–201.

18. Brodsky S, Cutler S, Weiner D, et al: Hepatotoxicity due to treatment with verapamil. *Ann Intern Med* 1981;94:490–491.

19. Enyeart J, Price W, Hoffman D, et al: Profound hyperglycemia and metabolic acidosis after verapamil overdose. *J Am Coll Cardiol* 1983;2:1228–1231.

20. Koike Y, Shimamura K, Shudo I, et al: Pharmacokinetics of verapamil in man. *Res Commun Chem Pathol Pharmacol* 1979;24:37–47.

21. Lewis J: Adverse reactions to calcium antagonists. *Drugs* 1983;25:196–222.

22. Krebs R: Adverse reactions with calcium antagonists. *Hypertension* 1983;5(suppl II):125–129.

23. Lander R: Verapamil/β blocker interaction. *Mo Med* 1983;80:626–629.

24. Lown B: The future clinical role of nifedipine. *Am J Cardiol* 1979;44:839–841.

25. Zangerie K, Wolford R: Syncope and conduction disturbances following sublingual nifedipine for hypertension. *Ann Emerg Med* 1985;14:1005–1006.

26. Gelbke H, Schlicht H, Schmidt G: Fatal poisoning with verapamil. *Arch Toxicol* 1977;37:89–94.

27. Immonen P, Linkola A, Waris E: Three cases of severe verapamil poisoning. *Int J Cardiol* 1981;1:101–105.

28. Silva O, Melo R, Filho J: Verapamil acute self poisoning. *Clin Toxicol* 1979;14:361–367.

29. Moroni F, Mannaioni P, Dolara A, et al: Calcium gluconate and hypertonic sodium chloride in a case of massive verapamil poisoning. *Clin Toxicol* 1980;17:395–400.

30. Strubelt O, Diederich K: Experimental investigations on the antidotal treatment of nifedipine overdosage. *Clin Toxicol* 1986;24:135–149.

31. Lipman J, Jardine I, Roos C, et al: Intravenous calcium chloride as an antidote to verapamil-induced hypotension. *Intensive Care Med* 1982;8:55–57.

32. Passal D, Crespin F: Verapamil poisoning in an infant. *Pediatrics* 1984;73:543–545.

ADDITIONAL SELECTED REFERENCES

Dominic J, Bourne D, Tan T, et al: The pharmacology of verapamil: Part III: Pharmacokinetics in normal subjects after intravenous drug administration. *J Cardiovasc Pharmacol* 1981;3:25–38.

Giannini A, Houser V, Loiselle R, et al: Antimanic effects of verapamil. *Am J Psychiatr* 1984;141:1602–1603.

Hughes W, Ruedy J: Should calcium be used in cardiac arrest? *Am J Med* 1986;81:285–294.

Pedrinelli R, Fouad F, Tarazi R, et al: Nitrendipine, a calcium entry blocker. *Arch Intern Med* 1986;146:62–65.

Raftery E: Cardiovascular drug withdrawal syndromes: A potential problem with calcium antagonists? *Drugs* 1984;28:371–374.

Schiffl H, Ziupa J, Schollmeyer P: Clinical features and management of nifedipine overdosage in a patient with renal insufficiency. *Clin Toxicol* 1984;22:387–395.

Secher C, Brofeldt S, Mygind N: Intranasal verapamil in allergen-induced rhinitis. *Allergy* 1983;38:565–570.

Zaloga G, Malcolm D, Holaday J, et al: Verapamil reverses calcium cardiotoxicity. *Ann Emerg Med* 1987;16:637–639.

part V

AGENTS THAT BURN

chapter 17

Acids and Alkalis

There is a wide variety of materials that burn. Although they have different properties, they all share the ability to cause direct injury to tissues that may lead to cellular death.[1] These agents do not necessarily burn by hyperthermic activity but cause injury to tissue by various mechanisms.[1-5]

Chemicals that burn can be divided into agents that cause

- corrosion (lye and phosphorus)
- reduction (hydrochloric acid and nitric acid)
- salt formation (picric, acetic, and formic acids)
- desiccation (sulfuric acid)
- oxidation (chromic acid and potassium permanganate)
- metabolic competition (oxalic and hydrofluoric acids)
- vesication (mustard gas and cantharides)
- nonspecific protoplasmic poisoning and lacrimation (mace) (Table 17-1).

Thus chemicals that burn are classified according to their chemical activity or according to whether they are alkalis and acids.[2] This chapter discusses the various alkalis and acids that cause burns as well as the treatment of ingestions or exposures to these agents. Chapter 18 discusses other chemicals that burn because of properties other than pH.[4]

Most serious ingestions of caustic agents involve strong acids or alkalis. Although the initial presentations and treatments of such ingestions are similar, acids and alkalis differ in the type of injury that is produced both acutely and chronically.[6,7]

ALKALIS

The term caustic has traditionally been associated with alkalis,[8,9] but any chemical that injures the gastrointestinal tract is defined as a caustic agent. Caustic therefore refers to both acids and alkalis.[10] The term corrosive poison encompasses substances that can cause tissue destruction when they come in contact with mucous membranes.[5]

THE ALKALIS

Corrosive Agents

Corrosive agents consist of certain acids and alkalis as well as other compounds and are responsible for significant immediate and long-term morbidity. They are among the most dangerous commercial products found in the home.[11,12] These substances are used widely as raw materials and for cleaning, curing, extract-

Table 17-1 Chemical Agents That Cause Burns

Corrosive Substances
Lyes (sodium or potassium hydroxide)
Lime (calcium oxide)
Alkaline batteries
Phenol (carbolic acid)
Cresol
White phosphorus
Reducing Substances
Alkyl mercuric compounds
Hydrochloric acid (muriatic acid)
Nitric acid
Salt Forming Agents
Tungstic acid
Picric acid
Sulfosalicylic acid
Tannic acid
Trichloroacetic acid
Cresylic acid
Acetic acid
Formic acid
Desiccants
Sulfuric acid
Oxidizing Agents
Dichromate salts
Sodium hypochlorite (bleach)
Potassium permanganate
Metabolic Competitors
Oxalic acid
Hydrofluoric acid
Vesicants
Cantharides (Spanish fly)
Dimethylsulfoxide
Mustard gas
Lewisite
Miscellaneous
Mace

Table 17-2 Sources of Alkalis

Lye (Sodium, Potassium, Calcium, and Lithium Hydroxide)
Ammonium hydroxide
Calcium hydroxide
Calcium oxide
Lithium hydroxide
Sodium carbonate
Sodium hydroxide
Potassium carbonate
Potassium hydroxide
Lime
Calcium oxide
Disinfectants
Quaternary ammonium compounds
Sodium hypochlorite (Clorox®)
Calcium hypochlorite
Phosphates
Potassium permanganate
Hexachlorobenzene
Phenol
Pine oil
Toilet Bowl Cleaners (Vanish®, Saniflush®, Vansol®)
Sodium metasilicate
Soda ash
Paint Removers
Sodium hydroxide
Methylene chloride
Phenols
Cresols
Hair Dyes, Tints, and Bleaches
Ammonia
Hydrogen peroxide
Automatic Dishwasher Detergents (Electrosol®, Cascade®)
Trisodium phosphate
Sodium metasilicate
Sodium carbonate
Portland Cement
Calcium oxide
Low-Phosphate Detergents
Sodium metasilicate

ing, and preserving in industry as well as in the home.

Corrosive agents are so called because of the extensiveness of denaturization that they cause in tissue protein.[2] The corrosive agents include sodium metals and lyes, phenols and cresols, and white phosphorus (Table 17-1).

Sodium Metals and Lyes

Alkalis are substances that dissociate in water to yield an excess of hydroxyl ions, producing a pH above 7.0. The strong corrosive alkalis that are termed lyes include sodium, potassium, calcium, ammonium, lithium, and barium hydroxide; sodium and potassium carbonate; phosphates; and sodium metal.[2]

Sources of lye or strong corrosive alkalis include lime, Clinitest® tablets, bleaches, disinfectants, oven cleaners, drain cleaners, toilet bowl cleaners, and the other agents listed in Table 17-2.[2] Although modern household products are less concentrated than products sold in previous years, highly concentrated, industrial-strength alkali products are still available.[13–15]

Potassium Hydroxide and Sodium Hydroxide

Potassium hydroxide (caustic potash) and sodium hydroxide (caustic soda) are commonly available as white lumps, rods, or pellets. They are two of the strongest alkalis and are extremely corrosive. Potassium and sodium hydroxide are found in drain cleaners, oven cleaners, Clinitest® tablets, and alkaline batteries (Table 17-3).

Lithium Hydroxide (Lithium Hydrate)

Lithium hydroxide is a white, strongly alkaline powder that forms an irritating dust; it has been used to absorb carbon dioxide from the air in space capsules. Lithium hydride and related compounds react vigorously on contact with moisture to generate lithium hydroxide and hydrogen gas, which may ignite spontaneously.

Calcium Hydroxide (Calcium Hydrate, Slaked Lime, Hydrated Lime)

Calcium hydroxide is a white powdered or granular solid that is used in making mortar, plaster, cement, and whitewash. It is a typical lye and may cause major burns (see below).

Lime (Calcium Oxide, Quicklime, Burnt Lime, Unslaked Lime)

Lime is a substance found in various cements and is converted by water, with the evolution of heat, to calcium hydroxide, which is an alkali with a pH of 11 to 13.[16] The mixture of compounds will set to a hard product by the admixture of water. Hydration of this mixture will yield calcium hydroxide from the lime content and sodium and potassium hydroxide from the corresponding alkali oxides.[17] The pH of the

---

Table 17-3 Products That Contain Sodium or Potassium Hydroxide

---

Alkaline batteries
Clinitest® tablets
Detergents
Drain cleaners (Draino®, Liquid Plumr®)
Oven cleaners (Easy-off®)
Paint removers

---

mixture is usually about 12. The material is hazardous, especially in its fresh form, and perspiration and skin moisture may be sufficient to initiate the reaction.[1] The resultant burn, which is both thermal and chemical, is often serious because the material may remain in contact with the skin for a prolonged period. Hardening of cement causes any residual surface calcium hydroxide to react with carbon dioxide from the atmosphere and become a relatively inert material.

Concrete, a mixture of sand and gravel that is added to wet cement, is abrasive as well as caustic. In addition to these dermatologic problems cement often contains hexavalent chromate salts as a contaminant, and these can cause an allergic dermatitis in cement handlers who have become sensitive to this metallic salt.[16]

Cement burns result from prolonged direct contact of the material with the skin or contact with wet saturated clothing that remains on the skin. Cement burns usually occur on the lower extremities because the individual has walked or knelt in the wet cement. The knees, pretibial areas, and ankles are the areas most often affected. Some of these burns have resulted in deep necrotic ulcerations, sometimes requiring extensive hospitalization and skin grafts.[1,16]

Ammonium Hydroxide

Ammonia is produced as a by-product in the distillation of coal, by the action of steam on cyanamide, and by the catalytic combination of nitrogen and hydrogen gases at high temperature and pressure. It also results from the decomposition of nitrogenous materials and is released in fires from the combustion of wool, silk, and nylon, but its concentration is low in most ordinary building fires.

Ammonia is a colorless gas that is readily liquified and is highly soluble in water, with which it combines to form ammonium hydroxide. Ammonium hydroxide in various concentrations is used in a number of products such as cleaning agents, liniments, and aromatic spirits. It is also used extensively in refrigeration, petroleum refining, and the manufacturing of fertilizers, nitric acid, explosives, dyes, plastics, and other chemicals (Table 17-4). The strongest solution of ammonium hydroxide commonly available contains 28% ammonia. A 10% solu-

Table 17-4 Sources of Ammonia

Toilet bowl cleaners
Window cleaners
Metal cleaners
Hair dyes
Antirust agents
Jewelry cleaners
Aromatic spirits

Table 17-5 Active Chemicals in Low-Phosphate Laundry and Dishwasher Detergents

Sodium borate
Sodium carbonate
Sodium metasilicate
Sodium silicate
Sodium sulfate
Trisodium polyphosphate

tion is also in common use, and so-called household ammonia ranges in concentration from 5% to 10% ammonia.[5]

Ammonium hydroxide differs from other alkalis in its volatility because the vapor, even in low concentrations, is extremely irritating to skin, eyes, and respiratory passages. Inhalation of ammonia in high concentrations has caused pulmonary edema. This is the most frequent cause of death after exposure to ammonia.

The ingestion of commercial strength ammonia solutions produces effects similar to ingestions of other corrosive alkalis. In addition, respiratory signs and symptoms should be anticipated after ingestion as a consequence of aspiration of the solution or inhalation of the vapors.

Low-Phosphate Laundry and Dishwasher Detergents

Modern synthetic detergents are used in large quantities as household and industrial cleaners.[18] Many of the older detergents contained phosphates, which by themselves have only a moderate toxicity. The new, low-phosphate detergents contain active chemicals such as carbonates or metasilicates that react with metals in water to "soften" the water. Large quantities of high concentrations of these reactive anions are necessary for this purpose.[19]

Most commercially available nonphosphate detergents are highly alkaline, with *p*H values of 10.5 to 12.0. They commonly contain combinations of sodium metasilicate, sodium borate, sodium silicate, and sodium carbonate (Table 17-5). Sodium metasilicate is the most alkaline and corrosive substance found in such products; a weak solution has a *p*H of approximately 12.5.

Highly alkaline nonphosphate chemicals have caustic effects similar to the commonly recognized alkalis, with corrosive esophagitis, severe gastric erosion, permanent injury, and death as a consequence of ingestion.[19] In addition, alkaline soap solutions administered as an enema have produced inflammatory colitis and resulted in severe serosanguineous fluid loss, rectal gangrene, colonic stricture, and even death.[20] Recently, low-phosphate and nonphosphate detergents have been balanced with other builders to reduce their alkalinity.[8]

Clinitest® Tablets

Clinitest® tablets, which are used commonly by diabetics to check their urine, are alkaline agents that cause significant thermal as well as caustic injury to the esophagus.[21] Clinitest® tablets are white with green-blue flecks of copper sulfate, citric acid, sodium hydroxide, and sodium carbonate.[22,23] Accidental ingestion of Clinitest® tablets by adults is more common than suicidal ingestion because the tablets may be mistaken for an oral medication.[22,23] A single tablet is considered extremely dangerous and may cause a devastatingly deep burn that may progress to stricture formation. The ingested tablet mixes with saliva in the mouth and usually sticks in the upper third of the esophagus because of thermal coagulation of the mucosa. Because of this, ingestion of Clinitest® tablets results in a high incidence of major morbidity.[8]

Alkaline Batteries

Alkaline disk batteries are used to power watches, cameras, games, computers, calculators, and hearing aids, and their use has increased.[8,9] There are many chemicals in such batteries. Their major ingredients are alkalis such as sodium or potassium hydroxide, and their ingestion results in delivery of caustic material to the gastrointestinal tract without obvious accompanying oropharyngeal lesions.[8,24] In addition, these batteries contain heavy metals such as mercury, zinc, silver, nickel, lithium, or cadmium, which may be systemically absorbed.[25] The major forms of mercury in these batteries are mercuric oxide and elemental mercury.[9,26] Toxicity of the battery depends on leakage from its casing,[26] duration of contact with the mucosa, location in the gastrointestinal tract, and inherent toxicity of the chemicals.[27–29]

Alkaline disk batteries are constructed with an electrolyte-soaked fabric inserted between a cathode can and an anode top.[30–32] In an ingestion, a small percentage of batteries may spontaneously leak electrolyte solution.[27] In addition, pressure necrosis may occur if the battery is lodged in the gastrointestinal tract. Because placing a battery in an electrolyte solution produces electrolysis, the acid medium of the stomach and the alkaline medium of the intestine may provide a potential for dissolution.

Batteries larger than 18 mm in diameter are likely to be caught in the esophagus.[33] Fatalities have resulted when the battery was wedged in the esophagus at the thoracic inlet with resulting esophageal perforation.[28]

Phenol (Carbolic Acid, Phenic Acid, Phenylic Acid)

Phenols are commercially available as disinfectants, deodorants, and sanitizers. In dilute aqueous solution, phenol has been used as an antiseptic and a topical anesthetic. The phenols are used in industry as bases for plastics and organic polymers.

Phenol is an aromatic alcohol derived from coal tar that is a highly reactive, corrosive contact poison.[4] It is also a general protoplasmic poison and is toxic to all cells.[34] It can be obtained as pure crystals or in a solution. Ten percent solutions of phenol regularly produce corrosion, and occasionally skin necrosis is seen with solutions as dilute as 1%.[2]

Phenols in strong concentrations rapidly produce a brown or whitish stain that turns to a greenish-black or copper-colored eschar. Concentrated solutions of phenol cause second- and third-degree burns of the skin unless very promptly removed. Formation of a coagulation necrosis of the dermis delays absorption, but this delay is only temporary. If skin absorption is significant, it may result in toxic effects on the CNS and the cardiovascular system.

Cresols (Tricresol, Cresylic Acid)

Like phenol, cresol is a derivative of coal tar. The cresols are the most important alkyl derivatives of phenol, and they occur as three isomers, orthocresol, metacresol, and paracresol; there are other cresol-like compounds as well (Table 17-6). The ortho and para isomers are even more toxic than phenol. The bacteriocidal potency of the cresols is about three times that of phenol; consequently, cresol solutions are used widely as disinfectants. Other commonly used compounds that are closely related are creosote, which is a distillate of coal and wood tars and is used as a wood preservative and also as an expectorant[34]; resorcinol, which is often used in bacteriocidal and fungicidal ointments; hexylresorcinol, which is used as an antiseptic[1]; thymol, which is used as a fungicide; and hexachlorophene, which is used as an antiseptic.

The corrosive action of cresols is slightly greater than that of the phenols, whereas the systemic effects appear to be a little milder be-

Table 17-6 Uses of Cresol and Cresol-Like Compounds

Compound	Use
Cresol (orthocresol, metacresol, paracresol)	Bacteriocide
Creosote	Wood preservative, expectorant
Resorcinol	Bacteriocide, fungicide
Hexylresorcinol	Antiseptic
Thymol	Fungicide
Hexachlorophene	Antiseptic

cause of cresol's slower absorption. The extent of the burn and necrosis that may follow an ingestion or exposure depends on the concentration of cresol in the agent. The systemic effects depend on the amount absorbed, which is dependent on the area of contact and the duration of contact. There may be prominent CNS effects with depression of consciousness (Table 17-7).[35] There may also be central lobular necrosis of the liver with jaundice, kidney damage, and Heinz-body anemias.[36]

Phosphorus

The properties of phosphorus as they relate to toxicology are discussed in Chapter 43.

MECHANISM OF TOXICITY OF CORROSIVE ALKALIS

Lyes are extremely corrosive and penetrating as a function of their ability to saponify lipids and to cause soap formation with subsequent epithelial sloughing and dehydration of tissue cells.[6] The term liquefaction necrosis is often associated with lye injury because a soft, gelatinous, friable, often brownish eschar is produced.[9,37] As these organic complexes penetrate further into the body, they carry unattached alkali molecules and continue to destroy tissue. Hemorrhage, thrombosis, and a marked inflammatory response with significant edema are seen within the first 24 hours of injury. Depending on the extent of the burn inflammation may extend through the muscle layer, and perforation may occur. Tissue destruction with lye is more intense than with acids.[38]

The closer to 14 the pH measures, the more destructive the caustic agent.[10] The critical pH that causes esophageal stricture and ulcer is approximately 12.5. Most lye solution concentrations and commercial lye products have a pH of 14.[39] Nonlye solutions known to cause esophageal ulceration have a pH in the range of 12.5 to 13.5, but most cases of deep ulcer developing into stricture formation involve lye solutions of pH 14.[39] A pH less than 11.4 is rarely associated with more than superficial mucosal burns.[9,10] This is true for common household bleach, for example.

Caustic material ingested accidentally or in a suicide attempt produces a wide array of injuries to the proximal gastrointestinal tract. The form (liquid or solid), pH, concentration, and chemical nature of the ingested material are important in the caustic agent's ability to damage delicate mucosa (Table 17-8).[12,40]

There are multiple points of normal anatomical narrowing in the esophagus. These are the cricopharyngeal area, the impression of the aortic arch and the left main bronchus, and the area of the lower esophageal sphincter or diaphragmatic hiatus.[37] These are also the most common points of stasis for ingested material passing through the esophagus and therefore the areas where ingested corrosive agents cause the most significant burns.[41]

Small quantities of alkali are sufficient to produce major esophageal injuries without even reaching the stomach. The gastric mucosa, however, is not preferentially resistant to alkaline destruction, and the neutralizing potential of the total gastric acid is insufficient when compared to even relatively small volumes of strong alkalis.

Table 17-7 Toxic Effects of Phenols and Cresols

Caustic burn
CNS depression
Hypotension
Intravascular hemolysis
Pulmonary edema
Central lobular necrosis of liver
Shock
Death

Table 17-8 Toxic Effects of Corrosive Alkalis

Form	Effects
Solid (crystalline)	Liquefaction necrosis of oropharynx, glossopharynx, palate, proximal esophagus
Liquid	Liquefaction necrosis of distal esophagus, stomach

Solid Caustic Agents

Solid crystalline caustics tend to adhere to moist surfaces and cause pain rapidly.[10,37,42] The oropharyngeal, glossopharyngeal, palatal, and proximal esophageal mucosa are usually involved, and deep, irregularly arranged burns may be produced.[40] Because the crystals adhere proximally, less necrosis occurs distally.[9] The limited areas of involvement show deeper penetration, with vascular thrombosis, ulceration, and frequently perforation.

Liquid Caustic Agents

High-density liquid caustics, because of their easy passage down the esophagus, usually pass rapidly through the oropharynx and upper esophagus and cause more significant damage to the lower esophagus and stomach.[10,37,40] There may therefore be minimal injury to the mouth and oropharynx with liquid caustics (Table 17-8).[9]

ACIDS

Acids are found in swimming pool cleaners, toilet bowl cleaners, batteries, metal cleaners, antirust agents, and disinfectants.[27,43] Automobile battery acid is usually about 28% sulfuric acid. Toilet bowl cleaners frequently contain sodium bisulfate, which forms sulfuric acid in water.[2] Similar products containing hydrochloric or phosphoric acids are also marketed. Soldering fluxes are often solutions or pastes of zinc chloride and hydrochloric acid. Gun barrel cleaning fluid may contain about 5% nitric acid (Table 17-9). Although the following substances are acids, they also have additional actions that classify them as reducing substances, salt forming agents, and desiccants.[2,3,5,10]

Reducing Agents

The reducing agents produce their effect by binding free electrons in tissue proteins, thereby producing protein denaturization.[2] Reducing substances include hydrochloric acid, nitric acid, and the alkyl mercuric agents.

Hydrochloric Acid

Hydrochloric acid is one of the most common acids and is a solution of hydrogen chloride in water. Concentrated hydrochloric acid is usually 38% hydrogen chloride; technical muriatic acid is usually 32%. Concentrated solutions of this reducing acid cause rapid conversion of surface protein to the chloride salt.[2] The resulting coagulum overlies a shallow ulcer. The process continues as long as active acid remains in contact with the nondenatured protein.

Alkyl Mercuric Agents

The many actions of the alkyl mercuric agents include skin irritation. This can progress to severe skin lesions and burns, which have been reported with both ethyl and methyl mercuric compounds.[2] The metallic mercury within the blister fluid can also be absorbed. These compounds are discussed further in Chapter 40.

Table 17-9 Sources of Acids

Swimming pool cleaners
  Sodium bisulfite
Toilet bowl cleaners
  Sodium bisulfite
  Hydrochloric acid
  Phosphoric acid
Batteries
  Sulfuric acid
Metal cleaners
  Nitric acid
Drain cleaners
  Hydrochloric acid
  Sulfuric acid
Antirust agents
  Hydrofluoric acid
  Oxalic acid
Disinfectants
Soldering flux
  Hydrochloric acid

Salt Forming Agents

This group of agents produces its detrimental effects by forming salts with proteins.[2] Among the protoplasmic poisons are the alkaloidal acids such as tungstic, picric, sulfosalicylic, tannic, trichloroacetic, acetic, and formic acids.[1]

Salt forming agents have wide industrial use. Most have pungent odors, frequently with a suffocating effect. Often they occur in crystalline form. When in contact with tissues, the material combines with a variety of functional groups to form additional products or to initiate polymerization. These agents form an eschar with some sparing of the underlying supporting structures. They are frequently absorbed, producing hepatic toxicity or nephrotoxicity.

Picric Acid (Trinitrophenol, Carbazotic Acid, Picronitric Acid)

Picric acid is a yellow crystalline solid used in the manufacture of explosives, fireworks, electric batteries, textiles, and colored glass (Table 17-10). Antiseptic solutions have been employed medically in 0.5% to 3% concentration. Picric acid and its salts are toxic by inhalation, ingestion, and percutaneous absorption.

Poisonings may manifest as severe gastroenteritis, hemorrhagic nephritis with anuria, intravascular hemolysis, acute hepatitis, progressive stupor, coma, and death. Picric acid is similar to

---

Table 17-10 Uses and Toxicity of Picric Acid

Uses
  Explosives
  Fireworks
  Electric batteries
  Textiles
  Colored glass
Toxic effects
  Burns
  Gastroenteritis
  Hemorrhagic nephritis
  Intravascular hemolysis
  Acute hepatitis
  Hyperthermia
  Uncoupling of oxidative phosphorylation
  Stupor
  Coma
  Death

---

dinitrophenol in that it accelerates body metabolism.

Acetic Acid

Vinegar and dilute acetic acid are about 4% to 6% acetic acid. Essence of vinegar is 14% acetic acid. Glacial acetic acid (100%) is highly corrosive, and its ingestion has produced penetrating lesions of the esophagus with stricture of the esophagus and pylorus. Permanent wave neutralizers may contain acetic acid. Vapors are capable of producing bronchial constriction with a clinical picture similar to that produced by other irritant gases and vapors.

Sulfosalicylic Acid (Trichloroacetic Acid)

Sulfosalicyclic acid is a corrosive organic acid that rapidly penetrates and fixes tissues. Systemic effects are presumably secondary to gastrointestinal damage and to acidosis and not due to the trichloroacetate ion, except in large doses.

Tannic Acid

Tannic acids are produced in plants from low–molecular weight polyphenols as a result of tissue injury to the plant.[44] They serve to protect the plant from potential infection by ''tanning'' an invading virus or fungus. Medicinal tannic acid is an extract containing various concentrations of polyphenol. This preparation had been used for years by radiologists to improve the contrast in barium sulfate diagnostic enemas.[45,46] Various plant extracts containing tannins have been used for centuries in the treatment of diarrhea and as astringents, antiseptics, and styptics on the skin and mucous membranes.

Tannic acid is readily absorbed from the gastrointestinal tract, and blood concentrations reach their peak in approximately 3 hours.[44] Tannic acid is a protoplasmic poison as well as a hepatotoxin,[45] and its toxic effects are dose related.

Desiccants

The deleterious effects of these agents are caused both by excessive heat production and by tissue dehydration.[2,38]

Sulfuric Acid (Oil of Vitriol, Battery Acid)

Sulfuric acid, when pure, is an odorless, colorless, oily liquid, but with slight impurities it becomes yellow or brown and may have an unpleasant odor. It is used in the steel industry for casting iron and steel.

The caustic and chemical properties of concentrated sulfuric acid differ greatly from those of diluted acid. Concentrated sulfuric acid appears to attach to the tissues chemically in a different and a more destructive manner than can be explained simply on the basis of hydrogen ion concentration. When the acid is diluted, the caustic and chemical properties become similar to those of simpler acids, such as hydrochloric acid. Sulfuric acid is an exceedingly potent desiccant that produces a hard eschar, under which an indolent, deep ulcer forms. Destruction of all carbon-containing tissue occurs, and considerable heat is released during the reaction.

Mechanism of Toxicity of Acids

Acid agents produce primarily a coagulation-type necrosis (Table 17-11).[2,6] The leathery eschar formed by reducing substances and desiccants usually stops acid penetration and typically results in damage limited to the mucosa. Although burns to the oropharynx and esophagus do occur, acids tend to produce less damage to the upper airway or the esophagus than alkalis because they pass rapidly through the esophagus.[3,6] There may be obvious burns to the mucosal surface of the lips, tongue, and mucosa

of the oropharynx. The epiglottis may be involved, although the larynx is usually spared.[43]

Acids usually produce necrotic gastric or proximal intestinal lesions with eschar formation.[46] Usually the lower two-thirds of the stomach is involved.[7] When the acid reaches the stomach, it progresses from the gastroesophageal junction along the lesser curvature to the pylorus.[6] Pylorospasm usually develops immediately, resulting in pooling of the acid in the antrum, where the greatest injury occurs.[38] The pooling of the agent caused by the pylorospasm may also cause acute gastric perforation, peritonitis, and death.[46] Long-term complications of acid ingestion include gastric scarring and pyloric stenosis with clinical obstruction. Acid ingestions, although less frequent than alkali ingestions, have a high complication rate.[27]

INFORMATION FOR BURN HISTORY

History should include the type of substance ingested, the time since ingestion, the quantity taken, and whether or not vomiting has occurred; the pH of the emesis should also be determined (Table 17-12). In addition, the presence of pain and its location, any difficulty in swallowing or breathing, and whether or not hematemesis has occurred should be ascertained.[5] Nevertheless, it is not possible on the basis of history or physical examination to predict the degree of esophageal involvement in many patients who have ingested a caustic or corrosive substance.[37,40,47]

Table 17-11 Differences in Toxic Properties between Alkalis and Acids

Property	Alkalis	Acids
Type of injury	Liquefaction necrosis	Coagulation necrosis
	Saponification of fats	Eschar formation
	Intense tissue destruction	Limited tissue involvement
Typical location of injury	Mouth	Stomach
	Pharynx	
	Esophagus	
Long-term effects	Esophageal stricture	Pyloric stenosis
		Gastric scarring

Table 17-12 Information for Burn History and Clinical Manifestations of Burns

History
  Type of substance ingested
  Estimated quantity of substance ingested
  Time since ingestion
  ? Emesis
  Determination of emesis pH
Clinical manifestations
  Ingestion
    Dysphagia
    Hypersalivation
    Drooling
    White or black mucous membranes
    Acute respiratory distress
    Pain
      Tongue
      Lips
      Palate
      Substernum
      Abdomen
      Back
    Edema
      Tongue
      Lips
      Palate
      Oral mucosa
    Dyspnea
    Hematemesis
  Inhalation
    Dyspnea
    Cyanosis
    Pulmonary edema
    Hemoptysis
  Ocular contact
    Conjunctivitis
    Pain
    Lacrimation
    Photophobia
    Corneal abrasion

CLINICAL MANIFESTATIONS OF ACID AND ALKALI BURNS

Clinical manifestations may include dysphagia; hypersalivation with drooling; pain; and edema of the tongue, oral mucosa, lips, or palate.[10] Drooling and the inability to clear secretions are indicative of significant posterior pharyngeal or upper esophageal injury.[8] Drooling may cause the solid caustic to drain over the chin so that circumoral burns develop.[10,48] Examination of the mouth may reveal soapy, white mucous membranes that might later become edematous.

Acute respiratory distress may occur as a result of posterior pharyngeal edema or spillage of the caustic agent into the upper airway. The patient may also complain of burning substernal, back, and abdominal pain and may vomit copious amounts of bloody material. There are patients, however, who are asymptomatic and have no oral burns but who are subsequently shown to have esophageal injuries.[8,10,40] The absence of oral burns therefore does not rule out the possibility of significant esophageal burns.[13,37,49] Symptoms that suggest severe injury include dyspnea, dysphagia, chest pain, and hematemesis.[9]

Eye Involvement

Alkali

Alkali damages the eye by increasing the hydroxyl ion concentration beyond the limits of protein stability.[4] This results in the formation of alkaline proteinates that react with the lipid cellular membranes, causing them to saponify and lyse. By this process the alkali rapidly penetrates the ocular tissue. A strong corrosive spilled into the eye may produce immediate whitening of the cornea and sclera. The anterior chamber pH rises within 2 to 3 minutes, causing damage to the iris, lens, and ciliary body. This may lead to irreversible loss of vision within minutes.[1] If the burn is mild, only the epithelium will be lost; this is equivalent to a corneal abrasion and can be seen on fluorescein staining.[50]

Large volumes or higher concentrations of alkali readily penetrate the corneal stroma, causing injury of the endothelium with resultant corneal edema. Initially there is intense pain generated from the stimulation of free nerve endings, especially in the epithelium. The pain is enhanced by a sudden rise of the intraocular pressure induced by the direct effect of the alkali. This rise in intraocular pressure is prolonged as a result of prostaglandin release within the eye.

Acids

As a rule, acids produce less severe ocular injury than alkalis because they coagulate the corneal epithelium, which then serves as a barrier to further penetration. Hydrofluoric, sulfuric, sulphurous, and chromic acids are exceptions to this rule.[1]

Chemical burns of the eye, like burns of the skin, are more devastating from alkalis than from acids. Long-term sequelae secondary to significant chemical eye burns include corneal perforation or ulceration, iritis, lens damage, cataracts, and possible atrophy of the globe.

Acute and Long-Term Complications of Orally Ingested Caustic Agents

Acute complications of orally ingested caustic agents include airway obstruction,[51] esophageal ulcers, and esophageal, gastric, or intestinal perforation leading to mediastinitis or peritonitis (Table 17-13). Gastric ulcerations may occur, but they are less common in alkali ingestion than in acid ingestion. Mediastinitis may occur without frank perforation owing to bacterial invasion through the damaged mucosa.[38]

Stricture formation is a common sequela of lye ingestion.[9,47] Late stricture formation is related to the agent ingested. Some substances

such as household ammonia and bleaches may produce marked mucosal edema but rarely penetrate deeply enough to injure the submucosa or muscularis propia. There are isolated reports, however, of household-strength (3% to 10%) ammonia causing severe mucosal burns.[5]

Other complications include circulatory failure and shock, asphyxia from glottic or laryngeal edema,[51] intercurrent infection, inanition, and pulmonary complications. Squamous cell carcinoma of the esophagus has been reported and may develop more than 10 to 20 years after ingestion; this sequela occurs most commonly in patients who have sustained esophageal damage from lye.[52]

Late achlorhydria has been noted with acid burns and may be due to antral destruction, effectively producing a physiologic antrectomy. The achlorhydria is usually but not always permanent.[46] Disseminated intravascular coagulation has been described in patients who have ingested acid. The major tissue damage to the stomach and hemorrhage from the damaged gastrointestinal tract may be contributing factors to this condition.

LABORATORY EXAMINATION IN CAUSTIC INGESTIONS

Chest and abdominal roentgenograms, including upright films, are usually indicated to check for signs of pulmonary injury or aspiration, evidence of free intra-abdominal air secondary to gastric perforation,[48] or pneumomediastinum secondary to esophageal perforation or to locate an ingested disk battery (Table 17-14).[3,38] Contrast radiological studies of

Table 17-13 Acute and Long-Term Complications of Significant Caustic Burns

Local
 Airway obstruction
 Asphyxia
 Laryngeal edema
 Glottic edema
Esophageal (alkalis>acids)
 Ulceration
 Perforation
 Stricture
 Carcinoma (late sequelae)
Gastric (acids>alkalis)
 Perforation
 Ulceration
 Achlorhydria
Systemic
 Mediastinitis
 Peritonitis
 Circulatory failure
 Shock
 Infection
 Pulmonary complications
 Disseminated intravascular coagulation

Table 17-14 Laboratory Work-Up in Caustic Ingestion

Upright chest roentgenogram
Upright abdominal roentgenogram
Complete blood count
Serum electrolytes
Blood urea nitrogen
Serum glucose
Blood type and cross-match
Toxicologic screen
Heavy metal concentrations

the upper gastrointestinal tract are not helpful acutely and in fact frequently underestimate the extent of injury.[9] They have value in the recovery stage, when evaluation of stricture formation is important.[38] Routine baseline studies such as a complete blood count and measurement of electrolytes, blood urea nitrogen, and glucose should be obtained in the symptomatic individual. If necessary, blood should be typed and cross-matched and a drug screen obtained.[5] Heavy metal concentrations should be obtained in blood and urine in those patients who have ingested a disk battery if it is not passing quickly through the gastrointestinal tract.

TREATMENT OF ALKALI AND ACID BURNS

Much of the difficulty in managing patients who have ingested a caustic substance is related to the rapid onset of tissue damage. Although many other forms of poisoning can be treated effectively after an initial delay, measures instituted at the hospital for caustic ingestion may have little or no effect on the extent of tissue damage or outcome. Treatment, therefore, must be administered as soon as possible after ingestion to have the best chance of lessening the destructive potential of caustic agents.[10]

Initial treatment for ingestion of all caustic agents is directed at minimizing the extent of tissue damage and then preventing and treating both short- and long-term complications (Table 17-15). In general, this consists of immediate dilution and subsequent direct examination of involved tissue, usually by endoscopy.[48]

Cutaneous Burns

If the material is on the skin, removal by irrigating the area with copious amounts of water under low pressure for long periods of time is indicated. Particulate matter should be débrided from the wound before or during irrigation. Clothing and protective garments must be removed to prevent further injury to the patient. Cutaneous burns are like thermal injuries in that they require cleansing with soap, the application of a topical antibiotic such as silver sulfadiazine (Silvadene®), and tetanus prophylaxis.

Table 17-15 Treatment of Caustic Burns

Cutaneous
   Copious irrigation with water
   Removal of particulate matter
   Topical antibiotic
   Tetanus prophylaxis
Eye
   Continuous irrigation with water
   Tetanus prophylaxis
   Careful follow-up
Gastrointestinal
   Adequate ventilation
   Intravenous infusion of crystalloid solution
   Nothing by mouth (except for dilution)
   Medication for relief of pain
   Emesis or lavage (contraindicated)
   Charcoal and cathartic (contraindicated)
   Blood type and cross-match (for hematemesis)
   Dilution with water or milk
   Neutralization (contraindicated)
   Esophagoscopy (within 24 hours)
   Prophylactic antibiotics (withhold)
   Tetanus prophylaxis
   Steroids (withhold)
   Parenteral nutrition

Eye Burns

Burns of the eye can be treated by flooding the eye with water if this is started within seconds of contact with the caustic. The importance of time so outweighs other considerations that the first water, or innocuous watery solution at hand, should be used.[50] Time should not be wasted in looking for some special irrigation fluid. A lid speculum may be necessary to open the eyes before irrigation. Irrigation can continue in the emergency department through a small-bore catheter fixed in the palpebral sulcus until the pH of the cul-de-sac returns to neutrality.[50] Tetanus prophylaxis is also indicated, as is careful follow-up.

For the patient's comfort, a drop of local anesthetic and slightly warmed water can be applied to the injured eye.[9] The duration of irrigation depends on the nature of the chemical and on the concentration and quantity involved. Common practice calls for prolonged irrigation, at least 20 to 30 minutes, to be sure of thorough cleansing.

The rise of intraocular pressure that occurs after the burn frequently responds to the oral administration of carbonic anhydrase inhibitors such as acetazolamide (Diamox®, 125 mg four times a day). Soft contact lenses may facilitate re-epithelialization by covering and protecting fresh epithelium from exposure to the air and by reducing the shearing stress of blinking.[50]

Gastrointestinal Burns

The first step in treating gastrointestinal burns is to rinse the mouth with water or milk, which is then expectorated. This may prevent swallowing of crystals that adhere to the oral cavity.[3,10]

As with any acute intoxication, the first issue in management is to ensure that the patient has the ability to maintain adequate ventilation and that the cardiovascular status is acceptable.[42] Because respiratory tract involvement suggests significant injury, control of the airway may be necessary.[3] Blind nasotracheal intubation is contraindicated because of the risk of inducing tracheal or pharyngeal perforation. Oral endotracheal intubation under direct visualization is the preferred procedure, but cricothyrotomy may be performed in the patient requiring airway control who cannot be intubated. Although airway obstruction is not common, laryngeal edema or edema of the base of the tongue may produce significant airway obstruction that requires careful intubation.

Intravenous access should be initiated immediately, and hypotension should be treated initially with crystalloid solution through multiple large-bore intravenous lines. If the clinical picture suggests impending perforation, blood should be typed and cross-matched in preparation for emergency surgical intervention. Once the diagnosis is confirmed, narcotic analgesic should be given in adequate doses to control pain.[10]

The importance of adequate nutrition cannot be overemphasized. Patients with significant esophageal injury should receive parenteral nutrition early in their course. In a child, the clinician should look for other injuries, such as cigarette burns, scars, and other signs of body and head trauma, so as to exclude the possibility of child abuse.

Emesis, Lavage, or Charcoal and Cathartic

Gastric lavage and emesis are contraindicated in caustic ingestions because they may lead to iatrogenic esophageal perforation, cause an aspiration, or cause another burn as the material is passed back through the esophagus.[38] Oral fluids, therefore, should never be forced to the point of emesis, and patients with a caustic injury should not receive oral fluids until they are able to swallow their own saliva.[3] The primary focus of initial management should be to prevent vomiting.[42]

Activated charcoal and cathartics are contraindicated for caustic ingestions for a number of reasons. The instantaneous nature of the injury negates any benefit from the use of these substances, and in addition charcoal is a poor adsorbent of caustic agents. Charcoal may also interfere with the subsequent use of the endoscope, and, most important, the administration of activated charcoal may cause an emesis. This emesis may reintroduce the corrosive material on the epiglottis, vocal cords, and larynx, leading to more severe injury, edema, and acute airway obstruction. Additionally, regurgitated materials may be aspirated, leading to potentially severe chemical pneumonitis.

Dilution

Although water is widely recommended as a diluent in patients who have ingested caustic substances, there are no data to support its efficacy. Despite this, water is relatively benign if aspirated and may be effective in diluting residual alkali or acid (Table 17-16). Accordingly, it is not unreasonable to consider its use in small quantities immediately after a caustic substance has been ingested.[42,53] If diluents are to be used, the clinician must recognize the inherent dangers of the induction of vomiting and the potential for aspiration and must weigh these factors against the lack of demonstrated effi-

Table 17-16 Dilution of Caustic Agents

Agents of choice
 Water
 Milk
Contraindications
 Emesis
 Acute airway obstruction
 Perforation of esophagus, stomach, or intestine

cacy.[9] Dilution is contraindicated in patients with acute airway swelling and obstruction or in those who have clinical evidence of esophageal, gastric, or intestinal perforation.

Neutralization

Many product labels inappropriately suggest neutralization of the caustic.[53] Neutralizing a chemical burn often produces an exothermic reaction, in which a thermal burn is added to the chemical burn.[4] Mild acids or alkalis that are administered to neutralize ingested caustics should therefore not be used because they may aggravate the chemical burn by the further production of heat.[38,42,53]

Esophagoscopy

Direct examination of the esophagus is essential in determining the medical management of each case. The role of endoscopy in caustic ingestion has changed considerably. This is mainly due to a change from the rigid endoscope, which may cause a perforation as it passes damaged mucosa, to the use of the flexible fiberoptic endoscope, which allows for the safe visualization of the esophagus and stomach.[40] Unless the patient is unstable or pharyngeal injury precludes the study, esophagoscopy with a flexible endoscope should be performed within the first 12 to 24 hours.[9,37,48] Delaying beyond 48 hours will cause the procedure to coincide with the period when the injured wall is at its weakest. All adult patients, especially those who have attempted suicide, and children with a reliable history of significant ingestion should be evaluated by esophagoscopy. The level of the first significant injury should be visualized to establish the presence of lesions requiring treatment.[42]

Endoscopic findings may be classified as superficial, transmucosal, or transmural and are classified in the same manner as burns of the skin (Table 17-17).[37] Superficial lesions are mild and show nonulcerative esophagitis and hyperemia of the mucosa but no loss of tissue. A superficial lesion is analogous to a first-degree burn with hyperemia, superficial sloughing of the mucosa, and mucosal edema.[48] A transmucosal or second-degree burn demonstrates mild to moderate transmucosal involvement

Table 17-17 Esophagoscopy in the Evaluation of a Chemical Burn

Examination
  First 24 hours after ingestion
  Flexible esophagoscope
Findings
  Superficial (first-degree burn)
    Mild, nonulcerative lesions
    Hyperemia of mucosa
  Transmucosal (second-degree burn)
    Shallow ulcers with involvement of muscular layer
  Transmural (third-degree burn)
    Ulcerative lesions
    Severe, widespread tissue destruction
    Possible mediastinitis and abscess formation
Contraindications
  Significant posterior pharyngeal burns
  Laryngeal burns
  Respiratory distress

with shallow ulcers or deep craters and involvement of the muscle layer. Blistering, exudate, and loss of mucosa may also be noted. A transmural or third-degree burn is described as ulcerative and severe with widespread tissue destruction. Erosion through the esophagus into the periesophageal tissues may ensue, leading to mediastinitis,[48] abscess formation, and peritonitis.[9]

The findings at endoscopy enable appropriate management to be determined.[13] If no burns are noted, the patient may be saved an expensive and unnecessary hospitalization. First-degree injuries do not progress to stricture,[37] but second-degree burns may stenose (although this is rare). A great majority of third-degree injuries produce a clinically significant esophageal stricture, especially when they are of the circumferential type.[37] In addition, if perforation is found surgical management is mandatory. In severe cases, this may involve total resection of the esophagus. In those patients with severe esophageal or gastric injury, close follow-up by a medical team is essential. Patients are hospitalized in an intensive care environment with frequent daily observations. In those patients with mild esophagitis or gastritis, less intensive observation and early hospital discharge are usually appropriate. Endoscopic re-evaluation of all second- and third-degree burns should be performed 2 to 3 weeks after the initial injury.

The presence of significant posterior pharyngeal burns with edema is a contraindication to early esophagoscopy because of the risk of airway obstruction. Other contraindications include burns involving the larynx and evidence of respiratory distress, frank shock, or mediastinitis.[37]

Antibiotics

Use of antibiotics is controversial. Because of the low risk of infection in uncomplicated esophageal burns, prophylactic antibiotics should generally be avoided but certainly instituted at the first sign of infection. Prophylactic antibiotics have not been shown to diminish the infection rate or to improve overall patient survival rate.[40] Nevertheless, two widely accepted indications for antibiotics are the presence of a perforation and the need for prophylaxis against infection when steroids are to be used.[10,37,38]

Steroids

The goal of the use of steroids is to decrease stricture formation without hindering the healing process of the esophageal mucosa. Nonetheless, the lack of adequately controlled clinical trials of steroids prevents any conclusion about their efficacy.[3,10,27] Studies have shown that steroids given in pharmacologic doses impair wound healing, depress the body's immune defense, and mask important physical findings of infection and visceral perforation.[40] In addition, superficial esophageal burns rarely proceed to stricture formation even in the absence of medical intervention. Transmural esophageal burns with concomitant tissue necrosis are likely to proceed to perforation, and steroid therapy may aggravate an already serious situation. Transmucosal injuries may benefit from steroid therapy, but this has yet to be shown conclusively.[3]

Steroids are recommended by some clinicians for patients with circumferential esophageal burns.[37] Methylprednisolone[54] (2 mg/kg/day) has been considered the intravenous steroid of choice once esophagoscopy is completed.[9] The recommended dosage is 40 mg every 8 hours in patients older than 2 years and half that dose for younger patients.[10]

TREATMENT OF ALKALINE BATTERY INGESTION

Clinical experience indicates that in most cases of battery ingestion the battery is eventually passed through the gastrointestinal tract without incident. The degree of medical intervention remains a matter of judgment. Most ingestions result in subclinical tissue damage as the battery moves through the digestive tract. Detection of impediment to a normal transit through the gastrointestinal tract or lodging of the battery in the esophagus are indications for prophylactic, aggressive removal.

Patients who ingest disk batteries should undergo an initial roentgenogram to confirm the diagnosis and to determine the location of the battery (Table 17-18).[30–32] If the battery has passed beyond the esophagus, if the patient is asymptomatic, and if there is no radiological evidence of leakage, the patient may be discharged with serial roentgenographic follow-up and with instructions to return to the hospital if fever, abdominal pain, vomiting, tarried or bloody stools, or decreased appetite ensue. Stools should also be checked for evidence of the battery.[31]

Ipecac-induced emesis is usually unsuccessful in removing an ingested battery and should not be attempted.[9,31,33] Activated charcoal, which has been advocated as a marker, should not be administered because it may obscure examination of the stool.

Table 17-18 Treatment of Battery Ingestion

Chest roentgenogram
Emesis (ineffective)
Activated charcoal (withhold)
Locate by roentgenogram
  Esophagus, remove
  Stomach, remove after 24 hours or observe until
    24 hours
  Respiratory tract, remove
Serial roentgenogram
Examination of stool for passage
Operative indications
  Mediastinitis
  Bowel perforation
  Leakage of battery contents

If the battery is in the esophagus or respiratory tract, immediate removal by endoscopy is indicated because there is a high risk of burns and perforation associated with esophageal lodgement.[9,24,30–33] Esophageal lodgement is further implicated by the rapid development of symptoms such as dysphagia, vomiting, anorexia, and fever. If signs or symptoms suggesting esophageal or bowel perforation develop, operative intervention is recommended.[55] Endoscopy may also be performed to remove a battery in the stomach, or it may be allowed to pass through the pylorus. If the battery remains in the stomach for more than 24 hours, it should be removed.[24] If the battery appears to lodge in a diverticulum,[9,23,31] surgical removal is also indicated. Spontaneous passage without morbidity may take as long as 7 days.[33]

In theory, administration of cimetidine (Tagamet®), antacids, or metoclopramide (Reglan®) to minimize corrosion of the battery case by gastric acid may be of some additional value. These recommendations, however, require confirmation.

REFERENCES

1. Stewart C: Chemical skin burns. *Am Fam Physician* 1985;31:149–157.

2. Jelenko C: Chemicals that "burn." *J Trauma* 1974;14:65–72.

3. Nelson R, Walson P, Kelley M: Caustic ingestion. *Ann Emerg Med* 1983;12:559–562.

4. Rodenheaver G, Hiebert J, Edlich R: Initial treatment of chemical skin and eye burns. *Compr Ther* 1982;8:37–43.

5. Klein M: Addressing the controversies of caustic ingestions. *Emerg Med Rep* 1983;4:155–160.

6. Penner G: Acid ingestion: Toxicology and treatment. *Ann Emerg Med* 1980;9:374–379.

7. Zamir O, Hod G, Lernau O, et al: Corrosive injury to the stomach due to acid ingestion. *Am Surg* 1985;51:170–173.

8. Wason S: The emergency management of caustic ingestions. *J Emerg Med* 1985;2:175–182.

9. Howell J: Alkaline ingestions. *Ann Emerg Med* 1986;15:820–825.

10. Ulin L: Caustic ingestions. *Curr Top Emerg Med* 1981;3:1–5.

11. Leape L, Ashcraft K, Scarpelli D, et al: Hazard to health—Liquid lye. *N Engl J Med* 1971;284:578–581.

12. Maull K, Osmand A, Mauli C: Liquid caustic ingestions: An in vitro study of the effects of buffer, neutralization, and dilution. *Ann Emerg Med* 1985;14:1160–1162.

13. Adam J, Birck H: Pediatric caustic ingestion. *Ann Otol Rhinol Laryngol* 1982;91:656–658.

14. Ashcraft K, Padula R: The effect of dilute corrosives on the esophagus. *Pediatrics* 1974;53:226–232.

15. Edmonson M: Caustic alkali ingestions by farm children. *Pediatrics* 1987;79:413–416.

16. Skiendzielewski J: Cement burns. *Ann Emerg Med* 1980;9:316–318.

17. Early S, Simpson R: Caustic burns from contact with wet cement. *JAMA* 1985;254:528–529.

18. Mercurius-Taylor L, Jayaraj A, Clark C: Is chronic detergent ingestion harmful to the gut? *Br J Indust Med* 1984;40:279–281.

19. Scharph L, Hill I, Kelly R: Relative eye-injury potential of heavy-duty phosphate and non-phosphate laundry detergents. *Food Cosmet Toxicol* 1972;10:829–837.

20. Kirchner S, Buckspan G, O'Neill J, et al: Detergent enema: A cause of caustic colitis. *Pediatr Radiol* 1977;6:141–146.

21. Burrington J: Clinitest burns of the esophagus. *Ann Thorac Surg* 1975;20:400–404.

22. O'Conner H, Grant A, Axon A, et al: Fatal accidental ingestion of Clinitest in an adult. *J R Soc Med* 1984;77:963–965.

23. Lacouture P, Gaudreault P, Lovejoy F: Clinitest tablet ingestion: An in vitro investigation concerned with initial emergency management. *Ann Emerg Med* 1986;15:143–146.

24. Mofenson H, Greensher H, Caraccio T, et al: Ingestion of small flat disc batteries. *Ann Emerg Med* 1983;12:88–90.

25. Kulig K, Rumack C, Rumack B, et al: Disc battery ingestion. *JAMA* 1983;249:2502–2504.

26. Temple D, McNeese M: Hazards of battery ingestion. *Pediatrics* 1983;71:100–103.

27. Levine D, Surawicz C: Severe intestinal damage following acid ingestion with minimal findings on early endoscopy. *Gastrointest Endosc* 1984;30:247–249.

28. Levine M, Jacob H, Rubin M: Battery ingestion: A potential form of alkaline injury to the gastrointestinal tract. *Ann Emerg Med* 1984;13:143–145.

29. Yasui T: Hazardous effects due to alkaline button battery ingestion: An experimental study. *Ann Emerg Med* 1986;15:910–916.

30. Litovitz T: Button battery ingestions. *JAMA* 1983;249:2495–2500.

31. Litovitz T: Battery ingestions: Product accessibility and clinical course. *Pediatrics* 1985;75:469–476.

32. Litovitz T, Butterfield A, Holloway R, et al: Button battery ingestion: Assessment of therapeutic modalities and battery discharge state. *J Pediatr* 1984;105:868–873.

33. Rumack B, Rumack C: Disc battery ingestion. *JAMA* 1983;249:2509–2511.

34. Bowman C, Muhleman M, Walters E: A fatal case of creosote poisoning. *Postgrad Med J* 1984;60:499–500.

35. Pegg S, Campbell D: Children's burns due to cresol. *Burns* 1985;11:294–296.

36. Cote M, Lyonnais J, Leblond P: Acute Heinz-body anemia due to severe cresol poisoning: Successful treatment with erythrocytapheresis. *Can Med Assoc J* 1984;130:1319–1322.

37. Buntain W, Cain W: Caustic injuries to the esophagus: A pediatric overview. *South Med J* 1981;74:590–593.

38. Friedman E, Lovejoy F: The emergency management of caustic ingestions. *Emerg Med Clin North Am* 1984;2:77–86.

39. Vancura E, Clinton J, Ruiz E, et al: Toxicity of alkaline solutions. *Ann Emerg Med* 1980;9:118–122.

40. Cello J, Fogel R, Boland R: Liquid caustic ingestion. *Arch Intern Med* 1980;140:501–504.

41. Tucker J, Yarington C: The treatment of caustic ingestion. *Otolaryngol Clin North Am* 1979;12:343–351.

42. Wasserman R, Ginsburg C: Caustic substance injuries. *J Pediatr* 1985;107:169–174.

43. Jena G, Lazarus C: Acid corrosive gastritis. *S Afr Med J* 1985;67:473–474.

44. Boyd E, Bereczky K, Godi I: The acute toxicity of tannic acid administered intragastrically. *Can Med Assoc J* 1965;92:1292–1297.

45. Eschar J, Friedman G: Acute hepatotoxicity of tannic acid added to barium enemas. *Dig Dis* 1974;19:825–829.

46. McAuley C, Steed D, Webster M: Late sequelae of gastric acid injury. *Am J Surg* 1985;149:412–415.

47. Gaudreault P, Parent M, McGuigan M, et al: Predictability of esophageal injury from signs and symptoms: A study of caustic ingestion in 378 children. *Pediatrics* 1983;71:767–770.

48. Kirsh M, Ritter F: Caustic ingestion and subsequent damage to the oropharyngeal and digestive passages. *Ann Thorac Surg* 1976;21:74–82.

49. Crain E, Gershel J, Mezey A: Caustic ingestions. *Am J Dis Child* 1984;138:863–865.

50. Pfister R, Koski J: Alkali burns of the eye: Pathophysiology and treatment. *South Med J* 1982;75:417–422.

51. Williams D: Acute respiratory obstruction caused by ingestion of a caustic substance. *Br Med J* 1985;291:313–314.

52. Appleqvist P, Salmo M: Lye corrosion carcinoma of the esophagus. *Cancer* 1980;45:2655–2658.

53. Rumack B, Burrington J: Caustic ingestions: A rational look at diluents. *Clin Toxicol* 1977;11:27–34.

54. Hawkins D, Demeter M, Barnett T: Caustic ingestion: Controversies in management. A review of 214 cases. *Laryngoscope* 1980;90:98–109.

55. Votteler T, Nash J, Rutledge J: The hazard of ingested alkaline disc batteries in children. *JAMA* 1983;249:2504–2506.

ADDITIONAL SELECTED REFERENCES

Davis L, Raffensperger J, Novak G: Necrosis of the stomach secondary to ingestion of corrosive agents. *Chest* 1972;62:48–51.

Ellis E, Brouhard B, Lynch R, et al: Effects of hemodialysis and dimercaprol in acute dichromate poisoning. *J Toxicol Clin Toxicol* 1982;19:249–258.

Fitzpatrick K, Moylan J: Emergency care of chemical burns. *Postgrad Med J* 1985;78:189–194.

Hardin J: Caustic burns of the esophagus. *Am J Surg* 1956;91:742–748.

Michel L, Grillo H, Malt R: Esophageal perforation. *Ann Thorac Surg* 1982;33:202–210.

Oakes D, Sherck J, Mark J: Lye ingestion. *J Thorac Cardiovasc Surg* 1982;83:194–204.

Okonek S, Bierbach H, Atzpodien W: Unexpected metabolic acidosis in severe lye poisoning. *Clin Toxicol* 1981;18:225–230.

chapter 18

Other Chemicals That Burn

The agents discussed in this chapter have in common their ability to cause local effects resembling a chemical burn as well as additional systemic effects. These agents consist of (1) oxidizing agents such as the dichromates, hypochlorites, and potassium permanganate; (2) metabolic competitors such as oxalic acid and hydrofluoric acid; (3) vesicants such as cantharides, dimethylsulfoxide, mustard gas, and lewisite; and (4) miscellaneous compounds such as mace (Table 18-1).

OXIDIZING AGENTS

The most commonly encountered oxidizing agents are the dichromates, sodium hypochlorite, and potassium permanganate. These agents produce damage because they become oxidized when in contact with body tissue, which often releases a toxic moiety.

Dichromates

Dichromate salts of sodium, potassium, and ammonium are water-soluble, crystalline substances that are highly corrosive to skin and mucosa.[1] Accidental poisoning with dichromates is not uncommon, particularly in industrial settings.[2]

Dichromates are derived from chromite ($FeCr_2O_4$), a chromium-containing ore.[3] Potassium and sodium dichromate are strong oxidizing agents that exist in the hexavalent form but are highly reactive and spontaneously convert to the trivalent form in vivo.[1,3] Although aqueous suspensions of dichromic acid salts are generally of intermediate pH, solutions containing dichromate may range in pH from 0.5 (chromic acid) to 13 (ammonium dichromate). Thus the toxicity of dichromate-containing compounds may be attributed in part to their caustic potential as well as to the powerful oxidizing action of the hexavalent molecule.[4]

Table 18-1 Miscellaneous Chemicals That Burn

Oxidizing agents
  Dichromate salts
  Sodium hypochlorite (bleach)
  Potassium permanganate
Metabolic competitors
  Oxalic acid
  Hydrofluoric acid
Vesicants
  Cantharides (Spanish fly)
  Dimethylsulfoxide
  Mustard gas
  Lewisite
Miscellaneous
  Mace

Chromium is required in glucose and lipid metabolism, and the total body burden of chromium in a 70-kg person is less than 6 mg. In the trivalent state, chromium is strongly bound to plasma proteins. The metabolic effects of toxic amounts of chromium are not fully understood.[3] Toxic tissue accumulation of chromium has been reported in kidney, liver, brain, spleen, lung, bone marrow, and muscle. The major excretory route for chromium is through the kidney,[3] and approximately 60% is excreted through the kidneys within 8 hours after ingestion; elimination through the intestine and in breast milk may also occur.

Potassium dichromate (also called chromic acid, dichromic acid, potassium bichromate, chromium trioxide, and chromic oxide) is a common industrial and laboratory reagent. It is used in electroplating, aircraft building, ship building, dye casting, metal cleaning, and tanning.[3] A pungent yellow liquid, it is a powerful oxidizing agent and is explosive when it comes in contact with small quantities of alcohol, ether, glycerin, and other organic substances.[5] Potassium dichromate is dangerous because of its oxidizing potency, not its acidity. As little as 0.5 to 1 g is considered a lethal dose.

Sodium dichromate is also extremely toxic, with an estimated oral lethal dose between 1 to 10 g in an adult. Fatalities often result from poisonings with this compound as well as with potassium dichromate despite various therapies.[3]

Ammonium dichromate is used in pyrotechnics, photography, and dyeing, in the glassmaking and tanning industries, and in photoengraving.[6] Ammonium dichromate is a powerful irritant when it comes in contact with the skin. When the skin is broken and frequent contact is established, chronic chromic sores or ulcers develop. Deaths from ammonium dichromate are unusual; reports of fatalities primarily involve sodium and potassium dichromate.

Manifestations of Dichromate Exposure

Manifestations of oral dichromate poisoning are immediate and include oral burns, nausea, vomiting, diarrhea, gastrointestinal hemorrhage, esophageal and gastric necrosis, and shock (Table 18-2).[5] Renal failure due to tubular damage, with glycosuria and gross and micro-

Table 18-2 Toxic Effects of Dichromates

Gastrointestinal
  Caustic burns
  Nausea
  Vomiting
  Diarrhea
  Gastrointestinal hemorrhage
  Esophageal necrosis
Hematologic
  Thrombocytopenia
  Intravascular hemolysis
  Hemorrhage
Neurologic
  Vertigo
  Coma
  Myalgia
Inhalation
  Rhinitis
  Nasal septum perforation
  Bronchitis
Miscellaneous
  Methemoglobinemia
  Liver damage
  Renal damage
  Peripheral vascular collapse

scopic hematuria, may also be noted. In addition, thrombocytopenia, intravascular hemolysis, and hemorrhagic diathesis have been seen as well as toxic hepatitis and encephalopathy.

Contact with chromium and its salts may cause diffuse dermatitis in hypersensitive individuals and can also cause deep perforating ulcers known as "chrome holes." Protein coagulation with ulcer and blister formation occurs after cutaneous contact. If inhaled, chromic dusts cause rhinitis and ulcers of the nasal septum and may also cause bronchitis, gastritis, and other inflammatory conditions. Peripheral vascular collapse, vertigo, muscle cramps, coma, and liver damage have also been reported. The dichromates may cause methemoglobinemia because they oxidize hemoglobin to methemoglobin.[2]

Morbidity and mortality rates in dichromate poisoning appear to be biphasic, with early multisystem involvement leading to shock and death. If the patient survives the initial phase, hepatic and renal failure may occur 8 to 10 days after ingestion.[3]

Treatment

Treatment for dichromate poisoning should center on early supportive measures. Dialysis may be warranted when renal failure occurs, but because it does not remove large quantities of chromium it is ineffective in the treatment of systemic dichromate toxicity.[3] Various agents have been suggested for the treatment of dichromate poisoning,[1] including dimercaprol and other chelating agents, but their efficacy has not been shown.

Hypochlorites

Hypochlorite salts (sodium, potassium, calcium, and magnesium) serve as bleaches, disinfectants, deodorizers, and water purifiers.[7] Dilute hypochlorites are found in almost every home in the form of laundry bleach (such as Clorox®), which is usually about 5% sodium hypochlorite. Ingestion of household bleach may include mild mucosal burns and edema, but extensive necrosis and stricture formation do not usually occur, although rare cases have been reported.[8] Products intended for industrial use may have much higher hypochlorite concentrations, but in these products the active ingredient is usually calcium hypochlorite.

Hypochlorite toxicity arises from the material's corrosive activity on skin and mucous membranes. This corrosiveness stems from the oxidizing potency of the hypochlorite ion, which is measured in terms of available chlorine.[5] The effects of ingested hypochlorite are related to concentration rather than dose. Solutions with 4% to 6% available chlorine, such as Clorox®, are not usually seriously toxic. Higher concentrations, as found in commercially available solutions of hypochlorite, are more dangerous because the free chlorine that is released coagulates cutaneous proteins as well as the protein of mucous membranes. Ingestion of these stronger compounds often leads to esophageal stricture as a late complication.

The risk of significant esophageal injury after ingestion of household bleach is low. Typically, erythema is the only problem. Immediate dilution is therefore the only therapy required in most cases. Because of the extremely low incidence of stricture formation, the decision to perform endoscopy after a bleach ingestion should be made on clinical grounds.[9] Symptomatic patients with pain on swallowing, shortness of breath, significant oropharyngeal burns, or chest pain should undergo endoscopy.[8,10]

Potassium Permanganate

Poisoning by ingestion of potassium permanganate is rare and generally occurs mainly in infants or as a result of a suicide attempt.[11] Potassium permanganate is a powerful oxidizing agent that is used as an abortifacient, a topical astringent, and an antiseptic agent in aqueous solution. As an astringent, it is diluted 1:500 to 1:10,000. Dilute solutions (1% to 3%) may be only mildly irritating, and the patient may experience burning in the throat, nausea, vomiting, moderate gastroenteritis, and some difficulty in swallowing (Table 18-3).[11,12] Concentrated solutions or the dry crystals are highly corrosive. In addition, concentrated solutions (8%) may result in some renal toxicity, hematochezia, hepatic dysfunction, and circulatory collapse. Because the material is poorly absorbed, systemic effects are typically not of great concern.[5] If absorption does occur, delayed neurological and gastrointestinal effects may be noted. Treatment consists of careful observation and supportive care.

METABOLIC COMPETITORS

Metabolic competitors produce their detrimental effects by binding or inhibiting calcium

Table 18-3 Symptoms of Potassium Permanganate Intoxication

Burning of the throat
Nausea and vomiting
Dysphagia
Hematochezia
Hepatic dysfunction
Renal impairment
Circulatory collapse

or other inorganic ions necessary for tissue viability and function. Metabolic competitors and inhibitors include oxalic acid and hydrofluoric acid.

Oxalic Acid

Oxalic acid is used for removing ink stains and iron mold and for cleaning leather (Table 18-4). It is found in disinfectants, household bleach, antirust products, furniture polishes, and metal cleaners. Many plants contain oxalate, notably rhubarb leaves, dieffenbachia, beets, and spinach. Other potential metabolic sources of oxalate include ethylene glycol, glyoxylic acid, and glycolic acid.

In dilute solution oxalic acid and its salts act by binding ionizable calcium from blood and tissues, thereby inactivating or poisoning protoplasm, preventing muscle contraction, and at times causing symptomatic hypocalcemia. Strong solutions of the acid are corrosive to the alimentary tract mucosa.

Table 18-4 Uses, Sources, and Toxic Effects of Oxalic Acid

Uses
  Removal of ink stains
  Leather cleaning
  Antirust agent
  Metal polish
  Cleaning agents
Sources
  Plants
    Rhubarb leaves
    Dieffenbachia
    Beets
    Spinach
    Marigold
  Other sources
    Ethylene glycol
    Glyoxylic acid
    Glycolic acid
    Furniture polish
Toxic effects
  Burns
  Muscular tremors
  Hypocalcemia
  Seizures
  Vascular collapse

In acute poisoning from ingestion there is local irritation and corrosion of the mouth, esophagus, and stomach; pain and vomiting are followed quickly by muscular tremors, convulsions, and collapse. Death may occur within a few minutes. Treatment consists of establishing an intravenous line and placing the patient on a cardiac monitor. A 12-lead electrocardiogram should be obtained, and serum calcium should be measured. Symptomatic hypocalcemia should be treated with calcium chloride (10 mL of 10% solution in adults).

Hydrofluoric Acid

Hydrofluoric acid is one of the strongest inorganic acids known[13] and has a number of chemical and industrial applications, such as in the production of fluorides, glass and silicon etching and frosting, semiconductor manufacturing, and the production of plastics and dyes (Table 18-5).[14–16] Many rust removal agents contain hydrofluoric acid. It is also used as a catalyst in alkylation units in the petroleum industry[17,18] as well as in the dental laboratories to clean and etch castings that are fused with porcelain.[19–21] Hydrofluoric acid is also used in the pesticide and fertilizer industries and in the production of refrigerants, aerosol propellants, fire extinguishers, aluminum germicides, and tanning agents.

At room temperature, fluorine is a pale yellow gas that is corrosive and reactive.[22] When combined with hydrogen, it forms violently explosive mixtures. Hydrogen fluoride completely dissociates in water to form hydrofluoric acid, a weak and unstable acid. Hydrofluoric acid is therefore the inorganic acid of elemental

---

Table 18-5 Uses of Hydrofluoric Acid

Glass etching
Petroleum refining
Dental work
Rust removal
Fertilizers
Manufacturing of fire extinguishers, dyes, tanning
  agents, refrigerants, aerosol propellents, plastics

---

fluorine. The fluoride ion has a strong affinity with apatite crystals, which are present in all calcified tissue. Thus on direct contact hydrofluoric acid causes liquefaction necrosis by disrupting the horny layer of the skin and immediately destroys the subcutaneous tissue.[13]

Hydrogen fluoride solutions are more damaging than the stronger halogen acids (hydroiodic, hydrobromic, and hydrochloric acids).[16] It is available as a liquid in various concentrations, from dilute solutions in erusticators (<10%) to highly concentrated solutions (70%). This exceedingly corrosive material is lethal in small quantities, even at low concentrations.[14,20,23]

Effects of Hydrofluoric Acid

Hydrofluoric acid produces burns by two mechanisms[24]: the hydrogen ion causes an initial corrosive burn that is identical to other acid burns, or the fluoride ion penetrates the skin and subcutaneous tissues.[22,23] As the fluoride ions penetrate deeper tissues they complex with calcium and magnesium to form insoluble fluoride salts (Table 18-6).[13,17] This destruction continues until the hydrogen fluoride is precipitated as calcium or magnesium fluoride by natural tissue magnesium or calcium compounds or by compounds administered medically.[16] This process can produce hypocalcemia and hypomagnesemia.

Fluoride ion also acts as a general enzyme inhibitor and inhibits cellular metabolism and the glycolytic enzymes, interferes with electrical membrane function, and decalcifies bone.[14] It appears that the fluoride ion binds the calcium on the cell membrane, leading to increased permeability of the membrane to potassium and thus to altered membrane potential and spontaneous depolarization; this produces pain and necrosis.[23] Severe hydrofluoric acid burns have been associated with systemic fluoride poisoning sometimes resulting in death.[25] One hydrofluoric acid death was caused by the electrolyte abnormalities described above from a burn involving 2.5% of the body surface.[26]

On the skin, concentrated hydrofluoric acid produces lesions that may be immediately and intensely painful;[16] the onset of lesions and pain may be delayed with weaker solutions. Some patients may not seek medical treatment for 18 to 24 hours,[22] which may lead to severe tissue destruction. Lesions may gradually become more severe, especially in the fingertips. Exposure of nail beds may produce permanent nail disfigurement and oncholysis.[13] After a latent period, painful, deep ulcers may be noted beneath an exceedingly tough coagulum. The salts formed by this destruction are soluble, and the fluoride released continues to destroy tissue.

The vapor of hydrofluoric acid is also intensely irritating to the lungs and conjunctivae and may itself produce skin burns. In addition, inhalation has produced oropharyngeal, airway, and lower respiratory tract damage with respiratory distress and pulmonary edema.[27] Deaths have been reported from inhalation of hydrofluoric acid vapors.[20,21,26]

Laboratory Determinations

After a significant exposure to hydrofluoric acid, blood should be drawn immediately for a complete blood cell count, to determine liver function, and to measure blood urea nitrogen, electrolytes, and serum creatinine, calcium, magnesium, and fluoride concentrations. The electrocardiogram should be monitored continuously for prolongation of the QT interval (Table 18-7).

Nonspecific Treatment

Initial treatment of hydrofluoric acid poisoning consists of the rapid removal of acid from the skin surface through good decontamination techniques (Table 18-8). Because the fluoride ion penetrates deeply into tissues and continues its destruction, decontamination with water alone is

---

Table 18-6 Effects of Hydrofluoric Acid

Corrosive-type burn (onset may be delayed)
Complexion with cations (may result in hypocalcemia
 or hypomagnesemia)
Bone decalcification
Increased cellular permeability to potassium
 Altered membrane potential
 Increased spontaneous depolarization
Interference with glycolytic enzymes, cellular
 metabolism, electrical membrane function
Systemic fluoride poisoning

Table 18-7 Laboratory Determinations in Hydrofluoric Acid Exposure

---

Complete blood cell count
Liver function studies
Blood urea nitrogen
Serum creatinine concentration
Serum electrolytes
Serum calcium concentration
Serum magnesium concentration
Serum fluoride concentration
Electrocardiogram

Table 18-8 Treatment of Hydrofluoric Acid Exposure

Nonspecific
  Decontamination
  Maintenance of electrolyte balance
  Monitoring for renal and hepatic toxicity
  Intravenous therapy
  Electrocardiographic monitoring
Specific
  Calcium gluconate gel (2.5%)
  Local calcium gluconate infiltration
  Intra-arterial calcium gluconate infusion

---

insufficient. The nails may need to be trimmed back to the nail bed to facilitate adequate decontamination in severe exposures because inadequate circulation in this area may prevent calcium from precipitating the fluoride ion.[21] Leather gloves and shoes cannot be decontaminated and must be destroyed.

Systemic therapy for the severely burned patient is generally supportive and includes maintenance of electrolyte balance, careful monitoring for signs of renal or hepatic toxicity, and maintenance of respiratory and cardiac function. Intravenous therapy should be initiated as soon as possible, and the electrocardiogram should be monitored continuously for evidence of hypocalcemia. The results of frequent electrolyte monitoring or clinical signs of hypocalcemia may indicate the need for intravenous calcium or magnesium (or both). Profound hypocalcemia may occur in the absence of clinical tetany.

Treatments no longer widely accepted for local hydrofluoric burns include topical steroids, systemic steroids, systemic calcium salts, and early surgical removal of affected tissue.

Specific Treatment

Authorities differ about the most effective specific treatment for hydrofluoric acid burns. Some suggest magnesium oxide ointment, topical or systemic calcium gluconate, and topical quaternary ammonium compounds.[23] The first two treatments depend on the precipitation of the fluoride ion into insoluble magnesium and calcium salts, respectively. The mechanism of action of the quaternary ammonium compounds is unknown, but it is postulated that ionized chloride is exchanged for the fluoride ion to produce a nonionized fluoride complex. It appears that calcium gluconate is more effective than other methods.

Calcium gluconate gel. Calcium gluconate gel can be a useful first aid technique and in some cases may be all that is necessary.[23,28] Calcium gluconate gel (2.5%) made for this purpose can be gently massaged into the contaminated areas until the pain is relieved. This gel is commercially available in the United Kingdom[23] but is not commercially available in the United States. A procedure to prepare 4 oz (120 g) of 2.5% gel is as follows. Weigh out 3 g of calcium gluconate powder, combine with 5 mL of sterile water to form a smooth paste, and incorporate the paste into 120 g of K-Y Jelly®. The resulting mixture is a 2.5% (by weight) gel and contains a preservative of chlorhexidine gluconate.

Calcium gluconate infiltration. Calcium gluconate infiltration is thought of as the treatment of choice for hydrofluoric acid skin burns.[20,23] If used appropriately, local calcium gluconate infiltration may provide excellent symptomatic relief and prevent serious tissue destruction.[14] The primary disadvantage of local infiltration is the mechanical trauma and pain from the multiple tissue injections. This procedure requires good medical supervision and follow-up. The volume of calcium gluconate that may be injected is limited because of possible vascular compromise.

After vigorous flooding of the involved area with water, ampules of 10% calcium gluconate should be diluted with physiologic saline solution to obtain a 5% concentration of calcium gluconate. This solution may be injected into the burned areas with a 25- or 27-gauge needle to bind the fluoride ions. The usual recommendation is that injections be limited to 0.5 mL per square centimeter of involved tissue.[13,22,29] The administration of calcium gluconate in concentrations greater than 5% tends to produce severe irritation of the tissues, which may cause keloid development and scarring.

Because pain is an excellent indicator of the extent of tissue involvement, use of local anesthesia should be delayed until the calcium infiltrations are complete. When pain recurs after injection of calcium gluconate, it indicates that free fluoride ions are again present.

Intra-arterial infusion of calcium gluconate. If the burn is of suitable size (such as to a limb, hand, or foot), then an intra-arterial infusion of 10 mL of 20% calcium gluconate in 40 mL of normal saline by means of a pump over 4 hours should be considered.[30] If the burn is to the hand the infusion can be performed through the radial artery with the aid of digital subtraction if the patient is able to cooperate.[22] This has been shown to be of considerable benefit in significant exposures in that much greater amounts of calcium gluconate can be administered, which may then offset local calcium deficits and bind remaining fluoride ion.[31] Disadvantages of this technique involve the invasiveness of the vascular procedure and the expense associated with the long duration of treatment.[22]

VESICANTS

The vesicant agents produce their damage through a series of physiologic changes that results in blistering and edema. Frequently they liberate histamine or serotonin at the site of contact, and the net result is local production of ischemia and anoxic necrosis. Among the important vesicants are the cantharides (Spanish fly), dimethylsulfoxide (DMSO), mustard gas (dichlorodiethyl sulfide), and lewisite [dichloro(2-chlorovinyl)arsine].

Cantharides (Spanish Fly, Blister Beetle)

Cantharides can be obtained from dried *Cantharis vesicatoria*, the blister beetle, and contain cantharidin, which is an irritant and vesicant to

the skin. A dose of 1 mg, or contact with a single insect, can produce distressing symptoms that may commence immediately or be delayed for as long as 12 hours.

Preparations of cantharides have been employed externally as rubefacients, counterirritants, and vesicants. Two preparations containing cantharidin are Cantharone® and VerrCanth®. Cantharone® liquid is a preparation for the treatment of warts and contains 0.7% cantharidin in a vehicle of acetone and colloidin. More concentrated cantharides produce severe, partial-thickness lesions. Cantharides are frequently used by farmers as veterinary aphrodisiacs[5]; occasionally, human contact occurs as a result of the mistaken belief that the material has aphrodisiac effects in humans. On skin contact, because of a severe histaminic response, papular lesions may occur that may then result in the burns previously described.

After ingestion of a cantharide there may be burning pain in the throat and stomach with difficulty in swallowing, nausea, vomiting, colic, bloody diarrhea, tenesmus, renal pain, frequent urination, hematuria, syncope, and circulatory failure. Treatment is nonspecific and supportive.

Dimethylsulfoxide

Dimethylsulfoxide (DMSO) is a colorless, highly polar organic liquid that was discovered in 1866.[32,33] DMSO is an inexpensive by-product of paper manufacturing. It has a high dielectric constant and therefore exhibits exceptional solvent properties for both organic and inorganic chemicals; it is widely used as an industrial solvent for resins, fungicides, dyes, and pigments (Table 18-9). It is also used as a reaction medium to accelerate rates of chemical combination and as antifreeze, hydraulic fluid, paint remover, a cryopreservative for platelets, and as a transport medium to facilitate transcutaneous drug absorption.[33]

DMSO is reported to have various pharmacological actions, including membrane penetration, anti-inflammatory effects, local analgesia, weak bacteriostasis, diuresis, vasodilation, and dissolution of collagen.[34] Its one approved use in the United States is for inter-

Table 18-9 Uses of Dimethylsulfoxide (DMSO)

Nonmedicinal
    Industrial solvent for resins, fungicides, dyes,
        pigments
    Reactant for chemical synthesis
    Antifreeze
    Hydraulic fluid
    Paint remover
Medicinal
    Anti-inflammatory agent (not FDA approved)
    Treatment of cerebral edema (not FDA approved)
    Cryopreservative for platelets
    Treatment of interstitial cystitis (FDA approved)
    Treatment of scleroderma (approved for use in
        Canada)
    Transport medium for drug absorption (not FDA
        approved)

stitial cystitis, a urologic condition of unknown etiology that causes irritative voiding symptoms and suprapubic pain that usually improves after urination.[34,35] Three preparations—Demasorb®, Rimso-50®, and Rimso-100®—are available for use for this condition for intravesicular instillation; the last two of these are 50% and 100% sterile, pyrogen-free preparations. DMSO is also a potent osmotic agent and is gaining increasing acceptance as adjunctive therapy for severe cerebral edema secondary to massive stroke or head trauma.[36]

Nonapproved medical applications for DMSO include use as an analgesic and anti-inflammatory agent in musculoskeletal disorders by application to the skin,[36] but its value in specific diseases has not been shown. Topical DMSO has been used to treat arthritis, sports injuries, scleroderma, and keloids. A 90% solution is also approved as a veterinary medication for topical use. In Canada, DMSO is approved as a 70% solution for cutaneous use in patients with scleroderma.

Properties

DMSO is readily absorbed through the body surface and readily crosses most membranes without apparently destroying their integrity.[5] This is a result of reversible configurational changes of protein molecules due to temporary water substitution by DMSO. In other words, it is the movement of DMSO through the skin that influences the movement of other molecules through the skin. It is also readily absorbed by injection and by mouth.[17]

DMSO has come into use as a penetrating solvent to aid absorption of drugs through the skin, such as testosterone, corticosteroids, and salicylates. Impurities in DMSO preparations are also distributed systemically (it should be noted that the manufacturer makes no claim regarding the absence of contaminants). If the skin is contaminated with dirt or chemicals, DMSO may carry these compounds through the skin and into the circulation. Rubber gloves do not necessarily provide adequate protection from absorption of DMSO.

DMSO permeates body water, and serum concentrations reach their peak 4 hours after administration by mouth and 4 to 8 hours after percutaneous administration.[17] Most of a dose is converted to an odorless compound, but about 3% to 6% is converted to a malodorous dimethylsulfide and is excreted through the lungs. This gives a characteristic garlic odor to the breath.[34]

Toxicity

The rate of absorption of DMSO is directly related to the relative concentration. Large amounts of high concentrations applied to the skin may cause burning, discomfort, itching, erythema,[37] occasionally vesiculation, hemoglobinuria, hemolysis, and profound release of histamine and serotonin in the immediate area.[17] Severe tissue edema and ischemia may also result.[35,37] Long-term eye toxicity has included lens opacification in animals; this has not been documented in humans. A reddish discoloration of the urine may be secondary to the transient systemic hemolysis.[36] Despite the hemoglobinuria, no long-term renal damage has been demonstrated.[36] DMSO may also increase serum osmolality.[38] Treatment for DMSO consists of decontamination and supportive care.

Mustard Gas

Mustard gas is of scientific historic interest because it is the first substance observed to act by an akylation reaction, or by binding to tissue proteins. During World War I, mustard gas was used as a vesicant and for chemical warfare.[5] In an aqueous medium it rearranges into a form that is highly reactive with sulfhydryl acid, carboxyl acid, amino acids, proteins, and the hydroxyl ions of water. This rearrangement is very stable and alters the functional and physiochemical properties of enzymes and other proteins so that they are denatured or inactivated.

Although mustard gas reacts very quickly with tissues, delayed symptoms are characteristic; there may be no clinical indication of injury until after a period of several hours. Nevertheless, decontamination must be carried out within seconds of exposure to be effective in preventing injury.

Lewisite

Lewisite is an extremely toxic member of a group of arsenic compounds that produce lesions of the epithelium of the skin and respiratory system as a result of their vesicant action. It received considerable attention in World War I and World War II as a potential agent in chemical warfare. Lewisite reacts with thiol groups of tissue proteins, and an effective antidote known as British anti-lewisite (BAL) or dimercaprol was produced specifically for its actions.[5]

MISCELLANEOUS COMPOUNDS

Mace is the prototype of the nonexplosive, pressurized, solvent tear gas weapons. These agents have been used by law enforcement agencies for riot control, although private use of these agents has also become prevalent.

Although some 15 sensory irritants have been used on occasion, only four agents (CS, CN, DM, and BBC; see Table 18-10) have been used

---

Table 18-10 Lacrimatory Agents

CS—Chlorobenzmalononitrile
CN—Chloroacetophenone
DM—Diphenylaminechlorarsine
BBC—Bromobenzyl cyanide

---

extensively.[39] Of these agents, only CN and CS have been widely employed in the United States, and all but one of the over-the-counter products contain CN. These agents are primarily intended to incapacitate an individual without causing illness or permanent bodily harm.[40]

Both CN and CS are alkylating agents that react with sulfhydryl groups.[39] They were first synthesized during World War I for use as lacrimatory agents. CS is approximately ten times more potent than CN as an irritant and at the same time is less systemically toxic.[40]

Chemical mace consists of a potent lacrimator (usually CN) dissolved in a mixture of hydrocarbons resembling kerosene. The mixture is maintained in a metal container and released as a spray of small liquid droplets directed in a stream that may travel 6 to 10 feet. Most of the active ingredient is dispersed before it reaches the target. The droplets of oily spray very effectively wet and spread on the skin.[40]

Symptoms

The acute transient clinical effects of both CN and CS are similar (Table 18-11). Major symptoms involve the eyes and respiratory tract. Instantaneous conjunctivitis is characteristic and is accompanied by stinging and burning sensations in the eyes that induces outpouring of tears and involuntary closure of the lids. The burning and pain persists for 2 to 5 minutes and usually disappears abruptly.[39] Conjunctivitis remains intense for 25 to 30 minutes. Erythema of the eyelids occurs and may persist for 1 hour. The profuse lacrimation that invariably occurs usually continues for 12 to 15 minutes.

The nose may be painful, and there may be an associated rhinorrhea. Excessive salivation and irritation in the throat are common. A burning sensation in the chest associated with tightness, coughing, and occasionally dyspnea also may be noted. If the material is swallowed, some epigastric discomfort and eructation may develop later. Most symptoms usually clear within 20 minutes, although some may persist.[40]

Respiratory symptoms include a stinging sensation in the nose and mouth and breath holding. At times, the chemical injury to the respiratory tract has resulted in acute pulmonary edema and

Table 18-11 Symptoms of Exposure to Lacrimating Agents

Eyes
Conjunctivitis
Lacrimation
Blepharospasm
Chemosis
Nose
Rhinorrhea
Pain
Mouth and throat
Salivation
Irritation
Skin
Contact dermatitis
Respiratory system
Cough
Dyspnea
Pulmonary edema (rare)

death after exposure to high concentrations of CN gas. These effects may be delayed, and a symptom-free interval after exposure may be observed.[39]

Permanent eye injury has been reported with these agents, although most have been associated with exposure to explosive-type devices discharged close to the face. CN has been known to cause chemical injury to the cornea as well as chemosis. These effects are more likely to occur when the agent is in powder or liquid form.

Fatalities have been reported to occur from 4 hours up to 4 days after exposure to CN.[39] Common causes have been pulmonary edema, focal intra-alveolar hemorrhage, and early bronchopneumonia.[40]

In addition to the irritant effects of these agents, repeated exposure may result in a contact dermatitis consisting of erythema, edema, and pruritus within 48 hours after exposure.[41] Contact dermatitis is most common with CN. An allergic blepharitis has also been reported.

Treatment

Other than prompt withdrawal from the area in which the aerosol is present, specific treatment is not required and recovery is usually prompt.[39] In the management of the conjunctivitis, topical anesthetics are not recommended. Cutaneous reactions should be managed by decontamination with copious amounts of water. Prevention of secondary exposure of medical personnel through contact with residual aerosols on skin or clothing must also be considered, which means that rubber gloves should be worn and contaminated clothing should be placed in plastic bags.

Because of the delayed pulmonary symptoms with the inhalation of large amounts of these chemicals, all patients who have been exposed to high concentrations of tear gas should be carefully observed for several days.[42]

REFERENCES

1. Behari J, Tandon S: Chelation in metal intoxication: Part VIII: Removal of chromium from organs of potassium chromate–administered rats. *Clin Toxicol* 1980;16:33–40.

2. Iserson K, Banner W, Froede R, et al: Failure of dialysis therapy in potassium dichromate poisoning. *J Emerg Med* 1983;1:143–149.

3. Ellis E, Brouhard B, Lynch R, et al: Effects of hemodialysis and dimercaprol in acute dichromate poisoning. *J Toxicol Clin Toxicol* 1982;19:249–258.

4. Kaufman D, Dinicola W, McIntosh R: Acute potassium dichromate poisoning. *Am J Dis Child* 1970; 119:374–376.

5. Jelenko C: Chemicals that ''burn.'' *J Trauma* 1974; 14:65–72.

6. Reichelderfer T: Accidental death of an infant caused by ingestion of ammonium dichromate. *South Med J* 1968; 61:96–97.

7. Hoy R: Accidental systemic exposure to sodium hypochlorite during hemodialysis. *Am J Hosp Pharmacol* 1981;38:1512–1514.

8. French R, Tabb H, Rutledge L: Esophageal stenosis produced by ingestion of bleach. *South Med J* 1970; 63:1140–1144.

9. Landau G, Saunders W: The effect of chlorine bleach on the esophagus. *Arch Otolaryngol* 1964;80:174–176.

10. Howell J: Alkaline ingestions. *Ann Emerg Med* 1986; 15:820–825.

11. Holzgraefe M, Poser W, Kijewski H, et al: Chronic enteral poisoning caused by potassium permanganate. *Clin Toxicol* 1986;24:235–244.

12. Huntly A: Oral ingestion of potassium permanganate or aluminum acetate in two patients. *Arch Dermatol* 1984; 120:1363–1365.

13. Rodeheaver G, Herbert J, Edlich R: Initial treatment of chemical skin and eye burns. *Compr Ther* 1982;8:37–43.

14. Mayer T, Gross P: Fatal systemic fluorosis due to hydrofluoric acid burns. *Ann Emerg Med* 1985;14:149–153.

15. McCulley J, Whiting D, Petitt M, et al: Hydrofluoric acid burns of the eye. *J Occup Med* 1983;25:447–450.

16. Dibbel D, Iverson R, Jones W, et al: Hydrofluoric acid burns of the hand. *J Bone Joint Surg* 1970;52:931–936.

17. Brown F, Johns L, Mullan S: Dimethylsulfoxide in experimental brain injury, with comparison to mannitol. *J Neurosurg* 1980;53:58–62.

18. Brown M: Fluoride exposure from hydrofluoric acid in a motor gasoline alkylation unit. *Am Ind Hyg Assoc J* 1985;46:662–669.

19. Moore P, Manor R: Hydrofluoric acid burns. *J Prosthet Dent* 1982;47:338–339.

20. White J: Hydrofluoric acid burns. *Cutis* 1984; 34:241–244.

21. Wilson G, Sanger R, Boswick J: Accidental hydrofluoric acid burns of the hand. *J Am Dent Assoc* 1979; 99:57–58.

22. Vance M, Curry S, Kunkel D, et al: Digital hydrofluoric acid burns: Treatment with intraarterial calcium infusion. *Ann Emerg Med* 1986;15:890–896.

23. Bracken W, Cuppage F, McLaury R, et al: Comparative effectiveness of topical treatments for hydrofluoric acid burns. *J Occup Med* 1985;27:733–739.

24. Harris J, Rumack B, Bregman D: Comparative efficacy of injectable calcium and magnesium salts in the therapy of hydrofluoric acid burns. *Clin Toxicol* 1981; 18:1027–1032.

25. Menchel S, Dunn W: Hydrofluoric acid poisoning. *Am J Forensic Med Pathol* 1984;5:245–248.

26. Tepperman P: Fatality due to acute systemic fluoride poisoning following a hydrofluoric acid skin burn. *J Occup Med* 1980;22:691–692.

27. Braun J, Stob H, Zober A: Intoxication following the inhalation of hydrogen fluoride. *Arch Toxicol* 1984; 56:50–54.

28. Trevino M, Herrmann G, Sproutt W: Treatment of severe hydrofluoric acid exposures. *J Occup Med* 1983; 25:861–863.

29. Stewart C: Chemical skin burns. *Am Fam Physician* 1985;31:149–157.

30. Pegg S, Siu S, Gillett G: Intraarterial infusions in the treatment of hydrofluoric acid burns. *Burns* 1983; 11:440–443.

31. Velvart J: Arterial perfusion for hydrofluoric acid burns. *Hum Toxicol* 1983;2:233–238.

32. Friend C, Freedman H: Effects and possible mechanism of action of dimethylsulfoxide on friend cell differentiation. *Biochem Pharmacol* 1978;27:1309–1313.

33. Kligman A: Topical pharmacology and toxicology of dimethylsulfoxide—Part I. *JAMA* 1965;193:140–148.

34. Fowler J: Prospective study of intravesical dimethylsulfoxide in the treatment of suspected early interstitial cystitis. *Urology* 1981;18:21–26.

35. Ek A, Engberg A, Frodin L, et al: The use of dimethylsulfoxide (DMSO) in the treatment of interstitial cystitis. *Scand J Urol Nephrol* 1978;12:129–131.

36. Muther R, Bennett W: Effects of dimethylsulfoxide on renal function in man. *JAMA* 1980;244:2081–2083.

37. Jacob S, Wood D: Dimethylsulfoxide (DMSO): Toxicology, pharmacology, and clinical experience. *Am J Surg* 1967;114:414–426.

38. Runckel D, Swanson R: Effect of dimethylsulfoxide on serum osmolality. *Clin Chem* 1980;26:1745–1747.

39. Sanford J: Medical aspects of riot control agents. *Annu Rev Med* 1976;27:421–429.

40. Beswick F: Chemical agents used in riot control and warfare. *Hum Toxicol* 1983;2:247–256.

41. Penneys N, Israel R, Indgin S: Contact dermatitis due to 1-chloracetophenone and chemical mace. *N Engl J Med* 1969;281:413–415.

42. Park S, Giammona S: Toxic effects of tear gas on an infant following prolonged exposure. *Am J Dis Child* 1972; 123:245–246.

ADDITIONAL SELECTED REFERENCES

Engberg A, Frodin L, Jonsson G: The use of dimethylsulfoxide in the treatment of interstitial cystitis. *Scand J Urol Nephrol* 1978;12:129–131.

Goodfellow R: Hydrofluoric acid burns. *Br Med J* 1985; 290:937.

Iverson R, Laub D, Madison M: Hydrofluoric acid burns. *Plast Reconstruct Surg* 1971;48:107–112.

Pike D, Peabody J, Davis E, et al: A re-evaluation of the dangers of Clorox ingestion. *J Pediatr* 1963;63:303–305.

Sperling S, Larsen I: Toxicity of dimethylsulfoxide (DMSO) to human corneal endothelium in vitro. *Acta Ophthalmol* 1979;57:891–898.

part VI

GASES AND ABNORMAL HEMOGLOBIN FORMATION

chapter 19

Carbon Monoxide

Carbon monoxide contamination and poisoning dates back to the roots of civilization and industrialization.[1] It was mentioned as early as the ancient Roman era, and early Greek physicians stated that carbon monoxide was harmful to the human body. Carbon monoxide was used by both the Greeks and Romans to execute criminals.[2] In 1895, Haldane first demonstrated that carbon monoxide combined with hemoglobin to form carboxyhemoglobin, which blocks oxygen binding and thereby decreases the amount of hemoglobin available for oxygen transport.

Poisoning with carbon monoxide is common and is responsible for thousands of deaths annually; many deaths are accidental because as little as 0.1% [1000 parts per million (ppm)] of the gas in inspired air can be lethal.[3–5] Carbon monoxide is normally present in the atmosphere at a concentration of less than 0.001% (10 ppm).[6–8]

PHYSICAL PROPERTIES

Carbon monoxide is a combustible, colorless, tasteless, and odorless gas that is nonirritating to the respiratory tract. It readily mixes with air without stratification because it has about the same density as air. Because of these physical properties, carbon monoxide may give no warning of its presence.

Carbon monoxide binds to hemoglobin and the resultant compound, carboxyhemoglobin, is a completely reversible complex that appears and disappears from the body only through the lungs and only in the course of respiration. Less than 1% of carbon monoxide is oxidized within the body to carbon dioxide.[9,10]

SOURCES OF CARBON MONOXIDE

Carbon monoxide is ubiquitous in the environment and is formed exogenously as a by-product of the incomplete combustion of any carbonaceous solid, liquid, or gaseous material (Table 19-1). It is also produced endogenously from the metabolic degradation of hemoglobin.

Fires

The most obvious source of carbon monoxide intoxication is smoke from any type of fire, and since the beginning of the use of fires for heat carbon monoxide accumulation has been a problem. Smoke from fires may contain from 0.1% to 10% carbon monoxide.[9] Cyanide and other toxic inhalants may also be liberated.[7,11] Fireplaces with faulty flues may be sources of carbon monoxide.

Table 19-1 Sources of Carbon Monoxide

Exogenous
  Automobile exhaust
  Cigarette smoke
  Coal gas
  Fireplace with faulty flue
  Fires
  Charcoal-burning grills
  Incomplete combustion of any fuel
  Methylene chloride
  Natural gases
  Sea plants
  Sterno®
  Volcanic activity
  Water gas
Endogenous
  Hemolytic anemia

Fuels

Environmental pollution probably constitutes the most common source of carbon monoxide.[7] The exhaust from gasoline engines may contain 6% to 10% carbon monoxide and diesel engines up to 7% or 70,000 ppm.[8,9,12–15] Not only does the automobile contribute to the sublethal concentrations of carbon monoxide in the atmosphere, but it can be a source of high-level exposure to its occupants when exhaust fumes enter the passenger compartment and build to lethal concentrations. It has been shown that automobile exhaust can saturate a car's interior or the interior of a small garage with lethal amounts of carbon monoxide in less than 20 minutes.[16–17] The use of gas-powered ice-surfacing machines at skating rinks has led to carbon monoxide intoxication in those enclosed areas.[9]

Older household fuels such as coal gas and water gas are made from coke and contain up to 40% carbon monoxide, hydrogen, methane, and other hydrocarbons. Natural gas does not contain carbon monoxide, but if it is improperly or incompletely combusted the by-product may be carbon monoxide.[5,8,18,19] Ironically, there is now an increased potential for carbon monoxide poisoning resulting from improved home insulation as well as the increased use of space heaters because both space heaters and kerosene heaters produce variable amounts of carbon monoxide.[12] Water heaters are also a common source of carbon monoxide, which is formed when a flame touches a surface cooler than the ignition temperature of the gaseous portion of the flame.[20] If these heaters are not properly vented, the room atmosphere readily becomes contaminated. Sterno®, a canned fuel used to heat food, contains ethyl alcohol, methanol, and acetone and has also been shown to elevate carbon monoxide concentrations in the surrounding air.[5,21]

Cigarette Smoke

Inhaled smoke of most tobacco cigarettes contains approximately 400 ppm carbon monoxide.[13,22] Smoking of tobacco products can produce carboxyhemoglobin concentrations from 5% to 18%, depending on the number of cigarettes smoked. A moderate smoker may have a carboxyhemoglobin concentration of 5% to 8%, and a heavy smoker (two to three packs per day) may have concentrations as high as 18%.[5] These individuals are usually asymptomatic. Significant increases in carbon monoxide (concentrations higher than those observed with conventional cigarettes) have been noted with the smoking of nontobacco cigarettes. In smoke-filled environments, nonsmoking individuals or ''passive smokers'' are exposed to elevated carbon monoxide concentrations. In addition, ''sidestream'' smoke, which is emitted by the burning tip of a cigarette, contains two and a half times more carbon monoxide than ''mainstream'' inhaled smoke.[9]

Charcoal-Burning Grills

Deaths have occurred from the use of charcoal-burning grills because the incomplete combustion of charcoal briquets can produce high concentrations of carbon monoxide in poorly ventilated spaces.[9,13,23]

Methylene Chloride

Methylene chloride (dichloromethane) is usually considered one of the safest of the chlorinated hydrocarbons.[14,24] It has numerous industrial applications, such as a degreaser, an aerosol propellant, and a solvent for plastic films and cement.[25] Domestically it is used in furniture and paint stripping.

Using methylene chloride paint remover in an enclosed room may lead to absorption of a large amount of the solvent through the lungs.[9,14,26] The chemical is then released slowly from body tissues and is metabolized to carbon monoxide endogenously, which may result in significant poisoning.[5,13] The biological half-life of carbon monoxide formed from methylene chloride is two to two and a half times longer than that of carbon monoxide exposure taken into the body from the environment. This is because of the slow release of methylene chloride from endogenous tissue stores even after contact with the compound is terminated. Methylene chloride is therefore particularly hazardous because the carboxyhemoglobin concentration continues to increase after cessation of exposure.[26] The amount of carbon monoxide formed in the body is directly related to the amount of methylene chloride absorbed; the greater the minute respiratory volume or the poorer the room ventilation, the greater the absorption of methylene chloride and the higher the elevation of carboxyhemoglobin concentration.[27]

Natural Sources

Natural sources of carbon monoxide include forest fires, volcanic activity, natural gases, certain sea plants, and photochemical degradation of organic compounds. These and other natural sources are large producers of carbon monoxide and are estimated to produce greater amounts of carbon monoxide than all automobile and industrial sources combined.

Catabolism of hemoglobin and other heme-containing compounds to bilirubin and carbon monoxide accounts for a baseline carboxyhemoglobin level of 0.3% to 3.0% in nonsmokers.[8,9] In patients with hemolytic anemias the concentration may rise to 4% to 6%.[12,13,22]

MECHANISM OF TOXICITY

Carbon monoxide causes toxicity in three ways: (1) by the formation of carboxyhemoglobin, (2) by shifting the oxyhemoglobin dissociation curve to the left, and (3) by binding to other heme-containing proteins.

Formation of Carboxyhemoglobin

Each molecule of hemoglobin has four heme groups and can reversibly bind up to four oxygen or carbon monoxide molecules in any combination. Carbon monoxide competes with oxygen for these binding sites on the hemoglobin molecule, and its affinity for hemoglobin is approximately 240 times greater than that of oxygen.[5,9,28–30] Thus extremely low concentrations of carbon monoxide in the air may produce poisoning.[13] Carbon monoxide is incapable of binding oxygen, and because the oxygen-carrying capacity of the blood is solely limited by the amount of hemoglobin not bound by carbon monoxide this results in tissue hypoxia. Bonding one or more of the four hemes of the hemoglobin molecule to carbon monoxide also appears to increase the bond strength between the remaining hemes and oxygen in the same molecule. In other words, the presence of some carboxyhemoglobin in an erythrocyte causes the remaining hemoglobin in the same erythrocyte to hold oxygen much more tightly than normal (see discussion of oxyhemoglobin dissociation below).[5] Because this binding is reversible, carbon monoxide can be competitively removed from hemoglobin by high concentrations of oxygen.

The reduction in oxygen-carrying capacity of blood is proportional to the amount of carboxyhemoglobin formed. Because the affinity for carbon monoxide is so many times that of oxygen, a small concentration of carbon monoxide in inspired air can tie up a large proportion of circulating hemoglobin. For example, carboxyhemoglobin concentrations of 0.01%, 0.02%, 0.1%, and 1% eventually saturate 11%, 19%, 54%, and 92% of the hemoglobin, respectively.

Shift in Oxyhemoglobin Dissociation Curve

The formation of carboxyhemoglobin inhibits oxyhemoglobin dissociation by shifting the oxyhemoglobin saturation curve to the left as well as by altering the shape of the curve toward a more hyperbolic form (Fig. 19-1).[5,31]

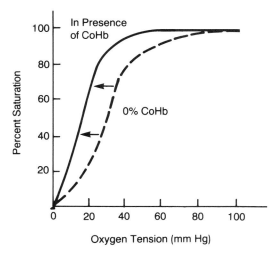

Figure 19-1 Oxyhemoglobin dissociation curve showing oxygen saturation in a patient with carbon monoxide poisoning. CoHb, carboxyhemoglobin. *Source*: Reproduced by permission from *Pediatrics* (1981;68:218), Copyright © 1981, American Academy of Pediatrics.

The leftward shift results in the availability of even less oxygen to the tissues than the carboxyhemoglobin saturation would suggest because of decreased unloading of oxygen at the tissues.[10,32] In other words, tissue oxygen tensions must become extremely low before the remaining oxyhemoglobin can give up its oxygen.[9] This effect is especially marked at carboxyhemoglobin concentrations greater than 45%.[12] Thus carbon monoxide results in a lower tissue end-capillary or venous oxygen tension.[33] In pathophysiologic terms, this means that carbon monoxide causes a hypoxemia that is similar to but more severe than anemic hypoxia. Carbon monoxide–induced hypoxemia, in contrast to hypoxic hypoxia, does not reduce arterial oxygen partial pressure and, in contrast to anemic hypoxia, does not lower blood viscosity.

Binding to Heme-Containing Proteins

Another important effect of carbon monoxide is its direct toxicity to the hemoproteins such as myoglobin, the peroxidases, the catalases, and the cytochromes.[5,34–36] Among the reactions with these proteins, the most significant are the reactions with cytochrome (a_3) oxidase, cytochrome P-450, and myoglobin.

The cytochromes are located in the mitochondria and are the seat of cellular respiration. The inhibitory effect of carbon monoxide on cytochrome oxidase therefore inhibits cellular respiration by competing with oxygen receptors in the cytochrome system. It is thought that the direct toxic effects on these cellular enzymes account for the often noted disparity between carboxyhemoglobin concentration and the patient's clinical condition, although this has not been shown. The affinity of the cytochrome system for oxygen is nine times that of carbon monoxide, so that, in adequately oxygenated individuals, carbon monoxide does not compete effectively for cytochrome oxidase.[9] This may be altered, however, during carbon monoxide exposure when tissue oxygen content may be severely reduced.

Except for hemoglobin, myoglobin is the most plentiful hemoprotein in the body and appears to act as a short-term oxygen store. Myoglobin also probably facilitates oxygen transport and diffusion across the cytoplasm from cell membrane to mitochondria. Carbon monoxide combines with myoglobin and interferes with this process. It binds to cardiac and skeletal muscle myoglobin, with cardiac muscle taking up about three times as much as skeletal muscle.[9] This indicates that in individuals with a carboxyhemoglobin concentration of 10% approximately 30% of cardiac myoglobin is saturated with carbon monoxide. This significantly decreases the oxygen reserve available to the myocardium.[37–39]

**MEASUREMENT OF
CARBOXYHEMOGLOBIN
CONCENTRATION**

Carboxyhemoglobin concentrations can be obtained from venous or arterial blood,[13] although the *p*H is better assessed with arterial samples and acidosis, which may be profound, is more adequately monitored by means of arterial blood gases.

Blood carboxyhemoglobin is usually expressed as percent saturation. The terms percent saturation and carboxyhemoglobin concentration are used interchangeably, and both imply the percentage of hemoglobin combined with carbon monoxide. Both are calculated with the following formula:

$$\frac{\text{Carboxyhemoglobin}}{\text{Concentration}} = \frac{\text{blood CO content}}{\text{blood CO capacity}} \times 100$$

The percentage of carboxyhemoglobin is the ratio of carboxyhemoglobin to hemoglobin. As an example, a carboxyhemoglobin concentration of 50% means that in a patient with 16 g of hemoglobin 8 g is carboxyhemoglobin. The percentage may be misleading, especially in the presence of anemia.

SIGNS AND SYMPTOMS OF CARBON MONOXIDE INTOXICATION

Carbon monoxide intoxication has symptoms referrable to those tissues or organs that are most sensitive to the disruption of aerobic metabolism (Table 19-2).[28,40] These tissues or organs are also those with the highest metabolic rates. Therefore the brain and heart are the organs most susceptible to the effects of carbon monoxide poisoning.[9,32,41,42] Children, because of their increased respiratory exchange requirements, may be more susceptible than adults to carbon monoxide intoxication.[12] Patients with coronary artery disease also are at high risk of developing cardiac symptoms after carbon monoxide exposure.[37,43] Sudden, acute exposure to a high atmospheric concentration of carbon monoxide may result in symptoms without elevated carboxyhemoglobin concentrations. Likewise, chronic exposure to carbon monoxide may result in elevated carboxyhemoglobin concentrations without symptoms.[43]

All factors that increase respiration and circulation accelerate this process and shorten the latent period before toxic signs and symptoms appear. Exercise, fever, and anemia increase the hazard from carbon monoxide. Symptoms of poisoning are therefore related to the blood carboxyhemoglobin concentration, which may be affected by (1) the amount of inspired carbon monoxide or the amount in the environment, (2) the degree of physical activity, (3) the duration of exposure or contact with the gas, (4) the degree of alveolar ventilation, (5) the level of cardiac output, and (6) the presence of cardiovascular or cerebrovascular disease (Table 19-3).[41,43]

Table 19-2 Effects of Carbon Monoxide Poisoning

Respiratory
Dyspnea on exertion
Hyperpnea
Respiratory failure
Neurologic
Headache
Giddiness
Irritability
Dizziness
Vomiting
Excitement
Hallucinations
Seizures
Stupor
Syncope
Coma
Cardiac
Angina pectoris
Myocardial infarction
Palpitations
Tachycardia
Bradycardia
Cutaneous
Dermatographia
Papules
Tropic erythema
Vesicles
Blistering
Visual
Blurred vision
Blindness
Flame-shaped hemorrhages
Paracentral scotoma
Papilledema
Visual field defects
Musculoskeletal
Rhabdomyolysis
Myoglobinemia
Myoglobinuria

Correlation between Symptoms and Carboxyhemoglobin Concentration

Although there are rough guidelines concerning carboxyhemoglobin concentrations and symptomatology, often the correlation between these two factors is poor. In addition, unless exposure to carbon monoxide is suspected, carboxyhemoglobin concentrations may not be measured because there are no pathognomic

Table 19-3 Conditions Affecting the Degree of Carbon Monoxide Intoxication

---

Concentration of inspired carbon monoxide
Degree of physical activity
Duration of exposure or contact with gas
Alveolar ventilation
Cardiac output
Pre-existing cardiovascular disease
Pre-existing cerebrovascular disease

---

symptoms, so that the presentation may easily imitate other illnesses. This may cause a dangerous delay in diagnosis. The possibility of carbon monoxide poisoning must therefore be considered when headache, nausea, dizziness, extreme fatigue, confusion, or collapse occur in an environment in which carbon monoxide could be present.

Only a few symptoms of carbon monoxide poisoning occur at carboxyhemoglobin concentrations of less than 10% to 13% (Table 19-4), although even low concentrations of carboxyhemoglobin significantly impair the delivery of oxygen to tissues. As an example, with blood carboxyhemoglobin concentrations of 1% to 4% myocardial blood flow increases, but no adverse effects are clearly demonstrable. At 5% to 9%, patients with coronary artery disease demonstrate a decreased threshold for exercise-induced angina.[38]

Typically the earliest symptom noted with carbon monoxide poisoning, with carboxyhemoglobin concentrations between 10% to

20%, is a slight headache or tightness across the forehead[35]; this concentration corresponds to 70 to 120 ppm carbon monoxide in the air. With concentrations between 20% to 30%, the headache may become more pronounced and be experienced as a throbbing pain.[1] Headache is presumed to be secondary to reflex cerebral vasodilation and increased cerebral blood flow resulting from relative tissue hypoxia. With carboxyhemoglobin concentrations of 30% to 40%, muscular weakness, palpitations, dizziness, dimness of vision, nausea, vomiting, and mental confusion may occur. Excitement and reckless behavior may also follow. These symptoms may progress to tachycardia and cardiovascular collapse when the carboxyhemoglobin concentration is in the range of 40% to 50%.[1] At concentrations greater than 50%, coma and intermittent seizures may appear. Concentrations greater than 60% may lead to death.[12] This corresponds to carbon monoxide concentrations as low as 0.1% inhaled for several minutes.

In addition, a particular carbon monoxide concentration can have a more profound effect on tissue oxygenation at high altitudes than at sea level because of the reduced oxygen partial pressures at high altitudes. The risk of carbon monoxide is also greater above 7000 feet than at sea level because the reduced amount of oxygen at high altitudes results in poor combustion of motor fuels, causing vehicles to emit much more carbon monoxide.

Carboxyhemoglobin concentrations may be within the normal range and not reflect the true

---

Table 19-4 Carboxyhemoglobin Concentration and Symptomatology

Carboxyhemoglobin Concentration (percent)	Carbon Monoxide in Air (percent)	Clinical Effect
0-10		None
10-20	0.007-0.012	Mild headache, fatigue
20-30	0.012-0.022	Throbbing headache, giddiness, blurred vision, dyspnea on exertion, irritability, impaired motor dexterity
30-40	0.022-0.035	Weakness, dizziness, nausea, vomiting, blurred vision, confusion, excitement, palpitations
40-50	0.035-0.052	Weakness, ataxia, tachypnea, syncope, tachycardia, confusion, hallucinations
50-60	0.052-0.080	Syncope, stupor, seizures, coma, hyperpnea
60-70	0.080-0.122	Coma, bradycardia, bradypnea, seizures, incontinence
>70	0.195	Respiratory failure, death

insult.[44-46] This may be particularly true when there is a significant delay between cessation of exposure and drawing of the blood sample or if supplemental oxygen has been administered. Some patients may have a circulating carboxyhemoglobin concentration of 25% and be severely acidotic and unconscious, whereas others with concentrations of 40% or more may be awake and alert and only manifest a headache.[43] A carboxyhemoglobin concentration that is within normal limits therefore does not rule out a significant case of carbon monoxide poisoning.[5,12,44,47] This is because the tissue concentration may more accurately reflect a degree of insult, a measurement that may have to be inferred from the clinical state and examination; the carboxyhemoglobin concentration is in such a case only one of many factors.

Respiratory Effects

The principal chemoreceptors that sense a reduction in oxygen and initiate cardiovascular and respiratory reflex responses are located in the carotid artery and the aortic bodies. With carbon monoxide intoxication, the partial pressure of oxygen in the blood is normal because blood is still in tension equilibrium with alveolar gas. The actual oxygen saturation is low, however. Because the carotid artery and aortic body chemoreceptors are sensitive to oxygen tension and not to the oxygen content of the arterial blood, no respiratory compensation for the tissue hypoxia occurs in most patients until very high blood concentrations of carbon monoxide are attained. Acute pulmonary edema has also been reported secondary to carbon monoxide intoxication.[48]

Neurologic Effects

Neurologic symptoms may include throbbing headache, excitability, confusion, visual complaints, seizures, and dizziness. Subtle neuropsychiatric symptoms may also be present after carbon monoxide poisoning (Table 19-5).[40] Physicians should be aware that signs of cortical dysfunction, particularly of the frontal and pa-

Table 19-5 Neurologic Effects Secondary to Carbon Monoxide Intoxication

Change in mental status
Coma
Decerebrate rigidity
Decreased comprehension
Decreased coordination
Decreased spatial reasoning
Decreased visual acuity
Extensor plantar responses
Short-term memory loss
Spatial disorientation
Transient cortical blindness

rietal lobes, may mimic psychiatric symptoms. In many cases the earliest and most common neurological accompaniment to the comatose state is a tonic disorder or decerebrate rigidity associated with increased deep tendon reflexes and extensor plantar responses. Cortical blindness is usually transitory and characterized by visual loss but intact pupillary reactions to light. Carbon monoxide poisoning may also result in cerebral edema secondary to hypoxia and interference with cellular respiration.[9]

Cardiac Effects

Carbon monoxide intoxication causes coronary artery vasodilation and an increase in coronary blood flow that is linearly related to the reduction in arterial oxygen content.[38,49,50] The heart may be unduly compromised with carbon monoxide poisoning because it must increase its output if peripheral oxygen transport is to be maintained, yet at the same time its own oxygen supply is compromised.[51] Therefore, in patients with ischemic heart disease, whose oxygen transport systems are marginal, very small increments in carboxyhemoglobin concentration can exacerbate symptoms. Exacerbation of angina pectoris with or without myocardial infarction is a well-established complication of carbon monoxide poisoning.[38,42] Electrocardiographic changes may include ST segment and T wave abnormalities suggestive of myocardial ischemia, or infarction, extrasystoles, and other dysrhythmias. Such abnormalities are sensitive indicators of myocardial damage.[8]

Cutaneous Effects

Cutaneous manifestations of carbon monoxide poisoning include dermatographia, papules, vesicles, blisters, and bullae,[52] which are often mistaken for burns or trauma in the unconscious patient.[9] The most common skin manifestation is tropic erythema, which may appear on the face and extremities and is not necessarily related to pressure areas.[53]

Because the formation of carboxyhemoglobin imparts a bright red color to the skin, patients may be profoundly hypoxic without manifesting cyanosis. Nevertheless the cherry-red appearance of the skin is relatively uncommon, occurring only in a minority of severe cases, and should therefore never be relied on for making the diagnosis.[5,54,55]

Visual Effects

Visual effects of carbon monoxide poisoning include temporary or permanent loss of vision, visual field defects, paracentral scotomas, decreased light sensitivity, and decreased dark adaptation.[13] Flame-shaped superficial retinal hemorrhages have been reported in long-term, subacute carbon monoxide poisoning.[9,56] Papilledema may also be seen on funduscopic examination. These visual changes may be permanent, even in the acute carbon monoxide exposure.

Musculoskeletal Effects

Although myonecrosis complicating carbon monoxide poisoning is uncommon, it has been recognized for many years.[53,57,58] In the comatose patient, the crushing effect of the patient's body on certain muscle groups leads to their injury; this has occurred both with and without coma. The resulting myoglobinuria may lead to acute renal failure with terminal hyperkalemia.[10,59] Although rhabdomyolysis can occur secondary to pressure necrosis, it may also be a result of a direct cellular toxic effect in patients with long-term exposure.[5]

Late Complications

Late complications of carbon monoxide poisoning are often not considered during initial management but can be more devastating than the effects of the original insult (Table 19-6).[31,54,60] Late complications include aspiration pneumonitis, myocardial damage, renal insufficiency, adult respiratory distress syndrome,[53] and, most important, neuropsychiatric disturbances (Table 19-7).[4,40,54,61] These complications may occur days to weeks after exposure, be varied and unpredictable, and occur after an initial period of recovery.[5]

Central nervous system damage resulting from carbon monoxide poisoning is similar to that from other severe hypoxic insults.[62–64] Postanoxic encephalopathy may begin 7 to

Table 19-6 Late Complications of Carbon Monoxide Intoxication

Adult respiratory distress syndrome
Aspiration pneumonitis
Myocardial damage
Neurologic abnormalities (see Table 19-7)
Ocular abnormalities
Renal insufficiency
Rhabdomyonecrosis

Table 19-7 Late Neurologic Sequelae of Carbon Monoxide Intoxication

Cerebral demyelination
Cortical blindness
Deafness
Dementia
Memory impairment
Mental retardation
Necrosis of globus pallidus
Necrosis of substantia nigra
Parietal lobe dysfunction
    Visual agnosia
    Temporospatial disorientation
    Constructional apraxia
    Dysnomia
Parkinsonism
Peripheral neuritis
Personality changes
Psychosis
Wernicke-Korsakoff syndrome

21 days after the initial insult and has been described only after episodes of severe CNS hypoxia.[40] Occasionally a victim may appear to recover but suffer a relapse of neurologic manifestations.

Delayed neurologic sequelae include a triad of gait disturbances, incontinence of urine, and mental deterioration. Long-term neuro-psychologic sequelae have included almost every type and degree of neurologic deficit, such as memory impairment, mental retardation, cortical blindness,[65] transient deafness, diabetes insipidus,[66] and Korsakoff's psychosis.[61] Personality alterations including irritability, impulsiveness, mood changes, violence, and verbal aggressiveness have also occurred. Occasional frank psychosis has ensued.[46] Specific signs of parietal lobe dysfunction such as visual agnosia, temporospatial disorientation, constructional apraxia, dysnomia, and dysgraphia may be noted. Parkinsonism,[67,68] chorea, spasticity, hyperreflexia, and polyneuritis have also been seen.[49] Demyelination with widespread foci of cellular degeneration in the cerebrum, cerebellum, and basal ganglia may be noted.

There are no clear clinical signs that accurately predict which patients presenting with carbon monoxide poisoning will have delayed neurologic effects. Mild cases may at times go on to delayed relapse.[50] The outcome of delayed neurologic sequelae is relatively good. Recovery rates vary from several days to as long as 8 months, with the highest cerebral functions being recovered last.[40] Neurologic symptoms may also worsen over time.[5]

Death

The major cause of death associated with acute carbon monoxide poisoning is cardiac dysrhythmias.[42,60,69] Carbon monoxide poisoning may also result in lethal cerebral edema as a consequence of cell death caused by hypoxia and interference with cellular respiration.[61]

Carbon Monoxide in Pregnancy

Carbon monoxide crosses the placenta, either by simple diffusion or mediated by a carrier, and enters the fetal blood supply.[2,70] Chronic exposure in pregnancy is usually a result of cigarette smoking by the mother, and there is a well-established, direct relationship between the number of cigarettes smoked per day and the decrease in birth weight. In addition, there is a reported increase in the rate of fetal wastage independent of birth weight as well as an increase in the rate of placenta previa, abruptio placentae, and premature rupture of membranes.[12,71,72] The fetus is more susceptible to carbon monoxide poisoning than the mother for two reasons: (1) fetal carboxyhemoglobin concentrations at equilibrium are higher than those of the mother by 10% to 15%,[2] and (2) the normal shift to the left of the fetal oxyhemoglobin dissociation curve accentuates the hemoglobin-binding properties of carbon monoxide.[2]

DIAGNOSIS OF CARBON MONOXIDE POISONING

The protean symptoms associated with carbon monoxide intoxication probably lead to a gross underestimation of its true incidence.[73] The most common misdiagnosis is a flu-like viral illness because of symptoms of headache, dizziness, nausea, vomiting, and shortness of breath.[9,74–77] Carbon monoxide poisoning should be considered in the differential diagnosis of an acute encephalopathic state. Appropriate settings for pathogenesis include a long automobile trip, smoke inhalation, and exposure to incompletely combusted domestic fuel; a history of suicidal thoughts or attempts is also grounds for suspecting carbon monoxide poisoning. Patients seen during winter months with severe headache, nausea, vomiting, unusual weakness, decreased cognitive function, new-onset angina pectoris, or exacerbation of chronic cardiopulmonary disorders should be questioned concerning similarly affected cohabitants of the home, faulty ventilation, defective heating, or the use of space heaters. Group exposures to carbon monoxide may be misdiagnosed as food poisoning, especially if vomiting is present.[9] An interesting practical point is that animals with high basal metabolic rates are particularly susceptible to carbon monoxide and frequently succumb before the development of symptoms in humans.[2,12,13]

Unless there is a diligent search for pathognomonic signs, findings on physical examination are of little specific help in the diagnosis. A thorough neurological examination should be performed so as not to miss the subtle signs that may be the only manifestation of poisoning. A funduscopic examination may reveal flame-shaped retinal hemorrhages, but this is a nonspecific indicator of subacute exposure to carbon monoxide.[74,78]

Psychometric assessments have shown that a patient's overall performance on a battery of tests decreases with increased carboxyhemoglobin levels. These tests involve comprehension, short-term memory, spatial orientation, visual motor speed and coordination, visual acuity, spatial reasoning, attentional ability, and fine motor control and are measures of cerebral functioning (Table 19-8). The mental status examination may also be a sensitive diagnostic indicator of carbon monoxide intoxication.

LABORATORY ANALYSIS

Routine laboratory studies (Table 19-9) may also offer no specific clues to the diagnosis. *Arterial blood gas* should be determined, but the values may be normal because the partial pressure of oxygen is a measure of the oxygen dissolved in plasma and is not affected by changes in hemoglobin saturation. An anion gap metabolic acidosis due to lactic acidosis may be seen in severely poisoned patients.

Many hospital laboratories calculate the oxygen saturation from the oxygen partial pressure by means of a slide rule nomogram. With carbon monoxide present the arterial oxygen partial pressure is normal if the patient is breathing normally, and calculated oxygen saturation may then be grossly incorrect. It is therefore mandatory to have a direct measurement of the oxygen saturation and to compare the calculated with the measured saturation.[5,44,74] A difference of more than 5% is considered significant, and carbon monoxide poisoning should be considered.[79]

An *electrocardiogram* may be abnormal, showing nonspecific ST-T wave changes. Atrial

Table 19-8 Psychometric Testing

Comprehension
Short-term memory
Spatial orientation
Visual motor speed
Coordination
Visual acuity
Spatial reasoning
Attentional ability
Fine motor control

Table 19-9 Laboratory Studies Suggested in Carbon Monoxide Poisoning

Arterial blood gas
Carboxyhemoglobin concentration
Chest roentgenogram
Electrocardiogram
Spirometry
Urinalysis

dysrhythmias and various conduction disturbances and occasionally evidence of myocardial infarction may also be noted.[8,38,42] Serial electrocardiograms and cardiac enzymes may be necessary to screen for immediate and delayed evidence of myocardial toxicity.

Spirometry can be a sensitive indicator of smoke inhalation. This may be indicated in cases where the diagnosis is unclear. Both the forced expiratory volume and the forced vital capacity may be abnormal.

A *chest roentgenogram* of acutely intoxicated patients may show a ground-glass appearance, perihilar haze, peribronchial and perivascular cuffing, and intra-alveolar edema. The ground-glass appearance can be considered parenchymal interstitial edema caused by tissue hypoxia or the toxic effects of carbon monoxide on alveolar membranes. Pulmonary edema may also be noted.

A *urinalysis* may be helpful in identifying myoglobinuria. Glycosuria and proteinuria may be seen secondary to renal tubular hypoxia. There are currently four *spot tests* for carboxyhemoglobin, but the presence of carboxyhemoglobin cannot be determined accurately by any of these tests; they should therefore be abandoned.[78]

There are relatively accurate *portable breath analyzers* for carbon monoxide that indicate immediately whether or not a patient has been exposed.[80–82] Other poisonous compounds do not appear to interfere with accurate carboxyhemoglobin readings from these instruments, which operate on the basis of an electrochemical principle. Estimates based on measurement of expired air, in parts per million, are less accurate than directly measuring carboxyhemoglobin concentrations.

The definitive diagnosis is made by measuring blood *carboxyhemoglobin* concentration; this measurement should therefore be made as early as possible. This can be done spectrophotometrically with a co-oximeter, which provides a rapid and accurate determination. This study is mandatory in all symptomatic patients to establish the diagnosis, to aid in determining the degree of intoxication, and to help plan the treatment needed.

It must again be emphasized that the carboxyhemoglobin concentration may not adequately reflect the diagnosis if supplemental oxygen therapy has been instituted or if there is a long period of time between exposure and drawing of a blood sample.[5,13] Consequently, patients can remain in a depressed clinical state even after the apparent elimination of carbon monoxide from the body. This situation may be the result of either an undetectable amount of carbon monoxide still bound in the tissues or a residual hypoxia.[83]

Computerized tomographic brain scanning of patients exposed to carbon monoxide has demonstrated symmetrical bilateral necrosis of the basal ganglia, most often the globus pallidus,[30,84,85] and of the red zone of the substantia nigra, many times with abnormal contrast enhancement of the pallidum.[40,62,86] This lesion is a pathological but nonspecific hallmark of carbon monoxide intoxication; barbiturate intoxication, cyanide poisoning, hydrogen sulfide poisoning, and hypoglycemia have a similar appearance.[87] Early evidence of low-density areas in the globus pallidus in comatose patients correlates with a high risk of death or poor neurological outcome.[9,13,50] Patients exposed to carbon monoxide who have normal tomographic scans have shown good recovery. An electroencephalogram may reveal diffuse frontal slow-wave activity consistent with a metabolic encephalopathy.[75]

TREATMENT

General

The management of carbon monoxide poisoning involves reversing the pathophysiologic process as quickly as possible. The first priority of treatment is removal of the patient from the poisoned environment and the administration of as much oxygen as possible.[9,38] Resuscitation of patients who have evidence of stupor, coma, or severe motor neurologic impairment may require intubation with sedation or curarization and fluid restriction. In addition, treatment should include ruling out other causes of symptomatology. If the patient presents with an altered mental state, dextrose in water, thiamine, and naloxone should be administered. Cardiac rhythm should be monitored during transport and in the emergency department.[9] There is no specific treatment for the patient presenting with delayed neurologic sequelae secondary to carbon monoxide poisoning.[12,13]

Fluid and Electrolyte Balance

Fluid and electrolyte balance should be carefully maintained to guard against overhydration and further pulmonary complications. Positive end expiratory pressure may be helpful in raising the functional residual capacity. Although some authorities suggest not treating a mild acidosis[5,8] because of the shift of the oxyhemoglobin dissociation curve to the right, care should be taken in the patient with myonecrosis because this condition decreases excretion of the toxin.[88,89] If ventilatory assistance is required, the use of a volume respirator is recommended because of increased airway resistance and decreased patient compliance.

Steroids

Steroids have been recommended by some investigators to combat cerebral edema. To date, there is no convincing evidence that steroids improve the prognosis for patients with diffuse cerebral edema. This is still an area of controversy. If steroids are used, they should be administered early in the course as a single, large intravenous bolus.

Oxygen

Oxygen therapy is the mainstay of treatment for carbon monoxide poisoning and should be instituted as quickly as possible with the greatest concentration available. Hyperbaric oxygen may be indicated, but when there are no hyperbaric oxygen facilities available or when there is no clinical indication for hyperbaric oxygen and the patient is cooperative, a tightly fitting face mask should be used to administer 100% oxygen. The plastic "rebreather" mask typically used in emergency departments may not deliver 100% oxygen, even at a flow rate of 10 L/min[90]. Furthermore, the unconscious or uncooperative patient may require intubation and mechanical ventilation to receive 100% oxygen. Supplementation with 5% carbon dioxide has been suggested because carbon dioxide shifts the oxyhemoglobin dissociation curve to the right, which tends to negate the carbon monoxide–induced shift.[12] This therapy is not recommended, however.[5,8]

Comparison of Oxygen Therapies

Carbon monoxide is eliminated from the body with different half-lives, depending on the percentage of inspired oxygen and atmospheric pressure. There are conflicting reports on the actual half-life of carbon monoxide in different environmental atmospheres. The half-life of carbon monoxide in the blood of healthy volunteers breathing room air is approximately 320 minutes, with a range of 120 minutes to 400 minutes (Table 19-10). It is decreased to approximately 80 to 90 minutes with a tight-fitting mask and the patient breathing 100% oxygen. Hyperbaric oxygen at three atmospheres decreases the half-life of carbon monoxide to less than 30 minutes.[5] Although these times may be different in the symptomatic patient in a clinical setting, there is no question that carboxyhemoglobin

Table 19-10 Half-Life of Carbon Monoxide in Blood

Source	Half-Life (Minutes)
Room air	240–320
100% oxygen	80–100
Hyperbaric oxygen (three atmospheres)	20–30

concentrations decrease dramatically when oxygen is administered.[54]

Hyperbaric Oxygen Therapy

Hyperbaric oxygen therapy has been suggested as the optimal treatment for cases of significant carbon monoxide poisoning.[3,4,61] Availability of hyperbaric oxygen chambers, although still limited, has improved with the use of helicopters and other air transport.[90] It is important that personnel establish liaison with the hyperbaric treatment facilities in their communities so that referral can be expeditiously accomplished when needed.[39]

There are two kinds of hyperbaric oxygen chambers available: monoplace chambers and multiplace chambers.[3] A multiplace chamber is large enough to accommodate the patient as well as medical staff; ongoing critical care can thus be administered while hyperbaric oxygen is being administered by mask. The monoplace chambers do not have this capability and are not used for the critically unstable patient. The monoplace chamber is the more commonly used.[91]

Among the beneficial effects of hyperbaric oxygen are (1) a greatly diminished carboxyhemoglobin half-life, (2) enhanced tissue clearance of residual carbon monoxide, (3) reduced cerebral edema, and (4) reversal of cytochrome oxidase inhibition.[30] Carbon monoxide is considered as a category one indication for hyperbaric oxygen, which essentially means that research and clinical experience have left little doubt about the efficacy of this therapy.[90] Hyperbaric oxygen decreases the period of symptoms and may also reduce the incidence of long-term sequelae.[41,92,93] Although the results of animal studies appear to confirm this latter effect,[94] no controlled clinical studies with humans have done so.[46] It has not been ascertained whether 100% oxygen or hyperbaric oxygen treatment can alter the long-term sequelae of carbon monoxide poisoning.[6]

Mechanism of Action of Hyperbaric Oxygen

Hyperbaric oxygen therapy provides a patient with breathing oxygen at pressures greater than one atmosphere so that high alveolar partial pressures of oxygen are attained. It is considered that three atmospheres (66 feet below sea level) of oxygen is the maximum safe pressure to which humans may be exposed for any considerable length of time.

The mode of action of hyperbaric oxygen treatment follows the laws of mass action: high concentrations of oxygen drive carbon monoxide from hemoglobin, the cytochromes, and myoglobin. With increased amounts of oxygen available the ratio of oxygen to carbon monoxide is increased, and the carbon monoxide is driven off more quickly.[3,4] In addition, tissue oxygenation is improved as a result of the increased amount of dissolved oxygen in plasma because hyperbaric oxygen provides oxygen independent of hemoglobin.

For example, at standard pressure plasma can dissolve a maximum of 0.3 volume-percent of oxygen. At 100% oxygen the dissolved oxygen is 2 volume-percent; this meets approximately one-third the oxygen needs of the body.[5] For every increase of one atmosphere, 2.3 volume-percent of oxygen can be dissolved in the plasma.[3,4,52,60,61] Three atmospheres amounts to 6.9 volume-percent of dissolved oxygen in the plasma, which is very nearly equal the amount of oxygen normally extracted from blood and almost meets the oxygen needs of the body without the use of any of the oxygen bound to hemoglobin.[13] Because 10% to 15% of carbon monoxide may be present in extravascular tissues, higher than normal tissue concentrations of oxygen physically dilute the carbon monoxide in blood and tissues and essentially halt the movement of carbon monoxide from hemoglobin to myoglobin and the cytochrome enzymes.

Another beneficial effect of hyperbaric oxygen is the reduction in intracranial pressure that occurs in a few minutes after the patient begins to breathe oxygen at pressure. This is due to the vasoconstrictive effect of oxygen and its consequent contraction of the intracranial vascular space.[3,4]

Criteria for Hyperbaric Oxygen Therapy

The criteria for selection of patients for hyperbaric oxygen therapy should take into account the availability of a hyperbaric facility.[12,13] Some investigators recommend that where a hyperbaric oxygen chamber facility exists all patients with carboxyhemoglobin saturation of 25% or more should be treated by hyperbaric oxygen regardless of symptoms. The rationale for this is partly because at this level electrocardiographic signs of myocardial ischemia begin to appear.[54] Others consider carboxyhemoglobin concentrations greater than 30% or 40% as the cut-off point for hyperbaric oxygen therapy, regardless of the patient's symptoms. In addition, any level of carboxyhemoglobin is an indication for hyperbaric oxygen therapy if the patient is comatose, irrespective of whether he or she is conscious on admission to the hospital.[3,4]

Other evidence of neurologic sequelae such as a clouded sensorium, posturing, or the inability to perform serial sevens or threes are also indications for hyperbaric oxygen (Table 19-11).[41] Mild headache and nausea by themselves are not indications for therapy. The pregnant patient should be considered for hyperbaric oxygen therapy for the reasons stated earlier. Finally, if there is evidence of acute electrocardiographic changes, symptoms of angina, or evidence of a metabolic acidosis,[12] hyperbaric oxygen therapy is indicated.

Table 19-11 Criteria for Hyperbaric Oxygen Therapy in Carbon Monoxide Poisoning

---

Availability of hyperbaric oxygen chamber
Carboxyhemoglobin concentration greater than 25, 35, or 40%
Any carboxyhemoglobin concentration with neurologic sequelae (coma, posturing, clouded sensorium)
Acute electrocardiographic changes
Symptoms of angina
Metabolic acidosis

Procedure for Hyperbaric Oxygen Therapy

The general procedure for hyperbaric oxygen therapy is to administer 100% oxygen at 2.5 to 3.0 atmospheres for 40 to 45 minutes.[91,95] Depending on the patient's response, this period may be extended but interspersed with breaks. Patients who remain unconscious are given a second hyperbaric oxygen treatment 6 to 7 hours later.[3,61] The goal of hyperbaric oxygen is to reduce the carboxyhemoglobin concentration to less than 5% to 10% in addition to providing complete symptomatic relief as quickly as possible.

Complications of Hyperbaric Oxygen Therapy

Complications associated with hyperbaric oxygen therapy are minimal (Table 19-12). The most common problem is ear barotrauma, but this is usually minor.[12] Occasionally a myringotomy may be necessary, but it should not delay definitive treatment.[3] Other complications include decompression sickness due to intravascular and intracellular expansion of dissolved nitrogen with formation of bubbles, oxygen toxicity with resultant seizures, cerebral gas embolism, and the potential to increase the size of a small pneumothorax.[13] Air embolism may also occur from holding the breath during the decompression phase.

The risk of fire or explosion in the oxygen-rich atmosphere can be diminished by keeping the humidity high, and vomiting, especially during decompression, can best be avoided by routine emptying of the patient's stomach before treatment. Retrolental fibroplasia may be a complica-

Table 19-12 Complications of Hyperbaric Oxygen Therapy

Cerebral gas embolism
Decompression sickness
Emesis
Explosion
Fire
Increasing size of pneumothorax
Oxygen toxicity
Retrolental fibroplasia (fetal)
Rupture of tympanic membrane

tion of hyperbaric oxygen therapy for the fetus. Major complications of hyperbaric oxygen are rare.

The risks of hyperbaric therapy should be carefully weighed against the possible benefits, particularly in cases of chronic sinusitis, history of spontaneous pneumothorax, upper respiratory infection, epilepsy, emphysema with carbon dioxide retention, and history of ear surgery. Untreated pneumothorax is an absolute contraindication.

Exchange Transfusion

Although some reports suggest treatment of carbon monoxide poisoning by exchange transfusion,[13,45] the cornerstone of treatment remains immediate therapy with as high a level of inspired oxygen as is available. Because of the ability of 100% inspired oxygen to decrease the half-life of carboxyhemoglobin, oxygen therapy must be viewed as a more rapid and effective treatment than attempting exchange transfusion for any patient with clinically significant carbon monoxide poisoning.

REFERENCES

1. Somogyi E, Balogh I, Rubanyi G, et al: New findings concerning the pathogenesis of acute carbon monoxide (CO) poisoning. *Am J Forensic Med Pathol* 1981;2:31–39.

2. Longo L: The biological effects of carbon monoxide on the pregnant woman, fetus, and newborn infant. *Am J Obstet Gynecol* 1977;129:69–102.

3. Myers R: Carbon monoxide poisoning. *J Emerg Med* 1984;1:245–248.

4. Myers R, Messier L, Jones D, et al: New directions in the research and treatment of carbon monoxide exposure. *Am J Emerg Med* 1983;2:226–230.

5. Mofenson H, Caraccio T, Brody G: Carbon monoxide poisoning. *Am J Emerg Med* 1984;2:254–261.

6. Olson K: Carbon monoxide poisoning: Mechanisms, presentation, and controversies in management. *J Emerg Med* 1984;1:233–243.

7. Olson K, Becker C: Hyperbaric oxygen for carbon monoxide poisoning. *JAMA* 1982;248:172–173.

8. Zimmerman S, Truxal B: Carbon monoxide poisoning. *Pediatrics* 1981;68:215–224.

9. Dolan M: Carbon monoxide poisoning. *Can Med Assoc J* 1985;133:392–399.

10. Bessoudo R, Gray J: Carbon monoxide poisoning and nonoliguric acute renal failure. *Can Assoc Med J* 1978;119:41–44.

11. Clark C, Campbell D, Reid W: Blood carboxy-hemoglobin and cyanide levels in fire survivors. *Lancet* 1981;1:1332–1335.

12. Crocker P, Walker J: Pediatric carbon monoxide toxicity. *J Emerg Med* 1985;3:443–448.

13. Crocker P: Carbon monoxide poisoning, the clinical entity and its treatment: A review. *Mil Med* 1984;149:257–259.

14. Stewart R: The effect of carbon monoxide on humans. *J Occup Med* 1976;18:304–309.

15. Stewart R, Hake C: Paint-remover hazard. *JAMA* 1976;235:398–401.

16. Landers D: Unsuccessful suicide by carbon monoxide: A secondary benefit of emissions control. *West J Med* 1981;135:360–363.

17. Landa J, Avery W, Sackner M: Some physiologic observations in smoke inhalation. *Chest* 1972;61:62–63.

18. Heckerling P, Leikin J, Maturen A, et al: Predictors of occult carbon monoxide poisoning in patients with headache and dizziness. *Ann Intern Med* 1987;107:174–176.

19. Heckerling P: Occult carbon monoxide poisoning. *Am J Emerg Med* 1987;5:201–214.

20. Murray T: Carbon monoxide in the modern society. *Can Med Assoc J* 1978;118:758–760.

21. Murray T: Carbon monoxide poisoning from Sterno. *Can Med Assoc J* 1978;118:800–802.

22. Jackson D, Menges H: Accidental carbon monoxide poisoning. *JAMA* 1980;243:772–774.

23. Wilson E, Rich T, Messman H: The hazardous hibachi. *JAMA* 1972;221:405–406.

24. Stewart R, Fisher T, Hosko M, et al: Experimental human exposure to methylene chloride. *Arch Environ Health* 1972;25:342–348.

25. Ratney R, Wegman D, Elkins H: In vivo conversion of methylene chloride to carbon monoxide. *Arch Environ Health* 1974;28:223–226.

26. Fagin J, Bradley J, Williams D: Carbon monoxide poisoning secondary to inhaling methylene chloride. *Br Med J* 1980;281:1461.

27. Stewart R, Stewart S, Stamm W, et al: Rapid estimation of carboxyhemoglobin level in fire fighters. *JAMA* 1976;235:390–392.

28. Burney R, Wu S, Nemiroff M: Mass carbon monoxide poisoning: Clinical effects and results of treatment in 184 victims. *Ann Emerg Med* 1982;11:394–399.

29. Leikin J, Vogel S: Carbon monoxide levels in cardiac patients in an urban emergency department. *Am J Emerg Med* 1986;4:126–128.

30. Garland H, Pearce J: Neurological complications of carbon monoxide poisoning. *Q J Med* 1967;34:445–454.

31. Anderson E, Andelman R, Strauch J, et al: Effect of low level carbon monoxide exposure on onset and duration of angina pectoris. *Ann Intern Med* 1973;79:46–50.

32. Winter P, Miller J: Carbon monoxide poisoning. *JAMA* 1976;236:1502–1504.

33. Larkin J, Brahos G, Moylan J: Treatment of carbon monoxide poisoning: Prognostic factors. *J Trauma* 1976;16:111–114.

34. Goldbaum L, Orellano T, Dergal E: Mechanism of the toxic action of carbon monoxide. *Ann Clin Lab Sci* 1976;6:372–376.

35. Goldbaum L, Orellano T, Dergal E: Studies on the relation between carboxyhemoglobin concentration and toxicity. *Aviat Space Environ Med* 1977;48:969–970.

36. Goldbaum L, Ramirez R, Absalon K: What is the mechanism of carbon monoxide toxicity? *Aviat Space Environ Med* 1975;46:1289–1291.

37. Aronow W: Effect of cigarette smoking and of carbon monoxide on coronary heart disease. *Chest* 1976;71:514–518.

38. Aronow W, Isbell M: Carbon monoxide effect on exercise-induced angina pectoris. *Ann Intern Med* 1973;79:392–395.

39. Zeller W, Miele A, Suarez C: Accidental carbon monoxide poisoning. *Clin Pediatr* 1984;23:694–695.

40. Choi I: Delayed neurologic sequelae in carbon monoxide intoxication. *Arch Neurol* 1983;40:433–435.

41. Norkool D, Kirkpatrick J: Treatment of acute carbon monoxide poisoning with hyperbaric oxygen: A review of 115 cases. *Ann Emerg Med* 1985;14:1168–1171.

42. Scharf S, Thames M, Sargent R: Transmural myocardial infarction after exposure to carbon monoxide in coronary-artery disease. *N Engl J Med* 1974;291:85–87.

43. Davis S, Levy R: High carboxyhemoglobin level without acute or chronic findings. *J Emerg Med* 1984;1:539–542.

44. Crapo R: Smoke-inhalation injuries. *JAMA* 1981;246:1694–1696.

45. Yee L, Brandon G: Successful reversal of presumed carbon monoxide–induced semicoma. *Aviat Space Environ Med* 1983;54:641–643.

46. Huber J: Do awake patients with high carboxy-hemoglobin levels need hyperbaric oxygen? *J Emerg Med* 1984;1:555–556.

47. Fisher J: Occult carbon monoxide poisoning. *Arch Intern Med* 1982;142:1270–1271.

48. Naeije R, Peretz A, Cornil A: Acute pulmonary edema following carbon monoxide poisoning. *Intensive Care Med* 1980;6:189–191.

49. Ginsburg R, Romano J: Carbon monoxide encephalopathy: Need for appropriate treatment. *Am J Psychiatr* 1976;133:317–320.

50. Ginsberg M: Carbon monoxide intoxication: Clinical features, neuropathology and mechanism of injury. *Clin Toxicol* 1985;23:281–288.

51. Moar J: Early acute fatal carbon monoxide poisoning—Assessment of the survival period. *S Afr Med J* 1984;68:650–652.

52. Myers R, Snyder S, Majerus T: Cutaneous blisters and carbon monoxide poisoning. *Ann Emerg Med* 1985;14:603–606.

53. Nagy R, Greer K, Harman L: Cutaneous manifestations of acute carbon monoxide poisoning. *Cutis* 1979;24:381–383.

54. Anderson G: Treatment of carbon monoxide poisoning with hyperbaric oxygen. *Mil Med* 1978;143:538–541.

55. Anderson R, Allensworth D, deGroot W: Myocardial toxicity from carbon monoxide poisoning. *Ann Intern Med* 1967;67:1172–1182.

56. Kelley J, Sophocleus G: Retinal hemorrhages in subacute carbon monoxide poisoning. *JAMA* 1978;239:1515–1517.

57. Linton A, Adams J, Lawson D: Muscle necrosis and acute renal failure in carbon monoxide poisoning. *Postgrad Med J* 1968;44:338–341.

58. Loughridge L, Leader L, Bowen D: Acute renal failure due to muscle necrosis in carbon monoxide poisoning. *Lancet* 1958;2:349–351.

59. Howse A, Seddon H: Ischemic contracture of muscle associated with carbon monoxide and barbiturate poisoning. *Br Med J* 1966;1:192–195.

60. Myers R, Snyder S, Emhoff T: Subacute sequelae of carbon monoxide poisoning. *Ann Emerg Med* 1985;14:1163–1167.

61. Myers R, Snyder S, Lindberg S, et al: Value of hyperbaric oxygen in suspected carbon monoxide poisoning. *JAMA* 1981;246:2478–2480.

62. Lacey D: Neurologic sequelae of acute carbon monoxide intoxication. *Am J Dis Child* 1981;135:145–147.

63. Siesjo B: Oxygen deficiency and brain damage: Localization, evolution in time, and mechanisms of damage. *Clin Toxicol* 1985;23:267–280.

64. Siesjo B: Carbon monoxide poisoning: Mechanism of damage, late sequelae and therapy. *Clin Toxicol* 1985;23:247–248.

65. Werner B, Back W, Akerblom H, et al: Two cases of acute carbon monoxide poisoning with delayed neurological sequelae after a "free" interval. *Clin Toxicol* 1985;23:249–265.

66. Halebian P, Yurt R, Petito C, et al: Diabetes insipidus after carbon monoxide poisoning and smoke inhalation. *J Trauma* 1985;25:662–663.

67. Klawans H, Stein R, Tanner C, et al: A pure parkinsonian syndrome following acute carbon monoxide intoxication. *Arch Neurol* 1982;39:302–304.

68. Davous P, Rondot P, Marion M, et al: Severe chorea after acute carbon monoxide poisoning. *J Neurol Neurosurg Psychiatr* 1986;49:206–208.

69. Myers R, Linberg S, Cowley R, et al: Carbon monoxide poisoning: The injury and its treatment. *JACEP* 1979;8:479–484.

70. Goldstein DL: Carbon monoxide poisoning in pregnancy. *Am J Obstet Gynecol* 1965;92:526–528.

71. Copel J, Bowen F, Bolognese R: Carbon monoxide intoxication in early pregnancy. *Obstet Gynecol* 1982;59:26s–28s.

72. Venning H, Roberton D, Milner A: Carbon monoxide poisoning in an infant. *Br Med J* 1981;284:651.

73. Binder J, Roberts R: Carbon monoxide intoxication in children. *Clin Toxicol* 1980;16:287–295.

74. Grace T, Platt F: Subacute carbon monoxide poisoning. *JAMA* 1981;246:1698–1700.

75. Barret L, Danel V, Faure J: Carbon monoxide poisoning, a diagnosis frequently overlooked. *Clin Toxicol* 1985;23:309–313.

76. Castle S, Lapham S, Troutman W, et al: Carbon monoxide intoxication: Diagnostic considerations. *JAMA* 1984;251:2350.

77. Gemelli F, Cattani R: Carbon monoxide poisoning in childhood. *Br Med J* 1985;291:1197.

78. Otten E, Rosenberg J, Tasset J: An evaluation of carboxyhemoglobin spot tests. *Ann Emerg Med* 1985;14:850–852.

79. Hall A, Linden C, Kulig K, et al: Cyanide poisoning from Laetrile ingestion: Role of nitrite therapy. *Pediatrics* 1986;78:269–272.

80. Wald N, Idle M, Boreham J, et al: Carbon monoxide in breath in relation to smoking and carboxyhemoglobin levels. *Thorax* 1981;36:366–369.

81. Wald N, Idle M, Boreham J, et al: Inhaling habits among smokers of different types of cigarettes. *Thorax* 1980;35:925–928.

82. Vogt T, Selven S, Widdowson G, et al: Expired air carbon monoxide and serum thiocyanate as objective measures of cigarette exposure. *Am J Public Health* 1977;67:545–549.

83. Cramer C: Fetal death due to accidental maternal carbon monoxide poisoning. *J Toxicol Clin Toxicol* 1982;19:297–301.

84. Smith J, Brandon S: Acute carbon monoxide poisoning—3 years' experience in a defined population. *Postgrad Med J* 1970;46:65–70.

85. Smith J, Brandon S: Morbidity from acute carbon monoxide poisoning at three-year follow-up. *Br Med J* 1973;1:318–321.

86. Nardizzi L: Computerized tomographic correlate of carbon monoxide poisoning. *Arch Neurol* 1979;36:38–39.

87. Destee A, Courteville V, Devos P, et al: Computed tomography and acute carbon monoxide poisoning. *J Neurol Neurosurg Psychiatr* 1985;48:281–291.

88. Mendelsohn D, Hertzanu Y: Carbon monoxide poisoning. *S Afr Med J* 1983;64:751–752.

89. Finley J, VanBeek A, Glover J: Myonecrosis complicating carbon monoxide poisoning. *J Trauma* 1977;17:536–540.

90. Kindwall E: Hyperbaric treatment of carbon monoxide poisoning. *Ann Emerg Med* 1985;14:1233–1234.

91. Vorosmarti J: Hyperbaric oxygen therapy. *Am Fam Physician* 1981;23:169–173.

92. Ziser A, Shupak A, Halpern P, et al: Delayed hyperbaric oxygen treatment for acute carbon monoxide poisoning. *Br Med J* 1984;289:960.

93. Mathieu D, Nolf M, Durocher A, et al: Acute carbon monoxide poisoning: Risk of late sequelae and treatment by hyperbaric oxygen. *Clin Toxicol* 1985;23:315–324.

94. Goulon M, Barois A, Rapin M, et al: Carbon monoxide poisoning and acute anoxia due to breathing coal gas and hydrocarbons. *J Hyperbaric Med* 1986;1:23–41.

95. Hart G, Strauss M, Lennon P, et al: Treatment of smoke inhalation by hyperbaric oxygen. *J Emerg Med* 1985;3:211–215.

ADDITIONAL SELECTED REFERENCES

Benowitz N, Jacob P, Yu L, et al: Reduced tar, nicotine, and carbon monoxide exposure while smoking ultralow- but not low-yield cigarettes. *JAMA* 1986;256:241–246.

Buehler J, Berns A, Webster J, et al: Lactic acidosis from carboxyhemoglobinemia after smoke inhalation. *Ann Intern Med* 1975;82:803–805.

Castleden C, Cole P: Variations in carboxyhemoglobin levels in smokers. *Br Med J* 1974;4:736–738.

Cohen M, Guzzardi L: Inhalation of products of combustion. *Ann Emerg Med* 1983;12:628–632.

Cordasco E, VanOrdstrand H: Air pollution and COPD. *Postgrad Med J* 1977;62:124–127.

Dinman B: The management of acute carbon monoxide intoxication. *J Occup Med* 1974;16:662–664.

Flanagan N, Wootton D, Smith G, et al: An unusual case of carbon monoxide poisoning. *Med Sci Law* 1978;18:117–119.

Gold A, Burgess A, Clougherty E: Exposure of firefighters to toxic air contaminants. *Am Ind Hyg Assoc J* 1978;39:534–539.

Gozal D, Ziser A, Shupak A, et al: Accidental carbon monoxide poisoning. *Clin Pediatrics* 1985;24:132–135.

Hauck H, Neuberger M: Carbon monoxide uptake and the resulting carboxyhemoglobin in man. *Eur J Appl Physiol* 1984;53:186–190.

Jett G: Red retinal vein (Jett) sign. *Ann Emerg Med* 1984;13:2802–2803.

Kachulis C: Secondhand cigarette smoke. *Postgrad Med J* 1981;70:77–79.

Kizer K: Toxic inhalations. *Emerg Med Clin North Am* 1984;2:649–666.

Manning R: The serial sevens test. *Arch Intern Med* 1982;142:1192.

Neubauer R: Carbon monoxide and hyperbaric oxygen. *Arch Intern Med* 1979;139:829.

Pulst S, Walshe T, Romero J: Carbon monoxide poisoning with features of Gilles de la Tourette's syndrome. *Arch Neurol* 1983;40:443–444.

Remick R, Miles J: Carbon monoxide poisoning: Neurologic and psychiatric sequelae. *Can Med Assoc J* 1977;17:654–657.

Spiller D: Carbon monoxide exposure in the home: Source and epidemiology. *Vet Hum Toxicol* 1987;29:383–386.

Stevenson M, Cooper G, Chenoweth M: Effect on carboxyhemoglobin of exposure to aerosol spray paints with methylene chloride. *Clin Toxicol* 1978;12:551–561.

Stewart R, Peterson J, Fisher R, et al: Experimental human exposure to high concentrations of carbon monoxide. *Arch Environ Health* 1973;26:1–7.

Takahashi M, Maemura K, Sawada Y, et al: Hyperamylasemia in acute carbon monoxide poisoning. *J Trauma* 1982;22:311–314.

Terrill J, Montgomery R, Reinhardt C: Toxic gases from fires. *Science* 1978;200:1343–1347.

Utidjian H: The criteria for a recommended standard. I. Recommendations for a carbon monoxide standard: Occupation exposure to carbon monoxide. *J Occup Med* 1973;15:446–451.

Webster J, McCabe M, Karp M: Recognition and management of smoke inhalation. *JAMA* 1967;201:71–74.

Williams R: Vehicular carbon monoxide screening: Identification in a cross-cultural setting of a substantial public health risk factor. *Am J Public Health* 1985;75:85–86.

Zarem H, Rattenborg C, Harmel M: Carbon monoxide toxicity in human fire victims. *Arch Surg* 1973;107:851–853.

Zikria B, Weston G, Chodoff A, et al: Smoke and carbon monoxide poisoning in fire victims. *J Trauma* 1972;12:641–645.

chapter 20

Cyanide and Laetrile®

Cyanide is one of the oldest toxins known.[1] In ancient Egyptian documents, administering cyanogenic peach kernel preparations is mentioned as a form of execution. Ancient Greeks and Romans used a cherry laurel distillate for suicides, murders, and judicial executions.[2] In 1782 hydrogen cyanide liquid was isolated by the chemist Karl Wilhelm Scheele through the action of sulfuric acid on Prussian blue, from which the name prussic acid for hydrocyanic acid derives. Scheele died 4 years after his discovery from inhaling hydrogen cyanide gas when he accidently broke a beaker of the deadly acid.[3]

Although cyanide poisoning is very rarely encountered by clinicians, few poisons are more rapidly lethal. Furthermore, cyanide is one of the few poisons for which specific antidotes exist.[4] The inhalation of hydrogen cyanide commonly produces reactions within a few seconds and death within minutes, although patients may survive at sublethal doses with symptoms lasting several hours.[5] Chronic cyanide poisoning also occurs throughout the world secondary to intake of cyanogenic glycosides as part of normal diets. An increasing number of nonindustrial cases of cyanide poisoning are being reported; these are probably related to the increasing availability of Laetrile® and the release of cyanide gas from burning synthetic materials.

SOURCES AND USES OF CYANIDE

Cyanide is a fairly widespread potential hazard of industrial and nonindustrial environments (Tables 20-1 and 20-2). Hydrocyanic acid and sodium and potassium cyanide are found in vermicidal fumigants, insecticides, rodenticides, metal polishes (especially silver polish), and electroplating solutions.[6] Cyanide is used in metallurgy for the extraction of gold and silver metals from their ores, in chemicals used to remove hair from hides, in processing photographic film, and in chemical synthesis and research.

Hydrocyanic acid is an effective agent in the fumigation of ships, army posts, navy stations, large buildings, flour mills, private dwellings, freight cars, and airplanes that have become infested with rodents and insects. As a fumigant it is applied directly as a solution, or the gas is generated from one of the cyanide salts by the action of dilute mineral acid. Cyanide has also been used as an insecticide and in the process of soil sterilization. Potassium cyanide crystals may be used in coyote ''gitter'' traps: when an animal bites into the meat in the trap, a shell explodes and releases cyanide.[6] Human intoxication may occur if the unwary were to step on the cyanide or somehow to allow the cyanide to be released.

Table 20-1 Sources and Uses of Cyanide

Pest control
Vermicidal fumigant
Insecticide
Rodenticide
Soil sterilization
Coyote "gitter" traps
Industrial uses
Metal polish
Electroplating
Extracting silver and gold from ore
Removing hair from hides
Photography
Chemical synthesis
Plastics
Phencyclidine
Synthetic rubber
Laboratories
Cigarette smoke
Fires
Horsehair
Wool
Silk
Polyurethanes
Polyacrylonitriles
Plants and fruits
Cassava
Amygdalin (Laetrile®)
Pits and seeds
Sodium nitroprusside
Judicial executions

Table 20-2 Compounds Containing Cyanide

Calcium cyanide
Cyanamide
Cyanates
Cyanogen
Cyanogenic glycosides
Hydrogen cyanide
Isobornyl thiocyanoacetate
Nitriles
Nitroprusside
Potassium cyanide
Potassium ferricyanide
Prussic acid
Sodium cyanide

Cyanide is used in the production of nitriles and cyanohydrins, which are chemicals used in the manufacture of many plastics.[7] Incomplete combustion of products containing carbon and nitrogen may liberate cyanide. Fires where there is combustion of organic nitrogen-containing polymers, both natural (wool and silk) and synthetic (polyurethanes and polyacrylonitriles), which are used extensively in domestic furnishings, may therefore yield significant amounts of hydrogen cyanide.[4,7,8] Plastics of any type, such as the plastics in electrical wires, can also yield cyanide when heated.[8] This may have practical medical significance in the treatment of severe smoke inhalation.[9] Firefighters involved in nonfatal fires have been found to have elevated cyanide concentrations in their blood.[10] In addition, propionitrile (ethyl cyanide), which is used in organic synthesis and as a solvent, is toxic if ingested, inhaled, or absorbed through the skin.

Some microorganisms, notably *Pseudomonas aeruginosa*, have the ability to produce cyanide. These organisms may become a source of abnormally high cyanide concentrations in patients with an overwhelming infection, which can be a consequence of burns and sepsis. These cyanide concentrations, however, may be forensically misleading.[11]

Sodium nitroprusside at therapeutic doses has been shown to release cyanide in vivo by reaction with hemoglobin to form cyanomethemoglobin. Because each nitroprusside molecule contains five cyanide groups, and because nitroprusside is metabolized to cyanide,[12] if a patient requires prolonged nitroprusside treatment the need for higher and higher doses to achieve the same effect (tachyphylaxis) may lead to cyanide intoxication.[4,12–15] The cyanide concentration obtained from therapeutic doses does not typically lead to cyanide intoxication because of the rapid uptake of cyanide by erythrocytes, incorporation of cyanide into hydroxycobalamin (vitamin B_{12a}) to produce cyanocobalamin (vitamin B_{12}), and adequate hepatic metabolism of cyanide by mitochondrial sulfurtransferase (rhodanase) to thiocyanate, which is less toxic. Prolonged administration of nitroprusside or administration in large dosages (greater than 10 µg/kg/min) may result in cyanide intoxication.[12,16,17] Some investigators have recommended that total dosages of sodium nitroprusside should not exceed 1.5 mg/kg during short-term infusions.[12,18] In addition, deaths attributable to cyanide have been reported from the purposeful ingestion of nitroprusside.[15]

The cyanide ion may originate in vivo from hydrocyanic acid; salts and complexes of cyanide; biotransformations of cyanohydrins, aliphatic nitriles, thiocyanate, and nitrile glycosides; and even the interaction in the stomach of ingested chlorinogenic water purifiers (such as halazone tablets) and the amino acids of some foods.

Cigarette smokers have been found to have mean whole blood cyanide concentrations that are more than 2.5 times the mean for non-smokers. This is because of the natural cyanide found in tobacco.[6] In addition, smokers have elevated whole blood thiocyanate concentrations.

Potassium cyanide is necessary in the most commonly employed method of illicit synthesis of phencyclidine. In addition, improperly synthesized phencyclidine may be contaminated by an intermediary containing cyanide (cyclohexanecarbonitrile).

Cyanide was also used in the extermination centers operated by the Hitler regime during World War II, and the use of cyanide in judicial executions has been reinstituted as a form of capital punishment in some areas of the United States. Potassium cyanide was implicated in the deaths of more than 900 individuals in Jonestown, Guyana, as well as the 7 individuals who ingested contaminated acetaminophen tablets in the Chicago area.[19]

Cyanide in Plants

The natural environment contains various cyanogenic glycosides that can release hydrogen cyanide when exposed to acid or appropriate enzymes (Table 20-3). Certain plants produce free hydrocyanic acid or cyanogenic glycosides because they lack the ability to convert all the available amino acids into proteins. For these species the production of cyanogenic glycosides is a side reaction in protein metabolism.

There are at least 360 varieties of fruits and vegetables in 41 families that can yield hydrocyanic acid. Members of the family Rosaceae, including the plum, peach, pear, apple, apricot, cherry, and almond, contain various quantities of amygdalin (mandelonitrile-β-glucosido-6-β-glucoside), a glycoside of gentiobiose, hydrocyanide, and benzaldehyde.[20–22] Other species of this family, notably the cherry laurel, contain a related cyanogenic glycoside termed prunin,

Table 20-3 Plants Containing Cyanogenic Glycosides

Bamboo
Cassava
Elderberry
Hydrangea
Lima bean
Linum
Sorghum species

Source: Adapted with permission from "Clinical Toxicology of Cyanide" by A Hall and B Rumack in *Annals of Emergency Medicine* (1986;15:1068), Copyright © 1986, American College of Emergency Physicians.

which has also been responsible for a number of cyanide poisonings.[23] The bitter almond is not to be confused with the somewhat larger sweet almond, which is nontoxic. Another glycoside of this group, linamarin, has been responsible for a federal restriction on the importation of some varieties of lima bean into the United States.[12]

Cassava

Cassava is a carbohydrate staple in many tropical countries. This food provides more than 70% of the caloric intake in some diets in these regions. Cassava contains large amounts of linamarin in its outer layers, which acts as a pesticide. Incorrect preparation of cassava has resulted in chronic cyanide intoxication in humans. With continued ingestion over a period of time, individuals may develop neuropathy manifesting as optic atrophy, nerve deafness, and ataxia (Nigerian ataxic neuropathy) due to sensory spinal nerve involvement.[11,24–26] A neurotoxicological role for cyanide has been suggested in tobacco-associated amblyopia and in a report of amygdalin-associated peripheral neuropathy.

Amygdalin

Pits and seeds that contain amygdalin (Table 20-4) usually also contain a group of enzymes, the emulsin complex, which breaks the linkages of the amygdalin to yield hydrogen cyanide.[12,27] These enzymes are activated when the plant tissue is crushed or otherwise dis-

Table 20-4 Pits and Seeds of Fruits Containing Amygdalin (*Prunus* species)

Apple
Apricot
Bitter almond
Cherry
Cherry laurel
Peach
Pear
Pin cherry
Plum
Western chokecherry
Wild black cherry

---

rupted, such as in chewing. The cyanide content of amygdalin is approximately 6%, and it has been estimated that 15 to 60 varieties of seeds containing amygdalin can, when ingested, result in severe intoxication or death.[28] For example, the cyanide content of moist apricot pits varies from 8.9 mg to 409 mg per 100 g;[29] peach pits contain 88 mg per 100 g; and bitter almonds contain 469 mg per 100 g.[12] Amygdalin is only toxic by the oral route; when administered intravenously the parent compound is almost completely excreted in the urine.[25]

Laetrile®

Amygdalin was first used as an antineoplastic agent in the 1890s in Germany but was discarded after excessive toxicity and a lack of antineoplastic properties were found.[30] Amygdalin was reintroduced in the 1950s under the trade name Laetrile® as an anticancer agent that is still not approved by the FDA; this agent contains various cyanogenic glycosides, not a single chemical entity.[31] Laetrile® as originally developed was a natural substance derived from apricot pits. In recent years, pure amygdalin isolated from apricot kernels is used, although peach kernels have also been reported as a source.[25,32]

According to proponents of the use of Laetrile®, malignant cells convert the drug into hydrocyanic acid in greater concentrations than normal cells, which kills the malignant cells.[33] It has also been stated that tumor tissue is deficient in rhodanase, the enzyme that detoxifies cyanide; therefore, tumor tissue is selectively attacked by cyanide because normal cells contain a high concentration of rhodanase.[34] Although there are no studies showing beneficial effects of Laetrile® in this setting,[35–38] the drug has had great popularity with the public and lay practitioners, and its use is now rather widespread.[36]

The use of Laetrile® is legal in many states and is legal for use nationwide with a Federal court order.[38] A dose of Laetrile® contains from 30 to 150 mg of cyanide per tablet. Orally administered Laetrile® is marketed only in 500-mg tablets and is approximately 6% cyanide by weight.[12] Laetrile® and seeds are two of the most commonly reported sources of cyanide poisoning in the medical literature.[4,27,39,40] The toxic effects of oral ingestion of Laetrile® are presumably due to the action of gastric acids on the amygdalin, releasing hydrogen cyanide.[25] Although Laetrile® is a toxic drug, its toxicity is limited to oral ingestion because by intravenous administration there is no liberation of cyanide. The drug is rapidly cleared from the blood and largely excreted unchanged in the urine.[25]

The mechanism of toxic action of Laetrile® is similar to that of seeds and pits. The amygdalin in Laetrile® is broken down by the enzymes in vegetables (celery, lettuce, green peppers, carrots, mushrooms, and bean sprouts), nuts (almonds), and fruits (peaches and plums), so that cyanide can be released with the co-ingestion of the drug and these foods.[4] Also, hydrolysis by β-glucosidase can occur in the alkaline medium of the intestine and cause the same effect. Acute cyanide poisoning has also followed the administration of Laetrile® enemas.[4,41]

MECHANISM OF ACTION OF CYANIDE

Cyanide binds avidly to iron in the ferric (trivalent) state but not in the ferrous (divalent) state.[42] Cyanide therefore does not react with the iron in hemoglobin, which is ferrous. Any iron-containing enzymes that cycle between the ferric and ferrous states during reduction-oxidation reactions are particularly susceptible to inactivation by cyanide because the cyanoferric complex is relatively stable and the enzyme remains trapped in this form.

Cyanide produces a cellular hypoxia by inhibiting the reoxidation of cytochrome oxidase; this hemoprotein has iron in the ferric state. Essentially, cyanide combines reversibly with cytochrome oxidase (cytochrome aa_3), inhibiting the final step of oxidative phosphorylation and the transfer of electrons to oxygen, thereby inhibiting cellular respiration and preventing the formation of adenosine triphosphate.[39,42,43] This results in anaerobic metabolism.[4] Pyruvate, which can no longer be incorporated into the tricarboxylic acid cycle, is reduced to a lactate ion, which accumulates rapidly. Therefore, the mechanism of cyanide toxicity is to block aerobic metabolism, the major pathway of high-energy phosphate production.[39] The patient essentially suffocates not from the inability to obtain or transport oxygen but from the inability to use it.[4] Venous blood may retain the bright red color of oxyhemoglobin, and the patient will not usually appear to be cyanotic. This differs from carbon monoxide intoxication, in which hypoxia is due to decreased oxygen transport. The cytochrome oxidase–cyanide complex is dissociable, and if death does not intervene the mitochondrial enzyme sulfurtransferase mediates the transfer of sulfur from thiosulfate to the cyanide ion. Thus thiocyanate is formed, the respiratory enzyme is released, and cell respiration is restored.

Although cyanide preferentially binds to ferric iron, some cyanide binds to the ferrous iron of normal hemoglobin. This cyanohemoglobin cannot transport oxygen. Significant amounts of cyanohemoglobin may be indicated by a decrease in the measured percentage of arterial oxygen saturation, whereas the calculated percentage of oxygen saturation remains normal.[42]

Cyanide can also form complexes with other hematin compounds, such as catalase, peroxidase, cytochrome-peroxidase, and methemoglobin, as well as with nonhematin metal-bearing compounds, such as tyrosinase; ascorbic acid oxidase; xanthine oxidase; amino acid oxidase; succinic, lactic, and formic dehydrogenase; phosphatase; and hydroxycobalamin (a precursor of vitamin B_{12}). The acute pathophysiologic effects of cyanide, however, are attributable to its action on cytochrome oxidase alone. In contrast to higher mammals, bacteria are not harmed by cyanide and are able to utilize the nitrogen of the poison to make their proteins.[44]

In addition to multiple enzymes being affected by cyanide, there are differences in cytochrome oxidase in various organs. The predominant site of lethal effects of cyanide is the CNS because the cytochrome oxidase in the brain is the most susceptible to the toxic effects of cyanide.[1]

Absorption

Cell membranes are highly permeable to cyanide, and the compound is rapidly absorbed through any body surface such as the alveolar membranes, intestinal mucosa, or skin. Neither the liquid nor the vapor is irritating to the skin or membranes of the respiratory tract. A maximal effect is seen with either intravenous administration or inhalation of hydrocyanic acid vapors. Gas masks usually provide inadequate protection from poisoning.[4,8] The oral route is less rapid because of a slower rate of entry of cyanide into the circulation; it gains entry through the hepatic portal system and passes through the liver, which is the main site of the body's detoxification system.

Metabolism

There are five routes through which cyanide is metabolized, two of which have clinical import. Absorbed cyanide is excreted in small amounts unchanged by the lungs. In addition, a small amount is excreted in the urine. Cyanide is also oxidized to formate ion and carbon dioxide and is incorporated into methyl groups to produce choline and methionine. Approximately 15% of cyanide reacts with cystine and is excreted. These routes of excretion are not of clinical import in intoxication.

A minor route of detoxification, but one with clinical importance, is the incorporation of cyanide into hydroxycobalamin to form cyanocobalamin (vitamin B_{12}). This minor route is under investigation for exploitation as therapy for the cyanide-poisoned patient.

The major mechanism of detoxification, accounting for 80% of cyanide metabolism, is the conversion of cyanide to the relatively

Tachpnca
Seizures

harmless thiocyanate ion by an enzymatic reaction mediated by mitrochondrial enzyme rhodanase with thiosulfate as substrate. This enzyme is widely distributed in tissues, but the greatest amounts occur in the liver.[1] Rhodanase has a large capacity to combine with cyanide but is relatively slow with respect to elimination of a toxic overdose, so that the reaction may be limited by the endogenous supply of thiosulfate.[42] The resulting thiocyanate formed has some inherent toxicity but is rapidly excreted by the kidneys.

Toxicity

Clinical Features

Cyanide is a fast-acting poison and is capable of causing death in a matter of minutes. The manifestations of cyanide toxicity depend on the degree of tissue hypoxia: the more rapidly the individual acquires cyanide, the more acute are the signs and symptoms of poisoning and the smaller is the total absorbed dose required to produce toxicity. Short-term inhalation of 50 ppm of hydrogen cyanide causes acute symptoms of CNS, gastric, and respiratory tract disturbances, and inhalation of 130 ppm can be fatal.[24] The lethal dose of sodium or potassium cyanide is approximately 200 to 300 mg, and the lethal dose of hydrogen cyanide is 50 mg.[1,39,45]

Onset of symptoms depends on the form of cyanide ingested, the route of ingestion, and the amount ingested. In actual practice, the most rapidly acquired form of poisoning occurs from the inhalation of hydrogen cyanide vapor, with little difference noted between this and the intravenous route.

As with other chemical asphyxiants, the critical organs are those that are most sensitive to oxygen deprivation, notably the brain and the heart. In low concentrations, the cyanide ion stimulates respiration. The sites of action are the chemoreceptors of the carotid and aortic bodies, which respond to a decreased partial pressure of oxygen in the blood. This respiratory response may also be related to early, low-level lactic acid accumulation from cyanide inhibition of cellular respiration.[12] This stimulation of ventilation may actually worsen the effects of cyanide inha-

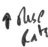
↑ *fluf*
fate

lation. The transient CNS stimulation is followed by CNS depression and finally hypoxic convulsions, with death due to respiratory arrest. Although the heart shows toxic effects, it usually continues to function for some minutes after respirations have ceased.

Recovery from cyanide poisoning may be complete or may be followed by sequelae due to hypoxic and hemodynamic brain damage similar to that seen after other hypoxic insults.

Inhaled and Intravenous Cyanide

Symptoms of intoxication from inhaled or intravenous cyanide in large amounts include a very brief sensation of dryness and burning in the throat from local irritation, a suffusing warmth, and air hunger. The first breath is followed immediately by hyperpnea, which is due to stimulation of the chemoreceptors in the carotid and aortic bodies. Apnea, coma, and seizures may occur in less than 1 minute and are often accompanied by cardiovascular failure.[6] As stated above, the heart may continue to beat with various irregularities and blocks for as long as 3 to 4 minutes after the last breath (Table 20-5).[8]

Ingested Cyanide

The most common mode of suicide involving cyanide is ingestion of salts of cyanide. The salts cause a less acute syndrome because they are absorbed slowly and variably from the gastrointestinal tract and because their toxicity is attenuated by passage through the liver.[4]

Central nervous system effects predominate from oral ingestion of cyanide. Within 1 to 5 minutes hyperpnea develops from chemore-

---

Table 20-5 Symptoms of Cyanide Overdose by Inhalation

Dryness of mouth
Air hunger
Hyperpnea
Apnea
Coma
Seizures
Cardiovascular collapse

---

ceptor stimulation (Table 20-6). Vomiting occurs secondary to central hypoxic stimulation and because the sodium and potassium salts of cyanide are strongly alkaline and therefore irritative to the gastric mucosa. Neurologic symptoms such as anxiety, confusion, vertigo, giddiness, headache, and generalized seizures and trismus often occur.[12] In addition within 5 to 20 minutes the patient may exhibit flushed, hot, and dry skin, a rapid, irregular pulse that may lead to bradycardia, and gasping respiratory efforts. This is followed by hypoxic dilatation of the pupils and vascular collapse.

Although Laetrile® may cause cyanide intoxication, after a toxic dose has been ingested there may be a delay in the development of symptoms because the enzyme emulsin does not normally hydrolyze amygdalin until it is transported into the alkaline environment of the small intestine.[46,47] This delay of symptomatology may last from 90 to 120 minutes after ingestion of the drug.[12,25]

An anion-gap metabolic acidosis has been associated with cyanide intoxication.[6] This is caused by lactic acidosis.[3,4] It is postulated that, because oxidative phosphorylation is blocked by cyanide, the rate of glycolysis is markedly increased, leading to lactic acidosis. There is decreased tissue perfusion associated with the circulatory effects of cyanide, which also contributes to a lactic acidosis.

lactic acidosis

Pulmonary edema has also been reported in oral cyanide intoxication.[3,4,12,48] This may be the result of the direct toxic effect of cyanide on capillary endothelia or an indirect neurogenic effect leading to increased pulmonary capillary permeability.[45,49]

DIAGNOSIS

Diagnosis of cyanide poisoning may be difficult because of a lack of a positive history (Table 20-7).[12] Exposure to cyanide may not be considered even when clinical and laboratory evidence are highly suggestive. The key to making a correct diagnosis of cyanide poisoning is having a high index of suspicion in patients with an altered level of consciousness and an otherwise unexplained metabolic acidosis.[4] High-risk groups, such as laboratory technicians, chemists, pharmacists, physicians, and others with easy access to cyanide and its compounds, should be considered.[4,12] Industrial accidents and fires may suggest cyanide as the causative factor of symptoms of toxicity.

The odor of hydrocyanic acid released into the air from solutions of sodium or potassium cyanide can be detected by most individuals, even in small concentrations, but it is estimated that 20% to 40% of the population is unable to detect cyanide by odor.[4,6,12,39,50] The odor and the taste of hydrocyanic acid have a characteristic musty quality that resembles that of bitter almonds or macaroons.[51]

odor

Because of poor oxygen utilization, venous blood may retain the bright red color of arterial blood; for example, retinal veins and arteries have been reported to be equally red when exam-

Red veins & used

Table 20-6 Symptoms of Cyanide Overdose by Ingestion

Gastrointestinal
  Nausea
  Vomiting
Neurologic
  Confusion
  Vertigo
  Giddiness
  Seizures
Cardiac
  Tachycardia
  Bradycardia
Respiratory
  Hyperpnea
  Respiratory depression
  Pulmonary edema

Table 20-7 Diagnostic Clues for Cyanide Poisoning

High index of suspicion
Appropriate clinical setting
Unexplained cardiac arrest
Odor of bitter almonds
Abolition of difference between arterial and venous
  oxygen saturation
Anion-gap metabolic acidosis
Absence of cyanotic appearance

Red veins in fundo scopie

ined on funduscopic examination,[6] yet this examination may be impractical in the emergency department.

Although the diagnosis of the comatose, hypotensive, apneic patient with dilated pupils presents a difficult problem, the associated features of bradycardia and the absence of cyanosis resulting from cellular inability to utilize oxygen could lead to a consideration of cyanide poisoning. Although poisoning by carbon monoxide may present a similar picture, including bradycardia and pink mucous membranes, the patient's history may reveal circumstances that might better suggest the diagnosis of cyanide poisoning.

Table 20-8 Blood Cyanide Concentrations and Associated Symptoms

Concentration (μg/mL)	Symptoms
0.2—0.5	None
0.5—1.0	Tachycardia, flushing
1.0—2.5	Depressed level of consciousness
2.5—3.0	Coma
>3.0	Death

Source: Adapted with permission from "Clinical Toxicology of Cyanide" by A Hall and B Rumack in *Annals of Emergency Medicine* (1986;15:1070), Copyright © 1986, American College of Emergency Physicians.

LABORATORY ANALYSIS

Not picked up on toxo screen

Routine toxicologic screens do not check for cyanide, so that the screen will be negative even in cases of pure cyanide ingestion. There are no readily available cyanide assays that confirm the poisoning within the time needed to treat an acutely poisoned patient. Confirmatory laboratory analysis specific for cyanide in the acute situation is seldom useful in prognosis or treatment and is also time consuming. Specimens should be saved, however, in case a chemical analysis is needed for legal purposes. Because the toxicity of cyanide is due to the intracellular concentration of cyanide, the actual blood concentration finally reported may be misleading.[52] As a result of the tight binding of cyanide to cytochrome oxidase, serious poisoning has occurred with only modest blood concentrations, especially several hours after ingestion.[53]

Cyanide concentration may be measured in whole blood, gastric contents, tissues, and urine. The usual technique is a colorimetric diffusion method, although measurement by a specific electrode can be performed (Table 20-8).[1,6,54] Whole blood cyanide concentration in nonsmokers is approximately 0.02 μg/mL and in smokers is 0.04 μg/mL[1]; this is measured from the cyanide found predominantly in vitamin B_{12} or intermediaries of 1-carbon metabolism.[3] Although difficult to measure and correlate with symptoms, the approximate toxic range is 0.1 to 0.2 μg/mL, and the fatal range is usually considered greater than 1 to 3 μg/mL in

whole blood.[1,4,55] Thiocyanate concentrations normally range from 1 to 4 μg/mL in nonsmokers and from 3 to 12 μg/mL in smokers.

Spectrophotometric and colorimetric methods for the estimation of blood cyanide concentration have adequate sensitivity but lack specificity because they react with thiocyanate as well as with cyanide and are also subject to interference with thiosulfate.[1] These substances may be present in blood samples obtained after cyanide intoxication if nitrite-thiosulfate therapy was administered.

Because sophisticated laboratory confirmation of cyanide is time consuming, a simple chemical test is available to measure cyanide concentration in gastric aspirate (Lee-Jones test).[6,56] This test is reported to detect as little as 50 mg of ingested cyanide. The test is based on the Prussian blue reaction and uses reagents that are stable and can be kept in the emergency department or an adjacent laboratory. A few small crystals of ferrous sulfate are added to 5 mL of gastric aspirate, and four to five drops of 20% sodium hydroxide solution are added to precipitate the iron. The mixture is boiled, cooled, and acidified with eight to ten drops of 10% hydrochloric acid. A greenish-blue precipitate, the color of which intensifies on standing, indicates the presence of cyanide. The reaction is not obtained with barbiturates, phenothiazines, benzodiazepines, or tricyclics, nor is the color reaction changed appreciably by the presence of these drugs in addition to cyanide. A color change does occur with salicylate, so that confusion with this substance could be a problem.[3,46,56]

An elevated anion-gap metabolic acidosis is usually present in acute poisoning but is not specific. Because of the possibility of lactic acidosis, arterial blood gas and blood lactate determinations should be obtained, if possible, in the cyanide-intoxicated patient; these measurements may provide both therapeutic and prognostic information (Table 20-9).[3] Abolition of the difference between atrial and venous oxygen saturation may be seen in moderate to severe intoxication.[6] Because of the small amount of cyanide that combines with ferrous iron in hemoglobin, there may be a "saturation gap" noted in cyanide intoxication similar to that in carbon monoxide intoxication.[6] A difference of greater than 5% between the calculated and measured oxygen saturation suggests that another agent is combining with hemoglobin; this agent may be carbon monoxide, methemoglobin, cyanide, and possibly hydrogen sulfide.[6]

TREATMENT

Initial treatment of cyanide poisoning should include airway support, oxygen therapy, cardiac monitoring, decontamination of the skin and clothing, gastric lavage if necessary, and sodium bicarbonate as indicated for severe acidosis (Table 20-10).[57] Rescuers entering a contaminated area to remove an individual should first protect themselves with rubber boots and gloves. If a gas mask is used, the cannister must be appropriate for hydrogen cyanide because the usual cannister does not protect against cyanide.[4,8]

Even if cyanide has been ingested, gastric lavage should follow, not precede, the initiation

Table 20-9 Laboratory Determinations for Cyanide Overdose

Arterial blood gas
Serum lactate concentration
Lee-Jones test
Cyanide concentration
Thiocyanate concentration

Table 20-10 Treatment of Cyanide Poisoning

Airway support
Oxygen
Cardiac monitoring
Decontamination
Amyl nitrite
Sodium nitrite
  Adult: 300 mg
  Child: 10 mg/kg
Sodium thiosulfate
  Adult: 12.5 g
  Child: 1.5 mL/kg
Methods not FDA-approved
  Dicobalt edetate
  Hydroxycobalamin
  Aminophenol
  Rhodanase
  Stroma-free methemoglobin

of more specific treatment for the symptomatic individual.[58] Patients have survived even when cardiac asystole has occurred, so that vigorous treatment should be instituted immediately. In mild cases of cyanide poisoning, in which the individual may present with weakness, vertigo, headache, nausea, and vomiting, it may be only necessary to remove the individual from exposure and administer supportive care. In severe cases, specific antidotal therapy may be indicated. In some cases patients who have ingested a potentially lethal dose of cyanide may survive with only nonspecific supportive measures.[4,6] One survivor of cyanide intoxication, who had a blood concentration of 2.9 µg/mL, was treated with supportive measures alone; this was the largest overdose of cyanide successfully treated in this way. Survival with antidotal therapy has been reported with cyanide concentrations of 3.2 to 16.3 µg/mL.[6,25,42]

Oxygen

The effect of oxygen therapy cannot be overemphasized; oxygen therapy has been shown experimentally to abolish the inspiratory gasp and improve the electroencephalographic and electrocardiographic abnormalities associated with cyanide poisoning.[4,39,59,60] Its low toxicity and ease of administration recommend it for use in any cyanide-intoxicated patient. The proposed salutary effect of oxygen is unexpected and may be based on a cyanide-oxygen interaction at the cytochrome level.[1,12] Cyanide may combine with reduced rather than oxidized cytochrome oxidase, thus allowing the possibility of oxygen competition with cyanide.

Dextrose, Thiamine, and Naloxone

Dextrose, thiamine, and naloxone should also be administered to any cyanide-intoxicated patient with an altered mental status. Naloxone should also be administered, both as a nonspecific agent when the diagnosis is unknown as well as when the diagnosis of cyanide poisoning has been made. This is because of the potential for naloxone to reverse the endorphin-induced respiratory depression that may also occur with cyanide intoxication.[61]

Antidotal Therapy

The decision to treat a potentially lethal ingestion of cyanide with a toxic treatment regimen many times rests on nonspecific circumstantial evidence. Yet it may be this quick recognition and treatment that is lifesaving.

The rational therapeutic approach to cyanide toxicity is to prevent the cyanide ion from binding to cytochrome oxidase or to reverse the binding once it has occurred. In the United States treatment of cyanide intoxication consists of two separate antidotes that, when used jointly, can potentiate each other's beneficial effect. One of these antidotes produces methemoglobin, an oxidation product of the normal blood pigment hemoglobin. Production of methemoglobin causes the ferric ion to act as an alternative site to cytochrome oxidase for cyanide binding.[4,62–65] Although the cyanomethemoglobin complex is less tightly bound than the cyanide–cytochrome oxidase complex, the relatively greater amounts of methemoglobin generated in this procedure favor the formation of cyanomethemoglobin.[19] The methemoglobin is capable of binding any cyanide in the plasma, but, more important, it can effectively compete for cyanide already bound to cytochrome oxidase.[66] Recent evi-

dence casts doubt on the traditionally proposed mechanism.[1,6]

At one time methylene blue was used for cyanide poisoning because of its ability to form methemoglobin.[4,67] It was determined, however, that methylene blue is not an efficient antidote because it forms methemoglobin poorly. Methylene blue more efficiently reverses the reaction and is an effective antidote in the treatment of methemoglobinemia.

Nitrite Therapy

The formation of methemoglobin is accomplished with the administration of nitrites.[62–65] The first nitrite employed to antagonize cyanide was amyl nitrite; sodium nitrite was used subsequently.

The suggested regimen for nitrite therapy in the United States consists of the application of amyl nitrite perles over the patient's nose or through positive-pressure breathing apparatus for 30 seconds of each minute (so that the patient can also be adequately oxygenated). Amyl nitrite is recommended because of the speed with which it can be administered. Amyl nitrite inhalation produces a relatively low concentration of methemoglobin and must be followed by intravenous sodium nitrite. If sodium nitrite is immediately available, amyl nitrite can be omitted.[12]

The goal of nitrite therapy is to attain a methemoglobin concentration that is approximately 10% to 40% of the patient's total hemoglobin.[6,66]

The recommended dose of sodium nitrite for adults is 300 mg or 10 mL of a 3% solution; for children the dose is 10 mg/kg or 0.2 mL/kg not to exceed 10 mL.[12] The nitrite solution should be administered at a rate not greater than 2.5 to 5 mL/min.[68]

Normal methemoglobin is approximately 1% of the total hemoglobin. The initial amyl nitrite inhalation may raise the methemoglobin concentration to approximately 5%.[4,12] The first dose of sodium nitrite should continue to raise the methemoglobin concentration to approximately 25%.[4] The resulting compound, cyanomethemoglobin, has relatively low toxicity. The methemoglobin thus produced is spontaneously reconverted to oxyhemoglobin by intraerythrocyte enzymes. The co-oximeter does not detect cyanomethemoglobin, and there is no readily available assay for this compound.[6] The methemoglobin concentration may not be accurately measured as a consequence.

Sodium Thiosulfate Therapy

Sodium thiosulfate produces the relatively nontoxic thiocyanate, which is then excreted by the kidneys. Sodium thiosulfate acts as a sulfur donor and provides a substrate for the liver enzyme rhodanase to convert cyanide released from methemoglobin to thiocyanate.[6,25] It is believed that three times more thiosulfate than cyanide must be present for successful detoxification.[52] Administration of sodium thiosulfate has no toxic effects.[3,46]

The dose of sodium thiosulfate for adults is 50 mL of a 25% solution (12.5 g) administered intravenously; for children the dose is 1.5 mL/kg.[12] A continuous intravenous infusion has also been suggested, but this is not yet widely accepted.[16]

Although nitrite and thiosulfate have approximately equal antidotal activity, when they are used together there is a potentiation of effect; the combination of nitrite and thiosulfate is therefore suggested. A kit is marketed for this purpose (Lilly).

A temporary improvement in the patient's condition after the initial medication may occur but does not ensure complete recovery. The patient should be closely monitored, and if symptoms recur both the nitrite and the thiosulfate should be administered at one-half the original dose.

Care should be taken to administer the correct dose of sodium nitrite to children because a fatal methemoglobinemia may result if too much is administered.[4] Although the pediatric dose of nitrite should ideally be based on the amount of hemoglobin, generally it is not feasible to wait while this is being determined. An initial dose of 10 mg/kg is safe, and blood should be drawn immediately to measure both hemoglobin and methemoglobin concentrations. Subsequent nitrite doses can be calculated on the basis of these values.[69–71]

Sodium nitrite should be administered slowly to lessen the chance of developing hypotension; nitrite can significantly decrease mean blood pressure when injected as a bolus. The toxicity of sodium thiosulfate is low, and doses of 12.5 to 50 g by intravenous injection are well tolerated.

Nitrite-Thiosulfate Therapy

Nitrite and thiosulfate are two distinct antidotes that are used for two distinct effects. The nitrite-thiosulfate kit is used to cause a methemoglobinemia to form, to which the cyanide ion attaches. Although this is not ideal, it may be lifesaving.[42] Recent studies suggest that methemoglobin formation by sodium nitrite may be only a partial explanation for the therapeutic benefit of nitrites in cyanide poisoning.[42] Nitrites may act through effects on the cardiovascular system or changes in blood flow to organs.[1] Certainly it seems that the mechanism of action of the nitrites is more complex than previously believed.[6,42] The effect of thiosulfate is a stimulation of what naturally takes place in the body, that is, the rhodanase system, which normally detoxifies cyanide. Because this detoxification is a relatively slow process, and because the rate-limiting factor is usually a limited supply of sulfur ions, sodium thiosulfate is administered so that more rhodanase may form and detoxify the cyanomethemoglobin. The thiocyanate thus formed is excreted through the kidney.[70]

A concentration of 30% methemoglobin does not usually produce significant symptoms; a concentration of 40% is considered to cause mild symptoms, and 70% is considered lethal.[4] Because 30% methemoglobin does not usually produce symptoms and because the lethal dose of sodium nitrite for an adult is about 2 g, a dose of 300 to 600 mg of sodium nitrite is well within safe limits.

Adjunctive therapy to nitrite-thiosulfate. Although the mechanism of action is not clear, as previously mentioned oxygen is often recommended as a therapeutic adjunct in cyanide poisoning.[58] In one study, oxygen alone even at hyperbaric pressures had only slight protective effect against cyanide in mice, but it dramatically potentiated the protective effects of thiosulfate alone or in combination with nitrite.

Hemodialysis has been shown to remove thiocyanate but not cyanide. It may therefore be indicated in the patient with renal failure after antidotal treatment is instituted.[12]

Limitations of nitrite-thiosulfate therapy. There are several disadvantages to the nitrite-thiosulfate combination. For example, the production of methemoglobin by nitrites is relatively slow. It has been reported that peak methemoglobin concentrations are attained in approximately 30 minutes.[66] In addition, the higher percentage of methemoglobin decreases the oxygen-carrying capacity of the blood, so that a profound hypotension can result from the rapid administration of nitrites.[42] Most important, however, the cyanide is not removed quickly from the body by this method but remains bound in the erythrocyte while awaiting conversion to thiocyanate.

Antidotes Not Approved by the FDA

Stroma-free methemoglobin. Stroma-free methemoglobin solution is made by oxidizing stroma-free hemoglobin solution, which is produced by releasing hemoglobin from erythrocytes. Stroma-free hemoglobin and methemoglobin solutions are free of membrane lipids. In theory, stroma-free methemoglobin binds cyanide, as does intracellular methemoglobin, but does not cause a reduction in the patient's oxygen-carrying capacity. It can also be administered intravenously.[45] This antidote has been tried experimentally and may offer advantages over the nitrite-thiosulfate combination.[39,45]

Rhodanase. Recent applications of crystalline rhodanase have been promising. This antidote may be of value in the future management of cyanide poisoning.

Aminophenols. The aminophenols have been used in Europe. They have a mechanism of action that is similar to that of the nitrates. 4-Dimethylaminophenol (DMAP) is a more rapid producer of methemoglobin than the nitrites and has been successfully used in animal models. DMAP has also been shown to be effective in sulfide and mercaptan poisonings because the mechanism of toxicity is similar to that of cyanide.[8] Some investigators have promoted the use of aminophenols over the nitrites because

they form methemoglobin more rapidly than the nitrites.[19]

Cobalt salts. Although the cobalt salts were among the earliest antidotes employed to antagonize the lethal effects of cyanide, they have not received widespread acceptance in the United States.[72] Despite their apparent lack of use, many toxicologists believe that cobaltous compounds either alone or in combination with sodium thiosulfate should be the primary antidote for cyanide poisoning.

Cobalt salts are believed to exert their detoxifying effect primarily by combining directly with cyanide ion as a chelate rather than indirectly by methemoglobin formation.[73] The reason for the preferential use of cobalt compounds is that cobaltous ion has a higher affinity for cyanide than either methemoglobin or cytochrome oxidase and can also bind cyanide more rapidly than nitrite can convert hemoglobin to methemoglobin for subsequent binding to cyanide. Furthermore, cobalt forms a stable, presumably nontoxic complex with the cyanide ion that is excreted within 24 hours. The inherent toxicity of cobalt compounds is considered less than that of the nitrite-thiosulfate combination, and the large amount of methemoglobin generated by sodium nitrite can be dangerous and has resulted in the death of at least one child.

It has been shown that cobaltous chloride in combination with sodium nitrite produces additive antidotal effects in experimental cyanide poisoning. More striking are the results that showed the combination of cobalt and sodium thiosulfate to be much more effective than the traditional nitrite-thiosulfate combination against the lethal effects of cyanide.[37]

Dicobalt edetate seems to be one of the most effective cobalt compounds and has had the most clinical use.[6,74] Dicobalt edetate is commercially available in Europe as Kelocyanor.[4] The kit consists of ampules, each containing 300 mg of dicobalt edetate in 20% glucose.[75] The manufacturer recommends injecting two ampules (40 mL) initially. If there is no response, two more doses are given. The product formed, presumably cobalticyanide, is considered stable and of low toxicity; the toxicity of dicobalt edetate is greater when it is not chelating cyanide.[4] Symptoms of intoxication may include hypertension, hypotension, cardiac dysrhythmias, and cardiac insufficiency.[6,25]

Hydroxycobalamin, vitamin B_{12a}, is another cobalt antidote shown to be effective against cyanide.[17,76,77] Hydroxycobalamin has been used for more than 15 years in France with very little associated toxicity.[7] It has also been suggested for use in combination with thiosulfate.[7,73]

Hydroxycobalamin contains a central cobalt atom in a porphyrin-like ring structure. It has one cyanide less than cyanocobalamin (vitamin B_{12}) and combines in equimolar amounts with cyanide to form cyanocobalamin,[24] which is extremely stable and is excreted in the urine.[7,52] It does this by giving up one hydroxyl group and binding one cyanyl group. Hydroxycobalamin has the advantage of low toxicity, with no toxic effects seen in moderate doses. It has a greater affinity for cyanide than cytochrome oxidase and can free the respiratory enzyme to resume its normal activity.[78]

Hydroxycobalamin is considered unsuitable for use in the United States because it is not manufactured in a sufficiently concentrated form. It is commercially available in a solution of 1 mg/mL. This concentration has been used experimentally to prevent cyanide accumulation during nitroprusside administration.[78] The recommended dose for cyanide intoxication is approximately 50 mg/kg.[4,6,12,78] Hydroxycobalamin is considered an orphan drug and is currently available in the United States under an investigational license as a powder in combination with sodium thiosulfate.[4,78] A proposed dose is 4 g combined with 8 g of sodium thiosulfate.[1,78]

As much as 50% of hydroxycobalamin is excreted unchanged in the urine,[77] but it may still play an active role in cyanide detoxification by binding cyanide to form vitamin B_{12}. The cyanide is excreted in this form or is later given up to rhodanase for complexing with thiocyanate; hydroxycobalamin is thereby regenerated.

Problems associated with the use of hydroxycobalamin include limited solubility in a reasonable volume, scarcity of the preparation, expense, and stability of the solution. Proper storage of the powder is necessary to maintain potency; otherwise deterioration will occur, liberating cobaltous ions.[17] Minor side effects reported from hydroxycobalamin include urticaria, which may be related to the vehicle in which the material is suspended. It may also cause a transient reddish-brown discoloration of the urine, skin, and mucous membranes.[1,78]

Further clinical investigations are necessary to evaluate the place of cobalt compounds in the treatment of cyanide poisoning. Although these agents appear to be promising, sodium nitrite–thiosulfate therapy should still be considered the treatment of choice in the United States. Perhaps the main use of cobalt compounds in the future will be in combination with sodium thiosulfate because, as mentioned above, cobalt compounds rapidly bind cyanide and then can be detoxified with thiosulfate.

Hyperbaric Oxygen Therapy

Hyperbaric oxygen therapy has been proposed as a treatment for cyanide poisoning, but evidence supporting the use of this modality is inconclusive.[39] In addition, animal studies have not shown that hyperbaric oxygen is more efficacious than the administration of 100% oxygen at one atmosphere.[6] Even in view of these studies, the Undersea Medical Society has classified cyanide as a category one condition, essentially stating that hyperbaric oxygen is mandatory for cyanide intoxication. If hyperbaric oxygen is readily available, it may be appropriate to administer it to cyanide-intoxicated patients who do not respond to supportive measures and antidotal therapy.[6,12] Because the accumulated evidence does not point to any clear-cut conclusions, however, hyperbaric oxygen should not be considered the standard of care for cyanide poisoning.[6]

REFERENCES

1. Becker C: The role of cyanide in fires. *Vet Hum Toxicol* 1985;27:487–490.

2. Peters C, Mundy J, Rayner P: Acute cyanide poisoning. *Anaesthesiology* 1982;37:582–586.

3. Graham D, Laman D, Theodore J, et al: Acute cyanide poisoning complicated by lactic acidosis and pulmonary edema. *Arch Intern Med* 1977;137:1051–1055.

4. Vogel S, Sultan T, Ten Eyck R: Cyanide poisoning. *Clin Toxicol* 1981;18:367–383.

5. Stewart R: Cyanide poisoning. *Clin Toxicol* 1974; 7:561–564.

6. Hall A, Rumack B: Clinical toxicology of cyanide. *Ann Emerg Med* 1986;15:1067–1074.

7. Bismuth C, Baud F, Djeghout H, et al: Cyanide poisoning from propionitrile exposure. *J Emerg Med* 1987; 5:191–195.

8. Weger N: Treatment of cyanide poisoning with 4-dimethylaminophenol (DMAP)—Experimental and clinical overview. *Fund Appl Toxicol* 1983;3:387–396.

9. Bell R, Stemmer K, Barkley W, et al: Cyanide toxicity from the thermal degradation of rigid polyurethane foam. *Ann Ind Hyg Assoc J* 1979;40:757–762.

10. Symington I, Anderson R, Oliver J, et al: Cyanide exposures in fires. *Lancet* 1978;2:91–92.

11. Way J: Cyanide antidotes. *Drug Ther* 1977; 7:99–100.

12. Litovitz T, Larkin R, Myers R: Cyanide poisoning treated with hyperbaric oxygen. *Am J Emerg Med* 1983; 1:94–101.

13. Atkins D: Cyanide toxicity following nitroprusside-induced hypotension. *Can Anaesth Soc J* 1977;24:651–660.

14. Perchau R, Modell J, Bright R, et al: Suspected sodium nitroprusside–induced cyanide intoxication. *Anesth Analg* 1977;56:533–537.

15. Smith R, Kruszyna H: Nitroprusside produces cyanide poisoning via a reaction with hemoglobin. *J Pharmacol Exp Ther* 1974;191:557–563.

16. Ivankovich A, Braverman B, Kanuru R, et al: Cyanide antidotes and methods of their administration in dogs: A comparative study. *Anesthesiology* 1980; 52:210–216.

17. Posner M, Tobey R, McElroy H: Hydroxycobalamin therapy of cyanide intoxication in guinea pigs. *Anesthesiology* 1976;44:157–160.

18. Vesey C, Cole P, Simpson P: Cyanide and thiocyanate concentrations following sodium nitroprusside infusion in man. *Br J Anaesth* 1976;48:651–660.

19. Wesson D, Foley R, Sabatini S, et al: Treatment of acute cyanide intoxication with hemodialysis. *Am J Nephrol* 1985;5:121–126.

20. Rubino M, Davidoff F: Cyanide poisoning from apricot seeds. *JAMA* 1979;241:359.

21. Sayre J, Kaymakcalan S: Cyanide poisoning from apricot seeds among children in central Turkey. *N Engl J Med* 1964;270:1113–1115.

22. Townsend W: Cyanide poisoning from ingestion of apricot kernels. *MMWR* 1975;24:8–10.

23. Pijoan M: Cyanide poisoning from chokecherry seeds. *Am J Med Sci* 1942;204:550–553.

24. Blanc P, Hogan M, Mallin K, et al: Cyanide intoxication among silver-reclaiming workers. *JAMA* 1985; 253:367–371.

25. Hall A, Linden C, Kulig K, et al: Cyanide poisoning from Laetrile ingestion: Role of nitrite therapy. *Pediatrics* 1986;78:269–272.

26. Freeman A: Chronic cyanide intoxication. *Br Med J* 1981;282:1321.

27. Humbert J, Tress J, Braico K: Fatal cyanide poisoning: Accidental ingestion of amygdalin. *JAMA* 1977; 238:482.

28. Schwarting A: Poisonous seeds and fruits. *Prog Chem Toxicol* 1963;1:385–401.

29. Grabois B: Exposure to hydrogen cyanide in the processing of apricot kernels. *NY State Dept Labor Mon Rev* 1974;33:33–36.

30. Jukes T: Laetrile for cancer. *JAMA* 1976;236: 1284–1286.

31. Lewis J: Laetrile. *West J Med* 1977;127:55–62.

32. Greenberg D: The vitamin fraud in cancer quackery. *West J Med* 1975;122:345–348.

33. Cassileth B: Sounding boards: After Laetrile, what? *N Engl J Med* 1982;306:1482–1484.

34. Levi L, French W, Bickis I, et al: Laetrile: A study of its physiochemical and biochemical properties. *Can Med Assoc J* 1965;92:1057–1061.

35. Baker J, Lokey J, Price N, et al: Against legalization of Laetrile. *N Engl J Med* 1976;295:679.

36. Moss M, Khabl N, Gray J: Deliberate self-poisoning with Laetrile. *CMAJ* 1981;125:1126–1127.

37. Moertel C, Fleming T, Rubin J, et al: A clinical trial of amygdalin (Laetrile) in the treatment of human cancer. *N Engl J Med* 1982;306:201–206.

38. Moertel C, Ames M, Kavach J, et al: A pharmacologic and toxicological study of amygdalin. *JAMA* 1981;245:591–594.

39. Krieg A, Saxena K: Cyanide poisoning from metal cleaning solutions. *Ann Intern Med* 1987;16:582–584.

40. Sadoff L, Fuchs K, Hollander J: Rapid death associated with Laetrile ingestion. *JAMA* 1978;239:1532.

41. Ortega J, Creek J: Acute cyanide poisoning following administration of Laetrile enemas. *J Pediatrics* 1978; 93:1059.

42. Hall A, Doutre W, Ludden T, et al: Nitrite/thiosulfate-treated acute cyanide poisoning: Estimated kinetics after antidote. *Clin Toxicol* 1987;25:121–133.

43. Burrows G, Liu D, Way J: Effect of oxygen on cyanide intoxication: Physiologic effects. *J Pharmacol Exp Ther* 1973;184:739–748.

44. Ware G, Painter H: Bacterial utilization of cyanide. *Nature (London)* 1955;175:900–902.

45. Ten Eyck R, Schaerdel A, Lynett J, et al: Stroma-free methemoglobin solution as an antidote for cyanide poisoning: A preliminary study. *Clin Toxicol* 1984;21:343–358.

46. Beamer W, Shealy R, Prough D: Acute cyanide poisoning from Laetrile ingestion. *Ann Emerg Med* 1983; 12:449–451.

47. Dorr R, Paxinos J: The current status of Laetrile. *Ann Intern Med* 1978;89:389–397.

48. Winek D: Cyanide poisoning as a mode of suicide. *Forensic Sci* 1978;11:51–55.

49. Shragg T, Albertson T, Fisher C: Cyanide poisoning after bitter almond ingestion. *West J Med* 1982;136:65–69.

50. Kirk R, Stenhouse N: Ability to smell solutions of potassium cyanide. *Nature (London)* 1953;171:698–699.

51. DeBusk R, Seidl L: Attempted suicide by cyanide: A report of two cases. *Calif Med* 1969;110:394–396.

52. Cottrell J, Casthely P, Brodie J, et al: Prevention of nitroprusside-induced cyanide toxicity with hydroxycobalamin. *N Engl J Med* 1978;298:809–811.

53. Soffer A: Chicken soup or Laetrile—Which would you prescribe? *Arch Intern Med* 1977;137:994–995.

54. Groff W, Stemler F, Kaminskis A, et al: Plasma-free cyanide and blood total cyanide: A rapid, completely automated microdistillation assay. *Clin Toxicol* 1985;23:133–163.

55. Marbury T, Sheppard J, Gibbons K, et al: Combined antidotal and hemodialysis treatments for nitroprusside-induced cyanide toxicity. *Clin Toxicol* 1982;19:475–482.

56. Lee-Jones M, Bennett M, Sherwell J: Cyanide self-poisoning. *Br Med J* 1970;4:780–781.

57. McKiernan M: Emergency treatment of cyanide poisoning. *Lancet* 1980;2:86.

58. Bain J, Knowles E: Successful treatment of cyanide poisoning. *Br Med J* 1967;2:763.

59. Cope C: The importance of oxygen in the treatment of cyanide poisoning. *JAMA* 1961;175:1061–1064.

60. Isom G, Way J: Effects of oxygen on the antagonism of cyanide intoxication: Cytochrome oxidase in vitro. *Toxicol Appl Pharmacol* 1984;74:57–62.

61. Leung P, Sylvenster D, Chiou F, et al: Stereospecific effect of naloxone hydrochloride on cyanide intoxication. *Toxicol Appl Pharmacol* 1986;83:525–530.

62. Chen K, Rose C, Clowes G: Amyl nitrite and cyanide poisoning. *JAMA* 1933;100:1920–1922.

63. Chen K, Rose C, Clowes G: Comparative values of several antidotes in cyanide poisoning. *Am J Med Sci* 1934;188:767–781.

64. Chen K, Rose C: Nitrite and thiosulfate therapy in cyanide poisoning. *JAMA* 1952;149:113–119.

65. Chen K, Rose C: Treatment of acute cyanide poisoning. *JAMA* 1956;162:1154–1155.

66. Ten Eyck R, Schaerdel A, Ottinger W: Comparison of nitrite treatment and stroma-free methemoglobin solution as antidotes for cyanide poisoning in a rat model. *Clin Toxicol* 1986;23:477–487.

67. Geiger J: Cyanide poisoning in San Francisco. *JAMA* 1932;99:1944–1945.

68. Wolfsie J, Shaffer C: Hydrogen cyanide: Hazards, toxicology, prevention and management of poisoning. *J Occup Med* 1959;1:281–288.

69. Berlin C: The treatment of cyanide poisoning in children. *Pediatrics* 1970;46:793–796.

70. Berlin C: Accidental childhood poisoning. *Pediatrics* 1971;47(6):1093.

71. Berlin C: Cyanide poisoning—A challenge. *Arch Intern Med* 1977;137:993–994.

72. Rose C, Worth R, Kikuchi K, et al: Cobalt salts in acute cyanide poisoning. *Proc Soc Exp Biol Med* 1965;120:780–783.

73. Evans C: Cobalt compounds as antidotes for hydrocyanic acid. *Br J Pharmacol* 1964;23:455–475.

74. Smith R: Cobalt salts: Effects in cyanide and sulfide poisoning and on methemoglobinemia. *Toxicol Appl Pharmacol* 1969;15:505–516.

75. Hillman B, Bardhan D, Bain J: The use of dicobalt edetate (Kelocyanor) in cyanide poisoning. *Postgrad Med J* 1974;581:171–174.

76. MacRae W, Owen M: Severe metabolic acidosis following hypotension induced with sodium nitroprusside: Case report. *Br J Anesth* 1975;46:795.

77. Wilson J, Linnell J, Matthews D: Plasma-cobalamins in neuro-ophthalomogical diseases. *Lancet* 1971;1:259.

78. Hall A, Rumack B: Hydroxycobalamin/sodium thiosulfate as a cyanide antidote. *J Emerg Med* 1987;5:115–121.

ADDITIONAL SELECTED REFERENCES

Ballantyne B, Bright J, Williams P: An experimental assessment of decreases in measurable cyanide levels in biological fluids. *J Forensic Sci* 1973;13:111–117.

Braico K, Humbert J, Terplan K, et al: Laetrile intoxication—Report of a fatal case. *N Engl J Med* 1979;300:238–240.

Brivet F, Delfraissy J, Duche M, et al: Acute cyanide poisoning: Recovery with nonspecific supportive therapy. *Intensive Care Med* 1983;9:33–35.

Buchanan I, Dhamee M, Griffiths F, et al: Abnormal fundal appearances in a case of poisoning by a cyanide capsule. *Med Sci Law* 1976;16:29–32.

Butler A, Glidewell C, McGinnis J, et al: Further investigations regarding the toxicity of sodium nitroprusside. *Clin Chem* 1987;490–492.

Crile G: Legalization of Laetrile—A suggestion. *N Engl J Med* 1976;295:116.

Dalderup L: Cyanide intoxication. *Lancet* 1973;2:625.

Goodman AG, Goodman LS, Gilman A (eds): *The Pharmacologic Basis of Therapeutics.* New York, MacMillan, 1975.

Gwilt J: The odour of potassium cyanide. *Medicolegal J* 1961;29:98–99.

Herbert V: Laetrile: The cult of cyanide—Promoting poison for profit. *Am J Clin Nutr* 1979;32:1121–1158.

Isom G, Way J: Cyanide intoxication: Protection with co-baltous chloride. *Toxicol Appl Pharmacol* 1973;24:449–456.

Jones G, Abramson N: Laetrile: What we know and what we do about it. *J Fla Med Assoc* 1979;66:548–552.

Khandekar J, Edelman H: Studies of amygdalin toxicity in rodents. *JAMA* 1979;242:169–171.

Morse D, Boros L, Findley P: More on cyanide poisoning from Laetrile. *N Engl J Med* 1980;301:892.

Pettersen J, Cohen S: Antagonism of cyanide poisoning by chlorpromazine and sodium thiosulfate. *Toxicol Appl Pharmacol* 1985;81:265–273.

Rosen G, Shorr R: Laetrile: A survey of judicial and administrative activity. *Ann Intern Med* 1981;94:530–533.

Schmidt E, Newton G, Sanders S, et al: Laetrile toxicity studies in dogs. *JAMA* 1978;239:943–947.

Tyrer F: Treatment of cyanide poisoning. *J Soc Occup Med* 1981;31:65–66.

Veatch R: Laetrile: The new medicine show? *Hosp Physician* 1976;12:15–16.

Vincent M, Vincent F, Marka C, et al: Cyanide and its relationship to nervous suffering: Physiological aspects of intoxication. *Clin Toxicol* 1981;18:1519–1527.

Worsley R: Hydrogen sulfide poisoning. *Can Med Assoc J* 1978;118:775–776.

chapter 21

Sulfide Poisoning

Sulfide poisoning usually occurs after exposure to hydrogen sulfide, carbon disulfide, one of the mercaptans, or a soluble salt of sulfide. Hydrogen sulfide and soluble salts of sulfides are potent poisons and have a toxicity comparable to that of cyanide.[1,2] The common soluble salts as well as the sulfur acids all produce nearly identical toxic syndromes, and in general the route of administration is not a critical determinant of the toxic effects.

PROPERTIES OF SULFIDES

Hydrogen Sulfide

Hydrogen sulfide is a nonflammable, colorless, irritating gas whose odor is similar to that of rotten eggs.[3–5] Hydrogen sulfide is heavier than air, and for this reason it accumulates in underground locations such as sewers and wells. Hydrogen sulfide gas usually occurs in the setting of degrading protein waste. Although it has a strong and identifiable odor, it causes olfactory fatigue after short exposure and at relatively low concentrations. Hydrogen sulfide is poorly soluble in water. The proposed safe air concentration is 10 parts per million (ppm).[6]

Hydrogen sulfide is used or encountered in diverse industries such as farming, glue making, rubber vulcanizing, and rayon manufacturing

(Table 21-1).[1,7] Farm workers may be exposed to fumes from liquid manure or from pouring hydrochloric acid into a farm well that has a high content of organic material. Large quantities of hydrogen sulfide are used in the production of elemental sulfur, sulfuric acid, and heavy water for nuclear reactors.[7,8] It is a natural constituent of volcanic gases and occurs in some deposits of natural gas and petroleum.[6] Hydrogen sulfide

Table 21-1 Sources of Sulfides

Hydrogen sulfide
Carbon disulfide
Mercaptans
  Sulfides found or used in:
    Sulfur springs
    Volcanic gases
    Liquid manure
    Insecticides
    Soil fumigants
    Petroleum industry
    Farm industry
    Jet fuels
    Metal refining
  Sulfides used in the manufacture of:
    Rubber
    Synthetic fabrics
    Heavy water
    Leather
    Plastics
    Asphalt

may also be encountered in mining and felt manufacturing.[9] A mixture of sulfuric acid and bleach can release hydrogen sulfide, as has an industrial cleaner with Plaster of Paris in a cast room.[6] Hydrogen sulfide is produced endogenously from sulfur-containing proteins in the alimentary canal of animals.

Sulfide Salts

Hydrogen sulfide is released in vivo from ingested or injected soluble inorganic sulfide salts. Sodium sulfide is therefore completely hydrolyzed in body fluids, and there is no toxicological distinction between it and hydrogen sulfide. Mixing liquid sodium sulfide with an acid-containing agent, mixing acid and alkaline drain cleaners, and breathing fumes from sodium sulfide have been responsible for cases of poisoning.[4] The leather industry uses substantial amounts of sodium sulfide in preparing hides for tanning.[7] Sodium sulfide monohydrate, a common commercial form of sulfide salt, is highly hydroscopic and corrosive.[10]

Carbon Disulfide

Carbon disulfide is a colorless liquid with a sweet odor that vaporizes at room temperature. Because of this, inhalation is the major route of entry. Hydrogen sulfide is necessary for the production of carbon disulfide.[10] Carbon disulfide is used widely as an insecticide, soil fumigant, and solvent for rubber, sulfur, phosphorus, lipids, and waxes. The production of carbon disulfide is most prominent in oil and gas exploration and processing.

Mercaptans

The mercaptans are toxic, flammable gases. There are two mercaptans of note: ethyl and methyl mercaptan. These compounds are used in the production of pesticides, jet fuels, and plastics. They are extremely foul-smelling agents and are added in very small concentrations as warning agents for the release of natural gases and other gases because their odor can be de-

tected well below the concentrations necessary to produce toxicity.

METABOLISM OF SULFIDES

Hydrogen sulfide and similar compounds may be detoxified spontaneously by various oxidative mechanisms with formation of nontoxic products such as polysulfides, thiosulfate, and sulfate, which are excreted by the kidneys.[2,5,11] These reactions are catalyzed by heavy metals, particularly in the presence of proteins; this occurs with low concentrations of the sulfide. Other modes of sulfide elimination whose significance is unknown include urinary excretion of unoxidized sulfide and pulmonary excretion of the gas.

MECHANISM OF TOXICITY

The sulfides are intracellular toxins; their mechanism of poisoning is similar to that of cyanide.[1,4,5] Both act as inhibitors of the ferric iron peroxidases and catalases. In addition, the sulfides inhibit succinic dehydrogenase, carbonic anhydrase, and other enzymes. The sulfides bind to iron in the trivalent or ferric states in cytochrome oxidase within the mitochondria and inhibit oxidative phosphorylation.[3] This inhibition blocks cellular respiration, leading to cellular anoxia.[2] Anaerobic metabolism and lactic acid accumulation result.[4,5]

In body fluids, dissociated and undissociated hydrogen sulfide exist in approximately equal proportions. The undissociated acid penetrates biologic membranes more rapidly than the hydrosulfide anion. It is thought that the hydrosulfide anion inhibits the cytochrome oxidase system by interrupting electron transport.[11] This is done by formation of a dissociable complex with ferric heme groups in cytochrome oxidase to produce sulfmethemoglobin. Sulfmethemoglobin is therefore analogous to cyanomethemoglobin. When the mitochondrial electron transport system is unable to function properly, cellular respiration continues anaerobically with production of organic acid by-products.

Two differences are recognized between cyanide binding to methemoglobin and sulfide binding to the same ferric heme sites. The first is that sulfmethemoglobin undergoes gradual auto-oxidation–reduction to ferrohemoglobin, and the second is that cyanide is bound more tenaciously than sulfide by a factor of 200.[10]

Sulfhemoglobin and Sulfmethemoglobin

There has been a great deal of confusion regarding the relationship between sulfhemoglobin and the toxicity associated with the sulfides.[8] Sulfmethemoglobin is unrelated to sulfhemoglobin, and even though many investigators refer to sulfhemoglobinemia as a cause of death in sulfide poisoning, no abnormal pigments including sulfhemoglobin are found in significant concentrations in those fatally poisoned by sulfide.[9,10]

Sulfhemoglobin is a bright green derivative of hemoglobin.[12] This derivative has a sulfur atom incorporated into the porphyrin ring. It is ineffective for oxygen transport.[13] Although it can be formed in vitro from oxyhemoglobin by various compounds that oxidize hemoglobin, it is rarely found in life.[13] Sulfhemoglobin, in contrast to sulfmethemoglobin, has rarely been encountered in those who survive sulfide poisoning, but its postmortem formation may be responsible for the various tissue discolorations noted.[9,10] Unlike carbon monoxide, the sulfides do not combine with hemoglobin during life. The formation of sulfmethemoglobinemia occurs after death as a result of decomposition of tissues. This sulfur-containing hemoglobin complex is thought to be responsible for the discoloration of tissues at autopsy. The many cases of sulfhemoglobin that are in the literature involve phenacetin, nitrites, nitrates, and sulfa drugs such as dapsone.[14–16] These drugs also cause methemoglobinemia, and this may very well be the pigment that is read as sulfhemoglobin. It has also been associated with drug abuse and exposure to polluted air.[13] This pigment may more precisely be called pseudosulfhemoglobin and may be a mixture of oxidized and denatured hemoglobin that may have formed abnormal disulfide bridges with sulfhydryl compounds.[9,10] Some investigators hold that sulfhemoglobinemia is probably a relatively nontoxic syndrome, if it truly exists.[13]

TOXICITY

Clinical Effects

The sulfides are absorbed by all routes, including through the skin. The intensity of exposure accounts for the highly diverse clinical patterns of hydrogen sulfide poisoning. Low concentrations of approximately 0.01% to 0.15% cause paralysis of the olfactory nerve.[5,6] At 0.02% (200 ppm), hydrogen sulfide depresses the CNS and may cause acute pulmonary edema. In moderate concentrations it stimulates the nervous system and respiration. At concentrations greater than 500 ppm, cardiovascular collapse may ensue. In high concentrations of 0.1% (1000 ppm) or more it directly paralyzes the CNS, including the respiratory center.[6] Although the CNS appears to experience the greatest adverse effects from sulfide exposure, the lungs are frequently affected. Death secondary to respiratory arrest may occur.[4]

Low Concentrations of Hydrogen Sulfide

At 25 ppm the odor of hydrogen sulfide may be detected.[11] Odor is considered unreliable, however, because as mentioned above concentrations of approximately 150 ppm or greater cause rapid paralysis of the olfactory nerve (Table 21-2).[5] At these low concentrations (50 ppm to 200 ppm), symptoms of sulfide intoxication are due chiefly to local tissue irritation of the eyes and respiratory tract rather than to systemic actions.[5] The gas is relatively harmless at low concentration except for its unpleasant odor and the irritation it causes to the eyes, respiratory tract, and gastrointestinal tract. The most characteristic effect is on the eye, where superficial injury to the conjunctiva and cornea may be noted. This keratoconjunctivitis is known as "gas eye" and is manifested after several hours or days of exposure as a scratchy, irritated sensation with tearing and burning.[9]

Other local reactions may include pharyngitis, bronchitis, and pneumonia. Hydrogen sulfide may also produce significant hyperpnea by direct chemostimulation of the carotid body. Nonspecific effects in mild poisonings may include

Table 21-2 Symptoms of Hydrogen Sulfide Intoxication

Low concentration
  Irritation
    Eye ("gas eye")
    Respiratory tract (pharyngitis, bronchitis)
    Gastrointestinal tract
  Headache
  Nausea
  Vomiting
  Weakness
High concentration
  Neurologic
    Agitation
    Coma
    Seizures
    Respiratory paralysis
  Cardiac
    Disorders of conduction
    Various dysrhythmias
  Local
    Caustic burn

---

headache, nausea, vomiting, and generalized weakness. As stated earlier, at approximately 200 ppm (0.02%) hydrogen sulfide depresses the CNS.

High Concentrations of Hydrogen Sulfide

In high concentrations (1000 ppm), a single breath or a few breaths can lead to various neurological alterations ranging from agitation to abrupt loss of consciousness, coma, and death.[8] It has been thought that the respiratory paralysis noted is due to central depression of the hypothalamic respiratory center.[6] Apnea is often followed by hypoxic seizures, cardiovascular collapse, and death. Once apnea has developed, breathing generally does not begin again spontaneously. Pulmonary edema may be noted in a significant number of individuals poisoned with sulfide.[4,7,9,10]

The direct toxic action of sulfide on the heart has been associated with various dysrhythmias, disorders of conduction, and disorders of ventricular repolarization. Carbon disulfide appears to have a greater affinity for the CNS and cardiovascular system than does hydrogen sulfide. Because soluble salts of sulfides are alkaline substances, they may cause a caustic burn.

Most deaths due to hydrogen sulfide intoxication occur at the site of exposure. Those patients arriving alive at a treatment facility generally experience complete recovery without sequelae.

LABORATORY DETERMINATIONS

Patients exposed to compounds that can cause sulfmethemoglobin should undergo tests for arterial blood gas, serum electrolytes, and complete blood count, and arterial saturation should be both measured and calculated (Table 21-3). Sulfhemoglobin concentrations may be obtained, but their significance is unclear. They should not be used to determine or guide therapy in hydrogen sulfide poisoning.[2] Sulfmethemoglobin concentration may be more appropriate to obtain, but this assay is not widely available.

TREATMENT

Initial treatment for patients intoxicated with sulfides involves vigorous prehospital and hospital care. Rapid removal from the toxic environment to fresh air is necessary (Table 21-4).[6,9,10] Because sulfide is so rapidly detoxified in the body, any decrease in the exposure intensity may result in a rapid and spontaneous revival.[3] Rescuers should be cautious and wear protective clothing and face masks because ill-advised rescue attempts often lead to their exposure. Decontamination methods should be performed, especially if the sulfide was on the skin. Providing 100% supplemental oxygen with assisted ventilation if required is important. Although the use of 100% oxygen by itself is not life-saving, the use of oxygen may encourage noncyto-

Table 21-3 Laboratory Determinations in Sulfide Intoxication

Arterial blood gas
  Calculated arterial oxygen saturation
  Measured arterial oxygen saturation
Carboxyhemoglobin concentration
Methemoglobin concentration
Serum electrolytes
Complete blood count

Table 21-4 Treatment of Sulfide Poisoning

Comment	Treatment
Acute exposure	Rapid removal from environment
	Oxygen
	Supportive care
	Decontamination
Seizures	Diazepam
Antidotes	Amyl nitrite
	Sodium nitrite
	Adult: 10 mL of 3% solution
	(300 mg)
	Child: 10 mg/kg of 3% solution

chrome oxidase–mediated aerobic cellular respiration.[9,17,18] Support of the vital signs including pulse and blood pressure by standard means is also necessary. Seizures should be treated with diazepam or a short-acting barbiturate. Patients should be monitored closely for development of pulmonary edema.[19]

Nitrite Therapy

Although advocated by many investigators, there is controversy surrounding the use of nitrites as sulfide antidotes.[2,4] Because of the similarity between sulfide and cyanide toxicity, and because of the formation of sulfmethemoglobin, the chemical induction of methemoglobinemia has been suggested as an effective antidotal procedure in acute sulfide poisoning.[2,6] Induction of methemoglobinemia with the nitrites is thought to reverse the effects of the sulfides by the competitive binding of methemoglobin with the hydrosulfide anion.[6] The important role of methemoglobin may be the trapping of free sulfide because methemoglobin has a greater affinity for sulfide than does cytochrome oxidase.[5] As sulfide is exchanged from cytochrome oxidase, aerobic metabolism returns.[4] The nontoxic sulfmethemoglobin is then degraded to nontoxic oxidized forms of sulfur, which are excreted primarily by the kidney.[6,8,9] It may also be that the nitrites act by mechanisms other than methemoglobin formation, such as vasodilation or a more direct effect on cytochrome oxidase.[4]

Although amyl nitrite perles may be used, if sodium nitrite is available then amyl nitrite is not necessary. Ten milliliters of a 3% solution (300 mg) of sodium nitrite can be injected intravenously at a rate of 2.5 to 5 mL per minute in an adult.[6,9] In a child, 10 mg/kg should be administered. If signs and symptoms of systemic poisoning recur, administration of half these doses is indicated.

If nitrites are used, methemoglobin concentrations should be monitored in the critically ill patient so as to ensure that no compromise of oxygen delivery occurs.[9,10] Even with all the controversial data concerning nitrite therapy, it is prudent to use this therapy when confronted with a comatose patient who is intoxicated with hydrogen sulfide.[5] It should be remembered, however, that the efficacy of antidotal therapy is controversial[1,3] and that there are serious side effects associated with the use of nitrites in this context.

Thiosulfate Therapy

Although thiosulfate appears to be an effective antidote for cyanide, it is not suggested in the case of sulfide poisoning. This is because rhodanase is necessary to convert cyanide to thiocyanate, but no comparable detoxification pathway is known to exist for sulfide.[9,10]

Other Antidotal Therapy

The effectiveness of hydroxycobalamin and other agents such as *p*-aminopropiophenone for the treatment of sulfide poisoning remains to be shown.[10]

Hyperbaric Oxygen Therapy

The use of hyperbaric oxygen in sulfide poisoning is another area of controversy, and its role has yet to be defined with certainty.[2] Hydrogen sulfide intoxication is considered a category two condition by the Undersea Medical Society, which means that there are insufficient data to assess the efficacy of hyperbaric oxygen for this condition.[4] At this time it should be reserved for the patient who does not respond to maximal supportive care, 100% oxygen, and sodium nitrite.

REFERENCES

1. Beck J, Bradbury C, Connors A, et al: Nitrite as an antidote for acute hydrogen sulfide intoxication? *Am Ind Hyg Assoc J* 1981;42:805–809.

2. Smilkstein M, Bronstein A, Pickett H, et al: Hyperbaric oxygen therapy for severe hydrogen sulfide poisoning. *J Emerg Med* 1985;3:27–30.

3. Burnett W, King E, Grace M, et al: Hydrogen sulfide poisoning: Review of 5 years' experience. *Can Med Assoc J* 1977;117:1277–1280.

4. Hoidal C, Hall A, Robinson M, et al: Hydrogen sulfide poisoning from toxic inhalations of roofing asphalt fumes. *Ann Emerg Med* 1986;15:826–830.

5. Stine R, Slosberg B, Beacham B: Hydrogen sulfide intoxication. *Ann Intern Med* 1976;85:756–758.

6. Peters J: Hydrogen sulfide poisoning in a hospital setting. *JAMA* 1981;246:1588–1589.

7. Deng J, Chang S: Hydrogen sulfide poisonings in hot spring reservoir cleaning: Two case reports. *Am J Ind Med* 1987;11:447–451.

8. Smith R, Gossellin R: Hydrogen sulfide poisoning. *J Occup Med* 1979;21:93–97.

9. Smith R: Hydrogen sulfide poisoning. *Can Med Assoc J* 1978;118:775–776.

10. Smith R, Kruszyna R, Kruszyna H: Management of acute sulfide poisoning: Effects of oxygen, thiosulfate and nitrite. *Arch Environ Health* 1976;31:166–169.

11. Whitcraft D, Bailey T, Hart B: Hydrogen sulfide poisoning treated with hyperbaric oxygen. *J Emerg Med* 1985; 3:23–25.

12. Nichol A, Hendry I, Morell D, et al: Mechanism of formation of sulphhaemoglobin. *Biochem Biophys Acta* 1968;156:97–108.

13. Park C, Nagel R, Blumberg W, et al: Sulfhemoglobin. *J Biol Chem* 1986;261:8805–8810.

14. Lim T, Lower D: "Enterogenous" cyanosis. *Am Rev Respir Dis* 1970;101:419–422.

15. Medeiros M, Bechara E, Naoum P: Oxygen toxicity and hemoglobin in subjects from a highly polluted town. *Arch Environ Health* 1983;38:11–16.

16. Lambert M, Sonnet J, Mathieu P, et al: Delayed sulfhemoglobinemia after acute dapsone intoxication. *J Toxicol Clin Toxicol* 1982;19:45–50.

17. Park C, Nagel R: Sulfhemoglobinemia. *N Engl J Med* 1984;310:1579–1584.

18. Carrico R, Blumberg W, Peisach J: The reversible binding of oxygen to sulfhemoglobin. *J Biol Chem* 1978; 253:7212–7215.

19. Thoman M: Sewer gas: Hydrogen sulfide intoxication. *Clin Toxicol* 1969;2:383–386.

ADDITIONAL SELECTED REFERENCES

Berzofsky J, Peisach J, Alben J: Carboxysulfmyoglobin: The relation between electron withdrawal from iron and ligand binding. *J Biol Chem* 1972;247: 3774–3782.

Berzofsky J, Peisach J, Alben J: Sulfheme proteins. *J Biol Chem* 1972;247:3774–3782.

Blum J, Coe F: Metabolic acidosis after sulfur ingestion. *N Engl J Med* 1977;297:869–870.

Zwart A, Buursma A, Kampen E, et al: Multicomponent analysis of hemoglobin derivatives with a reversed-optics spectrophotometer. *Clin Chem* 1984;30:373–379.

chapter 22

Drugs and Toxins Causing Methemoglobinemia

In biochemical terms, methemoglobin, or ferrihemoglobin, is an oxidation product and chemical analog of the normal blood pigment hemoglobin.[1] When iron is oxidized from the ferrous state in hemoglobin to the ferric state, methemoglobin is produced.[2] Oxygen bound to methemoglobin is so firmly attached that it is not available to tissues; consequently, methemoglobin is not an oxygen-transporting pigment.[3] Methemoglobin is normally present in a low concentration in red blood cells; total blood pigment is usually about 1% to 2% methemoglobin and the remainder is hemoglobin, with iron in the normal reduced state.[3–5] The percentage of methemoglobin is the ratio of methemoglobin to hemoglobin; for example a methemoglobin concentration of 50% means that in a patient with 16 g of hemoglobin 8 g is methemoglobin. The percentage can therefore be misleading, especially in the presence of anemia.

MECHANISMS FOR OXIDIZING METHEMOGLOBIN

Physiologically, within the red blood cell hemoglobin shifts continually from the reduced, functional, ferrous form to the oxidized, nonfunctional, ferric form (Fig. 22-1).[6,7] An equilibrium exists between hemoglobin and methemoglobin, the latter being continuously reduced in the cell. The most important mechanism for maintaining hemoglobin in the reduced form employs reduced nicotinamide adenine dinucleotide (NADH), which is formed from the oxidation of glucose, the electron donor.[2] Methemoglobin is reduced by NADH in the presence of the NADH-dependent enzyme methemoglobin reductase. Methemoglobin reductase is also known as diaphorase I or NADH-dehydrogenase. It is now known as NADH–cytochrome b_5 reductase and accounts for more than 95% of this reducing activity.[2]

Normal erythrocytes make use of a second mechanism for reducing hemoglobin by the generation of reduced nicotinamide adenine dinucleotide phosphate (NADPH). This is usually not an important mechanism because there is no endogenous electron acceptor, yet when the methemoglobin concentration in the cell rises to more than the physiologic 1% to 2% its activity can increase by up to a factor of 60. In addition, this mechanism may be activated by the presence of exogenously added electron carriers such as methylene blue.[2,8] Although this system plays no physiologic role, its therapeutic activation is an important procedure for the management of acute acquired methemoglobinemia.[9]

A third mechanism is nonenzymatic and involves glutathione and ascorbic acid. This reaction is normally slow. Under physiologic conditions, it is the NADH-dependent pathway that plays the major role in methemoglobin reduction.

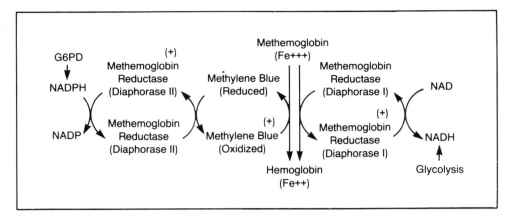

Figure 22-1 Mechanisms of methemoglobin reduction. G6PD indicates glucose-6-phosphate dehydrogenase; NADP, nicotinamide adenine dinucleotide phosphate; NADPH, nicotinamide adenine dinucleotide phosphate, reduced; NAD, nicotinamide adenine dinucleotide. *Source:* Reprinted with permission from *Journal of the American Medical Association* (1979;242:2871), Copyright © 1979, American Medical Association.

In methemoglobinemia the oxidized complexes do not bind oxygen, thus lowering hemoglobin's saturation without affecting arterial oxygen tension or arterial carbon dioxide pressure. Moreover, as with carbon monoxide, the remaining iron atoms in the hemoglobin tetramer bind oxygen more avidly in the presence of methemoglobin, causing a leftward shift in the oxyhemoglobin dissociation curve.[2,10,11] Both phenomena decrease oxygen delivery to the tissues.

Methemoglobinemia may result from (1) exposure to drugs or chemicals that accelerate the oxidation of hemoglobin beyond the reductive and protective capabilities of the cell, (2) deficiency in the ability to reduce methemoglobin (hereditary deficiency of NADH–methemoglobin reductase), and (3) the presence of a structural abnormality in hemoglobin.[3] This chapter deals only with exogenous substances that can cause an oxidation of hemoglobin (acquired methemoglobinemia).

ACQUIRED METHEMOGLOBINEMIA

Acquired methemoglobinemia results when the rate of formation of methemoglobin exceeds the rate of reduction secondary to the action of certain chemicals. A number of substances are capable of oxidizing hemoglobin directly to methemoglobin. In general, the cause of methemo-

globinemia relates to drugs, industrial exposure to certain chemicals, cultural dietary patterns, and recreational abuse of certain compounds. Compounds causing methemoglobinemia include the nitrites, chlorates, hydrogen peroxide, alloxan, the quinones, aniline dyes, local anesthetics, nitrobenzene, phenazopyridine, phenacetin, and others (Table 22-1).[1]

Nitrates and Nitrites

Nitrites are the chemicals that most frequently produce methemoglobinemia.[2] They are present in medicinal agents such as amyl nitrite, nitroglycerin,[11] and spirits of nitrite[12] as well as many other compounds.[13,14] Some of the nitrites are so toxic that only a small amount can rapidly cause intoxication that, if not treated, can lead to death.[15] Although the substances that contain nitrites are myriad, they may be divided into inorganic and organic compounds. The inorganic compounds are generally more toxic. These consist of sodium nitrite, potassium nitrite, bismuth subnitrate, and others. Organic nitrites include many drugs used in medicine.[15]

Because of its similarity in appearance to table salt and its use as a meat preservative and curing agent,[1] sodium nitrite is frequently the cause of methemoglobinemia associated with purposeful ingestion or with ingestion of contaminated food.[16] Methemoglobinemia has been caused by

Table 22-1 Causes of Acquired Methemoglobinemia

Nitrates and nitrites
  Bismuth subnitrate (Pepto-Bismol®)
  Nitrate-rich foods
  Nitrate-rich water
  Nitroglycerin
  Nitroprusside (Nipride®)
  Silver nitrate
  Sodium nitrite
  Volatile nitrites
    Amyl nitrite
    Butyl nitrite
    Isobutyl nitrite (Bolt®, Hardware®, Satan's scent®
      Locker room®, Quick silver®)
Local anesthetics
  Benzocaine (Unguentine®, Solarcaine®)
  Lidocaine (Xylocaine®)
  Prilocaine (Citanest®)
  Procaine (Novocain®)
Aromatic amino and nitroso compounds
  Aniline dyes (inks, shoe polishes)
  Nitrobenzene
  Nitrochlorobenzene
  Paranitroaniline
  Metachloroaniline
  Dinitrotoluene
  Phenazopyridine (Pyridium®)
Sulfonamides
  Dapsone
Miscellaneous
  Acetanalid
  Chlorates
  Methylene blue (large doses)
  Phenacetin
  Primaquine

---

nitrites added to sausage. Many times nearly maximum amounts of nitrite are added to meats because enhanced color is a desirable marketing technique.[17]

Methemoglobinemia has been reported in burn patients treated with silver nitrate.[18,19] The apparent mechanism for development of methemoglobinemia in these patients is nitrate reduction by bacteria on areas of granulation tissue with subsequent absorption of nitrite.[2,20]

There are many reports of nitrite-induced methemoglobinemia in infants fed well water contaminated with high concentrations of nitrates.[2,21–26] Nitrates are toxic only in amounts higher than those encountered in foods. The potential hazard of nitrate in water or food is its conversion to nitrite either before or after ingestion.[1] Methemoglobinemia has also been

reported in a home dialysis patient who was using well water high in nitrate concentration.[24]

Methemoglobinemia and Infants

Although persons of any age may be affected by methemoglobinemia, infants are particularly susceptible during the first 4 months of life.[1,24] Newborn infants normally have a low concentration of erythrocyte cytochrome b_5 reductase. The infant is also at risk from the ingestion of vegetables rich in nitrates, such as spinach, beets, carrots, turnips, and cabbage.[19,27] Nitrates do not directly oxidize hemoglobin to methemoglobin, but the nitrate can be converted by intestinal microflora to nitrite. It has been found that the nitrates normally present in these vegetables are reduced by bacteria, especially *Escherichia coli*, that colonize the upper gastrointestinal tract of some infants; these are introduced during preparation or storage of purees, soups, and stews.[2,15,19] Infants may be more susceptible to bacterial conversion because during the first few months of life they have a low gastric acidity, which can result in proliferation of bacterial species capable of reducing nitrate to nitrite.

Volatile Alkyl Nitrites

Although the volatile organic nitrites may cause methemoglobinemia, they are primarily inhaled as drugs of abuse.[7,28–32] For this reason, they are discussed with other chemical inhalants that are abused (see Chapter 33).

Miscellaneous Nitrite Compounds

Cases of methemoglobinemia that are due to nitrates have been reported after the use of bismuth subnitrate (Pepto-Bismol®), ammonium or potassium nitrate, and amyl nitrite and from the inhalation of nitrous gases by arc welders. Various reports list sublingual, oral, and intravenous nitroglycerin[33] as well as intravenous nitroprusside as causes of methemoglobinemia.

Local Anesthetics

Local anesthetics have induced methemoglobinemia. This has also been reported when benzocaine was applied as a gel to the gums of infants for the relief of teething pain.[2,34,35] Although prilocaine has been implicated most frequently,[36] topical procaine and lidocaine have also been noted to cause methemoglobinemia.[37] The case reports involving lidocaine all occurred in patients with enzyme deficiencies or some other condition predisposing them to methemoglobinemia.[38]

Aromatic Amino and Nitroso Compounds

Aniline Dyes and Nitrobenzene

Aniline, nitrobenzene, and their derivatives are found in many household products such as inks, shoe polishes, paints, and varnishes (Table 22-2). Aniline does not produce methemoglobinemia, but it is metabolized to active compounds in the body that are capable of forming methemoglobin. Three of these are the aminophenols, the phenylhydroxylamines, and the phenylenediamines. The most potent methemoglobin-generating metabolite is phenylhydroxylamine.[27] This compound is unstable and is readily oxidized to nitrosobenzene, which is the form that predominates in the circulation.[15]

Because aniline is a volatile liquid, it can gain access to the body by inhalation as well as by skin penetration.[39] When aniline dyes were in common use as laundry markers, dermal absorption from diaper markings caused numerous cases of methemoglobinemia.[2,12] In addition to methemoglobinemia, aniline has long been known to produce a Heinz-body hemolytic anemia.[27,40]

Phenazopyridine (Pyridium®)

Toxic reactions to phenazopyridine, an azo dye, appear to be exceedingly rare.[41] Both met-

hemoglobinemia and hemolytic anemia have been reported after an overdose of phenazopyridine as well as in patients with renal disease who were receiving the drug in therapeutic doses.[3,42] Patients with glucose-6-phosphate dehydrogenase deficiency have also been reported to develop methemoglobinemia after therapeutic doses of phenazopyridine.[43] Metabolism of phenazopyridine results in the formation of large quantities of aniline, and the production of methemoglobinemia by phenazopyridine is probably due to the aniline metabolites. Because the azo dye is deposited in the skin, a yellow skin pigmentation has been noted in cases of intoxication.[41,44]

The hemolysis secondary to the ingestion of phenazopyridine and other oxidizing agents may result in the appearance of bizarre red cell forms in the peripheral blood smear.[45] One such form has been named the ''bite cell'' or degmacyte because these red cells appear as though a bite has been taken out of them.[40]

Sulfonamides: Dapsone

Dapsone, a sulfonamide, has been used in the treatment of leprosy and dermatitis herpetiformis and for malaria prophylaxis in combination with other drugs. Common side effects include a dose-dependent hemolytic anemia and methemoglobinemia in normal individuals.[46,47]

The gastrointestinal absorption of dapsone is nearly complete. Concentrations in plasma reach their peak 1 to 3 hours after oral administration. The half-life of dapsone is 10 to 50 hours.

Miscellaneous Compounds: Chlorates

The chlorates (sodium and potassium) have occasionally been used therapeutically in mouth washes and gargles; they are also used in furniture polishes.[48] They are widely used in industry and as a nonselective weed killer. Because they have strong oxidizing properties, they have also been used commercially in the manufacture of explosives, matches, dyestuffs, tanning chemicals, and leather-finishing chemicals.[1] One of the characteristic features of chlorate poisoning is the great variability in toxic effects.

Table 22-2 Aniline Compounds

Coloring agents
Dyes
Inks
Laundry markers
Paints
Shoe polishes

The chlorates have three main actions: a local action that causes nausea, vomiting, and abdominal pain; the production of methemoglobinemia; and a late production of acute tubular necrosis.[48–50] The gastrointestinal symptoms are secondary to a direct action of the chlorates on the gastrointestinal tract. Because of their potent oxidizing action, methemoglobinemia may ensue.[51] The direct toxic effect on the red cell membrane may cause intense hemolysis.[52] The renal impairment appears to be due to a direct toxic effect on the proximal tubule with resultant anuria. This blocks the main route of elimination of the drug and prolongs the exposure time of the red blood cells to the oxidant effects.

SIGNS AND SYMPTOMS OF METHEMOGLOBINEMIA

Methemoglobinemia is manifested clinically by cyanosis. Because methemoglobin is incapable of binding with oxygen, the symptoms of methemoglobinemia are attributable to the hypoxia produced by the lowered oxygen-carrying capacity of the blood. As mentioned before, the oxygen-hemoglobin dissociation curve is also shifted to the left,[2,10] which makes the remaining oxyhemoglobin bind more tenaciously to the available oxygen. The severity of the symptoms is related to the quantity of methemoglobin present, the rapidity with which the methemoglobinemia develops, and the capacity of the patients' cardiorespiratory and hematopoietic system to adjust to hypoxia.

Methemoglobin is darker in color than unoxygenated hemoglobin and can produce a marked cyanosis even when present at concentrations that do not threaten life (Table 22-3). Symptoms of methemoglobinemia may vary from anxiety to headaches, fatigue, coma, and death. In patients without anemia, cyanosis first appears at methemoglobin concentrations of about 15%.[2] As the cyanosis increases, the lips, ears, and mucous membranes develop a violet cast that is unlike the bluish discoloration seen in oxygen desaturation.[2] This "chocolate cyanosis" is the hallmark of methemoglobinemia. In addition, methemoglobinemia-induced cyanosis im-

Table 22-3 Methemoglobin Concentrations and Symptomatology

Methemoglobin Concentration (percent)	Symptoms
10 to 15	Cyanosis "Chocolate cyanosis"
20 to 40	Headache Fatigue Weakness Dizziness
40 to 60	Lethargy Dyspnea Bradycardia Respiratory depression Stupor
60 to 80	Seizures Coma Death

proves little when even high concentrations of oxygen are administered.

In general, patients with acquired methemoglobinemia tolerate concentrations of methemoglobin up to 20% without ill effects.[53] At concentrations of 20% to 25%, symptoms such as headache, fatigue, tachycardia, weakness, and dizziness may appear. When methemoglobin concentrations reach 55% to 60%, oxygenation of tissues becomes inadequate; this may result in dyspnea, lethargy, metabolic acidosis, and sinus bradycardia and other dysrhythmias. Neurologic manifestations such as paralysis, coma, and seizures may also occur. Death occurs with concentrations greater than 70% and is due to heart failure from hypoxia.[1,2] The urine may be brown to black in color as a result of the presence of methemoglobin.

The toxic signs of acquired methemoglobinemia have been noted to be more severe than those produced by a corresponding degree of anemia. This is because methemoglobin, like carboxyhemoglobin, not only decreases the available oxygen-carrying pigment but also increases the affinity of the unaltered hemoglobin for oxygen, thus further impairing oxygen delivery.[1]

TOXIC EFFECTS UNRELATED TO METHEMOGLOBINEMIA

An acute toxic methemoglobinemia causes more pronounced symptoms than chronic methemoglobinemia. Methemoglobin concentrations that are relatively benign when caused by congenital defects are likely to produce more severe signs if induced by a chemical for two reasons. First, otherwise normal subjects do not have the compensatory mechanisms that develop over a lifetime, and second, a strong possibility always exists of additional toxic effects or side effects of the chemical agent. Any chemical agent used to generate methemoglobin may have additional toxic effects, which may make profound contributions to the toxic syndrome. Some aromatic amino and nitro compounds, such as aniline and nitrobenzene, have central and prominent cardiac effects. Chlorate salts produce intravascular hemolysis, gastroenteritis, and nephritis.[2] Inorganic salts of nitrite and organic nitrates and nitrites also act directly as peripheral vasodilators. It is doubtful that any chemical agent produces an otherwise uncomplicated methemoglobinemia. Therefore, it is inappropriate and misleading to suggest that there is a lethal concentration of methemoglobin without taking into account the particular agent involved.

DIAGNOSIS

The diagnosis of methemoglobinemia is not difficult to make if it is considered in the differential diagnosis of the cyanotic patient, particularly in the absence of cardiac or pulmonary disease and if the cyanosis is not promptly alleviated by oxygen therapy.[2] Direct measurements of methemoglobin will confirm the diagnosis.

About 5 g of deoxyhemoglobin per 100 mL of blood are required to produce visible cyanosis, but a comparable discoloration is produced by 1.5 to 2 g of methemoglobin per 100 mL.[1,10,42] The greater visible effects of this abnormal pigment are due to alterations in the absorption spectra.[6,7] A confirmation of the diagnosis can therefore be made by means of a spectrophotometric method, which measures the amount of methemoglobin present. Although methemoglobin concentrations expressed as a percentage of total hemoglobin in the methemoglobin form are reported, the total hemoglobin must always be taken into consideration.[2]

TREATMENT

Profound methemoglobinemia shares with narcotic overdose, hypoglycemia, organophosphate poisoning, and cyanide poisoning the need for treatment before a definitive diagnosis is made. Many times a decision must be made on the basis of strong clinical suspicion. Survival is possible with methemoglobinemia concentrations of 75% if immediate treatment with antidotal therapy is instituted (Table 22-4).

Acute overdose should be treated by inducing emesis or with gastric lavage followed by the administration of oral charcoal and a cathartic. Because some of the agents that cause methemoglobinemia can be percutaneously absorbed, a patient's contaminated clothing should be removed and the skin decontaminated by a thorough washing with soap and water.[2] Supplemental oxygen, even in the presence of normal oxygen partial pressure, is recommended, the aim being to saturate the remaining functional hemoglobin with oxygen.

In cases where the methemoglobin concentration is less than 45%, supportive care will usually suffice. In the absence of serious signs of hypoxia, removal of the offending chemical agent is the only therapy required because normal reducing mechanisms within the erythrocyte will usually convert methemoglobin to hemoglobin within 48 to 72 hours. Usually no specific

Table 22-4 Treatment of Acquired Methemoglobinemia

Condition	Modality
Acute ingestion	Emesis or lavage
	Charcoal and cathartic
	Naloxone or glucose
Dermal exposure	Decontamination
	Supplemental oxygen
Stupor or coma	Methylene blue (1 to 2 mg/kg of 1% sterile solution)

therapy is required unless stupor or coma is present.

Methylene Blue

When the degree of methemoglobinemia is so pronounced that semistupor or unconsciousness is present, an emergency exists and treatment must be prompt.[6] The chief feature of antidotal treatment consists of the intravenous injection of methylene blue (tetramethylthionine chloride).

It may seem to be paradoxical that methylene blue, which is a methemoglobin former, is effective in decreasing methemoglobinemia.[54] Actually, methylene blue is not a good methemoglobin former in vivo in humans. Doses much smaller than those that produce methemoglobin are capable of reducing methemoglobin because, in low concentrations, methylene blue forms a reversible oxidation-reduction system that can enhance erythrocyte reduction of methemoglobin.[2] In high concentrations, however, it can oxidize hemoglobin to methemoglobin and thus increase methemoglobinemia.[6] The enzymatic reduction of methemoglobin normally accounts for only a small portion of the methemoglobin-reducing activity of the red blood cell. When methylene blue is administered exogenously, this reaction is greatly accelerated. When methylene blue is administered in its oxidized form, it is reduced to a colorless, reduced form called leukomethylene blue. Leukomethylene blue acts as an electron donor and nonenzymatically reduces methemoglobin to hemoglobin.[2,6,8,12]

Methylene blue, when indicated, should be administered in a dose of 1 to 2 mg/kg intravenously as a 1% sterile aqueous or saline solution. It can be administered from a 10 mL syringe over 5 minutes; this is repeated in 1 to 2 hours if necessary.[3,6,10,15] The total dose should not exceed 7 mg/kg.[2]

Maximal response to methylene blue usually occurs within 30 to 60 minutes; therefore, methemoglobin concentrations should be monitored for approximately 1 hour after administration.[54] If the patient does not respond to methylene blue treatment within 30 to 60 minutes, other possibilities for the diagnosis should be considered.[55] For example, there may be an associated glucose-6-phosphate dehydrogenase deficiency that could lead to hemolysis, or there may be a subclinical deficiency in methemoglobin reductase, or the diagnosis may be incorrect.[56]

Methylene blue has been implicated as a cause of hemolytic anemia, but only in very large doses (usually greater than 7 mg/kg) or in the presence of glucose-6-phosphate dehydrogenase deficiency (Table 22-5). Nonspecific side effects of methylene blue seen with high doses include apprehension, precordial pain, dyspnea, restlessness, and tremors. Often the urine appears dark blue because some of the dye is present in the blue or oxidized form. Because of the irritating effect of this compound in the excreted form, dysuria may occur. Finally, as mentioned above, high concentrations of methylene blue may cause methemoglobinemia by directly oxidizing hemoglobin to methemoglobin.[57]

Ascorbic Acid

Although ascorbic acid can also reduce methemoglobin and has been used to treat hereditary methemoglobinemia, it has no place in the management of acquired methemoglobinemia because the rate at which it reduces methemoglobin is too slow to be of any benefit for severe poisoning.[37,58] In addition, it may produce a large number of Heinz bodies.

Exchange Transfusion

There has been only limited experience with exchange transfusion in methemoglobinemia.

Table 22-5 Side Effects of Methylene Blue

Precordial pain
Dyspnea
Restlessness
Apprehension
Tremors
Blue urine
Dysuria
Urinary frequency
Hemolytic anemia (with large doses in glucose-6-
  phosphate dehydrogenase deficiency)
Methemoglobinemia (with large doses)

As a treatment, it has the advantage of reducing blood concentrations of the offending chemical as well as restoring functional blood pigment. This advantage, however, must be weighed against the attendant risks of multiple blood transfusions.[27]

Hyperbaric Oxygen

Hyperbaric oxygen has been recommended for the treatment of chemically induced methemoglobinemia, but there is no evidence that it is effective and there has been little experience with its use.[59]

REFERENCES

1. Bodansky O: Methemoglobinemia and methemoglobin-producing compounds. *Pharmacol Rev* 1951; 3:144–196.

2. Curry S: Methemoglobinemia. *Ann Emerg Med* 1982;11:214–221.

3. Cohen B, Bovasso G: Acquired methemoglobinemia and hemolytic anemia following excessive pyridium (phenazopyridine hydrochloride) ingestion. *Clin Pediatr* 1971;10:537–540.

4. Fibuch E, Cecil W, Reed W: Methemoglobinemia associated with organic nitrate therapy. *Anesth Analg* 1979;58:521–523.

5. Smith R, Olson M: Drug-induced methemoglobinemia. *Semin Hematol* 1973;10:253–268.

6. Cohen R, Sachs J, Wicker D, et al: Methemoglobinemia provoked by malarial chemoprophylaxis in Vietnam. *N Engl J Med* 1968;279:1127–1131.

7. Cohen S: The volatile nitrites. *JAMA* 1979; 241:2077–2078.

8. Lukens J: The legacy of well-water methemoglobinemia. *JAMA* 1987;257:2793–2795.

9. Metz E, Balcerzak S, Sagone A: Mechanisms of methylene blue stimulation of the hexose monophosphate shunt in erythrocytes. *J Clin Invest* 1976;58:797–802.

10. Fibuch E, Cecil W, Reed W: Methemoglobinemia associated with organic nitrate therapy. *Anesth Analg* 1979;58:521–523.

11. Gibson G, Hunter J, Raabe D, et al: Methemoglobinemia produced by high-dose intravenous nitroglycerin. *Ann Intern Med* 1982;96:615–616.

12. Chilcote R, Williams B, Wolff L, et al: Sudden death in an infant from methemoglobinemia after administration of "sweet spirits of nitre." *Pediatrics* 1977;59:280–282.

13. Smith M, Stair T, Rolnick M: Butyl nitrite and a suicide attempt. *Ann Intern Med* 1980;92:719–720.

14. Smith R: The nitrite methemoglobin complex—Its significance in methemoglobin analyses and its possible role in methemoglobinemia. *Biochem Pharmacol* 1967;16:1655–1664.

15. Schimelman M, Soler J, Muller H: Methemoglobinemia: Nitrobenzene ingestion. *JACEP* 1978;7: 406–408.

16. Ten-Brink W, Wiezer J, Luijpen A, et al: Nitrate poisoning caused by food contaminated with cooling fluid. *J Toxicol Clin Toxicol* 1982;19:139–147.

17. Bakshi S, Fahey J, Pierce L: Sausage cyanosis—Acquired methemoglobinemic nitrite poisoning. *N Engl J Med* 1967;277:1082.

18. Cushing A, Smith S: Methemoglobinemia with silver nitrate therapy of a burn: Report of a case. *J Pediatr* 1967;74:613–615.

19. Geffner M, Powars D, Choctaw W: Acquired methemoglobinemia. *West J Med* 1981;134:7–10.

20. Strauch B, Buch W, Grey W: Successful treatment of methemoglobinemia secondary to silver nitrate therapy. *N Engl J Med* 1969;281:257–258.

21. Comly H: Cyanosis in infants caused by nitrates in well water. *JAMA* 1987;257:2788–2792.

22. Grant R: Well water nitrate poisoning review: A survey in Nebraska, 1973 to 1978. *Nebr Med J* 1981;66:197–200.

23. Johnson C, Bonrud P, Dosch T, et al: Fatal outcome of methemoglobinemia in an infant. *JAMA* 1987; 257:2796–2797.

24. Miller L: Methemoglobinemia associated with well water. *JAMA* 1971;216:1642–1643.

25. Shearer L, Goldsmith J, Young C, et al: Methemoglobin levels in infants in an area with high nitrate water supply. *Am J Public Health* 1972;62:1174–1180.

26. Vigil J, Warburton S, Haynes W, et al: Nitrates in municipal water supply cause methemoglobinemia in an infant. *Public Health Rep* 1965;80:1119–1121.

27. Kearney T, Manoguerra A, Dunford J: Chemically induced methemoglobinemia from aniline poisoning. *West J Med* 1984;140:282–286.

28. Dixon D, Reisch R, Santinga P: Fatal methemoglobinemia resulting from ingestion of isobutyl nitrite, a "room odorizer" widely used for recreational purposes. *J Forensic Sci* 1981;26:587–593.

29. Horne M, Waterman M, Simon L, et al: Methemoglobinemia from sniffing butyl nitrite. *Ann Intern Med* 1979;91:417–418.

30. Lowry T: Amyl nitrite and the EEG: A pilot study. *J Psychedelic Drugs* 1979;11:239–241.

31. Munjack D: Sex and drugs. *Clin Toxicol* 1979; 15:75–89.

32. Shesser R, Mitchell J, Edelstein S: Methemoglobinemia from isobutyl nitrite preparations. *Ann Emerg Med* 1981;10:262–264.

33. Marshall J, Ecklund R: Methemoglobinemia from overdose on nitroglycerin. *JAMA* 1980;244:330.

34. McGuigan M: Benzocaine-induced methemoglobinemia. *Can Med Assoc J* 1981;125:816.

35. O'Donohue W, Moss L, Angelillo V: Acute methemoglobinemia induced by topical benzocaine and lidocaine. *Arch Intern Med* 1980;140:1508–1509.

36. Ludwig S: Acute toxic methemoglobinemia following dental analgesia. *Ann Emerg Med* 1981;10:265–266.

37. Potter J, Hillman J: Benzocaine-induced methemoglobinemia. *JACEP* 1979;8:26–27.

38. Weiss L, Generalovich T, Heller M, et al: Methemoglobin levels following intravenous lidocaine administration. *Ann Emerg Med* 1987;16:323–325.

39. Harrison M: Toxic methemoglobinemia. *Anaesthesia* 1977;32:270–272.

40. Greenberg M: Heinz-body hemolytic anemia. *Arch Intern Med* 1976;136:153–155.

41. Alano F, Webster G: Acute renal failure and pigmentation due to phenazopyridine (Pyridium®). *Ann Intern Med* 1970;72:89–91.

42. Zimmerman R, Green E, Ghurabi W, et al: Methemoglobinemia from overdose of phenazopyridine hydrochloride. *Ann Emerg Med* 1980;9:147–149.

43. Jeffery W, Zelicoff A, Hardy W: Acquired methemoglobinemia and hemolytic anemia after usual doses of phenazopyridine. *Drug Intell Clin Pharmacol* 1982;16:157–159.

44. Eybel C, Armbruster K, Ing T: Skin pigmentation and acute renal failure in a patient receiving phenazopyridine therapy. *JAMA* 1974;228:1027–1028.

45. Nathan D, Siegel A, Bunn F: Acute methemoglobinemia and hemolytic anemia with phenazopyridine. *Arch Intern Med* 1977;137:1636–1638.

46. Cooke T: Dapsone poisoning. *Med J Aust* 1970;1:1158–1159.

47. Iserson K: Methemoglobinemia from dapsone therapy for a suspected brown spider bite. *J Emerg Med* 1985;3:285–288.

48. Steffen C, Seitz R: Severe chlorate poisoning: Report of a case. *Arch Toxicol* 1981;48:281–288.

49. Jackson R, Elder W, McDonnell H: Sodium chlorate poisoning. *Lancet* 1961;2:1381–1383.

50. Timperman J, Maes R: Suicidal poisoning by sodium chlorate. *J Forensic Med* 1966;13:123–129.

51. Sheahan B, Pugh D, Winstanley E: Experimental sodium chlorate poisoning in dogs. *Rev Vet Sci* 1971;12:387–389.

52. Stoodley B, Rowe D: Hematological complications of chlorate poisoning. *Br Med J* 1970;2:31–32.

53. Hall A, Kulig K, Rumack B: Drug and chemical induced methemoglobinemia. *Med Toxicol* 1986;1:253–260.

54. Sheehy M, Way J: Nitrite intoxication: Protection with methylene blue and oxygen. *Toxicol Appl Pharmacol* 1974;30:221–226.

55. Rosen P, Johnson C, McGehee W, et al: Failure of methylene blue treatment in toxic methemoglobinemia. *Ann Intern Med* 1971;75:83–86.

56. Harris J, Rumack B, Peterson R, et al: Methemoglobinemia resulting from absorption of nitrates. *JAMA* 1979;242:2869–2871.

57. Whitman J, Taylor A, White J: Potential hazard of methylene blue. *Anaesthesia* 1979;34:181–182.

58. Bolyai J, Smith R, Gray C: Ascorbic acid and chemically induced methemoglobinemia. *Toxicol Appl Pharmacol* 1972;21:176–185.

59. Goldstein G, Doull J: Treatment of nitrite-induced methemoglobinemia with hyperbaric oxygen. *Proc Soc Exp Biol Med* 1971;138:137–139.

ADDITIONAL SELECTED REFERENCES

Carlson D, Shapiro F: Methemoglobinemia from well water nitrates: A complication of home dialysis. *Ann Intern Med* 1970;73:757–759.

Chugh K, Singhal P, Sharma B: Methemoglobinemia in acute copper sulfate poisoning. *Ann Intern Med* 1975;82:226–229.

Clark D, Litchfield M: Role of inorganic nitrite in methemoglobin formation after nitrate ester administration to the rat. *Br J Pharmacol* 1973;48:162–168.

Clutton-Brock J: Two cases of poisoning by contamination of nitrous oxide with higher oxides of nitrogen during anaesthesia. *Br J Anesth* 1967;39:388–392.

Fisher A, Brancaccio R, Jelinek J: Facial dermatitis in men due to inhalation of butyl nitrite. *Cutis* 1981;27:146–153.

Goluboff N, Wheaton R: Methylene blue–induced cyanosis and acute hemolytic anemia complicating the treatment of methemoglobinemia. *J Pediatr* 1961;58:86–89.

Haley T: Review of the physiological effects of amyl, butyl, and isobutyl nitrites. *Clin Toxicol* 1980;16:317–329.

Harvey J, Keitt A: Studies of the efficacy and potential hazards of methylene blue therapy in aniline-induced methemoglobinemia. *Br J Haematol* 1983;54:29–41.

Keating J, Lell M, Strauss A, et al: Infantile methemoglobinemia caused by carrot juice. *N Engl J Med* 1973;288:824–826.

Lynn E, Walter R, Harris L, et al: Nitrous oxide: It's a gas. *J Psychedelic Drugs* 1972;5:1–7.

Wason S, Detsky A, Platt O, et al: Isobutyl nitrite toxicity by ingestion. *Ann Intern Med* 1980;92:637–638.

Yano S, Danish E, Hsia Y: Transient methemoglobinemia with acidosis in infants. *J Pediatr* 1982;100:415–418.

part VII

THE ALCOHOLS

chapter 23

Ethyl Alcohol

Probably the most frequent cause of a patient presenting to an emergency department with an altered mental status involves the acute ingestion of ethyl alcohol.[1,2] Ethanol is the most widely abused "drug" and is a component of overdose in up to 70% of cases.[3–6] In addition, physicians frequently encounter sequelae from the multi-system dysfunction caused by the chronic ingestion of ethanol.[7] Therefore, the physician must be aware of the effects expected from both the acute and chronic ingestion of ethyl alcohol or its substitutes.[2,4] Substitutes consist of methanol, ethylene glycol, and isopropyl alcohol (Table 23-1).[1] The emergency physician sees a large and increasing number of patients with problems related to alcohol and must be prepared to deal with these problems in an efficient and cost-effective manner.[5] The clinician must be able to identify and treat acute and chronic alcohol intoxication and acute ingestion of ethylene glycol and methanol and to use serum osmolality

and anion gap measurements in rendering a diagnosis of a toxic or medical disorder.[1]

The chapters in this section are devoted to a discussion of each of these alcohols and of the manner in which to evaluate the patient who may have ingested an alcohol substitute, an act that can lead to permanent organ damage. The alcohols of concern are ethyl alcohol (Chapter 23), isopropyl alcohol (Chapter 24), and ethylene glycol and methanol (Chapter 25). All are low–molecular weight, water-soluble substances with prominent multiorgan toxicity. Although they are related, each one has a separate toxicity.

ETHYL ALCOHOL (ETHANOL): SOURCES AND USES

Ethyl alcohol has many industrial and domestic uses. The consumer may encounter ethanol as a solvent in medicines or other pharmaceuticals or imbibe ethanol in alcoholic beverages (Table 23-2).

Ethanol As a Medicinal Agent

Ethanol is used as a solvent in many medicinal and nonmedicinal preparations, including antiseptics.[2,8–10] Applied locally, ethanol acts as an astringent and antimicrobial. It also acts as an

---

Table 23-1 The Alcohols

Ethyl alcohol (ethanol)
Ethylene glycol
Isopropyl alcohol (isopropanol)
Methyl alcohol (methanol)
Propylene glycol
Diethylene glycol

Table 23-2 Uses of Ethanol

Solvent
Antiseptic (local)
Astrigent (local)
Antimicrobial (local)
Nerve block
Treatment of methanol overdose
Treatment of ethylene glycol overdose

irritant. Ethyl alcohol is used externally as a solvent of many drugs as well as a skin disinfectant.[11] Ethanol is injected as a nerve block in the management of certain types of intractable pain, as with trigeminal neuralgia, inoperable cancer, and sciatica. Intravenous ethanol is also used for the treatment of methanol and ethylene glycol poisoning because of its ability to be preferentially metabolized by the common enzyme alcohol dehydrogenase.

Ethanol in Other Pharmaceuticals

Other easily available substances may contain ethanol, although the presence or the amount of ethanol may be unknown to the user. Household ethanol sources include perfumes, colognes, aftershaves, mouthwashes, antiseptics, elixirs, and food extracts (Table 23-3).[13] As an example, in the five most popular mouthwashes the

Table 23-3 Usual Concentration of Ethyl Alcohol in Common Products

Product	Concentration (percent)
Aftershave	15–80
Cements	7–30
Cough preparations	3–25
Elixirs	2–10
Extracts	40–90
Gasohol	10
Glass cleaners	10
Hair tonics	25–65
Liquid hand-washing detergent	1–10
Mouthwash	15–25
Paint stripper	25
Perfumes	25–95
Rubbing alcohol	70–90

concentration of ethanol ranges from 14% to 27%. Because mouthwashes are classified as cosmetics, they are not well regulated, are thought to be innocuous, and are often kept within easy reach of children. In addition, mouthwashes are frequently sold in containers large enough to supply a fatal dose of ethanol to a child.[14] Colognes and perfumes are more than 60% ethanol, and lemon extract is as much as 80% ethanol.[2] Most liquid-based oral medications contain some ethanol in widely variable concentrations. Liquid medications commonly prescribed for coughs, colds, congestion, and asthma usually contain ethanol in the range of 15% to 20%.

Ethanol in Beverages

The use of ethanol-containing beverages goes back almost to the beginning of recorded history. Wine is produced from the fermentation of grapes and other fruits, which causes the alcohol content of the fermentation liquid to rise from 12% to 18%.[2] Wines may be distilled to produce brandies with higher ethyl alcohol content or be fortified with added ethanol (Table 23-4).[12] Another source for ethanol-containing beverages is cereal grains. Corn produces bourbon, barley produces scotch, potatoes produce vodka, and molasses produces rum. Typically, beer and ale, which are produced from the fermentation of cereals, contain 3% to 6% ethanol; wine is 10% to 18% ethanol; brandy is approximately 40% ethanol; and hard liquors contain 40% to 50% ethanol.[2]

Table 23-4 Sources of Ethanol for Use As a Beverage

Beverage	Source	Alcohol content (percent)
Wine	Grapes	12–18
Brandy	Wine	40–50
Bourbon	Corn	40–50
Scotch	Barley	40–50
Vodka	Potatoes	40–50
Rum	Molasses	40–50
Beer	Cereals	3–6
Ale	Cereals	3–6

The strength of ethanol is usually stated in volume-percent, which indicates the volumes of ethanol in 100 volumes of fluid. The term proof indicates twice the concentration in volume-percent, so that 100 proof equals 50 volume-percent or 50% ethanol.[2]

Thirty milliliters (1 oz) of 80 proof whiskey can be expected to raise the serum ethanol concentration by approximately 25 to 30 mg/dL in a 70-kg individual.[1] A 12-oz can of beer and 4-oz glass of wine raise the ethanol as much as 1 oz of liquor.[2,13]

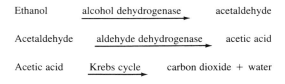

Figure 23-1 Metabolism of Ethanol

PHARMACOKINETICS

Blood ethanol concentrations after an ingestion of ethanol are affected by the rate of absorption from the gastrointestinal tract, the space of distribution in the body, and the rate of elimination.[15]

Ethyl alcohol is absorbed rapidly by diffusion mainly from the small intestine and to a lesser extent from the stomach and large intestine.[15] Concentrations reach a peak usually 30 to 60 minutes after ingestion.[16] There may be a delay if food is present in the stomach.[17] Carbonation appears to increase the rate of absorption of ethanol.[18] The volume of distribution of ethanol is 0.6 L/kg, which is approximately equal to that of total body water, so that ethanol diffuses freely in body tissues. It is neither accumulated to any extent by specific organs nor preferentially bound to cellular components.

METABOLISM

The metabolism of ethanol occurs principally through oxidative metabolism in the liver (Fig. 23-1).[15] Consequently, after an initial equilibrium phase the primary determinant of the duration and extent of ethanol's pharmacological actions is the rate of its oxidative metabolism by alcohol dehydrogenase to form acetaldehyde; this process requires nicotinamide adenine dinucleotide (NAD).[18] Acetaldehyde is then oxidized to acetate by the enzyme aldehyde dehydrogenase. Acetate (acetic acid) is then oxidized through the Krebs cycle, with the eventual production of carbon dioxide and water,

mostly in the peripheral tissues.[2,17] This first reaction, in which the enzyme alcohol dehydrogenase is used, essentially occurs by zero-order kinetics, with the rate of decay being constant and independent of concentration.[1,2]

There may be three separate pathways for metabolism of ethanol in the liver.[18] The alcohol dehydrogenase pathway is the predominant system, and this system has been found to contain a number of isoenzymes that appear to account for the great variability in metabolism among individuals. The second pathway is the microsomal ethanol-oxidizing system located in the endoplasmic reticulum. There is considerable controversy concerning the role of this system, which may be associated with the cytochrome P-450 mixed-function oxidase system in the liver.[19] The third system involves the catalases located in the perioxisomes.[18]

In most individuals, the rate of metabolism of ethanol is in the range of 15 to 25 mg/dL/hour regardless of the plasma concentration.[2,20] This variation parallels the history of ethanol use; it is approximately 12 mg/dL/hour in nondrinkers, 15 mg/dL/hour in social drinkers, and up to 30 mg/dL/hour in alcoholics.[16] In other words, it takes a 150-lb person approximately 1 hour to metabolize the amount of ethanol in 10 oz of beer.

Most authorities no longer hold that the rate of ethanol metabolism can be materially increased by the co-administration of other substances, such as fructose or other sugars, hormones, vitamins, or enzymatic cofactors.[21–25]

Intoxication from ethanol ingestion largely depends on how quickly a blood ethanol concentration has been attained as well as on the length of time it has been maintained.[26] Because ethyl alcohol is rapidly absorbed from the stomach, the blood concentration is usually at or near maximum on evaluation.

ACUTE INTOXICATION

Because alcohol often induces euphoria, it is frequently mistakenly classified as a stimulant rather than a depressant. This is because inhibitory synapses in the brain are depressed slightly earlier than are excitatory synapses with low doses of ethanol.[2] Ethanol, however, acts as a sedative-hypnotic throughout the entire CNS.

For the most part, the patient acutely poisoned by ethanol has intentionally ingested a large amount of ethanol. Occasionally the CNS depression may be a cause for the patient being brought to an emergency department, but usually the physician is evaluating a patient who has concomitant trauma or other medical problems, with ethanol ingestion being an additional finding.[27]

The acute ingestion of ethanol may result in decreased inhibitions, visual impairment, diplopia, nystagmus, muscular incoordination, slurred speech, ataxia, slowing of reaction time, tachycardia, vasodilation, hypoglycemia (especially in children), stupor, and depression of the deep tendon reflexes.[17,28–31] In severe stages, hypothermia, hypoventilation, hypotension, and possibly cardiovascular collapse may be seen.[32–34]

Blood concentrations greater than 50 mg/dL (0.05%) may be associated with some impairment, and concentrations greater than 100 mg/dL (0.1%) are generally used as evidence of driving while intoxicated. Interpretations of the physiologic effects of a particular blood alcohol concentration may be difficult because there is such wide variability among individuals. This is especially true in the individual who chronically ingests ethyl alcohol.[16] Despite large individual variation, if a patient is comatose at a blood concentration of 50 or 100 mg/dL, it is likely that another problem coexists. Ethanol concentrations in the range of 100 to 250 mg/dL generally cause mental confusion, ataxia, nystagmus, exaggerated emotional states, and incoordination. Most fatal intoxications are associated with ethanol concentrations greater than 400 mg/dL, although the highest reported concentration in a survivor was 1510 mg/dL.[35,36] The physiologic effects that may be expected in the occasional drinker are listed in Table 23-5.

Table 23-5 Ethanol Concentration and Acute Symptomatology

Concentration (milligrams per 100 mL)	Symptoms
50	Mild muscle incoordination
50–100	Incoordination Slow reaction time Decreased inhibitions Blurred vision
100–300	Diplopia Visual impairment Ataxia Hypoglycemia Slurred speech Decreased motor skills
300–400	Marked incoordination Stupor Hypoglycemia Hypothermia Seizures
>400	Coma Respiratory failure Death

LABORATORY ANALYSIS

When ethyl alcohol use is combined with multiple drug overdose, head injury, coma, major trauma, seizures, or psychosis, it is particularly important to obtain an ethanol concentration.[16,27,37] The most commonly used specimen for obtaining an ethanol level is the blood,[20] although the breath and occasionally the urine may be used. The saliva is infrequently used. Capillary and arterial blood most accurately indicate the brain ethanol concentrations; venous blood lags slightly in ethanol content during the absorption-distribution phase. The determination of serum ethanol concentration can be done in most hospital laboratories in 30 to 60 minutes. Postmortem blood is subject to putrefaction and fermentation, whereby the destruction and neoformation of ethyl alcohol is possible.

Techniques for the determination of serum ethanol include diffusion or distillation, oxidation of the alcohol, and osmometric, enzymatic, and gas chromatographic procedures. Early techniques for blood ethanol determination used distillation, aeration, or diffusion to separate the alcohol from plasma. This was a colorimetric method that was nonspecific and gave a reaction with all volatiles, including ketones. Osmometry by freezing-point depression was also nonspecific because all alcohols cause an osmolal gap. Enzymatic methods employ alcohol dehydrogenase, which reacts primarily with ethanol but not with methanol or acetone. This is a spectrophotometric method that is specific for ethanol. Gas chromatographic methods by flame ionization separate the alcohols on a chromatographic column and are specific for most alcohols. Laboratory differentiation of the alcohols should be performed with gas chromatography whenever possible.

The breath alcohol analyzer has been studied extensively and shown to be sufficiently accurate for clinical use.[16,38] The pocket-sized instrument measures the amount of ethyl alcohol in a sample of expired air by electrochemical oxidation and gives a digitally displayed reading of the equivalent blood ethanol. Breath is a reliable specimen for the measurement of ethanol because there is a fairly constant equilibrium of ethanol in blood and alveolar air. The breath analyzer should not be used within 15 minutes of the last drink because it gives a falsely high reading.[18]

Urine may be utilized as an alternative specimen, but the ethanol in a random urine specimen is not necessarily in equilibrium with that in the blood. This is because the bladder contents represent urine produced over a period of time, during which the blood ethanol concentration may have risen or fallen.[38]

TREATMENT

Although acute ethyl alcohol coma may be a potentially life-threatening situation, the treatment of the acute ingestion is relatively straightforward (Table 23-6). If the patient presents with an altered mental status, 2 mg of naloxone, 25 g of glucose, and 50 to 100 mg of thiamine should be administered.[17] If the patient responds to the dextrose, a continuous infusion of 10% dextrose should be administered. Unless concomitant ingestion of other drugs is suspected, ipecac or gastric lavage is

Table 23-6 Treatment of Ethyl Alcohol Overdose

Condition	Treatment
Altered mental status	Naloxone
	Glucose
	Thiamine
Hypoventilation	Mechanical ventilation
Ketoacidosis	Glucose
	Normal saline
Hypotension	Normal saline
	Trendelenburg's position
	Vasopressors

probably useful only if performed within 2 hours of ingestion of ethanol. There have been conflicting reports as to the adsorption of ethanol by charcoal. Some investigators have reported no significant adsorption, and others found moderate adsorption.[39]

If alveolar hypoventilation is present, a patent airway with supportive mechanical ventilation must be established. Correction of fluid deficits, acid-base disturbances, and hypothermia are important ancillary measures.

Ketoacidosis can be treated with glucose and saline. Insulin is not indicated, and bicarbonate therapy is usually not necessary. Hypotension generally responds well to volume replacement. Further treatment consists of treating any associated medical conditions. Analeptic agents are not only useless but dangerous and are to be avoided.

There have been many claims concerning the beneficial effect of fructose on accelerating the metabolism of ethyl alcohol and leading to a shortened clinical course. In theory, because ethyl alcohol requires NAD for its metabolism and because fructose can enhance the production of NAD by enhancing oxidation of NADH (the reduced form of NAD), enhanced alcohol metabolism results from administration of fructose. Nevertheless, because the rate of oxidation of alcohol is limited by the enzyme alcohol dehydrogenase and not by the availability of NAD, it is not surprising that this theory has not been substantiated.[21] Fructose, then, has not been shown to accelerate effectively the rate of ethanol metabolism or to decrease the amount of time of coma. In addition, the use of fructose has been associated with increased serum uric acid and lactate concentrations[23] leading to the increased likelihood of lactic acidosis.

Forced diuresis is ineffective in enhancing the removal of ethanol because most ethanol is eliminated by hepatic metabolism.[17] Hemodialysis increases ethanol elimination but is rarely required clinically because most patients can be effectively managed conservatively. The development of an alcohol antagonist may be helpful in the future for diagnosis of the inebriated patient with a concomitant medical condition.

ALCOHOL WITHDRAWAL

Because of the widespread abuse of ethyl alcohol, withdrawal from chronic ethanol consumption is the most common withdrawal syndrome encountered in the emergency department.[26,40–43] Ethanol is a cellular depressant, so that with its abrupt cessation a rebound neuronal hyperexcitability occurs, the severity of which is directly related to the amount of ethyl alcohol that was regularly consumed.[1,44]

The early stages of ethanol withdrawal are characterized by hyperactivity of the autonomic nervous system manifested by tachycardia and hypertension, diaphoresis, motor activity manifested by generalized tremulousness, and CNS hyperactivity manifested by insomnia and irritability.[45,46] These withdrawal symptoms begin within 12 to 24 hours after the cessation of ethanol ingestion and may last for 48 to 72 hours.

Acute ethanol withdrawal syndrome, with its inherent morbidity and mortality, can be complicated by its traditional pharmacologic management. Most patients experiencing acute alcohol withdrawal do not require pharmacologic intervention. A small percentage, however, may develop severe complications requiring pharmacologic intervention. Complications may include significant dysrhythmias or hypertension, seizures, hallucinations, and delirium tremens. In the past, sedative hypnotics such as barbiturates were used for withdrawal. These agents have their own inherent toxicity and their use was discouraged, but they are still advocated by some authorities.[47]

The benzodiazepines are now considered one of the safest classes of compounds for the treatment of alcohol withdrawal.[48] They are prescribed to alcoholics more often than any other psychoactive drug.[49] Not only are the benzodiazepines effective in suppressing the withdrawal symptoms and in treating or preventing seizures, but they also are of unequalled safety because of their minimal respiratory and cardiac depression.[49] These drugs may be abused by this group of patients, however.

In the last few years, clonidine has also been shown to be effective in reducing the adrenergic manifestations of both narcotic and alcohol withdrawal. The mechanism of action appears to be mediated through stimulation of centrally located α_2-adrenergic receptors. β-Blockers have also been used in alcohol withdrawal. Although they appear to be effective for the symptoms of withdrawal that are due to a hyperadrenergic state, they are of little value in preventing delirium or seizures. They may also be partially responsible for hallucinations.[49]

Withdrawal Seizures

Alcohol withdrawal seizures may be solitary or recurrent and usually respond to anticonvulsant therapy such as intravenous benzodiazepines.[1,50] Many patients with alcohol withdrawal seizure disorder are also treated with phenytoin, which in this instance is of questionable efficacy.[43] The development of status epilepticus has a high morbidity and mortality and should be aggressively treated.

Delirium Tremens

In the early stages of alcohol withdrawal, patients may have a mild disorientation of their sense of time with some impairment of memory. Few patients go on to have true delirium tremens.[51,52] Delirium tremens is the most advanced stage of alcohol withdrawal and includes hallucinatory behavior associated with severe tremors and autonomic hyperactivity. This stage occurs 2 to 3 days after cessation of alcohol and may last 3 to 5 days. Most significant complications occur during this phase and may include seizures, dysrhythmias, and hyperthermia.[48]

REFERENCES

1. Becker C: The alcoholic patient as a toxic emergency. *Emerg Clin North Am* 1984;2:47–61.

2. Tong T: The alcohols. *Crit Care Q* 1982;4:75–85.

3. Barnsley J, Sellers E: An interview study of hospitalized drug overdose patients. *Can Fam Physician* 1978; 24:850–855.

4. Patel A, Roy M, Wilson G: Self-poisoning and alcohol. *Lancet* 1972;2:1099–1102.

5. Rangno R, Dumont C, Sitar D: Effects of ethanol ingestion on outcome of drug overdose. *Crit Care Med* 1982;10:180–185.

6. Halpern J, Davis J: Use and abuse of alcohol: Further perspectives. *J Emerg Nurs* 1983;9:49–52.

7. Bernstein L, Tong T: Alcoholism. *Calif Pharm* 1979;6:26–30.

8. Cardoni A: The alcohol in liquid medicinals: Information for the pharmacist. *Guidelines Prof Pharm* 1978;5:1–2.

9. Varma B, Cincotta J: Mouthwash-induced hypoglycemia, editorial. *Am J Dis Child* 1978;132:930–931.

10. Weller-Fahy E, Berger L, Troutman W: Mouthwash: A source of acute ethanol intoxication. *Pediatrics* 1980;66:302–305.

11. Goldfinger T, Schaber D: A comparison of blood alcohol concentration using non-alcohol and alcohol containing skin antiseptics. *Ann Emerg Med* 1982;11:665–667.

12. Petroni N, Cardoni A: Alcohol content of liquid medicinals. *Drug Ther* 1978;8:72–93.

13. Rubinstein J: Beware of these drugs when you prescribe for a recovering alcoholic. *Resident Staff Physician* 1980;62–66.

14. Moore J, Christian P, Datz F, et al: Effect of wine on gastric emptying in humans. *Gastroenterology* 1981; 81:1072–1075.

15. Li T, Bosron W: Genetic variability of enzymes of alcohol metabolism in human beings. *Ann Emerg Med* 1986;15:997–1004.

16. Gibb K: Serum alcohol levels, toxicology screens, and use of the breath alcohol analyzer. *Ann Emerg Med* 1986;15:349–353.

17. Litovitz T: The alcohols: Ethanol, methanol, isopropanol, ethylene glycol. *Pediatr Toxicol* 1986; 33:311–323.

18. Lieber C: Metabolism and metabolic effects of alcohol. *Med Clin North Am* 1984;68:3–31.

19. Holtzman J, Gebhard R, Eckfeldt J, et al: The effects of several weeks of ethanol consumption on ethanol kinetics in normal men and women. *Clin Pharmacol Ther* 1985;38:157–163.

20. Jatlow P: Acute toxicology of ethanol ingestion—Role of the clinical laboratory. *Am J Clin Pathol* 1980;74: 721–724.

21. Crow K, Newland K, Batt R: The fructose effect. *N Z Med J* 1981;93:232–234.

22. Iber F: The effect of fructose on alcohol metabolism. *Arch Intern Med* 1977;137:1121.

23. Levy R, Elo T, Hanenson I: Intravenous fructose treatment of acute alcohol intoxication. *Arch Intern Med* 1977;137:1175–1177.

24. Meyer B, Mueller F, Hundt H: The effect of fructose on blood alcohol levels in man. *S Afr Med J* 1982; 62:719–721.

25. Sprandel U, Troger H, Liebhardt E, et al: Acceleration of ethanol elimination with fructose in man. *Nutr Metab* 1980;24:324–330.

26. Koch-Weser J, Sellers E, Kalant H: Alcohol intoxication and withdrawal. *N Engl J Med* 1976;294:757–762.

27. Bailey D: Comprehensive toxicology screening: The frequency of finding other drugs in addition to ethanol. *Clin Toxicol* 1984;22:463–471.

28. Madison L: Ethanol-induced hypoglycemia. *Adv Metabol Disord* 1968;3:85–109.

29. MacLaren N, Valman H, Levin B: Alcohol-induced hypoglycaemia in childhood. *Br Med J* 1970;1:278–280.

30. Miquel C, Rubies-Prat J: Effects of ethanol-induced hypoglycemia. *Br Med J* 1977;xx:1027.

31. Bittencourt P, Wade P, Richens A, et al: Blood alcohol and eye movements. *Lancet* 1980;2:981.

32. Hoppe P: Alcohol and the heart. *Ann Intern Med* 1983;97:109–110.

33. Abelmann W: Effects of alcohol on the cardiovascular system. *Hosp Pract* 1981;16:80A–80X.

34. Knochel J: Cardiovascular effects of alcohol. *Ann Intern Med* 1983;98:849–854.

35. Johnson C, Jackson D: Alcohol and sex. *Heart Lung* 1983;12:93–97.

36. Johnson R, Noll E, Rodney W: Survival after a serum ethanol concentration of 1½%. *Lancet* 1982;2:1394.

37. Pierce R: Stuporous alcoholics: Metabolic considerations. *South Med J* 1982;75:463–469.

38. Simpson G: Accuracy and precision of breath-alcohol measurements for a random subject in the postabsorptive state. *Clin Chem* 1987;33:261–268.

39. Minocha A, Herold D, Barth J, et al: Activated charcoal in oral ethanol absorption: Lack of effect in humans. *Clin Toxicol* 1986;24:225–234.

40. Knott D, Lerner W, Davis-Knott T, et al: Decision for alcohol detoxication—A method to standardize patient evaluation. *Postgrad Med* 1961;69:67–75.

41. Brown C: The alcohol withdrawal syndrome. *Ann Emerg Med* 1982;11:276–280.

42. Brown C: Alcohol. *Ann Emerg Med* 1986;15: 989–990.

43. Vance M: Drug withdrawal syndromes. *Top Emerg Med* 1985;7:63–68.

44. Rosenbloom A: Optimizing drug treatment of alcohol withdrawal. *Am J Med* 1986;81:900–904.

45. Baumgartner G, Rowen R: Clonidine vs chlordiazepoxide in the management of acute alcohol withdrawal syndrome. *Arch Intern Med* 1987;147:1223–1226.

46. Robertson C, Sellers E: Alcohol intoxication and the alcohol withdrawal syndrome. *Postgrad Med* 1978;64: 133–138.

47. Young G, Rores C, Murphy C, et al: Intravenous phenobarbital for alcohol withdrawal and convulsions. *Ann Emerg Med* 1987;16:847–850.

48. Liskow B, Goodwin G: Pharmacological treatment of alcohol intoxication, withdrawal and dependence: A critical review. *J Stid Alcohol* 1987;48:356–370.

49. Peachey J, Naranjo C: The role of drugs in the treatment of alcoholism. *Drugs* 1984;27:171–182.

50. Sellers E, Naranjo C, Giles H, et al: Intravenous diazepam and oral ethanol interaction. *Clin Pharmacol Ther* 1980;28:638–645.

51. West L, Maxwell D, Noble E, et al: Alcoholism. *Ann Intern Med* 1984;100:405–416.

52. Merrin E: Withdrawal states and alcoholic hallucinosis. *Am J Psychiatr* 1980;137:1280–1281.

ADDITIONAL SELECTED REFERENCES

Bennett W: Addenda to drug guidelines. *Ann Intern Med* 1977;87:794.

Elkins H: Basis of the maximum allowable concentrations for occupational exposure. *N Engl J Med* 1961; 265:335–336.

Ellinwood E, Linnoila M, Easler M, et al: Onset of peak impairment after diazepam and after alcohol. *Clin Pharmacol Ther* 1981;30:534–538.

Geokas M, Lieber C, French S, et al: Ethanol, the liver, and the gastrointestinal tract. *Ann Intern Med* 1981;95: 198–211.

Giannini A, DeFranco D: Metronidazole and alcohol— Potential for combinative abuse. *J Toxicol Clin Toxicol* 1983;20:509–515.

Goldstein D: Effect of alcohol on cellular membranes. *Ann Emerg Med* 1986;15:1013–1018.

Leevy C, Thompson A, Baker H: Vitamins and liver injury. *Am J Clin Nutr* 1970;23:493–499.

O'Keefe S, Marks V: Lunchtime gin and tonic—A cause of reactive hypoglycemia. *Lancet* 1977;1:1286–1288.

Olson E, McEnrue J, Greenbaum D: Alcohols and miscellaneous agents. *Heart Lung* 1983;12:127–130.

Rabins P, Mace N, Lucas MJ: Interaction of cimetidine and alcohol. *JAMA* 1983;249:351–352.

Ragan F, Samuels M, Hite S: Ethanol ingestion in children— A five-year review. *JAMA* 1979;242:2787–2788.

Schuckit M: Genetic aspects of alcoholism. *Ann Emerg Med* 1986;15:991–996.

Sheehan J: Alcohol and the heart, editorial. *Ann Intern Med* 1983;98:1022.

Tabakoff B, Cornell N, Hoffman P: Alcohol tolerance. *Ann Emerg Med* 1986;15:1005–1012.

chapter 24

Isopropyl Alcohol

Isopropyl alcohol (isopropanol or 2-propanol) is a three-carbon alcohol used as an industrial solvent and that also has found many uses in medicine. It is an ingredient in rubbing alcohol; various cosmetics such as aftershaves, perfumes, and colognes; skin disinfectants; aerosol products; deicing and antifreeze preparations; and hair tonics (Table 24-1).[1] Rubbing alcohol may contain either ethanol or isopropanol in concentrations of 70% to 90%.[2] Isopropyl alcohol is also an ingredient in mouthwashes and solvent mixtures. This alcohol is a clear, colorless, volatile liquid that has an odor different from that of ethanol and a distinctly disagreeable bitter taste except when highly diluted.[1,2]

Table 24-1 Sources and Concentrations of Isopropyl Alcohol

Source	Concentration (percent)
Antifreeze	40-55
Cements	5-20
Glass cleaners	3-15
Liquid detergents	5-12
Mouthwash	15-25
Paint stripper	2-10
Paint thinner	5-10
Rubbing alcohol	70-90
Windshield deicer	60-80

Isopropyl alcohol ingestion is relatively infrequent and is most often encountered in the alcoholic who has ingested rubbing alcohol or aftershave lotion as a substitute for ethanol.[3-6] N-propyl alcohol (1-propanol) appears to be more toxic than isopropyl alcohol. In the past this compound was mistaken for isopropyl alcohol, which led to a greater concern over isopropyl alcohol than was warranted.

Pharmacokinetics

The volume of distribution of isopropyl alcohol is 0.6 to 0.8 L/kg, which is similar to that of ethanol.[1] The half-life of isopropanol is 2.5 to 3 hours.[2] Although about 10% of isopropyl alcohol may be metabolized in the body to the glucuronide, the major metabolic pathway is first-order kinetics with the enzyme alcohol dehydrogenase acting to convert isopropanol to acetone, carbon dioxide, and water.[7] This is different from ethanol, which saturates its metabolic mechanisms at low levels and usually is eliminated independent of concentration (zero-order elimination). The rate of metabolism of isopropanol is thought to be approximately half that of ethanol.[8,9] The acetone formed is excreted predominantly by the kidney and in small amounts by the lungs. The acetone metabolite contributes to the CNS depression produced by isopropanol. Because of its higher molecular weight, isopropanol produces a smaller osmolal gap than a corresponding quantity of ethanol.[8] Concentrations of isopropyl alcohol in urine closely parallel those in the blood, which indicates that it is not substantially concentrated in the urine.

ABSORPTION

Isopropanol is absorbed easily through the gastrointestinal tract and, if not delayed by food, may be completely absorbed in less than 30 minutes.[1,2] Isopropanol is also absorbed by the lungs. It is not significantly absorbed through the skin.[2,6–8,10] Large amounts of isopropyl alcohol applied topically have little effect,[1] and, although there are reports of deep coma from the local application of isopropanol to the skin of infants, this appears to have been caused by inhalation of the alcohol during sponging procedures in poorly ventilated areas.[8,10–12] Concentrations greater than 120 mg/dL have been reported after sponging.[2] Isopropyl alcohol may also be absorbed by rectal mucosa.

ACUTE TOXICITY

Isopropyl alcohol is a CNS depressant with twice the potency of ethanol.[4,13] It has a longer duration of action (and thus intoxication) than ethanol because it is metabolized more slowly and because its major metabolite, acetone, is also a CNS depressant.[2,4,9,13] The initial phase of exhilaration that is noted with the ingestion of ethanol and is the usual reason for ingesting the material is not noted with isopropanol ingestion.[7]

Many of the same problems associated with ethanol overdose can be seen with isopropanol overdose (Table 24-2). It is much more irritating to the gastrointestinal tract and more likely to produce nausea, vomiting, and abdominal pain than ethanol.[2,14] In addition, pancreatitis, dizziness, confusion, and ataxia may be noted. Hematemesis and melena may appear early, and they are related to ulceration of the gastric mucosa.[1,15] Coma may occur with concentrations of approximately 120 mg/dL.[16–18] The pupil size is variable. Hypothermia, hypogly-

Table 24-2 Features of Isopropyl Alcohol Overdose

Gastrointestinal
  Nausea and vomiting
  Abdominal pain
  Gastritis
  Gastrointestinal hemorrhage
Neurologic
  Dizziness
  Confusion
  Ataxia
  Coma
Hypothermia
Hypotension
Hypoglycemia
Respiratory failure

cemia, and respiratory and renal failure are frequently reported with significant ingestions of isopropanol.[4,15,19] Hypotension, which may result from direct cardiac depression, may also occur and is considered a good prognosticator of a potentially fatal ingestion.[14] In the event of hypotension secondary to isopropyl alcohol, causes of volume depletion such as a gastrointestinal bleed should also be investigated. Death may occur from respiratory arrest.

Although isopropanol ingestion is a cause of ketosis, unlike the other ketones acetone is not an acid and does not cause a decreased bicarbonate or an elevated anion gap.[4,8,20,21] Where acidosis is noted, its etiology is probably lactic acid accumulation in the presence of isopropanol-induced hypotension. In addition, isopropanol is less toxic than both methanol and ethylene glycol and causes no permanent retinal injury or renal damage. When isopropanol is ingested in preparations not intended for ingestion, other volatile aromatics such as methyl salicylate, menthol, napthalene, and camphor may contribute to toxicity.[1,2]

DIAGNOSIS AND LABORATORY ANALYSIS

It is often difficult to make the diagnosis of isopropyl alcohol intoxication, even when it is the sole toxin involved.[1] A presumptive diagnosis of isopropanol ingestion can be made in the intoxicated-appearing patient who has acetonuria and acetonemia but no glycosuria, hyperglycemia, or acidemia.[21] The presence of the odor of acetone on the breath may aid in the diagnosis. In addition, an osmolal gap may be noted. In other words, if no history is available for a patient who has a normal anion gap associated with strongly positive serum ketones and normal serum bicarbonate and blood sugar concentrations, the diagnosis of isopropyl alcohol intoxication should be strongly considered.[20] Isopropyl alcohol intoxication differs from that of the alcohols because acidemia is not a part of the clinical picture.

The diagnosis of isopropyl alcohol ingestion can be confirmed by gas chromatography. As the concentration of isopropyl alcohol decreases, it can be expected that the serum acetone concentration will rise because of the continued production of this compound.[3,9,13] Enzymatic methods involving alcohol dehydrogenase may underestimate the amount of isopropyl alcohol. A breathalyzer for isopropyl alcohol is also unreliable.

Although these guidelines are not absolute, toxic symptoms have been noted to occur when isopropyl alcohol concentrations are approximately 50 mg/dL. Coma may be associated with concentrations of 120 mg/dL or more.[4] Depending on the method used, there may be a cross-reaction with ethanol measurements.

TREATMENT

The treatment of isopropanol overdose is essentially the same as that of ethanol and consists of naloxone, glucose, and thiamine if the patient presents with an altered mental status and, if appropriate, an attempt to prevent further absorption (Table 24-3). Although isopropyl alcohol has been demonstrated to be secreted into the stomach, it is not necessary to use continuous nasogastric suction. Supportive care should be instituted in much the same way as with ethanol intoxication. In the hypotensive patient, intravenous fluids should be administered. The patient should be placed in Trendelenburg's position. Vasoconstrictor agents such as dopamine or norepinephrine are usually not necessary. Usually with supportive care and artificial ventilation alone, even large doses of isopropyl alcohol can be survived. Dialysis can be effective but is only indicated in the rare instances when hypotension is present and the patient is unresponsive to alternate medical management.[1,8,14,16,17,22]

Table 24-3 Treatment of Isopropyl Alcohol Overdose

Condition	Treatment
Altered mental status	Glucose
	Thiamine
	Naloxone
	Oxygen
Hypotension	Normal saline
	Trendelenburg's position
	Vasopressors
	Dialysis
Hypoventilation	Mechanical ventilation

REFERENCES

1. Lacouture P, Wason S, Abrams A, et al: Acute isopropyl alcohol intoxication. *Am J Med* 1983;75:680–686.

2. Litovitz T: The alcohols: Ethanol, methanol, isopropanol, ethylene glycol. *Pediatr Clin North Am* 1986; 33:311–323.

3. Kelner M: Isopropanol ingestion: Interpretation of blood concentrations and clinical findings. *J Toxicol Clin Toxicol* 1983;20:497–507.

4. Adams S, Mathews J, Flaherty J: Alcoholic ketoacidosis. *Ann Emerg Med* 1987;16:90–97.

5. Scrimgeour E: Outbreak of methanol and isopropanol poisoning in New Britain, Papua New Guinea. *Med J Aust* 1980;1:36–38.

6. Tong T: The alcohols. *Crit Care Q* 1982;4:75–85.

7. Grant D: The pharmacology of isopropyl alcohol. *J Lab Clin Med* 1923;8:382–386.

8. Smith M: Solvent toxicity: Isopropanol, methanol, and ethylene glycol. *Ear Nose Throat J* 1983;62:126–135.

9. Lehman A, Schwerma H, Rickards E: Isopropyl alcohol: Rate of disappearance from the bloodstream of dogs after intravenous and oral administration. *J Pharmacol Exp Ther* 1944;82:196–201.

10. Moss M: Alcohol-induced hypoglycemia and coma produced by alcohol sponging. *Pediatrics* 1970; 46:445–447.

11. McFadden S, Haddow J: Coma produced by topical application of isopropanol. *Pediatrics* 1969;43:632–633.

12. Senz E, Goldfarb D: Coma in a child following use of isopropyl alcohol in sponging. *J Pediatr* 1958;53:323–324.

13. Lehman A, Chase H: The acute and chronic toxicity of isopropyl alcohol. *J Lab Clin Med* 1944;29:561–671.

14. Adelson L: Fatal intoxication with isopropyl alcohol. *Am J Clin Path* 1962;38:144–151.

15. Juncos L, Taguchi J: Isopropyl alcohol intoxication—Report of a case associated with myopathy, renal failure, and hemolytic anemia. *JAMA* 1968;204:732–734.

16. Freireich A, Cinque T, Xanthaley G, et al: Hemodialysis for isopropanol poisoning. *N Engl J Med* 1967; 277:699–700.

17. Mecikalski M, Depner T: Peritoneal dialysis for isopropanol poisoning. *West J Med* 1982;137:322–325.

18. Visudhiphan P, Kaufman H: Increased cerebrospinal fluid protein following isopropyl alcohol intoxication. *N Y State J Med* 1971;71:887–888.

19. Hawley P, Falko J: "Pseudo" renal failure after isopropyl alcohol intoxication. *South Med J* 1982;75:630–631.

20. Emmett M, Narins R: Clinical use of the anion gap. *Medicine* 1977;56:38–54.

21. Kreisberg R, Wood B: Drug- and chemical-induced metabolic acidosis. *Clin Endocrinol Metab* 1983; 21:391–411.

22. Rosansky S: Isopropyl alcohol poisoning treated with hemodialysis: Kinetics of isopropyl alcohol and acetone removal. *J Toxicol Clin Toxicol* 1982;19(3):265–271.

ADDITIONAL SELECTED REFERENCES

Goldfinger T, Schaber D: A comparison of blood alcohol concentration using non-alcohol and alcohol containing skin antiseptics. *Ann Emerg Med* 1982;11:665–667.

Schick J, Milstein J: Burn hazard of isopropyl alcohol in the neonate. *Pediatrics* 1981;68:587–588.

chapter 25

Ethylene Glycol and Methanol

THE GLYCOLS

Ethylene Glycol

Ethylene glycol (1,2-ethanediol), a bivalent aliphatic alcohol, is structurally similar to alcohol but contains a hydroxyl group on each carbon.[1] It was synthesized about 100 years ago and was considered of little commercial value until World War I, when a shortage of glycerin led to a widespread search for a practical nontoxic substitute to be used as a solvent for drugs.[2] Although it is now known that ethylene glycol is toxic, for many years it was believed to be nontoxic on the basis of two independent experiments 10 years apart, when two investigators drank small amounts of ethylene glycol without ill effects. For that reason, it has been included as a solvent in detergents, paints, lacquers, drugs, dyes, hydraulic brake fluid, polishes, cosmetics, and industrial solvents.[3,4] It also has been used as a glycerine substitute in enemas, as a coolant in the lunar module, and in the past as a preservative in juices and an ingredient in various early medicinals.[5] Its most familiar use as radiator antifreeze is based on its high boiling point and its ability to depress the freezing point of aqueous solutions (Table 25-1).

Intoxication by ethylene glycol is usually due to accidental ingestion, a suicide attempt, or consumption as a substitute for ethanol.[4,6–9] The compound's viscosity, warmth, sweet taste, and aromatic odor (which resemble the features of some liqueurs) in addition to its availability and low cost contribute to its popularity as a suicide agent or as a substitute for alcohol.[10,11]

Other Glycols

Among the various low–molecular weight ethylene glycol derivatives, the presence of an ether linkage appears to be the predisposing factor to intense renal damage. Glycols with an ether linkage include diethylene glycol; dipropylene glycol; dioxane; and monomethyl, ethyl, and butyl ethers of diethylene glycol. In contrast, the toxicity of simple esters resembles that of the parent glycol, to which they are hydrolyzed in the body.

Diethylene glycol, which consists of two ethylene glycol moieties connected through an ether

Table 25-1 Sources and Concentrations of Ethylene Glycol

Source	Concentration (percent)
Antifreeze	95
Brake fluid	70–95
Coolant	95
Windshield deicer	50

linkage, produces central necrosis of liver lobules as well as vacuolization of renal tubular cells and more severe renal damage than that produced by ethylene glycol.[1,12] Calcium oxalate crystals are not produced because oxalate is not an end-product of the metabolism of this compound as a result of the stable ether linkage.[13] Severe acidosis is also not a prominent feature of the clinical course with diethylene glycol poisoning. Dioxane, another glycol, is also not associated with a severe metabolic acidosis.

Propylene glycol (1,2-propanediol), a liquid, is another polyalcohol of low molecular weight that is considered safe for pharmacologic purposes and for use in food and cosmetics.[14] It has been widely used as a solvent in the preparation of oral and injectable drugs,[15] lotions, and ointments. It is generally considered a stable, pharmacologically inert substance with low systemic toxicity[15,16] because it enters the normal metabolic pathways of the body. It is approved by the FDA as a solvent for certain drugs, such as injectable phenytoin and diazepam (Table 25-2).[16–18] Studies have shown that propylene glycol is partly metabolized to lactic and pyruvic acids, which then enter the glycolytic pathway and are excreted as carbon dioxide and water.[1] It is theoretically possible, however, for lactic acidosis to occur, but this would be an extremely rare occurrence and would be noted only in a patient with impaired renal clearance of propylene glycol.[14,19]

Table 25-2 Commonly Used Drugs That Contain Propylene Glycol

Diazepam (injection)
Digoxin (injection)
Ergocalciferol (oral liquid)
Eucerin (cream)
Hydralazine (injection)
Multivitamin (injection)
Nembutal® (injection)
Nystatin® (ointment and cream)
Phenobarbital (injection)
Phenytoin (injection)
Sulfamethoxazole and trimethoprim (injection)

Source: Adapted with permission from *Pediatrics* (1987; 79:623), Copyright © 1987, American Academy of Pediatrics.

Although propylene glycol is generally considered nontoxic, there are reports of toxic effects in humans.[15] These are mostly secondary to intravenous administration and include cardiac dysrhythmias and asystole, renal damage, hemolysis, seizures, hepatic damage, and an increased osmolal gap.[17]

Pharmacokinetic Properties of Ethylene Glycol

Ethylene glycol is a colorless, odorless substance; it appears to have color because artificial coloring is added to the finished product.[20] Fluorescein, a fluorescent dye, is added to many commercial preparations of antifreeze to a final concentration of approximately 20 μg/mL. The high boiling point and low vapor pressure of ethylene glycol eliminates the danger of poisoning by inhalation. Ethylene glycol has a volume of distribution of approximately 0.7 L/kg,[21] a half-life of approximately 3 hours,[3,22,23] and a molecular weight of 62. Although the half-life of ethylene glycol has been reported to vary from 3 to 8 hours, its rate of elimination is more rapid than that of methanol, which means that the latent period for metabolic accumulation to toxic concentrations is usually shorter.

Absorption

There is no toxicity associated with skin absorption of ethylene glycol, nor is there toxicity secondary to its inhalation. Toxicity is limited to the ingestion of the compound. The estimated lethal dose is considered approximately 100 mL, although a much smaller amount has caused death.[5] Survival has been reported after ingestion of 400 mL.

Metabolism

Ethylene glycol intoxication may result in a profound, sometimes life-threatening metabolic acidosis, but in its original form the substance is relatively nontoxic and has no effect on respiration, the citric acid cycle, or other biochemical pathways. It is the metabolites and intermediaries that are formed that contribute to the toxicity associated with ethylene glycol.[11]

The major metabolites, in order of their appearance, are glycoaldehyde, glycolic acid, and glyoxylic acid (Figure 25-1).[24] The initial step in the metabolism of ethylene glycol is oxidation of one of the hydroxyl moieties to an aldehyde, resulting in glycoaldehyde. This oxidation is catalyzed by the hepatic enzyme alcohol dehydrogenase. Glycoaldehyde is then further oxidized to glycolic acid. The second hydroxyl group may then be oxidized, resulting in glyoxylic acid. Oxidation to formic acid and carbon dioxide occurs only to a small extent. A small fraction (3% to 10%) of the glyoxylic acid is converted to oxalic acid. Glycoaldehyde, glycolic acid, and glyoxylic acid are more toxic than the parent compound.

Other compounds contributing to a metabolic acidosis include hippuric and lactic acids.[3] These minor pathways are dependent on pyridoxal pyrophosphate and thiamine pyrophosphate[3,24,25] and occur primarily in the liver.

The role of oxalate. The role played by oxalate remains an unsolved problem in the etiology of ethylene glycol toxicity. It was once thought that oxalic acid was the major cause of the metabolic acidosis. Although oxalate is a minor metabolic product of ethylene glycol, oxalic acid may contribute to the organ damage noted in ethylene glycol intoxication.[26,27] Oxalate crystalluria can be a striking feature of ethylene glycol intoxication.[11] Oxalate rapidly precipitates as calcium oxalate (mainly in the monohydrate form), which is deposited in various tissues such as kidney, myocardium, brain, and pancreas. The exact mechanism of the renal necrosis and failure is not known, and as yet there appears to be a direct link between oxalate precipitation and the development of tubular necrosis.

The accumulation of oxalate has long been considered responsible for most of the clinical picture of ethylene glycol poisoning.[28] Although oxalate is a highly toxic compound and can by itself produce extensive renal damage, acidosis, and death, it does not account for all the effects of ethylene glycol.[3] Oxalic acid is an organic, dicarboxylic acid that is corrosive and has a marked affinity for calcium and magnesium.[29] Although calcium oxalate crystals have been shown in some cases to block physically the renal tubules, this may be an incidental finding; it may be the oxalic acid itself, among other intermediaries, that is toxic to cells by chelating calcium or magnesium intracellularly, leading to acute tubular necrosis.[30,31]

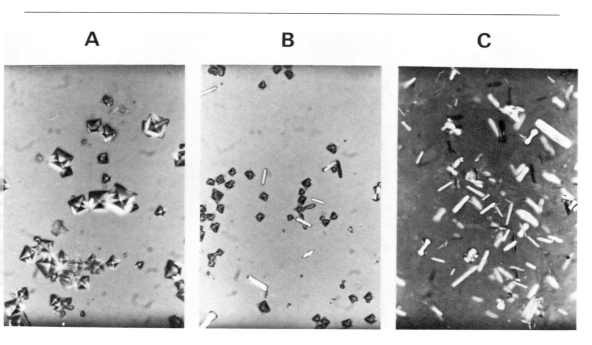

A   **B**   **C**

Figure 25-1 Pathways of ethylene glycol elimination. The **thick solid arrows** represent probable major pathways, the **thin solid arrows** less important pathways and the **broken arrows** indicate theoretic pathways. *Source:* Reprinted with permission from *American Journal of Medicine* (1988;84:146), Copyright © 1988, Technical Publishing Company.

Crystalluria. Two forms of urinary calcium oxalate crystals are now recognized (Figure 25-2).[32] The less prevalent form is the octahedral dihydrate or "envelope" form. On microscopic examination these crystals resemble a square containing an "x" that connects the vertices.[33] This form is present only at high concentrations of both calcium and oxalate. The monohydrate or needle-shaped crystal is seen more commonly because it is more thermodynamically stable under normal physiologic conditions.[26] This form was previously thought to be composed of hippuric acid crystals.[34] Hippuric acid crystals may be formed if patients consume antifreeze that contains benzoic acid as a preservative.[11] Although calcium oxalate crystals are considered an important diagnostic marker for ethylene glycol poisoning, in some cases they may be absent.[1,17] Tubular necrosis is usually severe and is believed to be irreversible, yet recovery from this condition has occurred.[17,35,36]

The anion gap in ethylene glycol intoxication is greater than that in any of the more common metabolic acidoses.[11] It has been shown that glycolic acid is the metabolite that accumulates in the highest concentrations in the blood.[4,26,27,37,38] This is because the rate of glycolic acid formation from ethylene glycol exceeds the rate of elimination.[39,40] This acid therefore appears to be the major contributing factor to the acute toxicity of ethylene glycol as well as the major determinant of the metabolic acidosis.[11,33] Serum and urine concentrations of glycolic acid have been found to correlate directly with clinical symptoms and mortality in poisoning cases, and glycolic acid may be found in the serum and urine longer than ethylene glycol.[4] Lactic acidosis may also be present as a result of inhibition of the citric acid cycle by glyoxylic acid as well as the increased cellular reduction:oxidation ratio, which favors the buildup of lactate over pyruvate.[11,26,27] The development of a concomitant lactic acidosis may be due

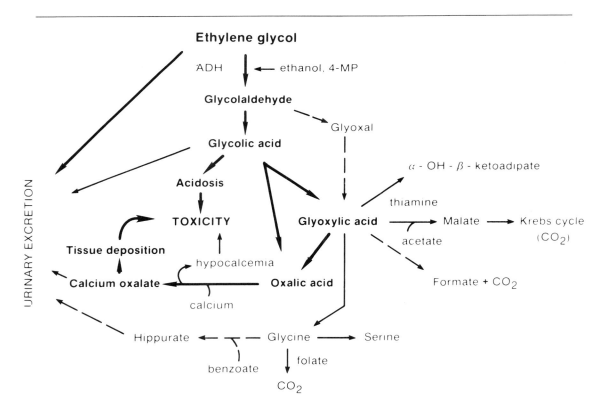

Figure 25-2 Crystalluria in ethylene glycol poisoning cause of metabolic acidosis. Envelope-shaped crystals are the dihydrate, whereas needle-shaped crystals are the monohydrate. *Source:* Reprinted with permission from *American Journal of Medicine* (1988;84:150), Copyright © 1988, Technical Publishing Company.

to circulatory failure and poor tissue perfusion.[11,39]

Acute Toxicity of Ethylene Glycol

Ethylene glycol has about the same CNS toxicity as ethanol and is rapidly absorbed and evenly distributed throughout the body tissues.[4] Blood concentrations reach their peak between 1 and 4 hours after ingestion.[10] The toxicity of ethylene glycol is due to the breakdown products. Classically, descriptions of ethylene glycol toxicity include three stages, but clinically patient presentations are rarely as well demarcated as the descriptions indicate.[27] These stages may be rather confluent, and the different latent periods before each stage depend on the amount of ethylene glycol and ethyl alcohol ingested. These three stages are the initial CNS, gastrointestinal, and metabolic stage, which is followed by the cardiopulmonary stage and then the renal stage. The severity and progression depend on the amount of compound ingested, the amount of ethylene glycol ingested, and therefore how quickly the parent compound is metabolized (Table 25-3). Early diagnosis is essential because removal of the toxin by dialysis and

---

Table 25-3 Stages of Ethylene Glycol Toxicity

Stage I (30 minutes to 12 hours)
 Intoxicated patient, no odor of alcohol
 Nausea and vomiting
 Metabolic acidosis
 Crystalluria
 Myoclonus
 Seizures
 Death
Stage II (12 to 24 hours)
 Tachypnea
 Tachycardia
 Hypertension
 Cyanosis
 Pulmonary edema
 Bronchopneumonia
 Cardiac enlargement
Stage III (36 to 48 hours)
 Crystalluria
 Costovertebral angle tenderness
 Acute tubular necrosis with oliguria
 Renal failure

---

reversal of the severe metabolic acidosis may be lifesaving.

Stage I

During the first 12 hours after ingestion of ethylene glycol, CNS manifestations predominate. These CNS manifestations are related to the aldehyde metabolites of ethylene glycol, which reach their maximal concentrations during this period.[39] The aldehydes are also toxic because they inhibit oxidative phosphorylation and glucose metabolism.

Clinically, the patient appears to be intoxicated with ethyl alcohol but the typical odor of alcohol is absent. Nausea, vomiting, and ataxia are common. This stage of intoxication is associated with the profound metabolic acidosis being produced in the metabolic degradation of ethylene glycol.

Generalized or focal seizures are relatively frequent, as is myoclonus or tetany secondary to hypocalcemia. Hypocalcemia is believed to be due to chelation of the calcium ion by oxalate, forming relatively insoluble calcium oxalate crystals.[27] Profuse calcium oxalate crystalluria, both before and after the period of anuria, is usually the hallmark of the renal sediment and may appear in the urine within 4 to 8 hours after ingestion.

Coma during this period is a frequent finding. Complete recovery from coma has occurred in a patient who was comatose for 17 days.[40] Coma may be due to cerebral oxalosis and cytotoxic damage, with secondary cerebral edema developing.[3]

Papilledema is seen and is usually due to cerebral edema, but occasionally it represents a toxic optic neuropathy with progressive loss of vision and optic atrophy similar to that seen in methanol ingestion.[5] In rare circumstances, abnormal eye findings consisting of nystagmus, ophthalmoplegia, and papilledema with subsequent optic atrophy are noted.[41] Although these eye findings have been reported on occasion, no methanol determinations were performed to rule out the possibility of methanol contamination of the liquid ingested.[27]

Death, if it occurs during this stage, is accompanied by cerebral edema. Examination of the cerebrospinal fluid characteristically reveals features of a meningoencephalitis with leukocytosis, xanthochromia, elevated cerebrospinal fluid pressure, and increased cerebrospinal fluid protein. On postmortem examination, calcium oxalate crystals can be found in the brain, leptomeninges, and perivascular spaces.[5] The aldehyde metabolite glycoaldehyde is thought to be responsible for much of the toxicity seen in this stage.

Stage II

The second or cardiopulmonary stage occurs between 12 and 24 hours after ingestion and has less well-defined symptoms. These consist of tachypnea, tachycardia, mild hypertension, cyanosis, and congestive heart failure or pulmonary edema.[39] Death, if it occurs, is associated with bronchopneumonia and cardiac enlargement. Fatalities in this stage are not as common as in the other stages.

The pathophysiology of the cardiopulmonary symptoms is not well known, but widespread capillary damage is assumed to be the primary lesion.

Stage III

Stage III, the renal stage, is noted 36 to 48 hours after ingestion. If the patient survives the initial 24 to 72 hours, renal failure usually becomes the predominant problem.[42] The renal damage may vary from temporary azotemia to anuria lasting for many weeks. Other abnormalities associated with renal involvement may include destruction of epithelial cells, interstitial edema, focal hemorrhagic necrosis of the cortex, extensive hydropic degeneration, numerous cellular casts, and oxalate crystals in the convoluted tubules.[39] Although oxaluria can occur during this stage, it can also be noted during stage I. If the patient is alert, he or she may complain of flank pain, and costovertebral angle tenderness may be noted. Acute tubular necrosis with oliguria and hematuria may eventually lead to renal failure.[36] Renal function may return to near normal if the patient survives.[39]

Laboratory Diagnosis

Diagnosis of ethylene glycol intoxication involves measuring serum electrolytes and arterial blood gas, urinalysis, Wood's lamp examination, measuring serum calcium and phosphorus concentrations, and measuring serum osmolality and calculating an osmolal gap (Table 25-4). The rise in the osmolal gap in ethylene glycol intoxication occurs only early in the poisoning, when unmetabolized ethylene glycol is present in the serum.[4] Serum calcium concentration may be low because of the precipitation of calcium by oxalate. This may also be reflected in evidence of hypocalcemia on the electrocardiogram.

Serum concentrations of ethylene glycol should also be measured in a known ethylene glycol ingestion. Most techniques presently available attempt to detect ethylene glycol in blood and urine. This approach can be unreliable in diagnosing the severity of the ingestion because of the rapid elimination of ethylene glycol by metabolic degradation or renal excretion.[4] The detection of high concentrations of glycolic acid when there has been an extended period of time between ingestion and admission is valuable in the diagnosis and treatment. In these cases, the major portion of ethylene glycol has been metabolized and may be detected in small quantities or not at all. Because high-performance liquid chromatography can detect both ethylene glycol and glycolic acid, it is important to have both concentrations reported, especially when there has been an extended period of time between ingestion and admission.[4]

An anion gap metabolic acidosis may be noted early after measuring serum electrolytes. A

Table 25-4 Laboratory Evaluation for Ethylene Glycol

Serum electrolytes
Arterial blood gas
Blood urea nitrogen
Serum creatinine
Urinalysis
Wood's lamp examination
Serum calcium
Serum phosphorus
Measured serum osmolality
Calculated serum osmolality
Serum ethylene glycol
Serum glycolic acid
Electrocardiogram

measurement of arterial blood gas may confirm this finding. Although the osmolal gap may be useful, it may not be present late in the course of an intoxication. The rise in the osmolal gap occurs only early in the poisoning when un-metabolized ethylene glycol is present in the serum and as ethylene glycol is metabolized and glycolic acid levels rise, there is an increase in the anion gap that corresponds to the amount of glycolic acid. The osmolal gap may not reflect this.[4]

A Wood's lamp examination of the urine or emesis may show fluorescence from the fluorescein coloring added to most ethylene glycol antifreeze (Snodgrass W, personal communication, 1987).

An approach to the workup of a patient potentially intoxicated with ethylene glycol is presented in greater detail in Chapter 26.

Treatment

The treatments for intoxication with ethylene glycol and methanol are similar enough that they can be discussed together (see below).

METHANOL

Methanol has been recognized as a serious toxic agent since the end of the 19th century. The classic method for producing methanol, or wood alcohol, relied on the distillation of hardwood, with fractionation yielding methanol, acetone, methylethylketone, and other products. With early distillation methods it produced such a vile odor and taste that it was not used as a substance of abuse. With the addition of deodorizing substances and the removal of many of the noxious impurities the product became more palatable, and the number of poisonings increased substantially.[43,44]

Uses

Methanol has been used as an adulterant or denaturant in other substances to discourage the oral use of that particular substance.[45–47] During the early part of this century in the United States,

it was legal to include methanol as a constituent of various spirits and whiskeys. In the past, it was not uncommon for "epidemics" of methanol poisoning to occur when methanol was ingested from a common contaminated source.[26,27,43,48,49] Methanol has also been used as an industrial solvent for shellac and paint thinners and in the manufacturing of rubber goods, synthetic textiles, antifreeze of the non-permanent type, duplicating fluid, printing solutions, and cleaning solutions, and it is commonly used as a windshield washing solution (Table 25-5).[50–52]

At present, many new uses of methyl alcohol are being proposed. These are primarily concerned with energy production or research on gasoline extenders, substitutes, and additives. Recently methanol has been used as a synthetic fuel for automobiles because it has excellent combustion mixing properties. Gasohol, the synthetic fuel, may contain 90% gasoline and 10% methanol or ethanol depending on local cost and availability. Sterno® (4% methanol) is marketed because of this combustion property.[51] Methanol is also used in the production of formaldehyde and methylated compounds such as methyl esters.[27]

In industry, methanol is produced in large quantities by the catalytic reaction of carbon monoxide or carbon dioxide with hydrogen. Methanol is a normal constituent of saliva and expired air and can be detected in the blood.

Table 25-5 Sources and Concentrations of Methanol

Source	Concentration (percent)
Sterno®	4
Carburetor fluid	99
Cements	1
Glass cleaners	1–40
Denatured ethanol	2–5
Duplicator fluid	60–90
Gasohol	10
Gas line antifreeze	100
Model engine fuel	45–75
Paint stripper	2–25
Pipe sweetener	75
Windshield deicer	4–90
Windshield washing solution	17–100

Dietary methanol arises in large part from fresh fruits and vegetables, where it occurs as free alcohol, methyl esters of fatty acids, or methoxy groups on polysaccharides such as pectin.

Aspartame (Nutrasweet®), a nutritive sweetener produced commercially from two amino acids (L-phenylalanine and L-aspartic acid), in theory has the ability to be converted to methanol. Studies have shown no increases in blood methanol with large doses (34 mg/kg), however, so that there is no concern of methanol intoxication from this artificial sweetener.[53]

Pharmacokinetics

Methanol is a colorless substance with an odor distinctly different from that of ethanol and a bitter taste.[43] This may often be difficult to recognize in the mixed liquids that cause poisonings.[26] Methanol has a low molecular weight, distributes throughout total body water, and has a volume of distribution of 0.6 L/kg.[54] Formate, the major metabolite that is responsible for toxicity, also has a low molecular weight and a volume of distribution of 0.5 L/kg.

Absorption

Absorption of methanol occurs by all routes. Methanol is rapidly absorbed from the gastrointestinal tract, with peak absorption occurring in 30 to 60 minutes. Blindness has been reported in a factory worker who accidentally spilled a gallon of methanol on a trouser leg,[51,52,55] and an infant died as a result of being wrapped in methanol-soaked towels.[56] Inhalation of vapors in excess of 200 parts per million (ppm) is associated with toxicity.[51] Ingestion of as little as 4 mL has caused blindness,[17,39,43] and as little as 15 mL has caused death.

Metabolism

Although some methanol is eliminated by the lungs in expired air, the main route of metabolism is through successive oxidation by alcohol dehydrogenase. Whereas ethanol is metabolized to carbon dioxide and water by alcohol dehydrogenase, 40% of a dose of methanol is metabolized by the same enzyme undergoing zero-order

kinetics to produce formic acid from formaldehyde.[57] This is the rate-limiting step in the metabolism of methanol.[58] The formaldehyde is then rapidly converted to formic acid and further metabolized by a folate-dependent process to carbon dioxide and water. The half-life of formaldehyde is 1 to 2 minutes, so that no accumulation is detectable.[26] The metabolism of methanol proceeds five times more slowly than that of ethanol, and approximately 30% of a dose of methanol remains unchanged in the body up to 48 hours after ingestion.[27] Formic acid, which is six times more toxic than methanol, is responsible for metabolic acidosis, anion gap, and ocular toxicity.[24,39,40,59–61]

Methanol is nontoxic, but its breakdown product, formic acid, may cause multisystem problems.[62] Susceptibility to methanol poisoning is regulated by the functioning of the folate systems in each species. Only humans and monkeys develop methanol poisoning because of the absence of a pathway allowing large amounts of formate to be metabolized into carbon dioxide.[27] The rate-limiting step for the production of formic acid, therefore, appears to be the availability of folic acid.[51] This may have clinical importance in the management of methanol intoxication, as will be discussed.[40,63]

There is individual variation in the clinical presentation of the methanol-intoxicated patient subject to such considerations as the amount of food in the patient's stomach, the quantity of methanol consumed, and the quantity of ethanol consumed. Individuals with folate deficiencies may be more susceptible to intoxication.

Acute Toxicity

Toxicity usually manifests itself in four systems: visual, CNS, gastrointestinal, and respiratory (Table 25-6).[64]

General Considerations

The initial period of inebriation is a disappointment to the intentional user because it is milder than expected, sometimes encouraging the user to ingest a greater quantity.[25,27,65,66] This is in contrast to the later stage, when coma

Table 25-6 Clinical Manifestations of Methanol Intoxication

General
  Mild inebriation
  Long latent period
  Metabolic acidosis
Gastrointestinal
  Nausea
  Vomiting
  Severe abdominal pain
Neurologic
  Headache
  Dizziness
  Seizures
  Stupor
  Coma
Visual
  Diminished sensation of light
  Reduced central vision
  Photophobia
  Blurred vision
  Retinal edema
  Hyperemia of optic disks

may occur as a result of the accumulation of metabolites. Early CNS depression after the ingestion of methanol may be due to the concomitant ingestion of ethanol.[26] An important part of the natural course of methanol intoxication is the relatively long latent period between ingestion and significant toxic findings.[65] A latent period of 6 to 72 hours, with an average of 24 hours between ingestion and toxic symptoms, is noted, and because the individual may be asymptomatic he or she may not seek medical attention until the toxic breakdown products have accumulated.[27,51] This latent period can be explained as the time required for methanol to be converted to the toxic metabolites responsible for the characteristic syndrome.[67,68] If ethanol is also ingested, the lag period before breakdown of the methanol is even longer.[27]

Visual Disorders

Visual disorders are very common.[57] There may be complaints of a diminished sensation of light; reduced central vision; photophobia; blurred or indistinct vision with a perception of dancing spots over the eyes; the sensation of "skin over the eyes"; flashes of gray, white, or yellow; or blindness.[69] On funduscopic exam-

ination retinal edema may be observed, which develops over 2 to 4 days and may persist for up to 2 weeks.[70] There may be dilated, sluggishly reactive pupils along with hyperemia of the optic disks.[69] In patients with severe visual damage, optic atrophy may develop with cupping of the optic disk.[71,72] The usual visual field defect is a central scotoma.[45,73] The patient's subjective complaints and actual eye findings very seldom correlate.[69]

Although in the past it was thought that formaldehyde caused optic toxicity, animal studies show unequivocally that visual impairment is caused by formic acid inhibiting cytochrome oxidase with resultant impairment of electron transport in the mitochondria.[27,69,74] As a result formation of adenosine triphosphate is defective, and stasis of nerve flow occurs in the optic nerve head rather than the retinal ganglia.[51] Axonal swelling develops because of the stasis, resulting in optic disk edema and leading to visual impairment.[69] Optic atrophy, if it occurs, is a late finding. Although recovery from partial loss of vision may occur,[43] the prognosis for recovery of vision from total blindness, if it occurs, is not favorable.

Metabolic Acidosis

In the early stages of methanol intoxication, formate accumulation is the main contributor to the metabolic acidosis. Lactic acidosis may appear at a late stage in severe methanol poisoning. This results mainly from formate inhibition of mitochondrial respiration, tissue hypoxia due to poor circulation, and altered lactate metabolism due to an increased ratio of NADH to NAD.[26,27,75]

Neurologic Abnormalities

Headache and dizziness are frequently found with methanol intoxication; weakness and malaise are seen less commonly. In severely intoxicated patients, seizures, stupor, and coma may also be present. Prognosis is poor if the patient has these neurologic findings in conjunction with signs of increased intracranial pressure, such as bradycardia, hypertension, and dilated, nonreactive pupils. White blood cells in the cerebral spinal fluid and xanthochromia have also been reported.[25] Survivors of serious methanol poisoning may be left with an extrapyramidal movement disorder due to permanent damage to the putamen.[26,51,76]

Gastrointestinal Effects

The local effects on the gastrointestinal tract may cause the individual to seek medical attention before a large amount of the compound is metabolized. Fifty percent of patients experience nausea and vomiting, which is usually persistent and violent. Approximately two-thirds of patients experience abdominal pain, which may be violent and colicky and, at times, may simulate an acute abdomen or renal colic. An elevated serum amylase concentration is a relatively frequent finding associated with the severe abdominal pain caused by methanol.[17,43,57]

Laboratory Analysis

Although there may be a poor correlation between blood methanol concentration and symptoms, a peak level greater than 50 mg/dL is considered toxic. Blood methanol concentrations are not as difficult to obtain as blood ethylene glycol concentrations; therefore, if the diagnosis of methanol poisoning is considered, serum concentrations should be measured. Further workup of the patient suspected of ingesting a methanol-containing compound is discussed more fully in Chapter 26.

TREATMENT FOR ETHYLENE GLYCOL AND METHANOL INTOXICATION

For the most part, the treatments of ethylene glycol overdose and methanol overdose are identical (Table 25-7). Treatment is directed first toward correcting the metabolic acidosis, then toward inhibiting the oxidation of the parent compound, and finally toward the removal of circulating amounts of the parent compound and its toxic metabolites. Because poisoning with these two alcohols causes such serious irreversible problems, treatment should be instituted as rapidly as possible, especially in patients who are symptomatic. Ethanol therapy may be

Table 25-7 Treatment of Ethylene Glycol and Methanol Overdose

Prevent further absorption
Ipecac or lavage
Charcoal
Cathartic
Alkalinization (2 to 3 mEq/kg)
Ethanol therapy (see Table 25-8)
Calcium (1 g of $CaCl_2$)
Thiamine (50 to 100 mg)—for ethylene glycol
Pyridoxine (2 to 5 g IV)—for ethylene glycol
Folic acid (50 to 100 mg IV)—for methanol
Dialysis

offered while waiting for positive laboratory confirmation of a suspected ingestion. This is especially true for ethylene glycol.[77]

Attempts to prevent further absorption by ipecac or lavage with subsequent administration of activated charcoal and a cathartic should be instituted. Skin decontamination should be performed in the methanol-exposed patient.

Alkali Therapy

If the patient is acidotic, intravenous alkali therapy should be started. It has been demonstrated that the mortality for methanol and ethylene glycol intoxication could be greatly influenced by prompt and generous sodium bicarbonate treatment, and it has been further shown that correction of metabolic acidosis alone significantly increases the patient's chance for survival.[11] Because methanol and ethylene glycol are responsible for the generation of organic acids as opposed to conditions that block excretion (such as uremia), large amounts of bicarbonate may be required.[78] In addition, unlike pure lactic acidosis or ketoacidosis, the anions generated in ethylene glycol and methanol intoxication are not metabolized to regenerate bicarbonate.

Bicarbonate therapy consists of continuous infusion of 5% sodium bicarbonate or administration of 2 to 3 mEq/kg of sodium bicarbonate, with frequent monitoring of electrolytes, arterial blood gases, and fluid status of the patient. Although large amounts of fluids may increase oxalate excretion, they may also increase the likelihood of pulmonary edema.

Ethyl Alcohol Therapy

Because it is the metabolic products of methanol and ethylene glycol that are toxic and not the parent compounds themselves, preventing the formation of these products will render these compounds nontoxic.[79,80] Ethyl alcohol is suggested in the management of ethylene glycol and methanol ingestion because it competes with alcohol dehydrogenase, the enzyme responsible for the critical first step in the metabolism of methanol and ethylene glycol.[81] Ethyl alcohol saturates this enzyme because its affinity for ethanol is 100 times greater than for either methanol or ethylene glycol.[5,25,81] Ethanol increases the half-life of ethylene glycol from 3 hours to 17 hours.[82,83] The administration of ethanol will therefore avoid a buildup of the toxic products of metabolism and allows for an increased excretion of unchanged parent compound through the kidneys. In theory, ethanol could be the only therapy for mild intoxication with these compounds. Severe intoxication requires more aggressive therapy.[11] If clinical suspicion of methanol or ethylene glycol poisoning is high, treatment with ethanol should not be delayed for the report of blood concentrations.

The aim of ethanol therapy is to saturate the enzyme system. This can be accomplished at approximately 100 mg/dL of ethanol.[5,82,83] At an ethanol concentration of 100 mg/dL, more than 75% of the metabolites of ethylene glycol is blocked. At ethanol concentrations up to 200 mg/dL, more than 95% is blocked.[5] To accomplish this goal, both a loading dose and a maintenance dose are necessary. Absolute ethanol or lesser concentrations of ethanol, administered either parenterally or orally, will produce the proper saturation of the enzyme. Advantages of oral administration of ethanol are the ease of administration and the ability to use a more concentrated solution than may comfortably be administered parenterally.[22,23,82] Parenteral administration, however, produces the desired blood level more quickly and obviates concern about prior intestinal absorption. Parenteral administration of ethanol may also be required for the patient who is vomiting. In a comatose patient or a patient with variable ethanol absorption (as occurs after activated charcoal administration), the intravenous route is preferred.

With absolute ethanol (95%), a loading dose of 1 mL/kg in 5% dextrose in water over 10 to 15 minutes brings the blood concentration to approximately 100 mg/dL.[5] A maintenance dosage consists of 0.1 mL/kg/hour, and therapy should be continued for 2 to 3 days (Table 25-8). Although absolute alcohol can be used, it should be diluted to approximately 10% for ease of parenteral administration[82] because concentrations greater than 10% are associated with local irritation. The hospital pharmacy may be able to prepare this solution from absolute alcohol.

Because of the relatively short half-life of ethylene glycol, ethyl alcohol therapy should be started within 4 to 6 hours after ingestion. It should also be started as soon as possible for methanol, although the rate of breakdown of methanol is much slower than that of ethylene glycol.

If dialysis is to be performed, increased amounts of maintenance ethanol should be administered because ethanol will also be eliminated in the dialysate.[5] Alternatives to absolute ethanol therapy, as well as the suggested dose if dialysis is instituted, are suggested in Table 25-8. Treatment with ethyl alcohol should be continued for 24 hours after the ethylene glycol is removed from the plasma because various

Table 25-8 Ethyl Alcohol Management of Ethylene Glycol and Methanol Overdose

Dose	95% Ethanol	40% Ethanol	10% Ethanol
Loading	1 mL/kg	2.5 mL/kg	10 mL/kg
Maintenance (without dialysis)	0.1 mL/kg/hour	0.3 mL/kg/hour	1 mL/kg/hour
Maintenance (with dialysis)	0.3 mL/kg/hour	1 mL/kg/hour	3 mL/kg/hour

Source: Adapted with permission from *Ear, Nose and Throat Journal* (1983;62:134), Copyright © 1983, Little, Brown & Company.

body tissues can act as reservoirs for the substance and release their contents even several days later.

Blood ethanol concentrations should also be routinely measured to assess whether dosage adjustments are needed to maintain the desired effect.[5] With prolonged ethanol administration, hypoglycemia may result, especially in children.[10]

Calcium

The suggested treatment for symptomatic hypocalcemic manifestations associated with ethylene glycol overdose is calcium chloride or calcium gluconate, but some investigators hold that the administration of calcium may increase the production of calcium oxalate crystals.[42]

Pyridoxine and Thiamine

Two of the most rapidly utilized cofactors in the enzymatic metabolism of ethylene glycol are thiamine and pyridoxine. Pyridoxine is an important cofactor in converting glyoxylate to glycine rather than to oxalate. Thiamine assists in the metabolization of glyoxalate to α-hydroxy-β-ketoadipate instead of to oxalate, although the importance of this pathway has recently been questioned.[11] Thiamine (50 to 100 mg) and pyridoxine (2 to 5 g) should therefore be given prophylactically.[3,10,84]

Folic Acid

Folic acid is suggested for the methanol-intoxicated individual because it enhances the oxidation of formic acid to carbon dioxide and water through a folate-dependent system.[51] Folic acid (1 mg/kg or 50 to 100 mg) administered intravenously every 4 hours for a total of six doses is the suggested dosage regimen.[85,86]

Pyrazole

Pyrazole compounds such as 4-methylpyrazole have been shown to be inhibitors of

alcohol dehydrogenase and thus of the oxidation of methanol.[87] It is an inhibitor of alcohol dehydrogenase rather than a competitive substrate like ethanol.[27] 4-Methylpyrazole has been used experimentally in animals for modifying ethanol metabolism with few toxic effects.[39,40,59,87] It does not appear to exert CNS depression and has a longer duration of action than ethanol because it is metabolized and eliminated more slowly. Although pyrazoles are still experimental, they may offer another approach to the treatment of methanol and ethylene glycol overdose.[51,85,86,88,89]

Dialysis

Dialysis is essential for the removal of both ethylene glycol and methanol (Table 25-9). Because these two alcohols have relatively small volumes of distribution and are freely water soluble, significant amounts can be removed by hemodialysis.[5] Hemodialysis is superior to peritoneal dialysis,[25,90–92] although either is effective for the removal of both the parent compounds as well as the metabolic breakdown products.[11,26,27,90,93] Dialysis not only removes these toxins but also permits infusion of alkali without the danger of overloading the circulation and increasing the likelihood of pulmonary edema. If dialysis is necessary, ethyl alcohol can be added to the dialysate bath at a concentration of 100 mg/dL, thus lowering the amount required for parenteral or oral admin-

Table 25-9 Substances Removed by Dialysis in Ethylene Glycol and Methanol Intoxication

Ethylene glycol
  Ethylene glycol
  Glycoaldehyde
  Glycolic acid
  Glyoxylic acid
  Oxalic acid
  Lactic acid
Methanol
  Methanol
  Formaldehyde
  Formic acid
  Lactic acid

istration.[4,77,81] In addition, hemodialysis aids in the correction of metabolic acidosis and other metabolic abnormalities while helping to maintain a therapeutic ethanol concentration.

Dialysis is indicated in ethylene glycol toxicity when a history of ingestion is obtained and the patient is symptomatic or when the patient is acidotic. If methanol is ingested, dialysis is indicated when the concentration exceeds 50 mg/dL or when the patient is symptomatic or has a metabolic acidosis (Table 25-10).

Table 25-10 Indications for Dialysis in Ethylene Glycol and Methanol Intoxication

Ethylene glycol
History of ingestion
Ethylene glycol concentration > 50 mg/dL *or*
Symptomatic patient *or*
Acidotic patient
Methanol
History of ingestion
Methanol concentration > 50 mg/dL *or*
Symptomatic patient *or*
Acidotic patient

Hemoperfusion

Although coated activated charcoal hemoperfusion removes ethylene glycol and methanol and their metabolites, the column becomes saturated in about 2 hours, which renders the process ineffective.

SUMMARY

Both ethylene glycol and methanol are dangerous compounds that may cause permanent injury or death. There should be little delay in making the diagnosis of intoxication, with aggressive treatment undertaken once the diagnosis is made.

Ethylene Glycol

Patients who have ingested ethylene glycol and are symptomatic or have a serum concentration greater than 50 mg/dL should be given the full therapeutic regimen of alkali therapy, ethanol, and dialysis.[20,77] With ethylene glycol concentrations less than 50 mg/dL, patients with normal renal function should be able to compensate and excrete the acids produced.[5]

Methanol

Patients who have ingested methanol, have blood concentrations less than 50 mg/dL, are asymptomatic, and are not acidotic should be treated with ethanol only.[93] For patients with concentrations greater than 50 mg/dL[90] who are symptomatic with mental, visual, or funduscopic abnormalities or who have a metabolic acidosis should undergo alkali, alcohol, and dialysis therapy (Figure 25-3).[17,25,57,77,90] A complete workup of the patient who may have ingested methanol or ethylene glycol is discussed in Chapter 26.

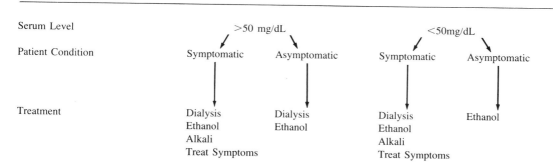

Figure 25-3 Summary of Treatment for Ethylene Glycol and Methanol Intoxication

REFERENCES

1. Turk J, Morrell J, Avioli L: Ethylene glycol intoxication. *Arch Intern Med* 1986;146:1601–1603.

2. Sangster B, Prenen J, De Groot G: Ethylene glycol poisoning. *N Engl J Med* 1980;302:465–466.

3. Parry M, Wallach R: Ethylene glycol poisoning. *Am J Med* 1974;57:143–150.

4. Hewlett T, McMartin K, Lauro A, et al: Ethylene glycol poisoning: The value of glycolic acid determinations for diagnosis and treatment. *Clin Toxicol* 1986;24:389–402.

5. Bobbitt W, Williams R, Freed C: Severe ethylene glycol intoxication with multisystem failure. *West J Med* 1985;144:225–228.

6. Bove K: Ethylene glycol toxicity. *Am J Clin Pathol* 1966;45:46–50.

7. Goldsher M, Better O: Antifreeze poisoning during the October 1973 war in the Middle-East: Case reports. *Mil Med* 1979;144:314–315.

8. Gordon H, Hunter J: Ethylene glycol poisoning—A case report. *Anaesthesia* 1982;37:332–338.

9. Haggarty R: Toxic hazards: Death from permanent antifreeze ingestion. *N Engl J Med* 1959;261:1296–1297.

10. Brown C, Trumbull D, Klein-Schwartz W, et al: Ethylene glycol poisoning. *Ann Emerg Med* 1983;12:501–506.

11. Gabow P, Clay K, Sullivan J, et al: Organic acids in ethylene glycol intoxication. *Ann Intern Med* 1986;105:16–20.

12. Cantarell M, Fort J, Camps J, et al: Acute intoxication due to topical application of diethylene glycol. *Ann Intern Med* 1987;106:478–479.

13. Winek C, Shingleton D, Shanor S: Ethylene and diethylene glycol toxicity. *Clin Toxicol* 1978;13:297–324.

14. Cate J, Hedreck R: Propylene glycol intoxication lactic acidosis. *N Engl J Med* 1980;303:1237.

15. Arulanantham K, Genel M: Central nervous system toxicity associated with ingestion of propylene glycol. *J Pediatr* 1978;93:515–516.

16. Gaunt I, Carpanini F, Grasso P, et al: Long-term toxicity of propylene glycol in rats. *Food Cosmet Toxicol* 1972;10:151–153.

17. Tong T: The alcohols. *Crit Care Q* 1982;4:75–85.

18. MacDonald M, Getson P, Glasgow A, et al: Propylene glycol: Increased incidence of seizures in low birth weight infants. *Pediatrics* 1987;79:622–625.

19. Bossaert L, Demey H: Propylene glycol intoxication. *Arch Intern Med* 1987;147:611–612.

20. Rothman A, Normann S, Manoguerra A, et al: Short-term hemodialysis in childhood ethylene glycol poisoning. *J Pediatr* 1986;108:153–155.

21. Jacobsen D, Bredesen J, Eide I, et al: Anion and osmolal gaps in the diagnosis of methanol and ethylene glycol poisoning. *Acta Med Scand* 1982;212:17–20.

22. Peterson C, Collins A, Himes J, et al: Ethylene glycol poisoning: Pharmacokinetics during therapy with ethanol and hemodialysis. *N Engl J Med* 1981;304:21–23.

23. Peterson D, Peterson J, Hardinge M, et al: Experimental treatment of ethylene glycol poisoning. *JAMA* 1963;186:955–957.

24. Smith M: Solvent toxicity: Isopropanol, methanol, and ethylene glycol. *Ear Nose Throat J* 1983;62:126–135.

25. Smith SR, Smith S, Buckley B: Lactate and formate in methanol poisoning. *Lancet* 1982;1:561–562.

26. Jacobsen D: Organic acids in ethylene glycol intoxication. *Ann Intern Med* 1986;105:799–800.

27. Jacobsen D, McMartin K: Methanol and ethylene glycol poisonings: Mechanism of toxicity, clinical course, diagnosis and treatment. *Med Toxicol* 1986;1:309–334.

28. Friedman E, Greenberg J, Merrill J, et al: Consequences of ethylene glycol poisoning. *Am J Med* 1962;32:891–902.

29. James L: Oxalate toxicosis. *Clin Toxicol* 1972;5:231–243.

30. Pons C, Custer R: Acute ethylene glycol poisoning: A clinico-pathologic report of eighteen fatal cases. *Am J Med Sci* 1946;211:544–552.

31. Underwood F, Bennett W: Ethylene glycol intoxication. *JAMA* 1973;226:1453–1454.

32. Terlinsky A, Grochowski J, Geoly K, et al: Identification of atypical calcium oxalate crystalluria following ethylene glycol ingestion. *Am J Clin Pathol* 1981;76:223–226.

33. Linnanvuo-Laitinen M, Huttunen K: Ethylene glycol intoxication. *Clin Toxicol* 1986;24:167–174.

34. Godolphin W, Meagher E, Sanders H, et al: Unusual calcium oxalate crystals in ethylene glycol poisoning. *Clin Toxicol* 1980;16:479–486.

35. Kahn H, Brotchner R: A recovery from ethylene glycol (antifreeze) intoxication: A case of survival and two fatalities from ethylene glycol including autopsy findings. *Ann Intern Med* 1950;32:284–294.

36. Collins J, Hennes D, Holzgang C, et al: Recovery after prolonged oliguria due to ethylene glycol intoxication. *Arch Intern Med* 1970;125:1059–1062.

37. Cadnapaphornchai P, Taher S, Bhathena D, et al: Ethylene glycol poisoning: Diagnosis based on high osmolal and anion gaps and crystalluria. *Ann Emerg Med* 1981;10:94–97.

38. Cheng J, Beysolow T, Kaul B, et al: Clearance of ethylene glycol by kidneys and hemodialysis. *Clin Toxicol* 1987;25:95–108.

39. Kreisberg R, Wood B: Drug- and chemical-induced metabolic acidosis. *Clin Endocrinol Metab* 1983;12:391–411.

40. Clay K, Murphy R: On the metabolic acidosis of ethylene glycol intoxication. *Toxicol Appl Pharmacol* 1977;39:39–49.

41. Ahmed M: Ocular effects of antifreeze poisoning. *Br J Ophthalmol* 1971;55:854–859.

42. Levy R: Renal failure secondary to ethylene glycol intoxication. *JAMA* 1976;173:1210–1213.

43. Bennett I, Cary F, Mitchell G, et al: Acute methyl poisoning: A review based on experiences in an outbreak of 323 cases. *Medicine* 1953;32:431–463.

44. Bohn G, Nicolson I, Owens J: A report of a fatal accidental methanol self-poisoning. *Med Sci Law* 1974;14: 219–221.

45. Scrimgeour E, Dethlefs R, Kevau I: Delayed recovery of vision after blindness caused by methanol poisonings. *Med J Aust* 1982;2:481–483.

46. Scrimgeour E: Outbreak of methanol and isopropanol poisoning in New Britain, Papua New Guinea. *Med J Aust* 1980;1:36–38.

47. Scully R, Galdabini J, McNeely B: Case 38-1979: Presentation of a case. *N Engl J Med* 1979;301:650–657.

48. Swartz R, Millman R, Billi J, et al: Epidemic methanol poisoning: Clinical and biochemical analysis of a recent episode. *Medicine* 1981;60:373–382.

49. Hashemy-Tonkabony S: Postmortem blood concentration of methanol in 17 cases of fatal poisoning from contraband vodka. *Forensic Sci* 1975;6:1–3.

50. Posner H: Biohazards of methanol in proposed new uses. *J Toxicol Environ Health* 1975;1:153–171.

51. Becker C: Methanol poisoning. *J Emerg Med* 1983; 1:51–58.

52. Becker C: The alcoholic patient as a toxic emergency. *Emerg Med Clin North Am* 1984;2:47–60.

53. Stegink L, Brummel M, McMartin K, et al: Blood methanol concentrations in normal adult subjects administered abuse doses of aspartame. *J Toxicol Environ Health* 1981;7:281–290.

54. Chinard F, Frisell W: Methanol intoxication: Biochemical and clinical aspects. *J Med Soc N J* 1976;73: 712–719.

55. Dutkiewicz B, Konezalik J, Karwacki W: Skin absorption of administration of methanol in man. *Int Arch Occup Environ Health* 1980;48:81–88.

56. Kahn A, Blum D: Methyl alcohol poisoning in an 8-month-old boy: An unusual route of intoxication. *J Pediatr* 1979;94:841–843.

57. Grufferman S, Morris D, Alvarez J: Methanol poisoning complicated by myoglobinuric renal failure. *West J Med* 1985;3:24–26.

58. Shahangian S, Ash K: Formic and lactic acidosis in a fatal case of methanol intoxication. *Clin Chem* 1986; 32:395–397.

59. McMartin K, Makar A, Martin A, et al: Methanol poisoning: The role of formic acid in the development of metabolic acidosis in the monkey and the reversal by 4-methylpyrazole. *Biochem Med* 1975;13:319–333.

60. McMartin K, Ambre J, Tephly T: Methanol poisoning in human subjects. *Am J Med* 1980;68:414–418.

61. Sejersted O, Jacobsen D, Ovrebo S, et al: Formate concentrations in plasma from patients poisoned with methanol. *Acta Med Scand* 1983;213:105–110.

62. Emmett M, Narins R: Clinical use of the anion gap. *Medicine* 1977;56:38–54.

63. Sharpe J, Hostovsky M, Bilbao J, et al: Methanol optic neuropathy: A histopathological study. *Neurology* 1982;32:1093–1100.

64. Martin D, Naughton J: Acute methanol poisoning: 'The Blind Drunk'. *West J Med* 1981;135:122–128.

65. Closs K, Solberg C: Methanol poisoning. *JAMA* 1970;211:497–499.

66. Fulop M: Methanol intoxication. *Lancet* 1982;1:338.

67. Heath A: Methanol poisoning. *Lancet* 1983;1: 1139–1140.

68. Keeney A, Mellinkoff S: Methyl alcohol poisoning. *Ann Intern Med* 1951;34:331–338.

69. Hayreh M, Hayreh S, Baumbach G, et al: Methyl alcohol poisoning: Ocular toxicity. *Arch Ophthalmol* 1977; 95:1851–1858.

70. Dethlefs R, Naraqi S: Ocular manifestations and complications of acute methyl alcohol intoxication. *Med J Aust* 1978;2:483–485.

71. Jacobsen D, Jansen H, Wiik-Larsen E, et al: Studies on methanol poisoning. *Acta Med Scand* 1982;212:5–10.

72. Jacobsen D, Ostby N, Bredesen J: Studies on ethylene glycol poisoning. *Acta Med Scand* 1982;212:11–15.

73. Baumbach G, Cancilla P, Martin-Amat G, et al: Methyl alcohol poisoning: Alterations of the morphological findings of the retina and optic nerve. *Arch Ophthalmol* 1977;95:1859–1865.

74. Olson E, McEnrue J, Greenbaum D: Alcohols and miscellaneous agents. *Heart Lung* 1983;12:127–130.

75. Martens J, Verberckmoes R, Westhovens R, et al: Recovery without sequelae from severe methanol intoxication. *Postgrad Med J* 1982;58:454–456.

76. McLean D, Jacobs H, Mielke B: Methanol poisoning: A clinical and pathological study. *Ann Neurol* 1980; 8:161–167.

77. Pappas S, Silverman M: Treatment of methanol poisoning with ethanol and hemodialysis. *Can Med Assoc J* 1982;126:1391–1394.

78. Chew W, Berger E, Brines O, et al: Alkali treatment in methyl alcohol poisoning. *JAMA* 1946;130:61–64.

79. Bergeron R, Cardinal J, Geadah D: Prevention of methanol toxicity by ethanol therapy. *N Engl J Med* 1982; 307:1528.

80. Wacker W, Haynes H, Druyan R, et al: Treatment of ethylene glycol poisoning with ethyl alcohol. *JAMA* 1965; 194:173–175.

81. Freed C, Bobbitt W, Williams R, et al: Ethanol for ethylene glycol poisoning. *N Engl J Med* 1981;304: 976–977.

82. Peterson C: Oral ethanol doses in patients with methanol poisoning. *Am J Hosp Pharmacol* 1981;38:1024–1027.

83. Peterson C, Collins A, Keane W, et al: Reply to Dr Freed et al, editorial. *N Engl J Med* 1981;304:977–978.

84. Robertson C, Sellers E: Alcohol intoxication and the alcohol withdrawal syndrome. *Postgrad Med* 1978; 64:133–138.

85. Noker P: Methanol toxicity: Treatment with folic acid and 5-formyl tetrahydrofolic acid. *Alcohol Clin Exp Res* 1980;4:378–383.

86. Noker P, Eels J, Tephly T: Methanol toxicity: Treatment with folic acid and 5-formyl tetrahydrofolic acid. *Alcoholism* 1980;4:378–383.

87. Van Stee E, Harris A, Horton M, et al: The treatment of ethylene glycol toxicosis with pyrazole. *J Pharmacol Exp Ther* 1975;192:251–259.

88. Narins R, Emmett M: Simple and mixed acid-base disorders: A practical approach. *Medicine* 1980;59:161–185.

89. Becker C: Acute methanol poisoning. *West J Med* 1981;135:122–128.

90. Gonda A, Gaunt H, Churchill D, et al: Hemodialysis for methanol intoxication. *Am J Med* 1978;64:749–759.

91. Keyvan-Larijarni H, Tannenberg A: Methanol intoxication: Comparison of peritoneal dialysis and hemodialysis treatment. *Arch Intern Med* 1974;134:293–296.

92. Vale J, Prior J, O'Hare J, et al: Treatment of ethylene glycol poisoning with peritoneal dialysis. *Br Med J* 1982;284:557.

93. Osterloh J, Pond S, Grady S, et al: Serum formate concentrations in methanol intoxication as a criterion for hemodialysis. *Ann Intern Med* 1986;104:200–203.

ADDITIONAL SELECTED REFERENCES

Ballantyne B, Myers R: The comparative acute toxicity and primary irritancy of the monohexyl ethers of ethylene and diethylene glycol. *Vet Hum Toxicol* 1987;29:361–366.

Baud F, Bismuth C, Garnier R, et al: 4-Methylpyrazole may be an alternative to ethanol therapy for ethylene glycol intoxication in man. *Clin Toxicol* 1987;24:463–483.

Boquist L, Lindqvist B, Oestberg Y, et al: Primary oxalosis. *Am J Med* 1973;54:673–681.

Clay K, Murphy R, Watkins W: Experimental methanol toxicity in the primate: Analysis of metabolic acidosis. *Toxicol Appl Pharmacol* 1975;34:49–61.

Hazra D, Seth H, Mathur K, et al: Electrocardiographic changes in acute methanol poisoning. *J Assoc Physician India* 1974;22:409–413.

Hussey H: Methanol poisoning. *JAMA* 1974;229:1335–1336.

Martin-Amat G, Tephly R, McMartin K, et al: Methyl alcohol poisoning: Development of a model for ocular toxicity in methyl alcohol poisoning using the rhesus monkey. *Arch Ophthalmol* 1977;95:1847–1850.

Michelis M, Mitchell B, Davis B: 'Bicarbonate-resistant' metabolic acidosis in association with ethylene glycol intoxication. *Clin Toxicol* 1976;9:53–60.

Okell R, Derbyshire D: Ethylene glycol poisoning. *Anaesthesia* 1983;38:168–170.

Seeff L, Hendler E, Hosten A, et al: Ethylene glycol poisoning. *Med Ann Dist Columbia* 1970;39:31–35.

Spector R: Methanol poisoning. *J Iowa Med Soc* 1983;73:60–64.

Stein Z, Barkin R, Lipscomb J, et al: Ethylene glycol toxicity and treatment. *Drug Intell Clin Pharm* 1983;17:376–377.

Stivrins T, Moore G: Ethylene glycol ingestion in a retarded young adult—A case report. *Nebr Med J* 1982;67:181–183.

Stokes J, Aueron F: Prevention of organ damage in massive ethylene glycol ingestion. *JAMA* 1980;243:2065–2066.

Tintinalli J: Of anions, osmols and methanol poisoning. *JACEP* 1977;6:417–421.

Wenger A: Methanol poisoning. *JAMA* 1975;232:906–907.

Younossi-Harstenstein A, Roth B, Iffland R, et al: Short-term hemodialysis for ethylene glycol poisoning. *J Pediatr* 1986;109:731–732.

Zoppi F, Montalbette N: Large-scale screening determination for formate as a tool for assessing severity of methanol intoxication. *Clin Chem* 1986;32:2002–2003.

chapter 26

Workup of the Patient with an Acid-Base Disorder

The preceding three chapters discussed the acute ingestion of ethanol and ethanol substitutes, many of which may offer the clinician a diagnostic challenge. This chapter discusses the workup of a patient with an acid-base disorder that may involve some of the toxins previously discussed. A systematic plan for the workup is presented.

ASSOCIATED MEDICAL CONDITIONS OF THE ALCOHOLIC

It is important to know the associated medical conditions of the patient group that may be more likely to be poisoned by ethanol and ethanol substitutes. Knowing what disorders to expect will aid in understanding the rationale for the suggested workup of the patient.

The patient who chronically ingests an alcohol-like substance may present to the emergency department with an episode of ethanol intoxication, but there may be any number of associated medical conditions (Table 26-1). The chronic alcoholic may have evidence of alcoholic liver disease, cirrhosis, or neurologic abnormalities associated with alcohol intake. Mental deterioration, nystagmus, and ophthalmoplegias suggestive of Wernicke-Korsakoff syndrome may also occur. The alcoholic has many nutritional deficiencies that should be considered. Multiple vitamin deficiencies, including decreases in folate, thiamine, and vitamin B_{12}, are common.[1] Complaints of abdominal pain may be secondary to liver disease, pancreatitis, gastritis, or Mallory-Weiss syndrome.[2] Hematologic disturbances may consist of bleeding diathesis, thrombocytopenia, pancytopenia, or anemia (either macrocytic or microcytic). Hypothermia may be a problem secondary to exposure. Infection and the sequelae of trauma should always be considered in the alcoholic.

A concomitant ingestion of any drug should be considered in any patient with an altered mental status, but consideration should especially be given to the ingestion of ethylene glycol, methanol, and isopropyl alcohol because these are substances that are considered substitutes for ethyl alcohol.[3,4]

The electrolyte disorders noted in this group can be varied and profound. Hypoglycemia may result from the depletion of glycogen stores and impairment of gluconeogenesis.[5] Normally, blood glucose is maintained by liver glycogen stores, by gluconeogenesis, and by the amount of carbohydrate intake. The nutritionally deficient alcoholic also has decreased glycogen stores and is dependent on gluconeogenesis to maintain a normal blood glucose concentration. Because alcohol inhibits gluconeogenesis, hypoglycemia may result.[6] This inhibitory effect appears to develop gradually, which accounts for the relatively slow decrease in serum glucose concentration and the late onset of symptoms of

Table 26-1 Associated Medical Conditions in the Alcoholic

Alcoholic liver disease with cirrhosis
Polyneuritis
Mental deterioration (Wernicke-Korsakoff syndrome)
Cardiac toxicity
Nutritional deficiencies
Abdominal pain
  Liver disease
  Pancreatitis
  Gastritis
  Mallory-Weiss syndrome
Hematologic disturbances
  Bleeding diathesis
  Thrombocytopenia
  Pancytopenia
  Anemia
    Macrocytic
    Microcytic
Hypothermia
Infection
Trauma
Overdose
  Ethylene glycol
  Methanol
  Isopropyl alcohol
  Other toxins
Electrolyte disorder
  Hypoglycemia
  Hypomagnesemia
  Hypophosphatemia
  Hypokalemia
Acid-base disorder
  Lactic acidosis
  Ketoacidosis
Alcohol withdrawal

---

hypoglycemia after ingestion of alcohol.[6] The ingestion of alcohol is the most common cause of profound, disabling, and lethal hypoglycemic coma in adults and children,[7] although there does not appear to be a direct relationship between the blood alcohol concentration and hypoglycemia.[8,9]

In normal adults, a fast of 42 to 72 hours is necessary to induce alcoholic hypoglycemia, whereas infants and children seem to be particularly susceptible to this condition. Both the period of fasting and the latent period from time of ingestion of ethanol to hypoglycemic coma are shorter in children than in adults; an overnight fast has been sufficient to cause hypoglycemia in healthy infants and children.[8–10] Although ethanol-induced hypoglycemia occurs most frequently in combination with malnutrition and chronic alcoholism, it also appears in both adult and adolescent ''binge'' drinkers.

Hypomagnesemia, hypophosphatemia, and hypokalemia may also be observed. These electrolyte disorders are thought to contribute to the dysrhythmias noted in the alcoholic population.[11] Atrial fibrillation is the most frequent conduction abnormality noted and is followed by atrial flutter and isolated premature contractions.[12] Alcoholic cardiomyopathy may also develop; this condition may have an insidious onset but may result in florid congestive failure.

Acid-base disturbances may be noted frequently, especially an anion gap metabolic acidosis secondary to lactic acidosis, ketoacidosis, or the concomitant ingestion of another drug causing an acidosis. Both lactic acidosis and ketoacidosis are related to the fact that alcohol depletes NAD during its metabolism, which leads to a buildup of NADH.[13] A functional block in NADH reoxidation also appears to exist, possibly because of the accumulation of acetaldehyde.[6] Lactic acidosis occurs because of inhibition of lactate transformation into pyruvate.[14–16] Ketoacidosis is produced through the increased oxidation of fatty acids to acetoacetic acid, which is consequently reduced to β-hydroxybutyric acid and then cannot be reoxidized to acetoacetic acid.[6,9] Because β-hydroxybutyric acid is not measured by Acetest® tablets or by a dipstick test (acetoacetate is the measured ketone), serum and urine ketones may be read as negative.[16] Many times patients have no measurable blood alcohol concentration because they stopped their alcohol intake 24 to 72 hours before presentation and at the same time consumed few calories.[5,6]

In addition to these disorders, alcoholic withdrawal and delirium tremens may present either as a life-threatening situation or a condition that requires medical intervention.

ITEMS IN THE WORKUP

The workup of the alcoholic patient presenting to the emergency department may consist of any or all of the following: electrolyte determinations, calculation of the anion gap, calculation of osmolal gap, urinalysis, measurement of serum concentrations of potential toxic substances, electrocardiography (if available), and other studies (Table 26-2).[3]

Serum Electrolytes

Electrolytes should be measured because imbalances are relatively common in the alcoholic, usually as a result of nutritional deficiencies and dehydration.[3] Serum electrolytes may also indicate an acid-base disorder.[2]

Anion Gap

The anion gap is an extremely useful aid in diagnosing disorders associated with both the alcoholic population and other groups with serious medical problems.[17,18] Results of the serum electrolytes are necessary for this calculation, which is based on the measured cations (sodium) and anions (chloride and bicarbonate).[19] Although the cation potassium has been used in some formulas, it does not significantly contribute to the calculation of anion gap and can be ignored.[6]

The formula for the calculation of the anion gap is

$$Na^+ - (Cl^- + HCO_3^-)$$

This calculation of anion gap is considered within normal limits if it is 8 to 12 mEq when potassium is not considered.[2,17,20] The number obtained from this calculation can signify the type of acid-base disorder. Sodium is the only cation included in the formula for simplicity; the other cations are relatively stable and present in small concentrations. If the calcium or magnesium concentrations change greatly, however, the anion gap may be significantly altered.[17] Even so, for all practical purposes laboratories do not routinely measure these cations because, in the normal state, sodium accounts for almost 90% of the extracellular cations. Chloride and bicarbonate account for 85% of the extracellular anions.[17,21] The unmeasured anions are albumin, which is an anion at physiologic pH, phosphate, sulfate, organic acids, and negatively charged proteins (Table 26-3).

Table 26-2 Laboratory Workup of the Alcohol-Intoxicated Patient

Electrolytes
Anion gap
Arterial blood gas
Amylase
Ketones
Osmolal gap
Urinalysis
Serum concentrations
Electrocardiogram
Liver function tests
Complete blood cell count
Clotting studies

Table 26-3 Cations and Anions Not Usually Measured

Anions
  Proteins
  Phosphate
  Sulfate
  Organic acids
Cations
  Magnesium
  Calcium

For the most part, a significantly increased anion gap signifies a metabolic acidosis, although small increases in the anion gap (2 to 3 mEq/L) can be caused by dehydration or starvation ketosis,[20] the administration of sodium salts such as sodium sulfate for hypercalcemia, or the administration of certain antibiotics containing large amounts of sodium such as disodium carbenicillin (in which the carbenicillin moiety acts as an anion and is not routinely measured).[18] In addition, respiratory alkalosis and hypocapnea may cause a slight increase in the anion gap.

In a patient who presents with an acid-base disorder, the type of acid-base disturbance that has occurred must be determined. If the bicarbonate is low and there is a gap, it is necessary to know whether this reflects a respiratory alkalosis or a metabolic acidosis. Respiratory acidosis causes an increased gap because the primary defect is the enhanced pulmonary excretion of carbon dioxide, which lowers the serum bicarbonate concentration. If the disorder is due to an anion gap metabolic acidosis, further examination of the cause is appropriate. Both drug and nondrug causes should be considered.[2,22] An acronym has been developed for causes of an anion gap metabolic acidosis (Table 26-4).[17,23]

Nondrug Causes of Anion Gap Metabolic Acidosis

Nondrug causes of an anion gap metabolic acidosis include lactic acidosis secondary to tissue hypoperfusion (as observed in hypotension and shock) or the body's inability to keep up with an increase in the metabolic demands (as seen in a grand mal seizure); diabetic ketoacidosis, in which the ketoacids contribute to the metabolic acidosis; alcoholic ketoacidosis in patients who are usually chronic alcoholics with a history of prolonged ethanol intake and a marked decrease in food intake before the development of the acidosis; and uremia due to the retention of sulfates, phosphates, urates, and unidentified acids.[5,18] Not all ketones produce an acidosis; in fact, only β-hydroxybutyric acid and acetoacetic acid lead to an acidosis. Acetone is a neutral ketone that does not change the serum bicarbonate or affect the anion gap.[5,17]

Drug Causes of Anion Gap Metabolic Acidosis

Drug causes of an anion gap metabolic acidosis include salicylates, which typically cause a respiratory alkalosis in adults (although a mixed acid-base picture can occur as well as an anion gap metabolic acidosis), iron, isoniazid, paraldehyde, toluene, Vacor®, carbon monoxide, and cyanide.[5]

Ethylene glycol can cause an anion gap metabolic acidosis because of the accumulation of glycolic acid and, to a lesser extent, glycoaldehyde, glyoxylic acid, oxalic acid, and hippuric acid.[23] Methanol causes an anion gap metabolic acidosis because of the formation of formic acid. Both ethylene glycol and methanol can interfere with the Krebs cycle, resulting in lactic acidosis.[5,18]

Osmolal Gap

In addition to the anion gap, the osmolal gap may also be helpful in making the diagnosis of an exogenous toxin.[23,24] Osmolality is a reflection of the number of molecules of solute dissolved in a solvent[25] or, in other words, of the total number of particles in a solution.[26] In clinical practice, solute concentrations are measured per liter of solution.[27] Usually sodium, urea, and glucose are the substances that primarily contribute to serum osmolality.[27] In the normal state, the dependence of serum osmolality on electrolyte concentration is essentially a function of sodium alone.[21]

The formula for the calculation of the serum osmolality[2,17,21,23,25,28–30] is

$$2(Na^+) + glucose/18 + blood\ urea\ nitrogen/2.8$$

The units for glucose and blood urea nitrogen are milligrams per deciliter. The coefficients (or denominators) for glucose and urea are used to convert these values to millimolar concentrations.[21] A normal serum osmolality is 280 to 295 mOsm per liter of water.[2,23] Normally the calculated value is within 10 mOsm/L of the measured value.[31] The calculated serum osmolality, however, does not take into account the possible presence of other osmotically active particles. When the measured value is greater than the calculated value by more than 10 mOsm, it is called an osmolal gap.[5,25,32] This implies the presence of one or more exogenous, low–molecular weight solutes in the blood. From a practical point of view the osmolal gap is normally less than 10 mOsm/L and consists mainly of calcium, lipids, proteins, and solutes not included in the formula.[26]

Table 26-4 Causes of Anion Gap Metabolic Acidosis (Acronym: A MUD PILE CAT)

A	Alcohol
M	Methyl alcohol
U	Uremia
D	Diabetic ketoacidosis
P	Paraldehyde
I	Iron, isoniazid
L	Lactic acidosis
E	Ethylene glycol
C	Carbon monoxide, cyanide
A	Aspirin
T	Toluene

An important reason for serum osmolality measurement is for detection of solute abnormalities when no primary disorder of sodium, glucose, or urea exists.[25] Specifically, it is the detection of the hyperosmolal state caused by the presence of an osmotically active substance ordinarily absent from the blood.[33] Typically, a substance contributes significantly to the osmolality of the serum only if it has a low molecular weight and achieves high blood concentrations.[28]

Practically speaking, few drugs or intoxicants with the exception of the alcohols affect plasma osmolality.[32] The alcohols that contribute in this regard are ethanol, methanol, ethylene glycol, and isopropanol (Table 26-5), with ethanol being the most commonly noted.[25,34] Because the molecular weight of methanol is so low, it can produce a profound osmolal gap that can be 50% greater than that produced by ethanol.[35] Since ethylene glycol has almost twice the molecular weight of methanol, the same amount of glycol produces only half the osmolal gap. An absence of an elevated osmolal gap with ethylene glycol, therefore, does not exclude the diagnosis of ethylene glycol intoxication, but detecting the presence of a gap can be crucial in making a rapid, accurate diagnosis.[24] In addition to these alcohols, glycerol, mannitol, sorbitol, diatrizoate (a dye used in intravenous pyelography), and acetone can also contribute to an osmolal gap.[27,33,36]

A lower than normal osmolal gap may be seen when water-insoluble substances are present in the blood; this is the case with hyperlipidemia or hyperproteinemia, in which the increase in plasma lipids or proteins in the serum causes an apparent reduction in the sodium and water concentration of the serum. Because globulins and lipids are not measured in osmolality, a low osmolal gap is reflected.

Two methods of osmolality measurement are freezing-point depression and vapor pressure. A vapor pressure osmometer is insensitive to the presence of volatile solutes in a sample, and the osmolality is not changed by these low–molecular weight organic compounds. The advantage of vapor pressure osmometers is that they can measure grossly lipemic serum. Nevertheless, most laboratories use freezing-point depression rather than vapor pressure for measuring serum osmolality.[23] A freezing-point depression osmometer responds with increased osmolality when volatiles such as alcohols are present in high concentrations.[26]

The osmolal gap is noted with all four alcohols. Its magnitude is proportional to the amount ingested and inversely proportional to the molecular weight (MW) of the alcohol (Table 26-6). Appropriate blood concentrations of each alcohol can be predicted from osmolality measurements by means of the following formula[2]:

$$\text{Predicted serum concentration} = (\text{osmolal gap} - 10) \times \text{MW}/10$$

The osmolal gap can also be used in the formula because it has been shown that for every 100 mg of ethanol per deciliter the osmolal gap increases by approximately 20 (Table 26-7). The amount of ethanol (in milligrams per deciliter) can therefore be divided by 5 to give an approximation of the amount of ethanol in the body. The same is true for other alcohols and alcohol-like substances. A serum methanol concentration of 100 mg/dL, for example, adds approximately 31 mOsm/L to the osmolal gap.[35]

Table 26-5 Substances That Cause an Osmolal Gap

Alcohols
  Ethanol
  Ethylene glycol
  Isopropanol
  Methanol
  Propylene glycol
Sugars
  Glycerol
  Mannitol
  Sorbitol
Diatrizoate
Acetone

Table 26-6 Molecular Weights of the Alcohols

Alcohol	Molecular Weight
Ethanol	46
Ethylene glycol	62
Isopropanol	60
Methanol	32

Only molecules that are unable to pass through a semipermeable membrane exert osmotic pressure. Any molecule that can freely diffuse through cellular membranes does not exert osmotic pressure. Solutes such as urea, ethyl alcohol, methanol, and ethylene glycol pass through cells freely; therefore, although they raise the osmolality, they do not cause any fluid shifts.[27] In contrast, accumulation of impermeable solutes such as sodium or glucose leads to water movement from cells, intracellular dehydration, and symptoms secondary to the fluid shifts.

The simplicity of osmolal analysis of serum permits rapid identification of the presence of a toxin in advance of formal quantitative toxicologic assay. All patients in whom there is a suspicion of alcohol intoxication, especially those who are comatose or acidemic, merit osmolal screening. When present, the osmolal gap must be reconciled with measured ethanol concentrations to determine whether there are additional or alternate toxins.

It is possible to use the osmolal gap to estimate the concentration of an osmotically active molecule.[21,23] For instance, if the measured serum osmolality is 380 mOsm/L and the calculated serum osmolality is 310 mOsm/L, the gap is 70. If the osmotically active substance is ethanol, the gap of 70 corresponds to a serum concentration of 300 mg/dL ($70 - 10 = 60$; $60 \times 5 = 300$ mg/dL). The concentrations of methanol, isopropanol, and ethylene glycol can also be calculated from this formula (Table 26-8).[31]

There may be several causes of an elevated anion gap or osmolal gap, but there are few conditions except the ingestion of methanol or ethylene glycol that will concomitantly elevate both anion and osmolal gaps.

Urinalysis

A urinalysis may be useful in a patient suspected of being intoxicated with an alcohol-like substance; analysis should be directed toward evidence of crystalluria, ketonuria, proteinuria, microscopic hematuria, and myoglobinuria. Calcium oxalate crystals appear in the urinary sediment of an ethylene glycol–intoxicated patient in octahedral (dihydrate or "envelope") form and, more commonly, in a monohydrate (dumbbell or rod) form. The monohydrate form has previously been misinterpreted as hippuric acid crystals.[23,37,38] These findings must not be overinterpreted, however, because oxalate crystals can be a normal constituent of urine, especially when certain foods such as rhubarb, spinach, tea, and cola drinks are ingested (Table 26-9).

Because of the fluorescein-based coloring added to ethylene glycol preparations, if a 30-mL volume of antifreeze is ingested 0.6 mg of fluorescein is also ingested. This may be noted on Wood's lamp examination of the emesis, gastric aspirate, or urine if performed in a timely fashion. This could be an adjunctive diagnostic test while awaiting definitive quantitation analy-

Table 26-7 Interpretation of Osmolal Gaps in the Presence of Alcohols

Alcohol (100 mg/dL increment)	Increase in Osmolal Gap
Ethanol	22
Methanol	31
Ethylene glycol	16
Isopropanol	17

Table 26-8 Coefficients Associated with the Alcohols for Use in Osmolal Gap Calculations

Alcohol	Coefficient
Ethanol	5
Methanol	3
Ethylene glycol	6
Isopropanol	6

Table 26-9 Oxalate-Rich Plants and Foods

Diffenbachia
Rhubarb
Spinach
Cola drinks
Beets
Tea

Table 26-10 Diagnostic Clues to the Presence of Toxins Commonly Ingested by Alcoholics

Substance/ condition	Eye findings	Anion gap metabolic acidosis	Distinct odor on breath	Urine crystals	Serum ketones	Osmolal gap
Ethanol	0	+	+	0	+	+
Methanol	+	+	0	0	0	+ +
Ethylene glycol	0	+	0	+	0	+
Isopropyl alcohol	0	0	+	0	+	+
Ketoacidosis	0	+	+	0	+	±

Source: Adapted with permission from "Clinical Use of the Anion Gap" by M Emmett and R Narins in *Medicine* (1977;56:46), Copyright © 1977, Williams & Wilkins Company.

sis of serum ethylene glycol concentration. (Snodgrass W, personal communication, 1987.)

Serum Concentrations of Various Agents

It may be necessary to measure serum concentrations to make a diagnosis of ingested agents that can cause an anion gap metabolic acidosis. Salicylate, iron (and iron-binding capacity), methanol, ethylene glycol, isopropyl alcohol, and ethanol should be measured if there is a suspicion of ingestion of any of these substances. Other more sophisticated toxicologic analysis may also be required.

Electrocardiogram

An electrocardiogram should be performed if there is a suspicion of ingestion of an alcohol-like substance to find evidence of hypocalcemia (ethylene glycol) or hypomagnesemia and hypokalemia (ethanol).[32]

Miscellaneous Studies

Liver function studies, a *complete blood cell count*, and *clotting studies* should also be per-

formed for baseline values in the patient who has ingested an alcohol or alcohol-like substance.

SUMMARY OF THE EFFECTS OF ALCOHOLS

Methanol typically produces eye findings usually late in the course of intoxication (Table 26-10). No characteristic odor of alcohol is noted on the breath. No urinary crystals or serum ketones are detected, and there is likely to be an osmolal gap.

Ethylene glycol typically produces no eye findings, and there is no characteristic ethyl alcohol odor on the patient's breath. Intoxication may exhibit one or both forms of calcium oxalate crystals in the urine. There are no serum ketones, and an osmolal gap occurs to a lesser extent than with methanol.

Isopropyl alcohol is not associated with eye findings or eye damage. There is a characteristic fruity odor from ketones on the breath. The urine contains no crystals but is positive for ketones. There may be an osmolal gap. The molecular weights of ethylene glycol and isopropyl alcohol are similar, and both these compounds raise the gap approximately half as much as methanol.

REFERENCES

1. Leevy C, Thompson A, Baker H: Vitamins and liver injury. *Am J Clin Nutr* 1970;23:493–499.

2. Becker C: The alcoholic patient as a toxic emergency. *Emerg Clin North Am* 1984;2:47–61.

3. Goldfrank L, Starke C: Metabolic acidosis in the alcoholic. *Hosp Physician* 1979;15:34–38.

4. Pierce R: Stuporous alcoholics: Metabolic considerations. *South Med J* 1982;75:463–469.

5. Adams S, Mathews J, Flaherty J: Alcoholic keto-acidosis. *Ann Emerg Med* 1987;16:90–97.

6. Duffens K, Marx J: Alcoholic ketoacidosis—A review. *J Emerg Med* 1987;5:399–406.

7. Seltzer H: Severe drug-induced hypoglycemia—A review. *Compr Ther* 1979;5:21–29.

8. Madison L: Ethanol-induced hypoglycemia. *Adv Metabol Disord* 1968;3:85–109.

9. Williams H: Alcoholic hypoglycemia and keto-acidosis. *Med Clin North Am* 1984;68:33–38.

10. MacLaren N, Valman H, Levin B: Alcohol-induced hypoglycemia in childhood. *Br Med J* 1970;1:278–280.

11. Sheehan J: Alcohol and the heart, editorial. *Ann Intern Med* 1983;98:1022.

12. Adelson L: Fatal intoxication with isopropyl alcohol. *Am J Clin Pathol* 1962;38:144–151.

13. Frommer J: Lactic acidosis. *Med Clin North Am* 1983;67:815–829.

14. Narins R, Rudnick M, Bastl C: Lactic acidosis and the elevated anion gap: Part I. *Hosp Pract* 1980;15:125–136.

15. Narins R, Rudnick M, Bastl C: Lactic acidosis and the elevated anion gap: Part II. *Hosp Pract* 1980;15:91–98.

16. Narins R, Emmett M: Simple and mixed acid-base disorders: A practical approach. *Medicine* 1980; 59:161–185.

17. Emmett M, Narins R: Clinical use of the anion gap. *Medicine* 1977;56:38–54.

18. Gabow P, Kaehny W, Fennessey P, et al: Diagnostic importance of an increased serum anion gap. *N Engl J Med* 1980;303:854–858.

19. Enger E: Acidosis, gaps and poisonings. *Acta Med Scand* 1982;212:1–3.

20. Scully R, Galdabini J, McNeely B: Case 38-1979: Presentation of a case. *N Engl J Med* 1979;301:650–657.

21. Dorwart W, Chalmers L: Comparison of methods for calculating serum osmolality from chemical concentrations, and the prognostic value of such calculations. *Clin Chem* 1975;21:190–194.

22. Kushner R, Sitrin M: Metabolic acidosis. *Arch Intern Med* 1986;146:343–345.

23. Epstein F: Osmolality. *Emerg Med Clin North Am* 1986;4:253–261.

24. Turk J, Morell L: Ethylene glycol intoxication. *Arch Intern Med* 1986;146:1601–1603.

25. Glasser L, Sternglanz P, Combie J, et al: Serum osmolality and its applicability to drug overdose. *Am J Clin Pathol* 1973;60:695–699.

26. Lund M, Banner W, Finley P, et al: Effect of alcohols and selected solvents on serum osmolality measurements. *J Toxicol Clin Toxicol* 1983;20:115–132.

27. Gennari F: Serum osmolality: Uses and limitations. *New Engl J Med* 1984;310:102–105.

28. Tintinalli J: Of anions, osmols and methanol poisoning. *JACEP* 1977;6:417–421.

29. Felts P: Ketoacidosis. *Med Clin North Am* 1983; 67:831–843.

30. Kreisberg R, Wood B: Drug- and chemical-induced metabolic acidosis. *Clin Endocrinol Metab* 1983; 12:391–411.

31. Cadnapaphornchai P, Taher S, Bhathena D, et al: Ethylene glycol poisoning: Diagnosis based on high osmolal and anion gaps and crystalluria. *Ann Emerg Med* 1981; 10:94–97.

32. Tong T: The alcohols. *Crit Care Q* 1982;4:75–85.

33. Jacobsen D, Bredesen J, Eide I, et al: Anion and osmolal gaps in the diagnosis of methanol and ethylene glycol poisoning. *Acta Med Scand* 1982;212:17–20.

34. Robinson A, Loeb J: Ethanol ingestion—Commonest cause of elevated plasma osmolality. *N Engl J Med* 1971;284:1253–1255.

35. Smith M: Solvent toxicity: Isopropanol, methanol, and ethylene glycol. *Ear Nose Throat J* 1983;62:126–135.

36. Stern E: Serum osmolality in cases of poisoning. *N Engl J Med* 1974;290:1026.

37. Godolphin W, Meagher E, Sanders H, et al: Unusual calcium oxalate crystals in ethylene glycol poisoning. *Clin Toxicol* 1980;16:479–486.

38. Terlinsky A, Grochowski J, Geoly K, et al: Identification of atypical calcium oxalate crystalluria following ethylene glycol ingestion. *Am J Clin Pathol* 1981;76:223–226.

ADDITIONAL SELECTED REFERENCES

Baud F, Bismuth C, Garnier R, et al: 4-Methylpyrazole may be an alternative to ethanol therapy for ethylene glycol intoxication in man. *Clin Toxicol* 1987;24:463–483.

Becker C: Methanol poisoning. *J Emerg Med* 1983;1:51–58.

Brown C, Trumbull D, Klein-Schwartz W, et al: Ethylene glycol poisoning. *Ann Emerg Med* 1983;12:501–506.

Evans J, Main J, Mitchell P, et al: Lactic acidosis and beer drinking. *Scott Med J* 1985;30:237–238.

Gamble J: In retrospect: A wrong turn in acid-base physiology. *Am J Med* 1986;81:125–126.

Heggarty H: Acute alcoholic hypoglycemia in two 4-year-olds. *Br Med J* 1970;1:280.

Lieber C: Metabolism and metabolic effects of alcohol. *Med Clin North Am* 1984;68:3–31.

Moss M: Alcohol-induced hypoglycemia and coma produced by alcohol sponging. *Pediatrics* 1970;46:445–447.

Ricci L, Hoffman S: Ethanol-induced hypoglycemic coma in a child. *Ann Emerg Med* 1982;11:202–204.

part VIII

DRUGS OF ABUSE

chapter 27

Drugs of Abuse: Overview

The use and misuse of mind-altering substances has existed since antiquity.[1,2] Drug abuse is now one of the major health problems in the United States and is implicated in many deaths, both directly from overdose and indirectly as a result of injuries sustained while the individual is intoxicated. Further, the number of available pharmaceuticals has increased greatly during the last few decades, as has societal use and dependence on medicines. Americans take prescription medications at an astonishing rate.[3,4] In addition, a large number of illicit drugs containing psychoactive substances are consumed each year.[5] The problems resulting from substance use and abuse appear to be more extensive in our modern society than ever before because of this increased availability and number of substances.[6] Also, there seems to be no limit to the type of material used to carry or disguise the drug or drug combination.[4] The United States seems to be at the forefront of the problem, but there are few countries whose youth are not involved.[7,8]

The definition of drug or substance abuse varies but is generally defined as the use of a chemical for a desired pharmacologic effect in a developmentally inappropriate way.[9] It may be considered an excessive and persistent self-administration of a drug without regard for medically or culturally accepted patterns of use. The use of the drug may interfere with the health and social functioning of an individual. The terms use and abuse are used interchangeably in this section.[10]

It is clear that, in discussing drugs of abuse, all sections of the community are involved—from the accidental ingestion of drugs by young children, to experimentation by youth, to the isolated individual for whom hallucinogens or hard drugs are part of a lifestyle, to the middle-aged "housewife" who is on the roller coaster of barbiturates or benzodiazepines and amphetamines, to the harried business executive who needs tranquilizers or alcohol to face the problems of his or her hectic world.[11–13]

Drugs of abuse include any substance or chemical used to alter an individual's mood, sense of well-being, or psychological conception of his or her relation to the environment.[5] Sometimes there is a fine line between where therapeutic use ends and abuse begins. Although there are major classes of drugs that are abused, such as stimulants, narcotics, sedative-hypnotics, and hallucinogens, there are also drugs that fit into no particular class. In this section drugs of abuse are discussed in separate chapters according to pharmacological class, and miscellaneous agents are also discussed separately.

Drug abusers may have a number of complaints referrable to many systems because they frequently abuse more than one substance and often ingest a large proportion of unknown diluents that are added without the observance of proper sterile precautions.[14] They may not know or may withhold valuable information. Usually, only the more severe and dramatic complications of drug misuse are seen in the emergency department. They may consist of toxic physiologic, psychological, and behavioral manifestations such as life-threatening reactions resulting from intentional and unintentional overdose and abstinence syndromes of varying intensity. The major drugs of misuse that bring patients to the clinician's attention are the opiates, sedative-hypnotics, alcohol, and CNS stimulants.[15]

This chapter serves as an overview of the problem of the misuse of drugs for recreational purposes. In general, those individuals who misuse drugs for this reason, especially when parenterally administered, suffer medical complications that can be severe to life threatening. The clinician should always suspect a coexisting medical or psychological problem in patients abusing drugs. In this regard, the heroin abuser may share the same type of problem as that seen with the intravenous cocaine user, and for that reason some of the medical complications of parenteral drug abuse are discussed in this chapter (Table 27-1).

Identification of the drugs used by an acutely intoxicated or overdosed patient usually depends on the clinical picture of the patient as well as a sound knowledge of various pharmacologic syndromes associated with drugs that are abused. It must be remembered that drugs of abuse may not be pharmacologically pure because of the adulterants or "cutting" substances used. Combinations meant to mimic or enhance a drug's effect may complicate and confuse diagnosis and treatment.[14]

ROUTES OF ADMINISTRATION

A drug of abuse can be administered by any means, including orally, by insufflation ("snorting"), by smoking, and by injection subcutaneously ("skin popping"), intramuscularly, or intravenously ("mainlining") (Table 27-2).[16] Administration into the web spaces of the fingers and toes, into the sublingual area, as well as by the dangerous internal jugular or subclavian route, has been attempted. This last is referred to as the "pocket shot" and is an attempt to obtain venous access by injecting into one of the large

Table 27-1 Complications of Parenteral Drug Abuse

Skin
  Necrotizing fasciitis
  Gangrene
  Thrombophlebitis
  Lymphedema
  Hyperpigmentation
  Cellulitis
  Abscess
Systemic
  Bacteremia
  Endocarditis
  "Cotton fever"
  Osteomyelitis
  Viral hepatitis
  Malaria
  Tetanus
  Acquired immune deficiency syndrome (AIDS)
Pulmonary
  Pneumonia
  Pulmonary edema
  Atelectasis
  Pulmonary embolism
  Tuberculosis
  Pulmonary hypertension
  Granuloma
  Pneumothorax
Neurologic
  Cerebral edema
  Transverse myelitis
  Horner's syndrome
  Cerebral infarction
  Intracerebral hemorrhage
  Polyarteritis
  Seizures
Renal
  Nephropathy
  Renal tubular acidosis
  Rhabdomyolysis
  Acute tubular necrosis
Eye
  Endophthalmitis
  Blindness
Metabolic
  Hypokalemia
  Metabolic acidosis
  Hypophosphatemia

veins in the neck.[17,18] This is used by long-term addicts who no longer have peripheral venous access. The patients inject themselves while looking in the mirror or have someone else perform the procedure.[19] Because of the proximity of the apical pleura to the internal jugular vein, this approach frequently causes a pneumothorax.[20]

Table 27-2 Routes of Administration of Drugs of Abuse

Oral
Insufflation ("snorting")
Smoking
Injection
    Subcutaneous ("skin popping")
    Intramuscular
    Intravenous ("mainlining")
    Intra-arterial ("pinkie")
    Web spaces fingers
    Web spaces toes
    Dorsal vein of penis
    Internal jugular vein ("pocket shot")
    Subclavian vein ("pocket shot")
    Sublingual
Mucosal membranes
    Vagina
    Penis

Drugs that are taken intravenously are usually heated in a spoon or bottle cap, drawn into a syringe or eye dropper through cotton or other homemade filters to remove large impurities, and then injected without cleaning the skin. Frequently the same syringe is used by several persons. It should be remembered that street drugs are impure substances. A dose may contain only 5% to 20% of the desired substance and 80% to 90% of "cutting" substances, many of which have significant actions of their own.[14,21,22]

ASSOCIATED MEDICAL CONDITIONS OF THE DRUG USER

Infections Secondary to Contamination

Intravenous drug abusers are subject to numerous infectious diseases, some of which may be life threatening.[23–25] Because of the lack of sterile technique among users, in addition to their custom of sharing paraphernalia, it is not surprising that the complications of intravenous drug abuse are often the result of serious infections, including localized cellulitis or abscess, bacteremia with septic arthritis, osteomyelitis, bacterial or fungal endocarditis, pneumonia, hepatitis, tuberculosis, and malaria.

Bacteremia is the most common hematologic complication of parenteral drug abuse.[26] This leads to "seeding" and infections in other organs. It has been shown that, in the febrile intravenous drug user, clinical data and clinical judgment on the part of the physician are not good predictors as to which patient may have a serious or life-threatening problem such as endocarditis. For this reason, a policy of admitting all febrile intravenous drug users with a thorough workup of the source of the fever is important.[27] Symptoms of chest pain and shortness of breath are common in intravenous drug users. The differential diagnoses of these complaints include a pulmonary embolus or septic pulmonary emboli, pneumothorax, pericarditis, pneumonia, and endocarditis. Malaria was first described as a complication of narcotic abuse more than 50 years ago.[28] Any of the naturally occurring forms of malaria may be seen in the abuser, and "epidemics" have been reported in various cities from shared needles. Recently this phenomenon has decreased, possibly owing to the quinine added as an adulterant. With the return of Viet Nam war veterans, an increase in the incidence of malaria was noted and was confined to the West Coast, where quinine was not in great use. In general, the most common side effect of parenteral drug use and shared needles is both acute and chronic hepatitis.[29]

Pulmonary Sequelae

Pulmonary abnormalities such as pneumonia, pulmonary edema, atelectasis, fibrosis, granuloma formation, and pulmonary embolism are frequently found.[16] Infarcts may progress to cavitation, abscess, or empyema formation.[30] Pneumonia is usually the result of infection with pneumococcus, *Hemophilus* species, or *Staphylococcus aureus* that is often unilateral and typically located in the right middle or lower lobe.[16,30,31] These pulmonary infections have been ascribed to the septicemia that accompanies the skin infections and right-sided endocarditis that occurs in the abuser. The roentgenographic appearance in this instance may be that of pulmonary consolidation.[28] In addition, the incidence of tuberculosis is increased in this population.[25,30]

Pneumothorax can be a traumatic complication of parenteral drug abuse because a growing number of long-term drug abusers are resorting to the use of central veins, particularly the jugular or subclavian veins, as preferred sites for venipuncture; these abusers gradually obliterate peripheral veins by an infectious or sclerotic process.[17,18]

Because marijuana may be contaminated with various fungi, various pulmonary fungal infections such as *Aspergillus pneumonitis* may be noted.[16]

Effects Secondary to "Filler" Substances

Because the addict often injects intravenous preparations intended for oral use, inert "fillers" are injected and may embolize to the lungs. The resultant angiothrombosis may eventually cause pulmonary hypertension and right ventricular failure.[16,32–34] The thromboses can be due to starch, talc, or other particulate matter.[34] This is commonly seen in patients who crush pills for injection that contain talc particles. Although many pills contain talc, tripelennamine and methylphenidate are two of the major substances that have been implicated as the causative agent of granulomas.[32,34]

"Cotton fever" may develop from the use of contaminated cotton to filter impurities. Fever may develop within 5 to 10 minutes after injection and may be a reaction to pyrogens in the cotton, transient bacteremia, multiple pulmonary microemboli, a pyrogenic reaction to heroin, or some other occult mechanism.

Noncardiogenic Pulmonary Edema

Noncardiogenic pulmonary edema is a frequently associated medical finding in the drug abuser, and the clinician should be on the lookout for signs such as cyanosis, diffuse rales, tachypnea, tachycardia, and foamy sputum.[35] Symptoms may occur after intoxication by any route of administration of most classes of illicitly used substances, including narcotics, cocaine, hydrocarbons, and sedative-hypnotics.[16] Individuals who develop pulmonary edema may do so almost instantaneously after injecting the substance; more commonly, the onset may be delayed up to 24 hours after administration.[16,36] Pulmonary edema is usually bilateral, although it may appear in one or only a part of one lung.[9,33,37] The chest roentgenogram may display fluffy, ill-defined densities in an alveolar pattern, radiating centrally to peripherally, with a normal-appearing heart.[38] Physical examination reveals rales and ronchi but absence of peripheral signs such as gallop heart sounds, increased jugular venous distension, or hepatomegaly. Swan-Ganz catheterization reveals a normal left ventricular end-diastolic pressure.[39]

Despite the fact that noncardiogenic pulmonary edema has been recognized for many years, a well-accepted mechanism for this entity is lacking. The pulmonary capillary wedge pressure is normal. The best explanation appears to be an increase in the capillary permeability, causing leakage of fluid into the alveoli. Management is supportive, and if uncomplicated by aspiration the edema usually resolves over a period of hours.[40]

Cardiac Sequelae

The highest rates of morbidity and mortality associated with drug abuse involve the cardiopulmonary system.[1] Endocarditis should be considered in any abuser presenting with fever of unknown etiology and especially in older addicts with heart murmurs, pulmonary infarction, splenomegaly, positive blood cultures, or systemic embolic phenomena.[25,41] In many cases, fever is the only indication of endocarditis.[42] Endocarditis, both right- and left-sided, may occur, although right-sided endocarditis is most common, sparing the pulmonic valve and attacking the previously normal tricuspid valve in almost all cases.[28] This is unusual for endocarditis from other causes, which usually affects the left side of the heart. Because right-sided endocarditis is more common, this group of patients may not have the classic signs or symptoms, and there is usually no history of predisposing heart disease.

The causative organism in right-sided endocarditis is not usually fungal in nature but typically *Staphylococcus aureus*.[25,41] Usually this is a "silent" problem, only seen by evidence of peripheral effects. The first clue to the presence of tricuspid regurgitation may be the existence of multiple or repeated septic pulmonary emboli that may simulate pneumonia.[41] This is in contrast to left-sided endocarditis, where physical signs of valvular disease are invariably apparent. Although the valve attacked has been usually previously normal, a left-sided endocarditis may be superimposed on old syphilitic, atherosclerotic, or rheumatic damage or on a prosthesis.

Staphylococcus aureus is the most common bacterial organism causing disease, although *Streptococcus* species, *Escherichia coli*, *Klebsiella* species, and *Pseudomonas* species are relatively common as well.[29] Fungal endocarditis is always due to *Candida albicans* and is almost always fatal.[25] Death from bacterial endocarditis is most frequently due to heart failure.

The abuser with bacterial endocarditis may present with peripheral embolization.[43] Physical findings most well recognized are Janeway's lesions of the fingers, splinter hemorrhages under the nails, petechiae of the conjunctivae, and Roth's spots in the fundi. Organisms may be cultured from these sites.[37]

Skin Lesions

Drug abusers are subject to several types of skin lesions, some of which are pathognomonic for drug abuse. Signs of venous injections vary from a subtle but definite hyperpigmentation over the injected area, usually antecubital, to the extreme "railroad tracks,"[28,44] which are cutaneous scars due to the repeated puncture of the skin overlying the accessible veins.[25] Because of the many adulterants in illicit opioids the veins eventually become sclerotic and grey, forming these tracks.[9] Tattoos may be imprinted over the course of veins in an attempt to hide the tracks. Hyperpigmentation or tattooing may also result from repeated carbon that is deposited by needles heated with a match before use.

Abscess formation at the site of injection is the most common skin infection encountered.[24] Another set of skin lesions is related to the administration of drugs by "skin popping" or subcutaneous injection, possibly leading to bacterial or chemical abscesses. Lesions secondary to subcutaneous administration may be round macular depressions with sharp borders, giving a "punched-out" appearance.[1] Another type of skin lesion is the rosette of a cigarette burn on the upper anterior chest wall, which is due to the addict "nodding out" with a lighted cigarette in the mouth.[25]

Other dermatologic abnormalities include cellulitis, lymphangitis, and thrombophlebitis. The "puffy hand syndrome," seen in those with longstanding addiction, is the result of occlusive thrombophlebitis, lymphatic obstruction, and lymphedema.[19,28] Necrotizing fasciitis has also been seen in the parenteral drug user.[31] It may begin in a manner similar to that of cellulitis but quickly spreads to a central zone of necrosis with eventual ulceration. It is important to differentiate this disorder from cellulitis so as to institute more appropriate treatment with antibiotics because *Bacteroides* species are frequent pathogens in necrotizing fasciitis. Gangrene, which is caused by intra-arterial injection, may be accompanied by intense pain distal to the injection site and is characterized by swelling, cyanosis, and coldness of the extremity.

The most common pathogens responsible for most of the soft tissue infections caused by a single bacterium are *Staphylococcus aureus* and β-hemolytic streptococci. Enteric gram-negative bacilli as well as normal flora may occasionally be noted. Tetanus, which is an uncommon disease in the United States, has a much greater incidence in the population of drug users than in any other group and often results from "skin popping" with resultant subcutaneous abscess formation.

Renal Involvement

Renal abnormalities include nephropathy, glomerulonephropathy, and rhabdomyolysis with acute tubular necrosis.

Acquired Immune Deficiency Syndrome (AIDS)

The acquired immune deficiency syndrome (AIDS) is a severe disorder first described in male and female drug abusers, hemophiliacs, Haitians, and homosexual men.[29] It is now known that it is not limited to any subgroup.[45] In AIDS, the depression of the individual's cellular immune system results in subsequent development of multiple opportunistic infections, unusual neoplasms, and an inability to mount a delayed hypersensitivity response. Patients with AIDS may exhibit lymphopenia, cutaneous anergy, hypergammaglobulinemia, and a reversal of the ratio of helper to suppressor T cells. These patients most often present with *Pneumocystis carinii* pneumonia, other unusual community-acquired opportunistic infections, and Kaposi's sarcoma.[31,45]

Bone and Joint Infections

Bone and joint infections, which are usually caused by *Pseudomonas aeruginosa*, may occur in the lumbar spine, sternoclavicular joint, and cervical spine. Low back pain may therefore be due to an infection of the disk space rather than to muscle strain. The technetium-99m bone scan is most helpful in localizing the site of infection before changes are visible in plain radiographs.

Neurologic Abnormalities

Neurologic abnormalities include cerebral edema and transverse myelitis; the mechanism for these is unclear. Horner's syndrome from injection into the neck has also been reported.[46] One common abnormality is an atraumatic mononeuropathy, which appears as a painless weakness shortly after injection. Cerebral infarction has been a sequela of intravenous drug abuse, either immediately after injection or hours later. This can be a direct result of the injection or secondary to infective endocarditis, with the cerebrovascular complications of embolization and subarachnoid hemorrhage being due to rupture of a mycotic aneurysm. Vascular changes due to polyarteritis (necrotizing angiitis) have been reported in persons who use amphetamines intravenously (principally methamphetamine).[31] These changes frequently result in cerebrovascular occlusion and intracerebral hemorrhage. CNS stimulants administered parenterally or orally may also cause intracerebral or subarachnoid hemorrhage.

Metabolic Abnormalities

Inhalation of paint and glue has been associated with severe metabolic abnormalities such as metabolic acidosis, often accompanied by hypokalemia, hypophosphatemia, renal tubular acidosis, and occasionally renal failure.[47] Liver necrosis has been reported as a complication of solvent abuse, whereas cardiac fibrillation has been associated with inhalation of the fluorinated hydrocarbons. Solvents such as methylethyl ketone and hexane can produce motor polyneuropathy.

Many abusers, because they know about the problems of associated infections, take nonprescribed antibiotics that are purchased on the street to prevent infections.[48] This may lead to a delay in proper treatment, may suppress bacterial growth in cultures, and may be a major factor promoting the development and spread of resistant organisms.[48]

Ophthalmic Abnormalities

Endophthalmitis is a serious and increasingly common ocular complication of intravenous drug abuse.[49] Endophthalmitis is an inflammation of the ocular tissues. Bacterial endophthalmitis, which consists of eye pain and redness, lid swelling, and decreased or blurred vision, may develop suddenly within 24 to 48 hours after drug use.[50] This condition should be suspected if pain, chemosis, lid edema, and anterior chamber and vitreous inflammation are present. Mycotic endophthalmitis has also been recognized as a complication of intravenous drug use. Species of *Candida*, *Aspergillus*, *Torulopsis*, *Helminthosporium*, and *Penicillium* have been reported to cause endophthalmitis secondary to intravenous drug use. The mycotic endophthalmitis, unlike bacterial endophthalmitis, has a slow, indolent course. In addition to endogenous metastatic endophthalmitis, talc retinopathy and ophthalmic manifestations of endocarditis may be caused by intravenous drug abuse.[50]

Blindness has been reported from quinine amblyopia. Although permanent blindness is rare, a permanent reduction of visual acuity is not uncommon.

CLASSIFICATION OF CONTROLLED SUBSTANCES

Although drugs of abuse can be classified in several ways, in this text they are classified according to their most prominent CNS effects. Classes include the narcotics and narcotic antagonists, sedative-hypnotics, stimulants, hallucinogens, phencyclidine, cannabinoids, volatile inhalants, and miscellaneous drugs (Table 27-3).

The Drug Enforcement Administration of the United States Department of Justice has categorized the controlled substances as narcotics, depressants, stimulants, hallucinogens, and cannabis; these categories reflect their medical utility and abuse potential. Many of the drugs of abuse fall under the Comprehensive Drug Abuse Prevention and Control Act of 1970, which is more familiarly known as the Controlled Substances Act. The Drug Enforcement Administration of the Department of Justice is responsible for enforcing the provisions of the Controlled Substances Act.

There are five categories or schedules that the government has compiled for many of the drugs of abuse; these rank drugs from those with high potential of abuse to those with very little potential for abuse.

Schedule I

The drugs listed in Schedule I are believed to have the highest potential for abuse and have no recognized medical use except for experimental purposes. Substances in Schedule I include heroin, marijuana, and the hallucinogen lysergic acid diethylamide (LSD). Because Schedule I drugs are almost always used within research institutions, there are no specific prescription requirements (Table 27-4).

Schedule II

These drugs have legitimate medical uses but have a high potential for abuse. Most narcotics are listed in Schedule II, along with barbiturates, amphetamines, and cocaine (Table 27-5).

Schedule III

Drugs in Schedule III, with moderate potential for abuse, include nonbarbiturate sedatives, nonamphetamine stimulants, and some narcotic preparations (Table 27-6).

Table 27-3 Classification of Drugs of Abuse

Narcotics
Sedative-hypnotics
CNS stimulants
Hallucinogens
Phencyclidine
Cannabinoids
Volatile inhalants
Miscellaneous agents

Table 27-4 Schedule I Drugs

Heroin
LSD
Marijuana (tetrahydrocannabinol)
Hashish
Methylene dioxyamphetamine
Methylene dioxymethamphetamine
Mescaline
Peyote
Psilocybin

Table 27-5 Schedule II Drugs

Amphetamine
Cocaine
Methylphenidate
Phenmetrazine
Amobarbital
Methaqualone
Pentobarbital
Secobarbital
Codeine
Fentanyl
Hydrocodone
Levorphanol
Meperidine
Methadone
Morphine
Opium
Oxycodone
Oxymorphone
Phencyclidine

Schedule IV

Drugs in Schedule IV have less abuse potential than those in Schedule III and have a limited likelihood of creating physical and psychological dependence. These include some sedatives and analgesics that do not contain narcotics (Table 27-7).

Schedule V

Drugs in Schedule V contain small amounts of narcotics and are used to control coughs and diarrhea. They have a low potential for abuse, may lead to limited physical and psychological dependence, and require the least amount of control and scrutiny.

"Designer Drugs"

"Designer drugs" are those created in illegal laboratories in attempts to circumvent the law by manufacturing substances that are not yet controlled. This is because the law currently requires that the chemical structure of a controlled substance be specified. Illegal laboratories create noncontrolled substances by altering the chemical structure of certain compounds.

Table 27-6 Schedule III Drugs

Benzphetamine
Glutethimide
Methyprylon
Acetaminophen with codeine
Aspirin, phenacetin, and caffeine (APC) with codeine
Acetylsalicylic acid (aspirin) with codeine
Paregoric

Table 27-7 Schedule IV Drugs

Diethylpropion
Phentermine
Chloral hydrate
Chlordiazepoxide
Clonazepam
Chlorazepam
Diazepam
Mephobarbital
Phenobarbital
Propoxyphene
Pentazocine
Meprobamate

Drugs manufactured in this way are of the amphetamine type with psychomimetic properties, such as methylene dioxymethamphetamine, the fentanyl derivatives, and the meperidine derivatives.

REFERENCES

1. Khantzian E, McKenna G: Acute toxic and withdrawal reactions associated with drug use and abuse. *Ann Intern Med* 1979;90:361–372.

2. McGuigan M: Toxicology of drug abuse. *Emerg Med Clin North Am* 1984;2:87–101.

3. Giannini A, Price W, Giannini M: Contemporary drugs of abuse. *Am Fam Physician* 1986;33:207–216.

4. Giannini A, DeFrance D: Metronidazole and alcohol—Potential for combinative abuse. *J Toxicol Clin Toxicol* 1983;20:509–515.

5. Vogel S, Leikin J: What's up (and down) in drug abuse: Street drugs. *Top Emerg Med* 1986;8:57–75.

6. Moriarty K, Alagna S, Lake C: Psychopharmacology. *Psychiatr Clin North Am* 1984;7:411–433.

7. Ficarra B: Toxicologic states treated in an emergency department. *Clin Toxicol* 1980;17:1–43.

8. Shulgin A: Drugs of abuse in the future. *Clin Toxicol* 1975;8:405–456.

9. Kulberg A: Substance abuse: Clinical identification and management. *Pediatr Clin North Am* 1986;33:325–361.

10. Montagne M: Drug-taking paraphernalia. *J Psychoactive Drugs* 1983;15:159–175.

11. Sanders J: Adolescents and substance abuse. *Pediatrics* 1985;76:630–632.

12. Smith H, Talbott G, Morrison M: Chemical abuse and dependence: An occupational hazard for health professionals. *Top Emerg Med* 1985;7:69–78.

13. Pope H, Ionescu-Pioggia M, Cole J: Drug use and life-styles among college undergraduates. *Arch Gen Psychiatr* 1981;38:588–591.

14. Klatt E, Montgomery S, Namiki T, et al: Misrepresentation of stimulant street drugs: A decade of experience in an analysis program. *Clin Toxicol* 1986;24:441–450.

15. Goldfrank L, Bresnitz E: Opioids. *Hosp Physician* 1978;14:26–37.

16. Glassroth J, Adama G, Schnoll S: The impact of substance abuse on the respiratory system. *Chest* 1987; 596–602.

17. Bell C, Borak J, Loeffler J: Pneumothorax in drug abusers: A complication of internal jugular venous injections. *Ann Emerg Med* 1983;12:167–170.

18. Lewis J, Groux N, Elliott J, et al: Complications of attempted central venous injections performed by drug abusers. *Chest* 1980;78:613–617.

19. Shuster M, Lewis M: Needle tracks in narcotic addicts. *NY State J Med* 1968;68:3129–3134.

20. Wisdom K, Nowak R, Richardson H, et al: Alternate therapy for traumatic pneumothorax in ''pocket shooters.'' *Ann Emerg Med* 1986;15:428–432.

21. Brown J, Malone M: Status of drug quality in the street-drug market: An update. *Clin Toxicol* 1976;9:145–168.

22. Brown J, Malone M: Legal highs—Constituents, activity, toxicology, and herbal folklore. *Clin Toxicol* 1978;12:1–31.

23. Orangio G, Latta P, Marino C, et al: Infections in parenteral drug abusers. *Am J Surg* 1983;146:738–740.

24. Orangio G, Pitlick S, Latta P: Soft tissue infections in parenteral drug abusers. *Ann Surg* 1984;199:97–100.

25. Sapira J: The narcotic addict as a medical patient. *Am J Med* 1968;45:555–588.

26. Kozel N, Adams E: Epidemiology of drug abuse: An overview. *Science* 1986;234:970–974.

27. Marantz P, Linzer M, Feiner C, et al: Inability to predict diagnosis in febrile intravenous drug abusers. *Ann Intern Med* 1987;106:823–828.

28. Sternbach G, Moran J, Eliastam M: Heroin addiction: Acute presentation of medical complications. *Ann Emerg Med* 1980;9:161–169.

29. Aston R: Drug abuse: Its relationship to dental practice. *Dent Clin North Am* 1984;28:595–610.

30. Gottlieb L, Boylen T: Pulmonary complications of drug abuse. *West J Med* 1974;120:8–16.

31. Jacobson J, Huschman S: Necrotizing fasciitis complicating intravenous drug abuse. *Arch Intern Med* 1982;142:634–635.

32. Krainer L, Berman E, Wishnick S: Parenteral calcium granulomatosis: A complication of narcotic addiction. *Lab Invest* 1962;11:671–675.

33. Kushner D, Szanto P: Heart failure, fever and splenomegaly in a morphine addict. *JAMA* 1958;166:2162–2165.

34. Lamb D, Roberts G: Starch and talc emboli in drug addicts' lungs. *J Clin Pathol* 1972;25:976–991.

35. Duberstein J, Kaufman D: A clinical study of an epidemic of heroin intoxication and heroin-induced pulmonary edema. *Am J Med* 1971;51:704–714.

36. Steinberg A, Karliner J: The clinical spectrum of heroin pulmonary edema. *Arch Intern Med* 1968;122:122–127.

37. Jaffe R, Koschmann E: Intravenous drug abuse: Pulmonary, cardiac and vascular complications. *Am J Roentgenol* 1970;109:107–120.

38. Frand U, Shim C, Williams M: Heroin-induced pulmonary edema. *Ann Intern Med* 1972;77:29–35.

39. Karliner J: Noncardiogenic forms of pulmonary edema. *Circulation* 1972;46:212–215.

40. Carlet J, Francoual M, Lhoste F, et al: Pharmacological treatment of pulmonary edema. *Intensive Care Med* 1980;6:113–122.

41. Banks T, Fletcher R, Ali N: Infective endocarditis in heroin addicts. *Am J Med* 1973;55:444–451.

42. Nicholi A: The nontherapeutic use of psychoactive drugs. *N Engl J Med* 1983;308:925–933.

43. Ramsey R, Gunnar R, Tobin J: Endocarditis in the drug addict. *Am J Cardiol* 1970;25:608–618.

44. Westerhof W, Wolters E, Brookbakker J, et al: Pigmented lesions of the tongue in heroin addicts: Fixed drug eruption. *Br J Dermatol* 1983;109:605–610.

45. Small C, Klein R, Friedland G: Community-acquired opportunistic infections and defective cellular immunity in heterosexual drug abusers and homosexual men. *Am J Med* 1983;74:433–441.

46. Hawkins K, Bruckstein A, Guthrie T: Percutaneous heroin injection causing Horner's syndrome. *JAMA* 1977;237:1963–1964.

47. Voigts A, Kaufman C: Acidosis and other abnormalities associated with paint sniffing. *South Med J* 1983;76:443–447.

48. Novick D, Ness G: Abuse of antibiotics by abusers of parenteral heroin or cocaine. *South Med J* 1984;77:302–303.

49. McLane N, Carroll D: Ocular manifestations of drug abuse. *Surv Ophthalmol* 1986;30:298–313.

50. Kreeger R, Pearson P, Bullock J, et al: Endophthalmitis associated with intravenous drug abuse. *Ann Emerg Med* 1987;16:585–587.

ADDITIONAL SELECTED REFERENCES

Dole V: Narcotic addiction, physical dependence and relapse. *N Engl J Med* 1972;286:988–992.

DuPont R: Substance abuse. *JAMA* 1985;254:2335–2337.

Dyment P: Drug misuse by adolescents. *Pediatr Clin North Am* 1982;29:1363–1367.

Krause G: Brown-Sequard syndrome following heroin injection. *Ann Emerg Med* 1983;12:581–583.

Menda K, Gorbach S: Favorable experience with bacterial endocarditis in heroin addicts. *Ann Intern Med* 1973;78:25–32.

Tsuang M, Simpson J, Kronfol Z: Subtypes of drug abuse with psychosis. *Arch Gen Psychiatr* 1982;39:141–147.

Vance M: Drug withdrawal syndromes. *Top Emerg Med* 1985;7:63–68.

White A: Medical disorder in drug addicts. *JAMA* 1973;223:1469–1471.

chapter 28

Narcotics

The term narcotic has a number of different meanings depending on the context in which it is used. Strictly speaking, narcotics are opiates, which are substances isolated from the opium poppy. Narcotics also include the semisynthetic opium derivatives, all of which produce tolerance and dependence and have the ability to suppress narcotic withdrawal. In the popular sense narcotics include any drug that can be substituted for heroin or morphine in abuse potential. This definition includes the synthetic opium derivatives, some of which are incapable of suppressing narcotic withdrawal. All these drugs are considered opioids. Endogenous opioids are released in response to stress, electrical brain stimulation, acupuncture, and exogenous opioid analgesics. Unless otherwise noted, the terms opioid, opiate, and narcotic are used interchangeably.

Many times emergency department personnel are approached by patients requesting drugs for symptoms such as headache, migraine, toothache, or other subjective complaints. The sophisticated user may also claim an allergy to agents of low potency and may even suggest what drug to prescribe.[1] Narcotics abusers may try to obtain meperidine, morphine, pentazocine, hydromorphone, oxycodone, and propoxyphene. This chapter is devoted to a discussion of the various legitimate narcotic agents that are available and yet may be abused as well as some of the "designer drugs" that have not found any accepted legitimate use.

CLINICAL USE OF OPIOIDS

A major use of the opioids is for relief of intense pain. Typically, there is a suppression of the perception of pain and a reduction in the response to pain without loss of consciousness. In addition to this major use, narcotics are also used as a cough suppressant (by their direct suppression of the cough centers in the medulla), for the treatment of diarrhea, and for the treatment of cardiogenic pulmonary edema. The opioids are also used preoperatively for sedation and as a supplement to anesthesia (Table 28-1).

ENDORPHINS AND ENKEPHALINS

The discovery of the endorphins, which are endogenous analgesic polypeptides, has led to

Table 28-1 Uses of Narcotic Agents

Relief of intense pain
Antitussive agents
Antidiarrheal agents
Cardiogenic pulmonary edema
Preoperative sedation

an enormous expansion of knowledge about opiate receptors in the brain and peripheral nervous system. These endogenous polypeptides act as specific neurotransmitters and, in the pituitary, as hormone modulators.[2] Thus they are involved in pain perception and analgesia, appetite regulation, respiration, temperature control, and the pathophysiology of shock.[3] A number of other opiate peptides have been identified, including the enkephalins, dynorphin, and casomorphine.[4–6] These peptides bind to several opiate receptors in the brain and peripheral nervous system to produce their physiologic actions, which affect virtually all functions of the body including opiate drug addiction, epilepsy, regulation of pancreatic secretions, and non–insulin-dependent diabetes (Table 28-2).[7] The naturally occurring alkaloids morphine and codeine, their semisynthetic derivatives, and other synthetic agents all either contain or mimic a piperidine ring structure, which is the active component.

Tolerance develops to synthetic enkephalins and endorphins because they appear to mimic morphine in every respect.[8] Enkephalin is rapidly destroyed in vivo, and endorphin is stable and has a long duration of action. The endorphins and enkephalins function as neurotransmitters by inhibition of sodium permeability in opiate receptors.[9] This decreases sodium conductance and permeability, thus inhibiting neuronal activity. Opioid antagonists, on the other hand, increase sodium permeability and cell firing.[9] In actuality, the mechanism may be much more complex and involve the calcium ion or cyclic AMP.[10]

Much work is now being done in the area of endorphins and opioid receptors. The relative analgesic potency of the various opioid drugs seems to parallel their affinity for specific binding sites. Early studies identified three opioid receptors on the basis of different syndromes produced by the prototype drugs. These receptors are localized in the substantia gelatinosa of the spinal cord as well as the brain stem, the reticular formation, the thalamus, and the limbic system.[5,6]

There appear to be at least three receptors that are of clinical importance: the μ, κ, and σ receptors.[11,12] Although other receptors have been postulated, little is known about their function.[3] The μ receptor is the classic morphine-like receptor, which mediates euphoria, physical dependence, respiratory depression, and supraspinal analgesia. These receptors are located mainly at supraspinal sites in the brain stem and limbic system (Table 28-3).

The κ receptors, which mediate pentazocine-like analgesia, sedation, and miosis and perhaps respiratory depression, are located in high density in the spinal cord.[10] Both the μ and κ agonists can produce tolerance and physical dependence, but the abstinence syndromes differ for different receptor agonists, and there is no cross-tolerance for the most part.[4]

The σ receptor appears to be responsible for dysphoria, hallucinations, respiratory and vasomotor stimulatory effects, and psychomimetic effects.[2,8] Many of the mixed agonist-antagonist analgesics act on this receptor (Table 28-4).[5]

In addition to the μ, κ, and σ receptors, δ receptors for the enkephalins and ϵ receptors for the endorphins have been proposed.[2]

Table 28-2 Physiologic Effects and Functions of Endogenous Opiates

---

Analgesia
Blood pressure regulation
Drinking regulation
Feeding behavior alteration
Hormone regulation
Mental function and memory alteration
Respiratory function alteration
Sexual function alteration
Temperature regulation

Source: Adapted with permission from *Journal of Clinical Psychiatry* (1984;45:20), Copyright © 1984, Physicians Postgraduate Press Inc.

Table 28-3 Location of Opiate Receptors

Amygdala
Area postrema of the chemoreceptor trigger zone
Medial thalamus solitary nucleus
Periacqueductal gray matter of the brain stem
Substantia gelatinosa
Vagal nerve fibers

Table 28-4 Opiate Receptor System

	μ	κ	σ
Agonists	Morphine Morphine-like analgesics	Pentazocine Nalorphine Cyclazocine	Pentazocine Nalorphine Cyclazocine
Antagonists	Pentazocine Cyclazocine Nalorphine Naloxone Naltrexone	Naloxone Naltrexone	Naloxone Naltrexone
Clinical Effects	Analgesia Euphoria Respiratory depression Miosis Physical dependence	Analgesia Sedation Miosis ?Respiratory depression	Dysphoria Delusions Hallucinations Respiratory stimulation Vasomotor stimulation

Source: Adapted with permission from *Drug Intelligence & Clinical Pharmacy* (1981;15), Copyright © 1981, Harvey Whitney Books.

EXOGENOUS OPIOIDS

The exogenous opioids are substances that mimic the action of the endogenous opioids.[13] These compounds bind to stereospecific receptors in the CNS and have at least some morphine-like activity.[14] Exogenously administered opioids are analgesic by acting like endogenous opioid peptides at opioid receptors.[13] Exogenously administered opioids also act in part by releasing endogenous opioid peptides.[2]

The morphine-like opioids exert their agonist effects primarily at the μ receptor and, to a lesser degree, the κ receptor. The agonist-antagonists are thought to bind to the μ receptor and to compete with agonists, but either they exert no action (competitive antagonism) or they exert only limited action (partial agonism).

Drugs can have activities at one or several of the receptors. They can also function as agonists, partial agonists, or competitive antagonists at one or more of these receptors (Tables 28-4 to 28-6). Nalorphine, for example, appears to be a competitive antagonist at the μ receptor, a partial agonist at the κ receptor, and an agonist at the σ receptor.

The mixed antagonists-agonists, such as pentazocine and cyclazocine, also produce analgesia but act mainly at the κ receptor in the spinal cord. Their addiction liability is low in

Table 28-5 Summary of Opioid Agonist and Antagonist Effects

Drug	Receptor		
	μ	κ	σ
Butorphanol	Antagonist	Agonist	Agonist
Morphine	Agonist	Agonist	
Nalbuphine	Antagonist	Agonist	Agonist
Nalorphine	Antagonist	Partial agonist	Agonist
Naloxone	Antagonist	Antagonist	Antagonist
Pentazocine	Antagonist	Agonist	Agonist

Source: Reprinted with permission from *Drug Intelligence & Clinical Pharmacy* (1983;17:411–417), Copyright © 1983, Harvey Whitney Books.

Table 28-6 Opiate Agonists, Partial Agonists, and Antagonists

Agonists	Partial Agonists	Antagonists
Alphaprodine	Butorphanol	Naloxone
Codeine	Levallorphan	Naltrexone
Fentanyl	Nalbuphine	
Hydrocodone	Nalorphine	
Hydromorphone	Pentazocine	
Levorphanol		
Meperidine		
Methadone		
Morphine		
Opium		
Oxycodone		
Oxymorphone		
Propoxyphene		

Table 28-7 Partial List of Natural, Semisynthetic, and Synthetic Narcotics

Natural	Semisynthetic	Synthetic
Opium	Heroin	Meperidine
Morphine	Hydromorphone	Methadone
Codeine	Oxymorphone	Levorphanol
Thebaine	Oxycodone	Butorphanol
		Pentazocine
		Paregoric
		Diphenoxylate
		Fentanyl
		Propoxyphene

Table 28-8 Trade Names of Selected Commonly Used Narcotics

Narcotic	Trade Name
Meperidine	Demerol
	Mepergan
	Pethadol
Propoxyphene	Darvon
	Darvon-N
	Dolene
	Pargesic
	Profene
Methadone	Dolophine
	Methadose
Oxymorphone	Numorphan
Butorphanol	Stadol
Hydrocodone	Entuss
	Hycodan
	Ru-Tuss
	Vicodin
Hydromorphone	Dilaudid
Pentazocine	Talwin
	Talwin Nx
Nalbuphine	Nubain
Opium	Pantopon
	Parepectolin
Oxycodone	Percocet
	Percodan
	Tylox

comparison to the μ activators because of their ability to block the agonistic tendency to develop tolerance.[9]

TYPES OF NARCOTICS

Narcotic drugs can be divided into three groups: natural, semisynthetic, and synthetic (Table 28-7). Aspects of the medical use of the narcotic drugs follow a typical life cycle. Each new drug is initially hailed as a potent nonaddictive analgesic agent that can safely be made available to medical practice and may even be useful in the treatment of pre-existing opiate addiction; such was the history of morphine and heroin. It should be considered that all the opioids have the potential for abuse and dependence.

Table 28-8 lists some of the commercially available narcotic preparations.

Naturally Occurring Narcotics

The naturally occurring narcotics include opium, morphine, codeine, and thebaine.

Opium

The poppy *Papaver somniferum* is the primary source of the nonsynthetic narcotics. It was grown in the Mediterranean region as early as

300 BC and is found in countries around the world, including Mexico, Hungary, Yugoslavia, Turkey, India, Burma, and China. The milky fluid that oozes from the unripe poppyseed

pod is air dried to form raw opium.[9] Clandestine laboratories then process the base drug to make morphine, codeine, or heroin in addition to the approximately 25 organic substances extractable from the parent compound.

Opium was an ingredient in old medicinals, and there were no legal restrictions on the importation or use of opium until the early 1900s.[15] At that time patent medicines often contained opium without any warning label. Today, although a small amount of opium is used to make antidiarrheal preparations such as paregoric, virtually all the opium imported into the United States is broken down into its alkaloid constituents, principally morphine and codeine. Paregoric, which consists of a combination of opium, camphor, benzoic acid, and anise oil, is still prescribed for diarrhea in children. The anise oil is used to flavor the medication, and the benzoic acid acts as a preservative. Paregoric has been reported to cause toxicity, including pulmonary edema,[16] so that there is little rationale for the use of this drug to treat gastrointestinal problems.[16]

Morphine

Morphine was isolated as early as 1803 and was named for Morpheus, the Greek god of dreams and sleep.[9] Morphine is a pure opiate agonist and is the principal constituent of opium, ranging from 4% to 20%. Although morphine produces many diverse effects, such as drowsiness, changes in mood, respiratory depression, decreased gastrointestinal motility, nausea, vomiting, and alterations of the endocrine and autonomic nervous system, its most important effect is analgesia. It is considered the prototype of the opiate agonists.[2] Morphine and some of its alkaloid surrogates act supraspinally at the μ receptor to produce analgesia; the effects at this locus also account for the addiction liability of these compounds.

Parenteral morphine is widely used in medicine both as an analgesic as well as in the treatment of cardiogenic pulmonary edema. Orally administered morphine is about one-third to one-sixth as potent as parenteral morphine because of a large first-pass effect by the liver, whereby only a small percentage of an oral dose reaches the systemic circulation. The analgesic effects of morphine are usually maximal within 1 hour after administration, regardless of route. After subcutaneous or intramuscular injection of morphine, plasma concentrations reach their peak within 30 minutes.

The major metabolite, morphine glucuronide, is inactive as an analgesic. Although codeine is a metabolite of morphine, the amounts produced appear to be small. A large amount of morphine is used in the manufacturing of codeine and hydromorphone. Morphine is not a widely abused drug.

Codeine

Codeine is a pure opiate agonist and, although it is a naturally occurring ingredient of raw opium (1% to 2%), most of it is produced from morphine. Codeine is approximately 20% as potent as morphine and is metabolized by enzymes in the liver to morphine, which then enters the brain and accounts for the pharmacological actions of the drug.[5] Codeine has great use as an analgesic in the relief of mild to moderate pain that is not alleviated by nonopiate agonists, and it is extensively used as an antitussive. Some liquid antitussive codeine preparations include Robitussin A-C®, Cheracol®, and elixir of terpin hydrate with codeine. It is as an antitussive that codeine is most frequently abused. In addition, codeine has found abuse as a constituent of "loads," which is a combination of glutethimide and codeine (see Chapter 30).

With routine use the most frequent adverse effects of codeine are gastrointestinal, with reports of abdominal pain, cramping, constipation, and occasional nausea and vomiting. Fatal intoxications due solely to the ingestion of codeine are rare but have occurred.[17] Deaths are more common when codeine is mixed with analgesics, antihistamines, or sedatives. Codeine is more stimulating to the spinal cord than other narcotics, and as a result delirium and seizures may occur during coma, although death occurs from respiratory depression.[17,18]

Thebaine

Thebaine is a minor constituent of opium and is not a drug of abuse, but it can be converted to other abusable drugs, including oxycodone, codeine, oxymorphone, and hydrocodone.

Semisynthetic Narcotics

The semisynthetic narcotics include heroin, hydromorphone, oxycodone, and oxymorphone and are produced through minor chemical alterations of the poppy plant.

Heroin

Heroin (3,6-diacetylmorphine) is one of the most popular narcotic drugs of abuse because of its intense euphoria and long-lasting effect.[19] It may be administered by all routes and has a rapid onset of action. Its duration of effect is approximately 3 to 5 hours.[14] Heroin has been reported to be about 2.5 times more potent than morphine. Heroin is faster in inducing pain relief and has a shorter duration of effect than morphine after parenteral administration.[19] These differences are from the rapid and extensive brain uptake of the more lipid-soluble heroin compared with morphine.[20] For this reason, it has the greatest addictive potential.[19]

Heroin has no legitimate use in the United States. It is produced by heating morphine in the presence of acetic acid and is nearly 10 times as potent as morphine.[21] Once in the body, heroin is converted back to 6-monoacetylmorphine in the liver, brain, kidney, and heart.[22,23] The 6-monoacetylmorphine is then slowly converted to morphine.[20] Morphine is then conjugated with glucuronic acid or excreted unchanged. Both the 6-monoacetylmorphine metabolite and morphine have metabolic activity.

Heroin, when in its pure form, is a white powder with a bitter taste. Illicit heroin varies in color because of impurities left from the manufacturing process or from additives such as food coloring, cocoa, or brown sugar, which act as "fillers."[14] A "bag" of heroin is a slang term for a single dosage unit, which may weigh approximately 100 mg and usually contains less than 10% pure heroin. Street heroin is usually 2% to 5% heroin, the remainder being adulterants.[14] In particular, quinine is a popular filler because it tastes bitter, like heroin.

Hydromorphone

Hydromorphone (Dilaudid®), a pure narcotic agonist, is a strong analgesic used in the relief of moderate to severe pain. It has 2 to 8 times the potency of morphine. Hydromorphone has a more rapid onset and shorter duration of action than morphine and is more sedative and less euphorant than morphine. Because of its greater potency, hydromorphone is a highly abused drug that is much sought after by narcotic addicts.

Oxycodone

Oxycodone, which is synthesized from thebaine, is similar in effect to codeine but is more potent and thus has a higher dependence potential. It is available only in combination products. Oxycodone is used to relieve moderate to moderately severe pain. Addicts take this drug orally as Percodan® or Tylox® or dissolve the tablets in water, filter out the insoluble material, and "mainline" the active drug.

Synthetic Narcotics

Although the synthetic narcotics are structurally unrelated to morphine, they have many of the same properties as the agonists. Synthetic narcotics include meperidine, methadone, propoxyphene, pentazocine, diphenoxylate, fentanyl, and butorphanol. These drugs are narcotic agonists or partial agonists, the latter of which may have dual effects.

Meperidine

Meperidine (Demerol®) is a pure narcotic agonist and was the first synthetic narcotic. It was initially synthesized as a substitute for atropine because of its anticholinergic effects.[24,25] It therefore has a different chemical structure from that of morphine. Because of a significant first-pass effect through the liver, it is less than one-half as effective when taken orally as when given parenterally.[26,27]

Meperidine is metabolized by the liver through two primary pathways: hydrolysis to meperidinic acid, and hydroxylation to normeperidine. Normeperidine is the only active metabolite. The half-life of normeperidine is 24 to 48 hours; hence, with repeated use, normeperidine accumulates.[27] Normeperidine has half the analgesic potency of meperidine yet has twice the neurotoxicity. Manifestations of toxicity include seizures, myoclonus, CNS stimulation, jitteriness, and tremors.[28] These signs generally appear after several days of meperidine use and are due either to the anticholinergic activity of the compound or to the accumulation of normeperidine.[28]

Meperidine differs from other narcotics in that it does not produce miosis and, in fact, may cause mydriasis or no pupillary changes secondary to its anticholinergic effect.[13]

Meperidine is a Schedule II controlled substance. MPPP is a little-known derivative of meperidine that has been used in the manufacture of industrial chemicals. It has recently surfaced as a "designer drug" of abuse.

MPPP is most often sold as heroin.[14] Street names include "synthetic heroin," "new heroin," and "synthetic Demerol." 1-Methyl-4-phenyl-1,2,5,6-tetrahydropyridine (MPTP) is a contaminant created during the faulty synthesis of MPPP (MPPP requires sophisticated laboratory procedures to ensure purity). The contaminant has produced destructive lesions of the substantia nigra and a clinical picture similar to that of parkinsonism. Although the mechanism is not completely understood, it appears that MPTP is only toxic to the substantia nigra when it is broken down by monoamine oxidase to MPP$^+$.

MPTP and its metabolites strongly resemble certain herbicides such as paraquat, which has also been associated with parkinsonism. Parkinsonism does not usually appear until 80% of the cells in the substantia nigra have been destroyed. The neurological damage of brain cells by MPTP is irreversible and worsens with time, especially if the user has repeated exposures.

Methadone

Methadone (Dolophine®) is a pure opiate agonist and was first synthesized by German scientists during World War II because of a shortage of morphine. It is structurally similar to propoxyphene. It is, along with heroin, one of the more frequently abused narcotics and may be made available to abusers by those enrolled in a methadone maintenance program.[22] As an analgesic, methadone has many advantages over some of the other narcotics in that it may be orally administered for a reasonable cost and has a prolonged duration of action with a mild abstinence syndrome on long-term usage. Methadone is used mainly in the detoxification and maintenance of opiate addicts.

A single dose of methadone produces less sedation and euphoria than morphine and has an extended duration of action (4 to 6 hours). Because of this long duration of action, depressant effects after overdosage may continue for 36 to 48 hours.[14] Such an extended action is possibly due to the drug's high degree of protein binding, which allows slow elimination. Because of this, methadone can be given once daily. As an analgesic, methadone may be used in the relief of severe pain but should not be used in narcotic withdrawal or maintenance unless the individual is enrolled in an approved withdrawal or maintenance program.[29]

Accidental methadone poisoning in children has been reported in relation to methadone maintenance programs because the drug is dispensed as a fruit-flavored solution to some patients, who then take the substance home and store it in the refrigerator.[30,31]

Propoxyphene

Propoxyphene is a pure opiate agonist that is structurally similar to methadone and contains the phenylpiperidine moiety found in all narcotic analgesics. It is a weaker analgesic than codeine or salicylate in single doses and is solely available as an oral preparation. Propoxyphene is a very dangerous drug, with the potential for inducing seizures and cardiac dysrhythmias in addition to its typical narcotic effects. Some of these toxic effects of propoxyphene are not explained by its opiate-like properties; it is believed that they are due to the local anesthetic action of propoxyphene and its metabolite norpropoxyphene.[32]

Propoxyphene is commercially available as the hydrochloride or napsylate salt. Toxic effects may develop more slowly with the napsylate salt because of its slower absorption, but, despite claims to the contrary, there is no evidence that the napsylate is any safer than the hydrochloride.

A 65-mg dose of the hydrochloride is equivalent to 100 mg of the napsylate. Propoxyphene has mild analgesic effects at the usual dosage and has no antipyretic action.

One reason why propoxyphene is considered a dangerous drug is that only 15 to 20 tablets or capsules are sufficient to cause death, and smaller amounts may be fatal in combination with ethanol or other CNS depressants. In addition, the metabolite norpropoxyphene has been shown to cause both cardiac and excitatory CNS effects because it has a local anesthetic effect similar to that of amitriptyline and other anti-dysrhythmic agents. Intracardiac conduction delays attributable to high concentrations of nor-propoxyphene may be of relatively long duration. Cardiac conduction disturbances reported include first-degree atrioventricular block, right and left bundle branch block, ventricular bigeminy, and ventricular fibrillation.[17] Grand mal seizures have also been attributable to the effects of norpropoxyphene.

In the past, propoxyphene has been abused by dissolving the hydrochloride pellets in water and injecting the solution intravenously. This practice has been discontinued because the manufacturer now disperses propoxyphene uniformly throughout the capsule.

Acute toxicity from propoxyphene overdosage results in symptoms similar to those of acute opiate intoxication; these may include miosis, coma, respiratory depression, circulatory collapse, and pulmonary edema (Table 28-9). Seizures, dysrhythmias, and bundle branch block occur frequently with propoxyphene intoxication and can be life threatening shortly after ingestion.[17] Cardiac failure is also responsible for many of the deaths.[33] Because of the rapid onset of action of propoxyphene, death may occur within the first hour, and a small number of deaths have occurred within the first 15 minutes. Although naloxone is effective as an antidote, large doses may be necessary. In addition, the action of propoxyphene may outlast that of naloxone. A temporary transvenous cardiac pacemaker may be necessary in some patients.[33]

Pentazocine

Pentazocine (Talwin®) is a synthetic opiate agonist with very weak antagonist effects. Pen-

Table 28-9 Clinical Effects of Propoxyphene

Miosis
Coma
Respiratory depression
Pulmonary edema
Circulatory depression
Grand mal seizures
First degree atrioventricular block
Bundle-branch block
Ventricular dysrhythmias
    Ventricular fibrillation
    Ventricular tachycardia

tazocine is a competitive antagonist of the μ receptor and an agonist of the κ and σ receptors. Orally administered pentazocine undergoes first-pass metabolism in the liver, and less than 20% of a dose reaches the systemic circulation unchanged.[34] Initially, pentazocine was developed with the intention of producing an analgesic with the potency of an opiate but with less potential for addiction because of its mixed agonist-antagonist properties. This was not the case, however.

The most common side effect of pentazocine is sedation with subsequent diaphoresis and dizziness. Psychologic side effects include hallucinations, depression, and psychosis. Pentazocine in large doses produces respiratory depression that may be reversed by naloxone. Because the affinity of naloxone for κ and σ receptors is less than that for μ receptors, large doses are frequently required to produce antidotal effects.

Pentazocine is often combined with tripelennamine, an antihistamine, to form a relatively common drug of abuse known as "T's and Blues."[14,35–37] T's and Blues, used intravenously, was first seen in the Chicago area in 1976 as an alternative to heroin, which was then in low supply there, and quickly spread to other major cities in the Midwest.[38] "T's" refers to the trade name Talwin®, and "Blues" is slang derived from the light blue color of the 50-mg tripelennamine tablet, an antihistamine of the ethylenediamine class that is marketed under the trade name Pyribenzamine®.[39–42]

Combinations of opioids and antihistamines have long been used as a "lytic cocktail," although there is no known mechanism to explain why this drug combination produces euphoric or heroin-like effects greater than those of pentazocine alone.[35,39,40] It is said that tripelennamine prolongs and heightens the duration of the euphoria of the pentazocine.[35,43,44] The reported injection of solutions of tripelennamine with or without narcotics dates back 20 years, when it was reported as a combination with heroin or paregoric known as "blue velvet."[35,42,45] As an antihistamine, tripelennamine can depress or stimulate the CNS. In patients with focal neurologic lesions, even small doses can precipitate seizures.[36,37,42] In an overdose of T's and Blues, there is usually a phase of CNS depression that is followed by CNS excitement and culminates in seizures. The simultaneous injection of tripelennamine with pentazocine greatly increases the frequency of this complication, although seizures have been reported with pentazocine alone.

The constituents of T's and Blues are sold in their legitimate commercial solid dosage forms, and various ratios of the two drugs are used.[37] The tablets are crushed and placed in a vial and allowed to dissolve in a small quantity of tap water. The resultant mixture is then filtered through cotton or a cigarette filter and then drawn into a syringe and injected intravenously.[39-41]

The effect of injection of a "dose," which is typically two or three tablets of pentazocine and one tablet of tripelennamine, may be coma, after which the patient awakens and experiences a euphoric effect; alternatively, the reaction may be an immediate "rush," which reportedly is indistinguishable from the heroin rush and lasts 5 to 10 minutes. For most users the rush is followed by dysphoria, so that the injection may be repeated.[37] The brief rush may be followed by a feeling of well-being lasting up to 2 hours, which then subsides over the next few hours.[37,43] Because of the purported intense feeling, alcohol or sometimes diazepam is frequently used as an additional drug. Tolerance develops to the repeated injections of the drug, and larger doses need to be injected for the same effect.

The oral dosage form of pentazocine was reformulated in 1983 to contain 0.5 mg of naloxone (Talwin Nx®). The reformulation to a yellow, oblong caplet, rather than the round peach-colored pill, was intended to eliminate the drug's misuse in T's and Blues.[46] Theoretically, because naloxone is inactive when administered orally in the amount present in this formulation, its presence does not affect the efficacy of oral pentazocine; however, if it is ground up, solubilized, and administered parenterally, the naloxone antagonizes the effects of pentazocine and precipitates withdrawl symptoms in the drug abuser.[41] Despite the theoretical validity of this formulation, Talwin Nx® in combination with tripelennamine continues to be abused. It may be that the dose of naloxone in the preparation is inadequate to block the combined effects of pentazocine and tripelennamine.[46] If the dose were effective, signs of neurologic toxicity after the administration of naloxone as an antidote in overdose would be secondary to the anticholinergic effects of the antihistamine.

The adverse effects of T's and Blues that are most often reported include nausea, vomiting, and headache (Table 28-10). More serious early effects of T's and Blues that are frequently reported are muscle tremors, myoclonus, and tonic-clonic seizures, which are possibly due to central excitation from tripelennamine.[36,41,43] The most frequent and serious reported complication involves the pulmonary system; symptoms may include shortness of breath and wheezing, sometimes leading to pulmonary hypertension and right-sided heart failure.[35] These symptoms are similar to those charac-

Table 28-10 Clinical Effects of T's and Blues

Gastrointestinal
  Nausea
  Vomiting
Neurologic
  Headache
  Coma
  Muscle tremors
  Myoclonus
  Seizures
Pulmonary
  Shortness of breath
  Bronchoconstriction
  Congestive heart failure
Psychiatric
  Dysphoria
  Depression
  Confusion
  Hallucinations

teristic of intoxication with blue velvet. Evidence suggests that these respiratory symptoms result from intravenous administration of insoluble particulates such as magnesium silicate (talc), which is found in tripelennamine, or microcrystalline cellulose, which is used as a binder for pentazocine. These may cause a granulomatous reaction that obliterates the smaller vessels in the lung, liver, kidneys, endocardium, and brain and lead to increased pulmonary artery resistance and pulmonary hypertension.[35,41–43,45,47] Other complications of embolization include angiothrombosis of pulmonary arterioles leading to pulmonary infiltrates. Psychiatric disturbances associated with the abuse of pentazocine in T's and Blues include dysphoria, depression, confusion, and hallucinations.

Diphenoxylate

Diphenoxylate is an ingredient in the antidiarrheal preparation Lomotil®, which contains 2.5 mg of diphenoxylate and 0.025 mg of atropine in each tablet or 5 mL of liquid preparation. Intoxication with this agent has been reported in children in both therapeutic administration and accidental ingestion. Adults do not appear to be as sensitive to the effects of overdose as young children.[48] Because of the combination of drugs contained in Lomotil®, effects can vary from narcotic-like to anticholinergic-like. Delayed effects of this drug have been noted with a lag of as long as 12 hours after ingestion.[48,49]

Fentanyl

Fentanyl is an opiate agonist related to the phenylpiperidines and is an ingredient in Sublimaze®. It was first introduced in 1968 as an intravenous analgesic anesthetic. After parenteral administration, fentanyl is more prompt and less prolonged in its action than morphine or meperidine. Fentanyl is estimated to be 50 to 100 times more potent as an analgesic than morphine. Large doses of fentanyl produce marked muscular rigidity and almost instantaneous respiratory arrest.

A methyl analog of fentanyl produced in clandestine laboratories has been sold along the West Coast as a "super heroin." α-Methyl fentanyl, known as "China White," is a synthetic opioid that may be as much as 200 times more potent than heroin. It was the first of more than ten "designer drugs" to appear on the street. 3-Methyl fentanyl is approximately 3000 times stronger than morphine sulfate.[41]

Other street names for fentanyl derivatives are "Synthetic Heroin," "Mexican Brown," and "Persian White." A pure white powder is sold as "Persian White." A light tan powder is sold as "China White" or "Synthetic Heroin." A light brown powder is sold as "Mexican Brown"; the brown color is acquired by carmelizing the lactose filler or using a dye. The fentanyl derivatives are normally diluted with large amounts of "cutting" substances. Because the active ingredient is present in small quantities, it is unrecognizable by color, odor, or taste.

Although the "designer" fentanyls have been sold in powder form, the most common route of administration is intravenous. Smoking and insufflation of fentanyl is growing in popularity because the compounds are highly lipid soluble. These drugs can cause very rapid onset of respiratory arrest or pulmonary edema. Large doses of naloxone may be necessary as an antidote for overdosage with any of the fentanyl narcotics.

Butorphanol

Butorphanol (Stadol®) is a partial agonist that is structurally related to morphine but pharmacologically similar to pentazocine. The analgesic effect is believed to result from a stimulation of κ and σ receptors in the CNS, and the antagonistic effect appears to result from competitive inhibition at the μ receptor. The analgesic activity is 4 to 7 times that of morphine. Although orally administered butorphanol is easily absorbed, because of significant first-pass metabolism only 17% of a dose reaches the circulation unchanged. Because the drug does not suppress the abstinence syndrome and may actually induce withdrawal in opiate-dependent patients, it cannot be substituted for opiate agonists after physical dependence has been established without prior detoxification.

Nalorphine

Nalorphine (Nalline®) is a partial narcotic agonist whose use has been supplanted by the pure narcotic antagonist naloxone. It is thought that nalorphine is antagonistic at the μ receptor and agonistic at the two remaining receptor sites. When administered to a patient who has ingested a narcotic, nalorphine reverses the narcotic effect, thereby acting as an antagonist. If no narcotic has been ingested, however, the agonist action of nalorphine is noted, with further CNS and respiratory depression. This makes the use of nalorphine potentially dangerous because it may induce respiratory depression and apnea.

"CUTTING" SUBSTANCES

Although there are classic effects that can be expected from the opiates, the effects seen are often unpredictable because the purity of the drug is usually unknown. Drugs obtained on the street are always mixed with "cutting" substances in a ratio of 20:1 to 100:1, and it may be those substances that cause adverse reactions. A number of agents are used as cutting substances, among which quinine is the most favored.

Quinine is a bitter-tasting white powder that was first used as a heroin adulterant when there was an epidemic of malaria in New York. Its use has continued, and for many drug dealers it is the preferred adulterant for two reasons: (1) its bitter taste prevents the buyer from being able to test the heroin content by tasting for bitterness, and (2) when injected intravenously, quinine produces a "flush" because of its vasodilator action, mimicking the effect of intravenously administered heroin. Quinine itself has gastrointestinal, auditory, neurologic, ophthalmic, and renal toxicity, and by itself it may be responsible for side effects and mortality.

In addition to quinine, cutting substances for heroin include sugars, local anesthetics, baking soda, starch, stimulants (including caffeine), CNS depressants (including barbiturates), powdered milk, and easily obtainable narcotic-like substances such as propoxyphene.

CLINICAL EFFECTS OF NARCOTICS

The clinical effects of opioids include euphoria, which is why this class of drugs is abused, as well as drowsiness, apathy, lethargy, and sedation. In addition, nausea and vomiting, constipation, miosis, sleep, and respiratory depression are seen.[14] Large doses of some opiate agonists, on the other hand, may induce excitation and seizures (Table 28-11). Nausea and vomiting are caused by stimulation of the chemoreceptor trigger zone in the medulla oblongata. After this initial stimulation the opiate agonists then depress the vomiting center, and subsequent doses of the drugs are unlikely to produce vomiting.

The classic triad for acute opiate intoxication is symmetrical pinpoint pupils, depressed respiratory rate, and coma.[14,25,50] In addition, there may be cardiovascular effects and pulmonary edema.[14,51,52] The onset of CNS depressant effects may occur immediately after intravenous administration of the substance. Absorption of the opiates by nasal insufflation or by the subcutaneous or oral route may be sufficiently slow that narcotic effects may not reach their peak for 2 or more hours.[25]

Normally, opiate-induced miosis is presumed to be due to an excitatory effect of the drug on the autonomic segment of the oculomotor nerve.[25] This effect may be antagonized by anticholinergic drugs such as atropine. Therefore, if a patient's pupils are dilated, opiate ingestion cannot be ruled out. This is because mydriasis can result if Lomotil® was ingested (from the atropine) or can be a direct effect of concurrently ingested nonnarcotic drugs if the patient is postictal or agitated or if asphyxia has occurred. Mydriasis can also result from an overdose of meperidine, a narcotic that causes a paradoxical pupillary response.

Table 28-11 Clinical Features of Narcotic Overdose

Apathy
Constipation
Drowsiness
Excitement
Lethargy
Miosis
Nausea
Pulmonary edema
Respiratory depression
Vomiting

LABORATORY ANALYSIS

There is usually no indication for determining serum concentrations of opiates in the clinical setting. It may be useful to know whether a narcotic was present, as can be determined from a qualitative drug screen, but concentrations of the particular narcotic are not helpful.

TREATMENT

Treatment of an overdose of any of the narcotics includes support of the patient's airway and establishing a patent intravenous line.[25] Naloxone (2 mg) should be administered and repeated as necessary.[52] This is of both diagnostic and therapeutic importance. Although the preferred route of administration is intravenous, naloxone can be administered intramuscularly or sublingually or placed down the endotracheal tube if an intravenous line cannot be established.[9,53–55]

If the offending drug has been taken orally, attempts to retrieve the material should be performed with gastric lavage if the patient has no gag reflex and has been previously intubated.

Treatment of noncardiogenic pulmonary edema, if it occurs, includes support of respiration and oxygen. Positive end-expiratory pressure may be added if oxygenation cannot be maintained, but it is seldom required and its use has certain hazards. If it is necessary to use mechanical ventilation, a volume-cycled respirator is recommended. The use of furosemide has also been suggested for this condition but has not been shown to be of benefit. Intravenous fluid administration should be kept to a minimum. Other customary components of pulmonary therapy are neither effective nor necessary. Response is usually dramatic, and physical findings usually clear within 1 day, with radiologic changes reverting to normal within 72 to 96 hours.

Cardiac dysrhythmias and hypotension rarely require specific treatment when caused by a narcotic and usually respond to effective ventilation and naloxone. Dialysis, diuresis, and hemoperfusion also should not be attempted for narcotic overdose because there is no evidence that any of these methods is beneficial.

TOLERANCE AND THE ABSTINENCE SYNDROME FROM NARCOTICS

All the narcotics produce both physical and psychological dependence. Physical dependence refers to an alteration of the normal functions of the body necessitating the continued presence of a drug to prevent the withdrawal or abstinence syndrome. The abstinence syndrome, then, is another facet of the drug abuser's problems that may be seen by emergency department personnel.[12] Although the withdrawal syndrome from narcotics may be dramatic and temporarily disabling, it represents the least life-threatening or permanently disabling danger when compared with withdrawal from other classes of drugs.[56]

Tolerance and withdrawal are also receptor phenomena. Because both enkephalins and opioid agonists decrease sodium permeability in opiate receptors, opioid administration decreases the baseline need for endogenous enkephalin production and secretion.[12] As endogenous production and secretion decreases, more exogenous narcotic can be tolerated without excessive adverse reaction. Sudden cessation of opioid administration does not allow adequate time for resumption of enkephalin production. The increasing sodium permeability results in neuronal excitability and symptoms of withdrawal.[9] The rate of metabolism of narcotics does not increase with prolonged usage, yet tolerance to the analgesic, sedative, and euphoric effects does. Tolerance does not develop to respiratory depression, which is the most common cause of death.

The onset and duration of opiate withdrawal symptoms are directly related to the pharmacological and biological half-life of the abused drug.[56] Several weeks of continuous high-dose narcotic abuse are necessary before withdrawal symptoms may manifest. There may be times where street narcotics may not be concentrated enough to cause tolerance and dependency.

Some investigators consider opiate withdrawal a model for conditions such as naturally occurring anxiety or panic states in humans and have suggested that it is mediated by a major noradrenergic nucleus in the locus coeruleus in the brain.[57,58] Narcotic withdrawal usually begins to appear close to the time when the individual would have been taking the next dose and gradually intensifies to peak severity at about 48 hours. It then diminishes until no overt signs remain 7 to 10 days after the last dose (Table 28-12).

Clinical Manifestations of Narcotic Withdrawal

Early signs and symptoms of narcotic withdrawal include yawning, lacrimation, rhinorrhea, and sweating about 8 to 10 hours after the last dose. Thereafter, the addict may fall into a restless sleep. As the abstinence syndrome continues, symptoms may progress to piloerection (''gooseflesh''), restlessness, irritability, anorexia, flushing, diaphoresis, tachycardia, tremor, and mydriasis. The term ''cold turkey'' is derived from the gooseflesh that is part of narcotic withdrawal. Later in the course of withdrawal, the individual may experience fever, nausea, vomiting, and abdominal pain as well as diarrhea, spontaneous ejaculation (in males), and involuntary muscle spasms (from which the term ''kicking the habit'' derives).[14] The patient is weak and depressed, may be socially withdrawn, and at this point may become suicidal.

In a medical sense, the withdrawal from narcotics generally is not life threatening.[14] Seizures do not occur as a part of opiate withdrawal unless the abuser was continually supplied with a sedative-hypnotic as part of the narcotic. In that case, the seizure is secondary to the withdrawal of the sedative-hypnotic.[56]

Treatment of Narcotic Withdrawal

Not all cases of narcotic withdrawal require treatment, and without treatment the syndrome eventually runs its course. Although the signs and symptoms of narcotic withdrawal can be

Table 28-12 Signs and Symptoms of Narcotic Withdrawal

Body aches	Sneezing
Diarrhea	Abdominal cramps
Gooseflesh	Fever
Loss of appetite	Diaphoresis
Nausea/vomiting	Yawning
Nervousness	Irritability
Rhinorrhea	Tachycardia
Trembling	Kicking movements

reversed by another narcotic, the administration of a narcotic for withdrawal is strictly proscribed by law.[50] Although some patients prefer to detoxify without the use of medications, most are frightened of the withdrawal syndrome and prefer treatment and medication. If treatment is deemed necessary, it should be symptomatic and supportive and treat the acute physical discomfort experienced by the patient. A phenothiazine may be administered for nausea and vomiting and a nonnarcotic pain medication given for pain relief. A nonnarcotic antidiarrheal agent can also be administered.

Clonidine and Narcotic Withdrawal

The administration of clonidine (Catapres®), an α_2 receptor stimulator, has been proposed to eliminate objective and subjective symptoms of withdrawal; its effects last for 4 to 6 hours after oral administration.[59–64] It has been proposed that this drug works directly on the locus coeruleus in the brain to inhibit many of the symptoms of withdrawal.[57,59] Although it may be used on an acute basis in the emergency setting, it is doubtful that it would be of great benefit to those who may require days or weeks of outpatient therapy.[56] Clonidine should be used in an inpatient setting because of its associated effects of dizziness, postural hypotension, dyscoordination, and sedation.[62]

REFERENCES

1. Aston R: Drug abuse: Its relationship to dental practice. *Dent Clin North Am* 1984;28:595–610.

2. Adams M, Brase D, Welch S, et al: The role of endogenous peptides in the action of opioid analgesics. *Ann Emerg Med* 1986;15:1030–1035.

3. Dipalma J: Opiate antagonists: Naloxone. *Am Fam Physician* 1984;29:270–272.

4. Barsan W: Narcotic agents. *Ann Emerg Med* 1986;15:1019–1020.

5. Snyder D: Opiate receptors in the brain. *N Engl J Med* 1977;296:266–271.

6. Snyder S: The opiate receptor and morphine-like peptides in the brain. *Am J Psychiatr* 1978;135:645–652.

7. Atkinson R: Endocrine and metabolic effects of opiate antagonists. *J Clin Psychiatr* 1984;45:20–24.

8. Handal K, Schauben J, Salamone F: Naloxone. *Ann Emerg Med* 1983;12:438–445.

9. Wald P, Weisman R, Goldfrank L: Opioids. *Top Emerg Med* 1985;7:9–17.

10. Way E: Sites and mechanisms of basic narcotic receptor function based on current research. *Ann Emerg Med* 1986;15:1021–1025.

11. Zola E, McLeod D: Comparative effects and analgesic efficacy of the agonist-antagonist opioids. *Drug Intell Clin Pharmacol* 1983;17:411–417.

12. Martin W: Clinical evidence for different narcotic receptors and relevance for the clinician. *Ann Emerg Med* 1986;15:1026–1029.

13. McLane N, Caroll D: Ocular manifestations of drug abuse. *Surv Ophthalmol* 1986;30:298–313.

14. Kulburg A: Substance abuse: Clinical identification and management. *Pediatr Clin North Am* 1986;33:325–361.

15. Moriarty K, Alagna S, Lake C: Psychopharmacology. *Psychiatr Clin North Am* 1984;7:411–433.

16. Rice T: Paregoric intoxication with pulmonary edema in infancy. *Clin Pediatr* 1984;23:101–103.

17. Heaney R: Left bundle branch block associated with propoxyphene hydrochloride poisoning. *Ann Emerg Med* 1983;12:780–782.

18. Pearson M, Poklis A, Morrison R: A fatality due to the ingestion of (methyl morphine) codeine. *Clin Toxicol* 1979;15:267–271.

19. Sternbach G, Moran J, Eliastam M: Heroin addiction: Acute presentation of medical complications. *Ann Emerg Med* 1980;9:161–169.

20. Inturrisi C, Max M, Foley K: The pharmacokinetics of heroin in patients with chronic pain. *N Engl J Med* 1984;310:1213–1217.

21. Gay G, Inaba D: Treating acute heroin and methadone toxicity. *Anaesth Analg* 1976;55:607–610.

22. Goldfrank L, Bresnitz E: Opioids. *Hosp Physician* 1978;14:26–37.

23. Goldfrank L, Bresnitz E, Weisman R: Opioids and opiates. *Curr Top Emerg Med* 1983;3:1–7.

24. Batterman R, Himmelsbach C: Demerol—A new synthetic analgesic. *JAMA* 1943;122:222–226.

25. Cuddy P: Management of acute opioid intoxication. *Crit Care Q* 1982;4:65–74.

26. Brena S: Oral analgesics: Use and misuse. *Emerg Med Rep* 1983;4:139–146.

27. Goetting M, Thirman M: Neurotoxicity of meperidine. *Ann Emerg Med* 1985;14:1007–1009.

28. Szeto H, Inturrisi C, Houde R, et al: Accumulation of normeperidine, an active metabolite of meperidine in patients with renal failure or cancer. *Ann Intern Med* 1977;86:738–741.

29. Nanji A, Filipenko J: Rhabdomyolysis and acute myoglobinuric renal failure associated with methadone intoxication. *J Toxicol Clin Toxicol* 1983;20:353–356.

30. Roland E, Lockitch G, Dunn H, et al: Methadone poisoning due to accidental contamination of prescribed medication. *Can Med Assoc J* 1984;131:1357–1358.

31. Carin I, Glass L, Parekh A, et al: Neonatal methadone withdrawal. *Am J Dis Child* 1983;137:1166–1169.

32. Krantz T, Thisted B, Strom J, et al: Severe, acute propoxyphene overdose treated with dopamine. *Clin Toxicol* 1985;23:347–352.

33. Strom J, Haggmark S, Madsen P, et al: Cardiac pacing and central hemodynamics in experimental propoxyphene-induced shock. *Clin Toxicol* 1985;23:353–356.

34. Stahl S, Kasser I: Pentazocine overdose. *Ann Emerg Med* 1983;12:28–31.

35. Butch A, Yokel R, Sigell L, et al: Abuse and pulmonary complications of injecting pentazocine and tripelennamine tablets. *Clin Toxicol* 1979;14:301–306.

36. Showalter C: T's and Blues: Abuse of pentazocine and tripelennamine. *JAMA* 1981;244:1225–1227.

37. Showalter C, Moorer L: Abuse of pentazocine and tripelennamine. *JAMA* 1978;239:1610–1612.

38. Tagashira E, Kachur J, Carter W, et al: Pentazocine-tripelennamine ("T's and Blues") substitution studies in morphine-dependent rodents. *J Pharmacol Exp Ther* 1984;231:97–101.

39. Poklis A, Whyatt P: Current trends in the abuse of pentazocine and tripelennamine: The metropolitan St Louis experience. *J Forensic Sci* 1980;25:72–80.

40. Poklis A, Mackell M: Pentazocine and tripelennamine (T's and Blues) abuse: Toxicological findings in 39 cases. *J Anal Toxicol* 1982;6:109–114.

41. Vogel S, Leikin J: What's up (and down) in drug abuse: Street drugs. *Top Emerg Med* 1986;8:57–75.

42. Jackson C, Hart A, Robinson M: Fatal intracranial hemorrhage associated with phenylpropanolamine, pentazocine, and tripelennamine overdose. *J Emerg Med* 1985;3:127–132.

43. Caplan L, Thomas C, Banks G: Central nervous system complications of addiction to T's and Blues. *Neurology* 1982;32:623–628.

44. Driscoll W, Lindley G: Self-administration of tripelennamine by a narcotic addict. *N Engl J Med* 1957;257:376–378.

45. Wendt V, Puro H, Shapiro J, et al: Angiothrombotic pulmonary hypertension in addicts: "Blue Velvet" addiction. *JAMA* 1964;188:755–758.

46. Legros J, Khalili-Varasteh H, Margetts G: Pharmacological study of pentazocine-naloxone combination: Interest as a potentially nonabusable oral form of pentazocine. *Arch Intern Pharmacodyn* 1984;271:11–21.

47. Tomashefski J, Hirsch C, Jolly C: Microcrystalline cellulose pulmonary embolism and granulomatosis. *Arch Pathol Lab Med* 1981;105:89–93.

48. Rumack B, Temple A: Lomotil poisoning. *Pediatrics* 1974;53:495–500.

49. McGuigan M, Lovejoy F: Overdose of Lomotil, editorial. *Br Med J* 1978;1:990.

50. Khantzian E, McKeena G: Acute toxic and withdrawal reactions associated with drug use and abuse. *Ann Intern Med* 1979;90:361–372.

51. Frand U: Methadone-induced pulmonary edema. *Ann Intern Med* 1972;76:975–979.

52. Light R, Dunham R: Severe slowly resolving heroin-induced pulmonary edema. *Chest* 1975;67:61–64.

53. Maio R, Gaukel B, Freeman B: Intralingual naloxone injection for narcotic-induced respiratory depression. *Ann Emerg Med* 1987;16:572–573.

54. Maio R, Griener J, Clark M, et al: Intralingual naloxone reversal of morphine-induced respiratory depression in dogs. *Ann Emerg Med* 1984;13:1087–1091.

55. Tandberg D, Abercrombie D: Treatment of heroin overdose with endotracheal naloxone. *Ann Emerg Med* 1982;11:443–445.

56. Vance M: Drug withdrawal syndromes. *Top Emerg Med* 1985;7:63–68.

57. DiStefano P, Brown O: Biochemical correlates of morphine withdrawal: Part 1: Characterization in the adrenal medulla and locus coeruleus. *J Pharmacol Exp Ther* 1985;233:333–338.

58. DiStefano P, Brown O: Biochemical correlates of morphine withdrawal: Part 2: Effects of clonidine. *J Pharmacol Exp Ther* 1985;233:339–344.

59. Gold M, et al: Clonidine blocks acute opiate withdrawal symptoms. *Lancet* 1978;2:599–601.

60. Gold M, Redmond E, Kleber H: Clonidine in opiate withdrawal. *Lancet* 1978;2:929–930.

61. Gold M, Redmond E, Kleber H: Noradrenergic hyperactivity in opiate withdrawal supported by clonidine reversal of opiate withdrawal. *Am J Psychiatr* 1979;136:100–102.

62. Javel A: Mixed substance abuse withdrawal treated by clonidine. *J Med Soc N J* 1980;80:1035–1036.

63. Cami J, Torres S, San L, et al: Efficacy of clonidine and of methadone in the rapid detoxification of patients dependent on heroin. *Clin Pharmacol Ther* 1985;38:336–341.

64. Preston K, Bigelow G, Liebson I: Self-administration of clonidine, oxazepam, and hydromorphone by patients undergoing methadone detoxification. *Clin Pharmacol Ther* 1985;38:219–227.

ADDITIONAL SELECTED REFERENCES

Bailey D, Shaw R: Blood concentrations and clinical findings in nonfatal and fatal intoxications involving glutethimide and codeine. *Clin Toxicol* 1985;23:557–570.

Cicero T, et al: Function of the male sex organs in heroin and methadone users. *N Engl J Med* 1975;292:882–887.

Duberstein J, Kaufman D: A clinical study of an epidemic of heroin intoxication and heroin-induced pulmonary edema. *Am J Med* 1971;51:704–714.

Garriott J, Sturner W: Morphine concentrations and survival periods in acute heroin fatalities. *N Engl J Med* 1973;289:1276–1278.

Gillman M: Nitrous oxide, an opioid addictive agent. *Am J Med* 1986;81:97–102.

Goldman A, Enquist R: Methadone pulmonary edema. *Chest* 1973;63:275–276.

Greenstein R, Resnick R, Resnick E: Methadone and naltrexone in the treatment of heroin dependence. *Psychiatr Clin North Am* 1984;7:671–679.

Judson B, Goldstein A, Inturrisi C: Methadyl acetate (LAAM) in the treatment of heroin addicts. *Arch Gen Psychiatr* 1983;40:834–840.

Kozel N, Adams E: Epidemiology of drug abuse: An overview. *Science* 1986;234:970–974.

Kreeger R, Pearson P, Bullock J, et al: Endophthalmitis associated with intravenous drug abuse. *Ann Emerg Med* 1987;16:585–587.

Ling G, MacLeod J, Lee S, et al: Separation of morphine analgesia from physical dependence. *Science* 1984;226:462–464.

Marantz P, Linzer M, Feiner C, et al: Inability to predict diagnosis in febrile intravenous drug abusers. *Ann Intern Med* 1987;106:823–828.

Martin W: Naloxone. *Ann Intern Med* 1976;85:765–768.

Menda K, Gorbach S: Favorable experience with bacterial endocarditis in heroin addicts. *Ann Intern Med* 1973;78:25–32.

Michaelis L, Hickey P, Clark T, et al: Ventricular irritability associated with the use of naloxone hydrochloride. *Ann Thorac Surg* 1974;18:608–614.

Montagne M: Drug-taking paraphernalia. *J Psychoactive Drugs* 1983;15:159–175.

Moore R, Rumack B, Conner C, et al: Naloxone. *Am J Dis Child* 1980;134:156–158.

Perry D: Heroin and cocaine adulteration, editorial. *Clin Toxicol* 1975;8:239–243.

Perry S: Using narcotic analgesics to optimum effect: A modern view. *Emerg Room Rep* 1982;3:91–96.

Quigley A, Bredemeyer D, Seow S: A case of buprenorphine abuse. *Med J Aust* 1984;140:425–426.

Sapira J: The narcotic addict as a medical patient. *Am J Med* 1968;45:555–588.

Steinberg A, Karliner J: The clinical spectrum of heroin pulmonary edema. *Arch Intern Med* 1968;122:122–127.

Thornton W, Thornton B: Narcotic poisoning: A review of the literature. *Am J Psychiatr* 1974;131:867–869.

Tong T, Pond S, Kreek M, et al: Phenytoin-induced methadone withdrawal. *Ann Intern Med* 1981;94:349–351.

Triana E, Frances R, Stokes P: The relationship between endorphins and alcohol-induced subcortical activity. *Am J Psychiatr* 1980;137:491–493.

Vandam L: Butorphanol. *N Engl J Med* 1980;302:381–384.

Wisdom K, Nowak R, Richardson H, et al: Alternate therapy for traumatic pneumothorax in "pocket shooters." *Ann Emerg Med* 1986;15:428–432.

Zaks A, Jones T, Fink M, et al: Naloxone treatment of opiate dependence. *JAMA* 1971;215:2108–2110.

chapter 29

Narcotic Antagonists

Narcotic antagonists are drugs that tend to block and reverse the effects of narcotics. They can be partial or pure antagonists.

PARTIAL ANTAGONISTS

The development of drugs for clinical use that antagonize the effects of morphine-like drugs began more than 40 years ago with the preparation of nalorphine, a partial antagonist-agonist.[1-4] Other antagonists-agonists include levallorphan, pentazocine, butorphanol, and nalbuphine. Nalorphine and levallorphan act antagonistically at the μ receptor while exhibiting agonistic properties at the two remaining opiate receptor sites.[5,6] The major problems limiting the use of these drugs are the physical dependence noted after sustained use, an increase in respiratory depression and coma if a nonnarcotic was taken, and intense dysphoria.

PURE ANTAGONISTS

The pure antagonists are naloxone and the oral preparation naltrexone.[1-3,6-10] These exhibit antagonistic activities at all three receptors. The discussion of the pure narcotic antagonists is limited to these two drugs.

Naloxone

Naloxone (*N*-allyloxymorphone; Narcan®) is a synthetic compound of oxymorphone (Numorphan®) originally derived from thebaine. It is approved by the FDA for the treatment of narcotic overdose, narcotic depression of the newborn, and reversal of narcotic analgesia. It has also been used in the treatment of narcotic addiction. Naloxone is effective for virtually all narcotic and narcotic-like substances (Table 29-1)[3,11,12] and has even been reported to be of some value in nonnarcotic overdose.[3,13-16]

The sites of narcotic agonist and antagonist action are specific opiate receptors on the synaptic membranes of the amygdala, hypothalamus, and thalamus. Naloxone is believed to act by competing for these receptor sites and displacing the opiate agonists because it binds to the receptors with greater affinity than the agonist without causing their activation.[6] Although naloxone antagonizes the μ, κ, and σ receptors, it is bound less avidly by the latter two receptors. Because it has no agonist activity, naloxone does not cause respiratory depression even if given in excessive amounts or in the absence of narcotic overdose.[14,17] When the nature of the depression is not known, naloxone is the drug of choice because it will not cause further respiratory depression. Naloxone, like other narcotic antago-

Table 29-1 Agonists and Partial Agonists for Which Naloxone Is Effective

Agonists	Partial Agonists
Alphaprodine	Butorphanol
Anileridine	Cyclazocine
Codeine	Levallorphan
Diphenoxylate	Nalbuphine
Fentanyl	Nalorphine
Heroin	Pentazocine
Hydromorphone	
Levorphanol	
Meperidine	
Methadone	
Opium	
Oxymorphone	
Propoxyphene	

nists, is ineffective in the treatment of respiratory depression caused by other CNS depressants.

Method of Administration

Although the intravenous route is the preferred method for administration of naloxone, frequently the drug must be administered to patients with a scarcity of peripheral veins. Difficulty in obtaining venous access sometimes precludes the use of the intravenous technique. This problem may be encountered in the long-term drug abuser, obese patients, neonates, and children. Under these conditions, naloxone can be administered by the intramuscular or subcutaneous route; however, these routes provide less rapid, less predictable, and more erratic systemic absorption and therapeutic response. The sublingual and endotracheal routes, on the other hand, provide quick access to the systemic circulation.[18] The ventral lateral surface of the tongue is a highly vascular area with an abundance of capillary beds; even in situations of low cardiac output, the tongue maintains its ability to autoregulate blood flow and to absorb material quickly.[3,19,20]

In the past it was believed that many patients were given an insufficient amount of naloxone.[12] For that reason, large doses of naloxone are currently recommended. In any adult patient with an altered mental status with respiratory depression, 2 mg of naloxone should be administered. It has been suggested that for neonates and children 0.01 mg/kg be administered,[5,12] but the administration of a larger dose should cause no harm. The pupils should not be relied on as an indicator of whether naloxone should be administered.[21] If there is a partial response, the same dose can be administered up to a total of 10 mg.[11] In addition to naloxone, patients with an altered mental status should receive 50 mL of 50% dextrose intravenously, along with thiamine and oxygen.

The manufacturer of naloxone now makes two preparations of different concentrations. The first product marketed contained naloxone in a concentration of 0.4 mg in 1 mL. To give 2 mg required the administration of 5 ampules. The same manufacturer now makes a concentration of 1 mg/mL in a 2-mL ampule. These two preparations should not be confused. In addition, there is a preparation for multiple use as well as a neonatal preparation.

Naloxone can be administered by continuous intravenous infusion by a number of methods. One method consists of placing 4 mg of naloxone in 1 L of 5% dextrose in water at an infusion rate of approximately 100 mL/hour.[11,22] Another method for continuous infusion is to administer the bolus dose necessary to reverse the respiratory depressant effects of the opioid overdose and to follow that with an infusion of two-thirds the initial bolus dose each hour.[19] In this regimen, half the loading dose may be administered 15 to 20 minutes after the first dose because of the transient decrease in naloxone levels.[11] If a continuous infusion is to be used, patients should be monitored closely in an intensive care setting.[22]

Onset of Action

Naloxone has an onset of action of 1 to 2 minutes after intravenous administration and 5 to 10 minutes after intramuscular injection. The rapid onset of action is related to the drug's rapid entry into the brain as a result of its high degree of lipid solubility.[13] Its duration of action after intravenous administration is 45 to 90 minutes in adults and about 3 hours in neonates.[3,11,13,22,23] Oral administration is 2% as potent as parenteral administration because of a prominent first-pass effect by the liver.[3] Although oral administration of naloxone can be effective, large amounts are required.[24] Because the duration of action of naloxone is generally shorter than that of the opiate, the effects of the opiate may recur as the effects of naloxone disappear.[25]

A positive response from naloxone typically consists of increased respirations, increased alertness, and reversal of miosis (Table 29-2). In addition, naloxone reverses the cardiovascular, gastrointestinal, analgesic, and emetic effects of the narcotics.[26]

A patient may have only a partial response to naloxone for a number of reasons (Table 29-3). The patient may have had a seizure with a subsequent postictal period or may have a mixed overdose of narcotic and nonnarcotic agents. In addition, there may be a concurrent head injury, hypoglycemia, or hypoxia that require treatment before the patient can regain a normal level of consciousness.

Toxicity of Naloxone

The toxicity of naloxone is minimal. In those patients who are physically dependent on opiates, naloxone may cause an acute withdrawal.[26] This may include the newborns of mothers who are physically dependent on opioids. Nausea and vomiting have been reported in postoperative patients who received a dose greater than the recommended dose, but

such reports are rare. Up to 20 mg have been given to children without adverse effect.[3] Several investigators have reported naloxone-induced hypertension that is possibly due to catecholamine release.[27] Although a casual relationship to the drug has not been established, hypotension, coagulation disturbances, ventricular irritability, and pulmonary edema have been described after postoperative administration of naloxone, but these reports are also uncommon.[26–30] Naloxone, therefore, is the drug of choice when the nature of the depressant drug is not known because it will not cause further respiratory depression. If naloxone is used for long-term treatment of opiate dependence, an abstinence syndrome does not develop.[30] The main drawback to the use of naloxone remains its relatively short duration of action and poor absorption when administered orally.

Other Uses of Naloxone

Although naloxone has been used on an investigational basis for detection of chronic opiate abuse, chemical methods used to detect the presence of opiates in the urine are preferable because naloxone may precipitate abstinence symptoms in patients who are physically dependent on opiates.[26]

In addition to reversal of narcotic withdrawal, naloxone has been used investigationally in intoxicated patients to reverse alcohol-, diazepam-, and clonidine-induced coma and respiratory depression.[3,14–16] Even though alcohol may in part act by releasing endogenous endorphins, there has never been satisfactory evidence that naloxone reliably reverses alcohol-induced coma.[5,31,32] It has also been used investigationally in the management of high-altitude pulmonary edema, acute respiratory failure, senile dementia, ischemic neurologic deficits, and septic and cardiogenic shock.[33] The efficacy of naloxone under these conditions has not been established.[5,31,34]

Naltrexone

Naltrexone (*N*-cyclopropylmethylnoroxymorphone; Trexan®) is a long-lasting orally administered synthetic narcotic antagonist that

Table 29-2 Narcotic Effects That Naloxone Acts To Reverse

Respiratory depression
Cardiovascular depression
Gastrointestinal effects
CNS depression
Miosis
Analgesia
Psychomimetic effects of partial agonists

Table 29-3 Reasons for Partial Response to Naloxone

Postictal period
Mixed overdose
Concurrent head injury
Hypoglycemia
Hypoxia

has been recently approved for use in the United States. It is a structural analog of naloxone and is derived from thebaine. Naltrexone is almost ideal as an opiate antagonist in that it is long acting, active orally, does not cause physical dependence, antagonizes the euphoric effects of opiates, is not associated with tolerance, and has no serious side effects or toxicities.[1]

Naltrexone is a pure opioid antagonist that markedly attenuates or completely and reversibly blocks the subjective effects of opioids, including those with agonist and antagonist activity. It appears to block the effects of opioids by competitive binding at the three opioid receptors. The major action, like that of naloxone, is on the μ receptor. This makes the blockade potentially surmountable. Naltrexone appears to have a narcotic antagonist activity 2 to 9 times greater than that of naloxone,[1] so that the equivalent of 3 g of naloxone is required to achieve the same effect as 30 to 50 mg of naltrexone.

Pharmacokinetics

Naltrexone is rapidly and nearly completely absorbed from the gastrointestinal tract. Concentrations reach their peak 1 hour after oral administration.[1] Approximately 25% of naltrexone is bound to plasma proteins. It is rapidly and extensively metabolized by the liver. Naltrexone, like naloxone, undergoes extensive first-pass hepatic metabolism, but its major metabolite, 6-β-naltrexol, is also a pure antagonist and contributes to opioid receptor blockade. The half-lives of naltrexone and 6-β-naltrexol are 4 hours and 13 hours, respectively. Urinary excretion is the most important route of elimination of naltrexone and its metabolite.

Naltrexone (50 mg) will block the pharmacologic effects of 25 mg of heroin for as long as 24 hours. Doubling the dose of naltrexone provides blockade for 48 hours, and tripling the dose provides blockade for about 72 hours.[1]

Uses

Naltrexone has been approved for the long-term treatment of addiction to heroin and other opioids and can be used in those individuals who are highly motivated to stop taking a narcotic agent.[1] For such patients the antagonist offers excellent protection against the temptation to use

narcotics. Although naltrexone is an effective narcotic blocking agent, it does not block any other class of psychoactive substances.[35] Patients may elect to accept naltrexone therapy and still abuse other psychoactive substances. Unlike patients who stop taking methadone and have withdrawal symptoms, patients who stop taking naltrexone experience no withdrawal. Patient compliance is then a major factor.[1] In addition, although naltrexone blocks the effects of opioids it does not abolish the craving for narcotics.[36] It appears to be most useful in discouraging impulsive use of narcotics, which is an important cause of relapse. Self-administration of large doses of heroin or other narcotics can overcome the blockade and may cause serious injury, including coma and death.

Opiate antagonism correlates well with naltrexone plasma concentrations, and effective blockade of opiate effects can be expected at plasma concentrations of 2 ng/mL. The lack of readily available commercial assays that are reliably sensitive to 2 ng/mL with a suitable margin of error makes routine assessments of naltrexone plasma concentrations difficult.

Narcotic antagonists precipitate withdrawal in opiate-dependent individuals; therefore, a drug-free interval is necessary before induction. Typically, the treatment should not be attempted until the patient has remained opioid-free for 7 to 10 days.[35] Before the first dose of naltrexone, 2 mg of naloxone may be administered intravenously to determine the presence of residual dependence and to avoid precipitating more prolonged and severe withdrawal with naltrexone.[37] Clonidine has also been used before naltrexone for narcotic abstinence. Tolerance does not appear to develop to the opioid antagonistic properties of naltrexone for up to 2 years of treatment.[38]

Side Effects

Naltrexone causes few side effects that, when present, tend to be mild.[1] In opiate-dependent individuals, naltrexone may precipitate acute opiate withdrawal. In the non–opiate-dependent individual, gastrointestinal irritation and clinically insignificant increases in blood pressure have been reported. Dosages of up to 800 mg per day have been administered with no untoward effects.[1] Doses of about 5 times the usual dose for the opioid addict have caused increases in serum aminotransferase activity in some patients. These patients were clinically asymptomatic, and their enzyme abnormalities returned to normal in a few weeks. Naltrexone, therefore, should not be used in patients with acute hepatitis or hepatic failure.

Contraindications

Contraindications to the use of naltrexone include failure of a naloxone challenge, a positive urine screen for opioids, the presence of acute opioid withdrawal, or a history of sensitivity to naltrexone.

Dosage

Approximately 50 mg of naltrexone blocks the opiate receptor for 24 hours, and 100 to 150 mg provides a block for several days.[8] The usual dosage of naltrexone is 50 mg once daily or 350 mg per week in three divided doses. Sustained-release delivery systems for naltrexone to enhance compliance are currently under investigation.

REFERENCES

1. Crabtree B: Review of naltrexone, a long-acting opiate antagonist. *Clin Pharmacol* 1984;3:273–280.

2. Foldes F, Lunn J, Moore J, et al: N-Allylnoroxymorphone: A new potent narcotic antagonist. *Am J Med Sci* 1963;245:57–64.

3. Handal K, Schauben J, Salamone F: Naloxone. *Ann Emerg Med* 1983;12:438–445.

4. Zola E, McLeod D: Comparative effects and analgesic efficacy of the agonist-antagonist opioids. *Drug Intell Clin Pharmacol* 1983;17:411–417.

5. Dipalma J: Opiate antagonists: Naloxone. *Am Fam Physician* 1984;29:270–272.

6. Martin W: Naloxone. *Ann Intern Med* 1976;85:765–768.

7. Foldes F, Duncalf D, Kuwabara S: The respiratory, circulatory, and narcotic antagonistic effects of nalorphine, levallorphan, and naloxone in anaesthetized subjects. *Can Anaesth Soc J* 1969;16:151–161.

8. Greenstein R, Arndt I, McLellan T, et al: Naltrexone: A clinical perspective. *J Clin Psychiatr* 1984;45:25–28.

9. Greenstein R, Resnick R, Resnick E: Methadone and naltrexone in the treatment of heroin dependence. *Psychiatr Clin North Am* 1984;7:671–679.

10. Atkinson R: Endocrine and metabolic effects of opiate antagonists. *J Clin Psychiatr* 1984;45:20–24.

11. Goldfrank L, Weisman R, Errick J, et al: A dosing nomogram for continuous infusion of intravenous naloxone. *Ann Emerg Med* 1986;15:566–570.

12. Moore R, Rumack B, Conner C, et al: Naloxone. *Am J Dis Child* 1980;134:156–158.

13. Berkowitz B: The relationship of pharmacokinetics to pharmacological activity: Morphine, methadone and naloxone. *Clin Pharmacol* 1976;1:219–230.

14. Bell E: The use of naloxone in the treatment of diazepam poisoning. *J Pediatr* 1975;87:803–804.

15. Barros S, Rodriguez G: Naloxone as an antagonist in alcohol intoxication. *Anesthesiology* 1981;54:174.

16. Lyon L, Antony J: Reversal of alcoholic coma by naloxone. *Ann Intern Med* 1982;96:464–465.

17. Evans L, Swainson C, Roscoe P, et al: Treatment of drug overdosage with naloxone, a specific narcotic antagonist. *Lancet* 1973;1:452–455.

18. Tandberg D, Abercrombie D: Treatment of heroin overdose with endotracheal naloxone. *Ann Emerg Med* 1982;11:443–445.

19. Wald P, Weisman R, Goldfrand L: Opioids. *Top Emerg Med* 1985;7:9–17.

20. Maio R, Griener J, Clark M, et al: Intralingual naloxone reversal of morphine-induced respiratory depression in dogs. *Ann Emerg Med* 1984;13:1087–1091.

21. Lovejoy F: Indications for naloxone in Lomotil poisoning. *Pediatrics* 1974;53:658.

22. Kulberg A: Substance abuse: Clinical identification and management. *Pediatr Clin North Am* 1986;33:325–361.

23. Fossel M, Rosen P: Naloxone treatment for codeine-induced gastrointestinal symptoms. *J Emerg Med* 1984;2:107–110.

24. Frand U: Methadone-induced pulmonary edema. *Ann Intern Med* 1972;76:975–979.

25. Khantzian E, McKenna G: Acute toxic and withdrawal reactions associated with drug use and abuse. *Ann Intern Med* 1979;90:361–372.

26. Schwartz J, Koenigsberg M: Naloxone-induced pulmonary edema. *Ann Emerg Med* 1987;16:1294–1296.

27. Tanaka G: Hypertensive reaction to naloxone. *JAMA* 1974;228:25–26.

28. Michaelis L, Hickey P, Clark T, et al: Ventricular irritability associated with the use of naloxone hydrochloride. *Ann Thorac Surg* 1974;18:608–614.

29. Andree R: Sudden death following naloxone administration. *Anaesth Analg* 1980;59:782–784.

30. Zaks A, Jones T, Fink M, et al: Naloxone treatment of opiate dependence. *JAMA* 1971;215:2108–2110.

31. Banner W, Lund M, Clawson L: Failure of naloxone to reverse clonidine toxic effect. *Am J Dis Child* 1983;137:1170–1171.

32. Jeffcoate W, Hastings A, Cullen M, et al: Naloxone and ethanol antagonism. *Lancet* 1981;1:1052.

33. McNicolas L, Martin W: New and experimental therapeutic roles for naloxone and related opioid antagonists. *Drugs* 1984;27:81–93.

34. Mattila M, Neotto E, Seppala T: Naloxone is not an effective antagonist of ethanol. *Lancet* 1981;1:775–776.

35. O'Brien C, Childress A, McLellan A, et al: Use of naloxone to extinguish opioid-conditioned responses. *J Clin Psychiatr* 1984;45:53–56.

36. Judson B, Goldstein A: Naltrexone treatment of heroin addiction: One year follow-up. *Drug Alcohol Dependence* 1984;13:357–365.

37. Ginzburg H, MacDonald M: The role of naltrexone in the management of drug abuse. *Med Toxicol* 1987;2:83–92.

38. Kleber H, Kosten T, Gaspari J, et al: Nontolerance to the opioid antagonism of naltrexone. *Biol Psychiatr* 1985;20:66–72.

ADDITIONAL SELECTED REFERENCES

Cohen M, Cohen R, Pickar D, et al: Hormonal effects of high dose naloxone in humans. *Neuropeptides* 1985;6: 373–380.

DeFazio J, Verheugen C, Chetkowski R, et al: The effects of naloxone on hot flashes and gonadotropin secretion in postmenopausal women. *J Clin Endocrinol Metab* 1984;58:578–581.

Goldstein D, Keiser H: A case of episodic flushing and organic psychosis: Reversal by opiate antagonists. *Ann Intern Med* 1983;98:30–34.

Jasinski D, Martin W, Haertzen C: The human pharmacology and abuse potential of *N*-Allylnoroxymorphone (naloxone). *J Pharmacol Exp Ther* 1967;157:420–426.

Jeffcoate W, Cullen M, Herbert M, et al: Prevention of effects of alcohol intoxication by naloxone. *Lancet* 1979;2:1157–1159.

Rae H: Retrospective review of ethanol concentration measurements in patients with ethanol overdose treated with naloxone. *Curr Ther Res* 1986;40:960–964.

Stella L, Crescenti A, Torri G: Effect of naloxone on the loss of consciousness induced by IV anaesthetic agents in man. *Br J Anaesth* 1984;56:369–373.

chapter 30

Sedative-Hypnotics

The use of depressant compounds is as old as the use of alcohol, which is the oldest of the depressant agents. In earlier days, alcohol was held to be a remedy for practically all diseases and problems. Since then, many compounds other than alcohol have been manufactured for many of the same effects.

The sedative-hypnotic compounds are drugs that may have diverse chemical structures but have in common their ability to induce various degrees of behavioral depression.[1,2] Hypnotics are used to produce sleep, and sedatives are used to relieve anxiety, restlessness, irritability, and tension.[3] Often there is no sharp distinction between the two effects, and the same drug may have both actions, depending on the method of use and the dose employed. Other terms that describe these drugs include minor tranquilizers, anxiolytic drugs, and antianxiety agents. These terms are often used interchangeably because there is no clear distinction among many of the drugs and their effects. In large amounts, these drugs produce a state of intoxication similar to that induced by ethanol and can, in addition, produce sedation, tranquilization, hypnosis, and anesthesia.[2]

Sedative-hypnotics are generally categorized as one of three main types: (1) the barbiturates, (2) the nonbarbiturate-nonbenzodiazepines, and (3) the benzodiazepines. Drugs in the first two classes have a greater potential for serious sys-temic sequelae of misuse than those in the last group.[4] Although there are other drugs that have sedation as a property, such as the antihistamines, it is usually seen as a side effect. Such drugs are therefore not included in this discussion.

Many of the effects from the sedative-hypnotics are similar, and much of the treatment after an overdose is symptomatic. As with the narcotics, there are two areas of concern: the management of the overdosed patient, and the management of the withdrawal state, which is recognized as a medical emergency more serious than that of any other drug of abuse.

Low doses of the sedative-hypnotics produce mild sedation.[3] In high doses, the main cause of morbidity and mortality is the resulting coma and apnea. Tolerance to the intoxicating effects develops rapidly and may lead to a progressive narrowing of the margin of safety between an intoxicating and lethal dose of the drug. Drug abusers may be able to increase their daily dose up to 10 to 20 times the recommended therapeutic dose.[3]

Toxic reactions from the sedative-hypnotics involve a general slowing of mental functions, slurred speech, ataxia, and impairment in thinking, including poor comprehension, memory disturbance, increased reaction time, poor judgment, limited attention span, labile mood, and a release of aggressive impulses. In large doses, sleep, stupor, coma, and death from respiratory and circulatory depression are possible.

BARBITURATES

Barbiturates are among the drugs still very commonly prescribed to induce sedation and sleep. Barbiturates are derivatives of barbituric acid and are formed from the condensation of urea and malonic acid.[4] They acquire an alkyl or aryl group, which confers their sedative-hypnotic properties. The first barbiturates were prepared in 1864; since that time about 2500 derivatives of barbituric acid have been synthesized, but only about 15 remain in medical use. Barbiturates are capable of producing all levels of CNS depression, from mild sedation to hypnosis to deep coma and death. The degree of depression depends on dose, route of administration, and pharmacokinetics of the particular barbiturate.

Patterns of Abuse

Patterns of abuse of the barbiturates vary from intermittent recreational use to compulsive daily use with chronic intoxication. Most barbiturate poisonings in adults are suicide attempts.

Many of the barbiturates have street names related to their colors. Phenobarbital pills are called "purple hearts." Secobarbital is red, so that the terms "reds," "red devils," and "red birds" are used. Amobarbital is blue and goes by the terms "blues" and "blue devils." A combination of reds and blues, or amobarbital and secobarbital, is Tuinal® or "Christmas trees." Pentobarbital is yellow, so that the names "yellows" or "yellow jackets" are used.

Mechanism of Action

In the CNS, barbiturates facilitate inhibitory neurotransmission by inhibiting chemical neurotransmission across neuronal and neuroeffector junctions. This is similar to the action of γ-aminobutyric acid and the benzodiazepines.[4,5] Barbiturates thus facilitate inhibitory neurotransmission in the CNS with a subsequent decrease in the activity of postsynaptic cyclic guanosine monophosphate and cyclic AMP.[6]

Pharmacokinetics

Lipid solubility of the barbiturates is the dominant factor in their distribution through the body.[4] Barbiturates suitable for clinical use as anesthetics are those that are the most lipid soluble and can most rapidly penetrate all tissues. In general, the more lipid soluble the barbiturate, the more rapid the onset of its action, the shorter the duration of its effects, and the greater the degree of its hypnotic activity. The highly lipid-soluble drugs penetrate the blood-brain barrier rapidly. Less lipid-soluble drugs, such as phenobarbital, penetrate and leave the brain more slowly and thus have a slower onset and longer duration of action. Termination of action with these barbiturates depends more on redistribution than metabolism.

The duration of action of the barbiturates is multifactorial and depends on the rates of drug absorption, whether elimination is primarily by metabolic degradation or excretion, and the rate of removal of the active drug from the CNS. On the basis of these differences in the duration of action, barbiturates are classified into three categories: (1) ultrashort acting, (2) short and intermediate acting, and (3) long acting (Table 30-1).[4] The anticonvulsant primidone (Mysoline®) is metabolized to phenobarbital and thus should be considered a barbiturate.[5]

There appears to be little difference in duration of the hypnotic action among barbiturates used orally as hypnotics.[7] For this reason, barbiturates have recently been grouped according to their intended pharmacological action, sedative-hypnotic or anesthetic, rather than according to the duration of their action. Because of the convenience of categorizing barbiturates as to their duration of action, however, this method is used in this chapter.

Ultrashort-Acting Barbiturates

The ultrashort-acting barbiturates are thiopental, methohexital, buthabital, hexobarbital, and thiamylal. These drugs are not a source of abuse, and there should be no occasion to see an over-

Table 30-1 Classification of Barbiturates by Duration of Action

Ultrashort acting
  Thiopental
  Methohexital
  Buthabital
  Hexobarbital
  Thiamylal
Short and intermediate acting
  Amobarbital
  Aprobarbital
  Butabarbital
  Butalbital
  Pentobarbital
  Secobarbital
  Talbutal
Long acting
  Phenobarbital
  Mephobarbital
  Metharbital

Table 30-2 Selected Trade Names of Commonly Abused Barbiturates

Amobarbital
  Amytal
Aprobarbital
  Alurate
Butabarbital
  Butal
  Butalan
  Butapan
  Butazem
  Buticaps
  Butisol
  Soduben
Butalbital
  Fiorinal
Metharbital
  Bemonil
Pentobarbital
  Nembutal
  PBR/12
Phenobarbital
  Luminal
  Phen-Squar
  Sedadrops
Secobarbital
  Seconal
Talbutal
  Lotusate

dose with these drugs in an emergency department setting.

Short- and Intermediate-Acting Barbiturates

The short- and intermediate-acting barbiturates have an onset of action of 15 to 40 minutes and a duration of 6 hours. These drugs are the most widely used and abused barbiturates, both separately and in combination. They include, among others, pentobarbital, secobarbital, amobarbital, and butalbital (Table 30-2). Tuinal® is a combination of amobarbital and secobarbital and is a favored drug for abuse. Overdoses of the short-acting barbiturates have the highest mortality rate.[5,8]

Long-Acting Barbiturates

The long-acting barbiturates have an onset of action of approximately 1 hour and a duration of action of up to 16 hours. They are used as sedative-hypnotics, anticonvulsants, in treating gastrointestinal disorders, and as preanesthetic agents. Some of the drugs in this group (Table 30-2) are phenobarbital and drugs that act as or are converted to phenobarbital in the body, such as methylphenobarbital.[9,10] These drugs are also abused but not to the same extent as the short-acting barbiturates.[5]

Metabolism

To some degree, all barbiturates undergo metabolic degradation by the liver.[1,2] After ingestion, the short-acting barbiturates are initially and rapidly sequestered in the tissues so that their effects on the CNS are terminated rapidly. These agents are then mobilized slowly and immediately degraded by the liver, and their inactive products are excreted in urine. Long-acting drugs are metabolized by the slower process of urinary excretion. For example, 25% to 50% of a dose of phenobarbital is excreted unchanged in the urine.

Toxicity

Clinical Features

Mild to moderate barbiturate intoxication may mimic the clinical picture of alcohol intoxication. The neurologic examination may reveal general incoordination with nystagmus, slurred speech, dysmetria, and ataxia.

Low doses of the barbiturates depress the sensory cortex, decrease motor activity, and produce sedation and drowsiness. In some patients, drowsiness may be preceded by a period of transient elation, confusion, euphoria, or excitement. This may be particularly true for children and the elderly.[11]

The toxic dose of barbiturates varies considerably, but in general a severe reaction is likely to occur when the amount ingested is more than 10 times the usual oral hypnotic dose.[7] Overdosage produces CNS depression ranging from sleep to coma and death.[4] Respiratory depression may progress to Cheyne-Stokes respiration and central hypoventilation. Also noted are cyanosis; cold, clammy skin; areflexia; tachycardia; hypotension; anuria; and hypothermia. Hypothermia results from depression of the temperature-regulating mechanism in the pons. It is usually seen in fairly deeply unconscious patients who have been exposed for several hours. Patients with severe overdosage often experience typical shock syndrome such as apnea along with circulatory collapse. Barbiturates may have a direct toxic effect on the myocardium, but large doses are required to achieve this effect.[1,2] In addition, there may be a reduction in vasomotor tone of the smaller peripheral blood vessels with escape of fluid into the extravascular space, leading to hypotension and shock (Table 30-3). Because of the central and peripheral effects of the barbiturates, which often lead to hypoxia, hypotension, and shock, a lactic acidosis may ensue.

Short-acting barbiturates may cause respiratory depression as quickly as they produce unconsciousness. These agents are considered dangerous because many patients die before rescue efforts can be initiated.[10]

Barbiturate blisters were first described about 50 years ago, and although blisters do not affect the outcome of a barbiturate-intoxicated patient they can be of considerable diagnostic importance.[11] They can appear as early as 4 hours after ingestion and do not necessarily occur over areas of maximum pressure; rather, they most often occur where skin surfaces have been in contact with each other.[12] These lesions are usually multiple and consist of erythematous, indu-

Table 30-3 Clinical Features of Barbiturate Overdose

Neurologic
 Areflexia
 Cerebral edema
 Coma
 Hypothermia
 Sleep
Respiratory
 Apnea
 Cyanosis
 Respiratory depression
Cardiovascular
 Circulatory collapse
 Hypotension
 Pulmonary edema
 Tachycardia
Miscellaneous
 Blisters
 Acute tubular necrosis

rated, irregular patches progressing to bullous lesions. Their presence is not dependent on depth of coma or associated complications such as hypotension and respiratory insufficiency. These bullous cutaneous lesions may heal slowly. Although the precise mechanism of development of these lesions is unknown, a local toxic effect has been postulated.[13] These blisters are important in that, although barbiturates are just one of the drugs that can cause them, their presence may give a clue as to what was ingested (see Chapter 1).[14,15]

Serious Complications

The serious complications from barbiturate overdose include pulmonary complications such as aspiration, pneumonia, and pulmonary edema.[16] In addition, acute tubular necrosis subsequent to hypotension, hypovolemia, and cerebral edema has also been reported. A severe overdose of barbiturates can also cause hypotension, profound shock, ventilatory depression, coma, and death as a result of cardioventilatory failure from depression of the vital medullary centers.[16]

Laboratory Analysis

The serum barbiturate concentration is not regarded as an important indicator of the severity of poisoning because it is not necessarily closely related to the clinical state. It also has little prognostic value in determining depth or duration of coma.[17] This is particularly so in epileptic patients and others habituated to these drugs. Serum barbiturate determinations may be of benefit, however, in discerning the etiology of coma and can distinguish short- from long-acting agents. In assessing a patient with barbiturate poisoning, the serum concentration should always be considered in relation to the patient's history and clinical condition and should never take precedence over the latter.[18]

Treatment

Supportive Therapy

The treatment of the barbiturate overdose (Table 30-4) consists mainly of supportive therapy. Because most deaths are due to respiratory causes, attention to the airway is the immediate priority. Maintenance of an adequate airway, administration of oxygen, and assisted respiration if necessary are extremely important. There is no role for analeptic agents because they may result in severe CNS and cardiac toxicity. Measures to remove the remaining material from the gastrointestinal tract by ipecac or lavage or by administering activated charcoal and a cathartic should be instituted. Fluids should be administered for blood pressure support and for diuresis if necessary.[4] Often, the blood pressure may return to normal after dehydration has been corrected and adequate ventilation has been restored. Vasoconstrictors are usually not necessary for blood pressure support, and fluid administration is usually adequate to correct even severe hypotension.

Multiple-Dose Activated Charcoal

Recently it has been shown that multiple-dose activated charcoal is of great benefit for phenobarbital overdose by decreasing the half-life of the drug, enhancing the elimination, and shortening the duration of coma.[4,19,20] The charcoal can be administered either orally (if the patient is cooperative) or through a nasogastric tube every 2 to 6 hours.[21] Activated charcoal, by adsorbing phenobarbital in the gastrointestinal tract, sets up a gradient differential that allows more phenobarbital to diffuse from blood into the bowel, where it is subsequently adsorbed by the charcoal.[19] This is considered "intestinal dialysis."[22] In addition to its direct adsorptive properties, activated charcoal significantly shortens the elimination half-life and increases total body nonrenal clearance of the drug. The effectiveness of this procedure is comparable to forced alkaline diuresis or dialysis, and it can be promptly and easily initiated.[21,22]

Urinary Alkalinization

Urinary alkalinization promotes ionization of barbiturates, which prevents tubular reabsorption and thus traps the drug in the kidney for excretion. An alkaline diuresis may be useful in enhancing the excretion of only the long-acting barbiturates (phenobarbital) or drugs that are converted to phenobarbital in the body (primidone and mephobarbital). It is ineffective for the short- or intermediate-acting barbiturates.[23] Although an alkaline diuresis removes reasonable amounts of these long-acting barbiturates, it should be reserved for the severely poisoned patient because there are risks associated with this procedure.[24]

Extracorporeal Methods

Hemodialysis and, to a lesser extent, peritoneal dialysis also remove long-acting barbiturates in significant amounts in a severely poisoned patient.[23] Hemoperfusion has also been shown to decrease the duration of coma caused by the long-acting barbiturates.[25] The amounts of intermediate- and short-acting barbiturates

---

Table 30-4 Treatment of Barbiturate Overdose

Emesis or lavage
Activated charcoal and cathartic
Maintenance of patent airway
Fluid administration for blood pressure support
Forced alkaline diuresis (for long-acting barbiturate
  overdose)
Hemodialysis (for long-acting barbiturate overdose)
Hemoperfusion (for long-acting barbiturate overdose)

---

retrieved are not substantial, and dialysis should not be attempted in these situations. Extracorporeal measures should only be used if other measures are unsuccessful or in patients with impaired drug elimination due to renal failure. These methods should be necessary only in rare cases.[23]

NONBARBITURATES-NONBENZODIAZEPINES

Chloral Hydrate

Actions

Chloral hydrate (Cohidrate®, H-S Need®, Noctec®, Oradrate®, SK-Chloral Hydrate®, Aquachloral®) is one of the oldest of the sedative-hypnotics and was once a popular drug for inducing sedation and sleep.[26] It was the source of "knockout drops," also known as the "Mickey Finn," the effect of which was due to the additive effects of chloral hydrate and alcohol and was never as rapid as depicted in movies. Chloral hydrate has CNS depressant effects similar to those of barbiturates and was mainly used for children and the elderly, who tolerate barbiturates poorly, because it was thought that chloral hydrate produced less paradoxical excitement in these age groups.[7] Chloral hydrate has little analgesic activity, and patients who ingest the drug may respond to pain with delirium or excitement.

Chloral hydrate is converted by liver alcohol dehydrogenase through a large first-pass hepatic effect to an active metabolite, trichloroethanol, which has a longer duration of action than the parent compound. Chloral hydrate is not a street drug of choice, and its main misuse is by the elderly.[27]

Toxicity

Clinical features of intoxication with chloral hydrate are similar to those for barbiturates and alcohol and may include drowsiness, lethargy, stupor, hypotension, hypothermia, and respiratory depression, the last of which sometimes can occur shortly after ingestion.[27] These may be the direct results of the parent compound, whereas a prolonged coma appears to be the result of the active metabolite. Chloral hydrate is irritating to the gastric mucosa, and gastric necrosis has occurred after intoxicating doses.[26] In addition, hepatotoxicity, renal failure, and cardiac dysrhythmias may occur.[26] The dysrhythmias are generally atrial fibrillation, occasionally with aberrant conduction or premature ventricular contractions. Rare cases of ventricular tachycardia have been observed. Torsade de pointes has also been reported. Death may occur from respiratory failure or refractory hypotension or secondary to a dysrhythmia (Table 30-5).[27]

As with all sedative-hypnotics, clinical assessment of the patient's condition is more important and reliable than a plasma concentration because of the various degrees of tolerance to the drug among individuals.[26]

Treatment

Treatment for chloral hydrate ingestion is supportive and includes maintenance of an adequate airway, assisted respiration if necessary, oxygen administration, and maintenance of body temperature and circulation. Lidocaine or propranolol may be used for ventricular tachydysrhythmias. If torsade de pointes is present, overdrive pacing, isoproterenol, or atropine may be effective. Methods to enhance drug removal such as dialysis, diuresis, and hemoperfusion should not be attempted.[26]

Table 30-5 Clinical Features of Chloral Hydrate Overdose

Central nervous system
  Drowsiness
  Hypotension
  Hypothermia
  Lethargy
  Respiratory depression
  Stupor
Cardiac dysrhythmias
  Atrial fibrillation
  Premature ventricular contractions
  Torsade de pointes
  Ventricular tachycardia

Glutethimide

Actions

Glutethimide (Doriden®, Dormtabs®, Rolathimide®) was introduced in 1954 as one of the earliest of the "new" sedative-hypnotics.[7] The structure is virtually identical to that of the barbiturates except for one slight modification of the molecule. It is also similar structurally and in therapeutic activity to methyprylon, a nonbarbiturate sedative-hypnotic.

Since its introduction, glutethimide has been shown to have a mortality consistently greater than that of other sedative-hypnotics. Two of the reasons for this is its long duration of action and the fact that it is metabolized to another active compound, 4-hydroxy-2-ethyl-2-phenyl-glutarimide.[4,28] This metabolite has twice the activity and potency of glutethimide and also a duration of action that is more than twice that of glutethimide.[29,30] About half the parent compound is metabolized to the active metabolite.

Glutethimide stimulates the hepatic microsomal enzyme system and has pronounced anticholinergic activity.[30] The drug appears to be slowly and erratically absorbed from the gastrointestinal tract.[31] Co-administration with ethanol appears to increase the oral absorption of glutethimide dramatically. Because of its high lipid solubility, once absorbed there is extensive tissue localization, with high concentrations found in the brain and adipose tissue. Glutethimide has a volume of distribution of approximately 3 L/kg.[31] It produces hypnosis and has no analgesic, antitussive, or anticonvulsant activity.[29,30]

Toxicity

An overdose of glutethimide produces symptoms similar to those of other sedative-hypnotics and may include profound and prolonged coma, hypotension, respiratory depression, shock, and hypothermia.[4] There may be cyclic fluctuations in the depth of coma. There appears to be a poor correlation between the plasma concentration of glutethimide and its metabolite and the clinical course of the patient.[17,31–33] In addition, because of the anticholinergic activity, patients overdosed on this drug may exhibit mydriasis,

urinary retention, tachycardia, and hypertension (Table 30-6).

A prominent feature of glutethimide poisoning is a characteristic fluctuation in the level of consciousness. This may be due to the formation of the metabolite, but alternative explanations for this phenomenon include further absorption of the parent compound from the gastrointestinal tract after recovery from an ileus, enterohepatic circulation of glutethimide and its metabolite, and release of the drug from body fat. Most of the drug that is absorbed is deposited rapidly in body tissues, leaving only a small fraction to circulate freely in the bloodstream.

In recent years glutethimide has become increasingly popular among drug users when it is mixed with codeine.[31,32] The two drugs together have been termed "loads," "4's and Dors," or "setups."[33] This combination was reported more than a decade ago and is purported to produce a euphoria equal to that of heroin. It is also relatively inexpensive and is more readily available than heroin and can be taken orally. Also, because of the potent enzyme-inducing properties of glutethimide, more codeine may be converted to morphine than occurs with codeine alone. The effects may last for 3 to 12 hours (depending on the individual's degree of tolerance) without the side effects of intravenous administration. Although the typical intravenous "rush" is absent, it can be approximated when loads are taken on an empty stomach.[34,35] One "load" may consist of two 500 mg glutethimide tablets combined with four 60 mg codeine tablets, and abusers may take from 3 to 12 "loads"

Table 30-6 Clinical Features of Glutethimide Overdose

Sedative-hypnotic effects
  Coma
  Hypotension
  Hypothermia
  Respiratory depression
  Shock
Anticholinergic effects
  Hypertension
  Tachycardia
  Urinary retention

---

per day.[35] Intoxication is achieved within 20 minutes after ingestion, with the peak effect occurring after 40 minutes.[34]

Clinical features of loads overdose may be the same as those expected from a combination of a sedative-hypnotic and a narcotic agent and are characterized by alternating states of dreamlike euphoria and "nodding," sometimes associated with prolonged sensorimotor disturbances in the extremities.

The finding of glutethimide by history or on a drug screen should prompt a search for codeine and vice versa, particularly when the presence of either drug by itself does not explain the clinical condition of the patient.[32]

Treatment

Treatment for overdose of glutethimide or loads is directed toward supporting the patient and consists of attempts at removal of the drug by emesis or lavage, even many hours after ingestion, because it can remain in the gastrointestinal tract. Concretions may also form from a large amount of glutethimide. If a combination drug was ingested or if the patient exhibits an altered mental status, then naloxone should be administered. Dialysis, although initially thought to be of benefit, has been shown not to be clinically useful. This is due to the large volume of distribution of glutethimide and its high concentration in body fat.[33] Hemoperfusion and diuresis are also ineffective.

The question of effectiveness of multiple-dose activated charcoal remains unanswered, but the known enterohepatic circulation of some of the metabolites of glutethimide suggests that continued administration of charcoal may be of benefit.[32]

Methaqualone

Actions

Methaqualone (Quaalude®, Sopor®, Parest®, Mequin®) was originally marketed in the early 1970s as a safe, effective, nonaddicting substitute for barbiturates, but it was soon realized that the drug by itself or in combination could cause serious poisoning.[4] Mandrax® is a European trade name for methaqualone in combination with an antihistamine, diphenhydramine; in

Great Britain, the first death from this compound was reported within a few months of its commercial availability.[36,37]

In addition to sedative-hypnotic properties, methaqualone has anticonvulsant, antispasmodic, local anesthetic, and weak antihistaminic properties. The drug has antitussive properties comparable to those of codeine. In toxic doses, methaqualone may lead to a defect in platelet function and, because of this, to spontaneous bleeding.[38,39]

Popular notions of the qualities of methaqualone have made it a widespread drug of abuse for more than a decade.[7] Methaqualone was thought to have aphrodisiac qualities and has been referred to as the "love drug."[4,37] It is a low-potency sedative-hypnotic agent that appears to have an inordinate capacity to produce a dissociative "high" without sedation.[40] Users describe a loss of the perception of physical and mental "self." At certain doses, a state of disinhibition or euphoria results. During such disinhibition an individual may feel euphoric about sexual experiences, but, as with all other sedatives, sensation may be increased but performance may be impaired.[41] These effects may also be due to the drug's muscle relaxant qualities. Methaqualone also causes physiologic dependence and withdrawal.[40]

Most manufacturers have voluntarily suspended production of the drug because of its widespread abuse, although street forms are still available. Counterfeit "quaalude" tablets sold on the street do not necessarily contain methaqualone. They are prevalent on the illicit market and are similar in appearance to the well-known commercial product. Some patients have experienced necrotizing cystitis manifested by painful hematuria after ingestion of methaqualone purchased on the street. This reaction is believed to be due to orthotoluidine, which is a contaminant of the street drug.

Toxicity

Symptoms of overdosage with methaqualone include lethargy, coma, respiratory depression, and death (Table 30-7). In contrast to the coma of barbiturate overdose, the coma of severe methaqualone overdosage may be accompanied by pyramidal signs such as restlessness, excite-

Table 30-7 Clinical Features of Methaqualone Overdose

CNS depression
  Respiratory depression
  Coma
  Death
CNS stimulation
  Muscle hypertonicity
  Myoclonus
  Seizures
  Hyperreflexia
  Restlessness
Miscellaneous effects
  Bleeding
  Blisters

---

ment, muscle hypertonicity, myoclonus, and seizures.[41] In addition, the methaqualone-diphenhydramine combination has been reported to cause delirium, signs of extrapyramidal stimulation, and grand mal seizures. Bullous lesions, seen with barbiturates, have also been reported with methaqualone.

Treatment

Treatment for overdose is similar to that for overdoses of intermediate-acting barbiturates and includes adequate emptying of the gastrointestinal tract with subsequent administration of activated charcoal and a cathartic as well as support for blood pressure and respiration. Dialysis and hemoperfusion are not effective, and forced diuresis may increase the risk of pulmonary edema.

Ethchlorvynol

Actions

Ethchlorvynol (Placidyl®) is a tertiary acetylenic alcohol that was introduced in the mid-1950s as a sedative-hypnotic.[4] It is considered very dangerous. Its half-life is long, between 10 and 25 hours, and can increase to more than 100 hours if the patient ingests large amounts of the drug.[7] Ethchlorvynol is highly lipid soluble and has a large volume of distribution, approximately 4 L/kg, with extensive dis-

tribution in adipose and brain tissue. It has anticonvulsant and muscle relaxant properties as well as sedative-hypnotic activity.[42] Ethchlorvynol has a pungent, aromatic odor that is often detectable on the breath and in gastric fluid.[43] It has a rapid onset of action and a short duration of effect. Blood concentrations reach their peak 60 to 90 minutes after ingestion.[44]

Known on the street as "Mr Green Jeans," "Pickles," and "Jelly Beans," ethchlorvynol is a frequently abused drug with only a small margin of safety.

Toxicity

Symptoms of overdose with ethchlorvynol include coma (which can sometimes be prolonged, lasting days to weeks), respiratory depression, profound hypotension, hypothermia, and bradycardia despite the profound hypotension.[44] In addition, peripheral neuropathy, hemolysis, pancytopenia, and thrombocytopenia have been reported.[43] Ethchlorvynol may cause noncardiogenic pulmonary edema after illicit intravenous administration but also after oral administration.[4,42] Experimentally it has been shown that ethchlorvynol exerts a direct toxic action on the alveolar capillary membrane.[42] Death may result from respiratory failure or hypotension or as a complication of prolonged coma (Table 30-8).

Table 30-8 Clinical Features of Ethchlorvynol Overdose

CNS depression
  Coma
  Hypothermia
  Hypotension
  Bradycardia
  Respiratory depression
  Death
Hematologic effects
  Hemolysis
  Pancytopenia
  Thrombocytopenia
Miscellaneous
  Pulmonary edema
  Peripheral neuropathy

Treatment

Treatment for ethchlorvynol overdosage is supportive and includes maintenance of an adequate airway, assisted respiration, and oxygen administration. Hypotension should be treated with intravenous fluids. Because of the drug's large volume of distribution, dialysis, diuresis, and hemoperfusion are believed to be ineffective in its removal. There are reports of effective yields from resin hemoperfusion with Amberlite XAD-4, which is a styrene-divinylbenzene copolymer that acts as an uncharged exchange resin. Although this procedure may rid the body of the drug,[45] it has not been reported to alter the clinical course of the overdose. In addition, some of the complications of hemoperfusion include anemia, thrombocytopenia, hypocalcemia, and pancreatitis. Care should be taken not to overtreat this type of patient with fluids because this may increase the likelihood of pulmonary edema.

Meprobamate

Actions

Meprobamate (Bamate®, Equanil®, Mepripam®, Meprotabs®, Miltown®, Neuromate®, SK-Bamate®, Suronil®), which was first synthesized in 1950, is only one of a large number of carbamate derivatives currently on the market.[20,46,47] It is a drug that still may be used by the elderly and is usually not a drug of abuse chosen by the younger population. Meprobamate acts as an intermediate barbiturate except that it also has muscle relaxant properties. Meprobamate does not produce sleep at therapeutic doses.[4]

Toxicity

Overdosage of meprobamate produces symptoms that are similar to those of barbiturate overdosage; these may include drowsiness, stupor, ataxia, lethargy, coma, hypotension, shock, and respiratory depression. Hypotension may be marked, and pulmonary edema has been reported in a number of patients (Table 30-9). Large amounts of meprobamate may cause concretions. Because of this, clinical effects may be

Table 30-9 Clinical Features of Meprobamate Overdose

Ataxia
Coma
Drowsiness
Stupor
Hypotension
Lethargy
Pulmonary edema
Respiratory depression
Shock

prolonged until the gastrointestinal tract is adequately emptied.

Treatment

Treatment of meprobamate overdose consists of supportive care. Emesis or lavage should be followed by administration of activated charcoal and a cathartic. Hypotension should be treated with fluids. Dialysis, diuresis, and hemoperfusion do not enhance excretion and should not be used.

Long-Term Effects of Sedative-Hypnotics

Many of the sedative-hypnotics have actions and toxicities that are similar to those of the barbiturates. In this regard, all the sedative-hypnotics cause sedation, hypnosis, and deepening stages of coma leading to death from respiratory and cardiovascular collapse. Barbiturates stimulate the hepatic microsomal enzyme system in the liver; meprobamate, chloral hydrate, glutethimide, and methaqualone also stimulate this enzyme system (Table 30-10). The consequence

Table 30-10 Sedative-Hypnotics That Stimulate the Liver Microsomal Enzyme System

Barbiturates
Chloral hydrate
Glutethimide
Methaqualone
Meprobamate

is that an individual who has been taking any of these drugs chronically may need to increase the amount to achieve the same therapeutic effects. At the same time tolerance to the lethal dose does not change much, which causes greater morbidity and mortality than the safer alternatives, the benzodiazepines.

BENZODIAZEPINES

The first benzodiazepine, chlordiazepoxide, was introduced in 1960.[48] They are currently the drugs of choice for the pharmacologic treatment of anxiety because of their low lethality, even when taken in massive amounts, and the fact that they do not activate the liver microsomal enzymes, so that their rate of metabolism and that of other drugs that may be in concurrent use is unchanged.[49] When alcohol or other CNS depressants are not used concomitantly, the benzodiazepines are the safest of all currently available antianxiety and hypnotic agents. They also have a wide margin of safety in cases of overdosage.[50] Although they appear to have a low potential for abuse, these drugs are used by more Americans than any other single prescription item.

Clinical Uses

The benzodiazepines are used to treat sleep disorders, anxiety, alcohol withdrawal, and seizure disorders. They are also administered as anesthetics and before surgery. Although the benzodiazepines may be effective for musculoskeletal disorders, the required dose is higher than that currently used.[51]

Pharmacokinetics

The determinant for onset of action of orally administered benzodiazepines is the rate of gastrointestinal absorption, which is proportional to the lipophilicity of the drug.[52] Highly lipophilic benzodiazepines are rapidly absorbed and attain relatively high peak concentrations shortly after administration, causing rapid and intense single-dose effects. Diazepam and clorazepate are two of the most rapidly absorbed benzodiazepines; oxazepam and prazepam are the least rapidly absorbed.[53]

Most of the benzodiazepines are metabolized in the liver by oxidation. This pathway has important clinical implications if the drug's metabolite is active, especially if the active metabolite has a long elimination half-life, in which case both the parent compound and the active metabolite accumulate with multiple dosing (Table 30-11). The elimination half-life of the benzodiazepines is prolonged in the elderly because of the age-related decrease in the hepatic transformation for the compounds. Chlordiazepoxide, clorazepate, diazepam, halazepam, flurazepam, and prazepam are transformed to active metabolites that have longer half-lives than the parent drug.[4,54]

Mechanism of Action

A feature of benzodiazepines is their selective action on the CNS. In pharmacologic doses no direct effect on peripheral organs and tissues has been found; all changes induced by these drugs on peripheral functions are the result of their action on the CNS.

γ-Aminobutyric acid (GABA) is now recognized as the most important inhibitory neurotransmitter in the CNS.[55] GABA is stored in

---

Table 30-11 Classification of Benzodiazepines by Length of Half-Life

---

Short half-life
　Midazolam
　Triazolam
Intermediate half-life
　Alprazolam
　Clonazepam
　Lorazepam
　Oxazepam
　Temazepam
Long half-life
　Clorazepate
　Chlordiazepoxide
　Diazepam
　Flurazepam
　Halazepam
　Prazepam

---

synaptic vesicles in the neuronal terminals, where it is released by the effect of calcium ions that flow into the terminal during the action potential. The effect of benzodiazepines is indirectly to enhance or facilitate the inhibitory neuronal properties of GABA.[56] It is postulated that this effect is due to benzodiazepine antagonism of a protein that usually inhibits the binding of GABA to its receptor.[55,57] Binding of GABA to postsynaptic sites causes an increase in the chloride conductance, with resultant membrane hyperpolarization. Benzodiazepines cause no change in their conductance or any alteration in the synthesis, release, reuptake, or degradation of GABA. There is also no competitive binding at GABA receptors.[57]

Actions

The benzodiazepines are capable of producing all levels of CNS depression, from mild sedation to hypnosis and coma.[58] In addition, the benzodiazepines suppress the spread of seizure activity but do not abolish the abnormal discharge from a focus in epilepsy.

In therapeutic amounts, the benzodiazepines produce sedation and relief of anxiety and, at higher doses, muscle relaxation.[56] Thus the benzodiazepines are marketed variously as anticonvulsants, antianxiety drugs, and hypnotics, although all the benzodiazepines share these actions and no benzodiazepine has been shown to be superior to chlordiazepoxide or diazepam for the treatment of acute and chronic anxiety or insomnia.[55,59] The wide margin of safety of benzodiazepines permits their use in various clinical situations (Table 30-12).[59]

Toxicity

As mentioned above, there are many factors involved in the onset and duration of clinical effects of the benzodiazepines, including metabolism, distribution, degree of protein binding, lipid solubility, and half-life.[56] When taken alone, massive quantities of benzodiazepines can be ingested with little or no hazard of prolonged or serious CNS depression, and an overdose of benzodiazepines alone is rarely fatal.

Table 30-12 Selected List of Benzodiazepines

Antianxiety agents
 Alprazolam (Xanax®)
 Chlordiazepoxide (Librium®, Libritabs®, Murcel®, Reposans®, Tenax®, Zetran®)
 Clorazepate (Tranxene®)
 Diazepam (Valium®)
 Halazepam (Paxipam®)
 Lorazepam (Ativan®)
 Oxazepam (Serax®)
 Prazepam (Centrax®)
Anticonvulsants
 Clonazepam (Clonopin®)
 Clorazepate
 Diazepam
Hypnotic agents
 Flurazepam (Dalmane®)
 Midazolam (Versed®)
 Temazepam (Restoril®)
 Triazolam (Halcion®)

The combination of benzodiazepines and alcohol has been lethal, however.[49,53,57,59]

Symptoms of overdose of the benzodiazepines include drowsiness, ataxia, dizziness, delirium, somnolence, confusion, and occasionally aggression. Hypotension and respiratory depression rarely occur (Table 30-13).[56] If deep coma with marked hypotension or cardiovascular collapse is clinically present, the clinician should suspect ingestion of another CNS depressant.

Laboratory Analysis

Single values of the plasma concentration of many of the benzodiazepines are not closely

Table 30-13 Clinical Features of Benzodiazepine Overdose

Aggression
Ataxia
Confusion
Delirium
Dizziness
Drowsiness
Hypotension
Respiratory depression

related to their therapeutic or toxic effects because of the presence of metabolites as well as other factors.[18,60] Qualitative laboratory analysis may be useful, but quantitation is rarely of benefit.[59,60]

Treatment

Treatment for benzodiazepine overdose is supportive. Even after a significant overdose of benzodiazepines, mechanical ventilation is not usually required, although, rarely, coma may persist for up to 3 days. Diuresis, dialysis, and hemoperfusion are not indicated.[53,58,59]

Several compounds have been found to block selectively the interaction of benzodiazepines with their specific receptors in the CNS without producing the behavioral and neurological effects typical of benzodiazepines.[61] The agent most fully investigated to date is the imidazobenzodiazepine derivative called Ro 15-1788.[55] Outside the United States the drug has been marketed as Flumazenil®.[61] When this compound was administered in patient trials, patients who were intoxicated with benzodiazepines alone were fully awake and alert within 1 to 2 minutes.[61] In many patients, CNS depression may return 1 to 4 hours after administration because the half-life of the compound is approximately 50 minutes. No untoward effects and no acute withdrawal symptoms have been observed with the use of this agent.[55,61,62] Research is currently being performed to evaluate benzodiazepine antagonists, but the true impact of these agents clinically may be minimal because supportive care alone is usually successful.

SEDATIVE-HYPNOTIC WITHDRAWAL

The abrupt cessation or reduction of high doses of sedative-hypnotics may result in a characteristic withdrawal syndrome that closely resembles the alcohol withdrawal syndrome.[5,11] It should be recognized as a medical emergency that may be more serious than that of most other drugs of abuse (Table 30-14).[63] Long-term intoxication with the equivalent of 600 to 800 mg of pentobarbital or secobarbital is sufficient to

Table 30-14 Clinical Features of Sedative-Hypnotic Withdrawal

Abdominal cramps
Diaphoresis
Hallucinations
Insomnia
Myoclonus
Orthostatic hypotension
Restlessness
Seizures
Status epilepticus
Tremors
Vomiting
Weakness

produce clinically significant physical dependency, and the equivalent doses of any of the other sedative-hypnotics may also cause a severe abstinence syndrome, ranging from tremulousness and irritability to seizures, delirium, and death.[11,64]

The short-acting barbiturates, such as pentobarbital and secobarbital, and the short-acting benzodiazepines, such as triazolam, produce an acute withdrawal syndrome similar to that of ethanol.[64] The long-acting barbiturates as well as other benzodiazepines have a delayed onset of withdrawal symptoms.[56] Symptoms may begin 48 to 72 hours after the last dose, and the clinical course may be prolonged.[5]

Typically, withdrawal may manifest itself after 12 to 16 hours with symptoms of apprehension and weakness, tremors, insomnia, diaphoresis, and restlessness. Vomiting and abdominal cramps may develop.[65] With severe withdrawal, major symptoms and neurologic manifestations appear as well as orthostatic hypotension and seizures.[66] Symptoms usually peak during the second or third day of abstinence from the short-acting barbiturates or meprobamate, but this may be delayed until the seventh or eighth day of abstinence from the long-acting barbiturates or some of the benzodiazepines.[63] It is during this peak period that the major withdrawal symptoms usually occur. Myoclonic muscular contractions, spasmodic jerking of the extremities, and grand mal seizures may develop, sometimes leading to status epilepticus. Often after the seizure, hallucinations and delirium may develop.[20,66] The hallucinations are usually auditory and may be indistinguishable from those of delirium tremens associated with alcohol withdrawal.

Because of the serious nature of the withdrawal from sedative-hypnotics, patients should be under medical supervision.[66] Specific treatment of the withdrawal consists of replacing the sedative-hypnotic with a short- or long-acting barbiturate and gradually tapering this dose over a period of time.[67]

REFERENCES

1. Matthew H, Lawson A: Acute barbiturate poisoning: A review of two years' experience. *Q J Med* 1966;35: 539-550.

2. Gault F: A review of recent literature on barbiturate addiction and withdrawal. *Bol Estud Med Biol* 1976;29: 75-83.

3. Matthew H: Barbiturates. *Clin Toxicol* 1975;8: 495-513.

4. Bertino J, Reed M: Barbiturate and nonbarbiturate sedative-hypnotic intoxication in children. *Pediatr Clin North Am* 1986;33:703-722.

5. Baltarowich L: Barbiturates. *Top Emerg Med* 1985;7:46-54.

6. Robinson R, Gunnells J, Clapp J: Treatment of acute barbiturate intoxication. *Mod Treat* 1971;8:561-579.

7. Gary N, Tresznewsky O: Barbiturates and a potpourri of other sedatives, hypnotics, and tranquilizers. *Heart Lung* 1983;12:122-127.

8. Goldfrank L, Osborn H: The barbiturate overdose. *Hosp Physician* 1977;13:30-33.

9. Hooper W, Kunze H, Eadie M: Qualitative and quantitative studies of methylphenobarbital metabolism in man. *Drug Metab Dispos* 1981;9:381-385.

10. Hooper W, Kunze H, Eadie M: Pharmacokinetics and bioavailability of methylphenobarbital in man. *Ther Drug Monit* 1981;3:39-44.

11. Khantzian E, McKeena G: Acute toxic and withdrawal reactions associated with drug use and abuse. *Ann Intern Med* 1979;90:361-372.

12. Beveridge G, Lawson A; Occurrence of bullous lesions in acute barbiturate intoxication. *Br Med J* 1965;1: 835-837.

13. Groeschel D, Gerstein A, Rosenbaum J: Skin lesions as a diagnostic aid in barbiturate poisoning. *N Engl J Med* 1970;283:409-410.

14. Boyce M, Mason P: Blisters in unconscious patients. *Lancet* 1972;2:874.

15. Burdon J: "Barbiturate burns" caused by glutethimide. *Med J Aust* 1979;1:101-102.

16. Shubin H, Weil M: Shock associated with barbiturate intoxication. *JAMA* 1971;215:263-268.

17. Parker K, Elliott H, Wright J, et al: Blood and urine concentrations of subjects receiving barbiturates, meprobamate, glutethimide or diphenylhydantoin. *Clin Toxicol* 1970;3:131-145.

18. Drost R, Plomp T, Maes R: EMIT-ST drug detection system for screening of barbiturates and benzodiazepines in serum. *J Toxicol Clin Toxicol* 1982;19:303-312.

19. Goldberg M, Berlinger W: Treatment of phenobarbital overdose with activated charcoal. *JAMA* 1982;247: 2400-2401.

20. Preskorn S, Denner L: Benzodiazepines and withdrawal psychosis. *JAMA* 1977;237:36-38.

21. Berg M, Berlinger W, Goldberg M, et al: Acceleration of the body clearance of phenobarbital by oral activated charcoal. *N Engl J Med* 1982;307:642-644.

22. Pond S, Olson K, Osterloh H, et al: Randomized study of the treatment of phenobarbital overdose with repeated doses of activated charcoal. *JAMA* 1984;251: 3104-3108.

23. Setter J, Maher J, Schreiner G: Barbiturate intoxication: Evaluation of therapy including dialysis in a large series selectively referred because of severity. *Arch Intern Med* 1966;117:224-236.

24. Bloomer H: A critical evaluation of diuresis in the treatment of barbiturate intoxication. *J Lab Clin Med* 1966;67:898-905.

25. Yatzidis H: The use of ion-exchange resins and charcoal in acute barbiturate poisoning, in Matthew H (ed): *Acute Barbiturate Poisoning*. Amsterdam, Excerpta Medica, 1971, pp 223-232.

26. Stalker N, Gambertoglio J, Fukumitso C, et al: Acute massive chloral hydrate intoxication treated with hemodialysis: A clinical pharmacokinetic analysis. *J Clin Pharmacol* 1978;18:136.

27. Young J, Vanedermolen L, Pratt C, et al: Torsade de pointes: An unusual manifestation of chloral hydrate poisoning. *Am Heart J* 1986;112:181-184.

28. Crow J, Lain P, Bochner F, et al: Glutethimide and 4-OH glutethimide: Pharmacokinetics and effect on performance in man. *Clin Pharmacol Ther* 1977;22:458-464.

29. Hansen A, et al: Glutethimide poisoning. *N Engl J Med* 1975;292:250-252.

30. Hansen A, Kennedy K, Ambre J, et al: Glutethimide poisoning: A metabolite contributes to morbidity and mortality. *N Engl J Med* 1975;292:250-252.

31. Curry S, Hubbard J, Gerkin R, et al: Lack of correlation between plasma 4-hydroxyglutethimide and severity of coma in acute glutethimide poisoning. *Med Toxicol* 1987;2:309-316.

32. Chazan J, Cohen J: Clinical spectrum of glutethimide intoxication: Hemodialysis re-evaluated. *JAMA* 1969;208: 837-839.

33. Chazan J, Garella S: Glutethimide intoxication: A prospective study of 70 patients treated conservatively without hemodialysis. *Arch Intern Med* 1971;128:215-219.

34. Bailey D, Shaw R: Blood concentrations and clinical findings in nonfatal and fatal intoxications involving glutethimide and codeine. *Clin Toxicol* 1985;23:557–570.

35. Khajawall A, Sramek J: "Loads" alert. *West J Med* 1982;137:166–168.

36. Sanderson J, Corodele R, Higgins G: Fatal poisoning with methaqualone and diphenhydramine. *Lancet* 1966;2:803–804.

37. Inaba D, Gay G, Newmeyer J, et al: Methaqualone abuse. *JAMA* 1973;224:1505–1509.

38. Brown S, Goenechea S: Methaqualone: Metabolic, kinetic, and clinical pharmacologic observations. *Clin Pharmacol Ther* 1973;14:314–321.

39. Mills D: Effects of methaqualone on blood platelet function. *Clin Pharmacol Ther* 1978;23:685–691.

40. Pascarelli E: Methaqualone abuse: The quiet epidemic. *JAMA* 1973;224:1512–1514.

41. Wetli C: Changing patterns of methaqualone abuse. *JAMA* 1983;249:621–626.

42. Glauser F, Smith W, Caldwell A, et al: Ethchlorvynol-induced pulmonary edema. *Ann Intern Med* 1976;84:46–48.

43. Teehan B, et al: Acute ethchlorvynol intoxication. *Ann Intern Med* 1970;72:875–882.

44. Westervelt F: Ethchlorvynol (Placidyl) intoxication. *Ann Intern Med* 1966;64:1229–1236.

45. Lynn R, Honig C, Jatlow P, et al: Resin hemoperfusion for treatment of ethchlorvynol overdose. *Ann Intern Med* 1979;91:549–553.

46. Parry H, Balter M, Mellnger G, et al: National patterns of psychotherapeutic drug use. *Arch Gen Psychiatr* 1973;28:769–783.

47. Rickels K, Case G, Downing R, et al: Long-term diazepam therapy and clinical outcome. *JAMA* 1983;250:767–771.

48. Boyer R: Anticonvulsant properties of benzodiazepines: A review. *Dis Nerv Syst* 1966;27:35–42.

49. Greenblatt D, Allen M, Noel B, et al: Acute overdosage with benzodiazepine derivatives. *Clin Pharmacol Ther* 1977;21:497–500.

50. Greenblatt D, Shader R, Abernethy D: Current status of benzodiazepines: Part I. *N Engl J Med* 1983;309:354–358.

51. Greenblatt D, Shader R, Abernethy D: Current status of benzodiazepines: Part II. *N Engl J Med* 1983;309:410–416.

52. Greenblatt D, Shader R, Koch-Weser J: Slow absorption of intramuscular chlordiazepoxide. *N Engl J Med* 1974;291:1116–1118.

53. Greenblatt D, Shader R, Koch-Weser J: Flurazepam hydrochloride. *Clin Pharmacol Ther* 1975;17:1–14.

54. Gamble J, Dundee J, Assaf R: Plasma diazepam levels after single-dose oral and intramuscular administration. *Anaesthesia* 1975;30:164–169.

55. Haefely W: The biological basis of benzodiazepine actions. *J Psychoactive Drugs* 1983;15:19–39.

56. Schauben J: Benzodiazepines. *Top Emerg Med* 1985;7:39–45.

57. Tallman J: Benzodiazepines: From receptor to function in sleep. *Sleep* 1982;5:812–817.

58. Greenblatt D, Shader R, Koch-Weser J: Flurazepam hydrochloride, a benzodiazepine hypnotic. *Ann Intern Med* 1975;83:237–241.

59. Greenblatt D, Woo E, Allen M, et al: Rapid recovery from massive diazepam overdose. *JAMA* 1978;240:1872–1874.

60. Lister R, File S, Greenblatt D: The behavioral effects of lorazepam are poorly related to its concentration in the brain. *Life Sci* 1983;32:2033–2040.

61. Hofer P, Scollo-Lavizzari G: Benzodiazepine antagonist Ro 15-1788 in self-poisoning. *Arch Intern Med* 1985;145:663–664.

62. O'Sullivan G, Wade D: Flumazenil in the management of acute drug overdosage with benzodiazepines and other agents. *Clin Pharmacol Ther* 1987;42:254–259.

63. Vance M: Drug withdrawal syndromes. *Top Emerg Med* 1985;7:63–68.

64. Leung F, Guze P: Diazepam withdrawal. *West J Med* 1983;138:98–101.

65. Reveri M, Pyati S, Pildes R: Neonatal withdrawal symptoms associated with glutethimide (Doriden) addiction in the mother during pregnancy. *Clin Pediatr* 1977;16:424–425.

66. Abernethy D, Greenblatt D, Shader R: Treatment of diazepam withdrawal syndrome with propranolol. *Ann Intern Med* 1981;94:354–355.

67. Hollister L, et al: Withdrawal reactions from chlordiazepoxide. *Psychopharmacologia* 1961;2:63–68.

ADDITIONAL SELECTED REFERENCES

Costello J, Poklis A: Treatment of massive phenobarbital overdose with dopamine diuresis. *Arch Intern Med* 1981;141:938–940.

Faulkner T, Hayden J, Mehta C, et al: Dose-response studies on tolerance to multiple doses of secobarbital and methaqualone in a polydrug abuse population. *Clin Toxicol* 1979;15:23–37.

Hall S: Apnea after intravenous diazepam therapy. *JAMA* 1977;238:1052.

Hancock B: Acute barbiturate poisoning in young epileptics. *Postgrad Med J* 1974;50:242–244.

Kaplan S, Jack M, Alexander K, et al: Pharmacokinetic profile of diazepam in man following single intravenous and oral and chronic oral administrations. *J Pharmacol Sci* 1973;62:1789–1796.

Korttila K, Linnoila M: Absorption and sedative effects of diazepam after oral administration and intramuscular administration into the vastus lateralis muscle and the deltoid muscle. *Br J Anaesth* 1975;47:857–862.

Lightman S: Phenobarbital dyskinesia. *Postgrad Med J* 1978;54:114–115.

Maes V, Huyghens L, Dekeyser J, et al: Acute and chronic intoxication with carbromal preparations. *Clin Toxicol* 1985;23:341–346.

McGuigan M, Lovejoy F: Overdose of Lomotil, editorial. *Br Med J* 1978;1:990.

Murphy J, Sawasky F, Marquardt K, et al: Deaths in young children receiving nitrazepam. *J Pediatr* 1987;111:145–147.

Roytblat L, Bear R, Gesztes T: Seizures after pentazocine overdose. *Isr J Med Sci* 1986;22:385–386.

Sato S, Baud F, Bismuth C, et al: Arterial-venous plasma concentration differences of meprobamate in acute human poisonings. *Hum Toxicol* 1986;5:243–248.

chapter 31

Stimulants

Stimulants have been used for thousands of years and are still popular as a class for abuse. Users, many of whom do not realize that they are abusing drugs, tend to rely on stimulants to wake up in the morning, to be more alert and attentive, or to feel stronger, more decisive, and self-possessed. Although the problem of physical withdrawal from the drugs is minimal, the psychological dependence is strong.

The most prevalent and socially acceptable stimulants are nicotine in tobacco products and caffeine in coffee, tea, soft drinks, and combination medicines. The most toxic drugs in this group are the amphetamines, cocaine, and the "look-alike" drugs (Table 31-1).

All the stimulant drugs cause many similar effects, the most obvious of which affect the central and peripheral nervous systems and the cardiovascular system. Some of the other effects from the stimulants include a temporary sense of exhilaration and euphoria, increased feelings of

sexuality, hyperactivity, irritability, decreased fatigue, and extended wakefulness. Anorexia is also an effect of the stimulants, and it is this property that may initially attract some people to these drugs. At typical therapeutic doses, however, dysphoric reactions such as anxiety and apprehension can also occur.

Physical signs of stimulant use may include tremors, dizziness, dilated and reactive pupils, dry mouth, hyperreflexia, mild hypertension, and tachycardia. Many abusers "shoot" the drugs because, with intravenous administration, the effects are greatly intensified. Shortly after injection a sudden sensation known as a "flash" or "rush" is felt. This feeling is described by users as a "total body orgasm." The protracted use of stimulants is usually followed by a period of depression known as "crashing." This depression can be relieved by more stimulants, thereby setting up a cycle for the abuser.

Large doses may result in behavioral abnormalities such as repetitive grinding of the teeth, touching and picking the face and extremities, performing the same act over and over, preoccupation with one's own thought processes, suspiciousness, a feeling of being watched, and auditory and visual hallucinations. Physiologic abnormalities may include tachydysrhythmias, hypertensive crisis, cardiovascular collapse, renal failure, and death (Table 31-2).

Amphetamines and cocaine are similar in the effects that they produce, and both have the same

Table 31-1 Abused Stimulant Drugs

Nicotine
Caffeine
Amphetamines
Cocaine
Methylphenidate
Anorectic drugs
"Look-alike" drugs

Table 31-2 Clinical Effects of Stimulants

Neurological
  Hyperactivity
  Tremors
  Dizziness
  Xerostomia
  Hyperreflexia
Psychological
  Temporary sense of exhilaration
  Euphoria
  Decreased fatigue
  Superabundant energy
  Decreased appetite
  Anxiety
  Paranoia
  Hallucinations
Cardiovascular
  Hypertension
  Tachycardia
  Dysrhythmias
  Cardiovascular collapse

toxic manifestations. The main difference between the two stimulants is the duration of action and the degree of withdrawal. Whereas the effects of amphetamines may last for several hours, cocaine may be active in the body for only a few minutes because it is metabolized extremely rapidly by the liver. In addition, tolerance to cocaine does not appear to develop in the same manner as tolerance to amphetamines, and withdrawal symptoms (manifested by sleep disorders and profound depression on abrupt cessation of use) are usually less severe than with amphetamines.

COCAINE

The use of cocaine (benzoylmethylecgonine) began about 3000 years ago, according to Inca documents found in the area of what is now known as Peru and Bolivia.[1,2] Cocaine is a naturally occurring alkaloid extracted from the coca shrub *Erythroxylon coca*, which grows abundantly in the West Indies, Central and South America, and Mexico.[3–5] The coca plant should not be confused with the cocoa plant, which contains another stimulant, caffeine. The coca plant grows to a maximum of 7 or 8 feet in height, and the cocaine extracted represents roughly 1% of the dry weight of the coca leaf.[6,7]

During the time of the Incas, coca leaves were considered precious and were usually reserved for use by the nobility and for religious ceremonies, although they were used by others as well because of their energizing properties.

At the beginning of the 20th century, many patent medicines and soft drinks in the United States contained small amounts of cocaine. At one time Coca-Cola® contained cocaine, but shortly after the turn of the century the cocaine was replaced with caffeine.[4,8–10] Cocaine was indiscriminately included in over-the-counter medicines, tonics, and wines.[4,11] It has subsequently been deleted from all these products. Estimates today are that more than 4 million Indians in Peru and Bolivia use coca leaves on a regular basis. Illegally imported cocaine is usually in the form of the hydrochloride salt, which is produced by a process of alkaloid extraction and crystallization.[12]

Recent History

In the past cocaine was expensive, and its price served as a barrier to widespread use. In recent years cocaine has become less expensive, and its availability and purity have increased.[4] Although it was once a drug for the wealthy, cocaine now pervades all strata of society. Thus during the last 3 to 4 years the growing epidemic of cocaine abuse in the United States has resulted in widespread physical, psychiatric, and social problems. Although cocaine was once thought to be a relatively safe street drug, the incidence of cocaine-related deaths has been steadily rising.[4,13]

Pharmacokinetics

Cocaine is an ester of benzoic acid and the amino alcohol base ecgonine.[3] Ninety percent of a dose of cocaine is metabolized by plasma cholinesterase and hepatic enzymes.

Plasma cholinesterase activity is much lower in fetuses, infants, elderly men, patients with liver disease, pregnant women, and individuals who are homozygous for atypical cholinesterase activity (Table 31-3).[4,11,14] These individuals may be unusually sensitive to cocaine and have

Table 31-3 Populations in Which Plasma Cholinesterase Activity Is Decreased

Fetuses
Infants
Elderly individuals
Liver disease patients
Congenitally deficient individuals

an exaggerated response to otherwise low doses because of their decreased ability to hydrolyze the drug.[4] Cocaine is detoxified and excreted as benzoylecgonine, ecgonine, norbenzoyl-ecgonine, and norecgonine. The amount of unchanged cocaine in the urine is dependent on urinary *p*H.

Mechanism of Action

Cocaine has a major effect on the sympathetic division of the autonomic nervous system by preventing neuronal uptake of catecholamines as well as by increasing the release of these substances from adrenergic nerve terminals.[4] Cocaine therefore blocks the reuptake of dopamine and norepinephrine in the CNS, which results in euphoria, garrulousness, restlessness, and increased motor activity.[14] This mechanism appears to be involved in the physical and psychological dependence noted.[3] Cocaine causes an increase in heat production by stimulating muscular activity and decreasing heat loss through vasoconstriction. This can lead to marked hyperpyrexia.[14]

Medical Uses

Despite its legal classification as a narcotic, cocaine is actually a tropane related to the belladonna alkaloids and is the only naturally occurring local anesthetic. Cocaine acts as a local anesthetic by virtue of a blockade of nerve initiation and conduction after local application; this effect can last from 20 to 40 minutes.

Although cocaine has had many medical uses in the past, its use is now limited to that of a topical anesthetic for rhinoplasty and intranasal surgery. Cocaine is particularly useful for this type of surgery because of its ability to anesthetize as well as to cause local vasoconstriction and thus limit bleeding.[8,12,15] Although cocaine had been used in ophthalmic surgery as both a local anesthetic and vasoconstrictor, this use has now been discontinued.

Absorption

Cocaine is absorbed from most routes. It may be injected intravenously, swallowed, smoked, nasally insufflated, applied to oral or genital mucous membranes, or mixed with liquor to make a "liquid lady."[5,14,16] Although it is widely assumed that the drug is inactive when given orally because of hydrolysis by gastrointestinal acids, overwhelming evidence to the contrary exists.[5] The oral route results in far less toxicity than other routes of administration, but toxic effects are still detected with large ingestions. Generally cocaine is not taken orally for recreational purposes, but toxic reactions and death have been reported from "body packing" (ingestion of drug-filled balloons to avoid police detection).

The abuser of street cocaine usually obtains a 5% mixture that may range from 10 mg to 200 mg of cocaine per dose. The average "line" of cocaine is 25 mg, and 10 to 15 mg is usually administered by the intravenous route. The latter provides the equivalent of 10 mg of dextroamphetamine.

Forms of Administration

Nasal Insufflation

Typically, cocaine is distributed as a white crystalline powder cut into grams or "spoons" (a spoon is considered approximately 0.5 g). One gram of cocaine may produce 30 to 40 lines.[4] The most common method of administration is intranasally.[17] The cocaine is chopped with a razor blade into lines or columns on a smooth surface such as a piece of glass, and a line is inhaled or snorted through a plastic straw or rolled up currency.[4,11] This process is usually repeated with the other nostril. After insufflation approximately 60% of the drug is absorbed, and cocaine may be detected on the nasal mucosa for as long as 3 hours after application. Cocaine administered by insufflation limits its own absorption by causing vasoconstriction of the nasal mucosa, and the plasma drug concentration usually rises relatively slowly.

After insufflation, the drug's effects usually begin within 5 minutes, reach a maximum in 20 minutes, and may last for more than 30 to 60 minutes.[14,18]

Free Basing

Cocaine hydrochloride is not suitable for smoking because heat causes it to decompose. To be smoked, the cocaine hydrochloride must be made into a free base, which is then more heat stable.[5] Free base, or cocaine alkaloid, is a colorless, odorless, transparent substance that is soluble in alcohol, acetone, ether, oils, and water.[14] This free base is absorbed from all sites but primarily from the lungs.

Technique of free basing. Free basing, or "base-balling," is performed by one of two methods. The more dangerous method involves taking the hydrochloride salt of cocaine, mixing it with an alkaline solution such as ammonium chloride to convert it to a free base, and using ether as a solvent.[14] Street cocaine is dissolved in water, and then a base with a pH higher than that of cocaine is added. Ether is then added to this mixture, and the cocaine alkaloid remains in the ether layer. After the ether evaporates, the substance remaining contains purified alkaloid crystals, which are more volatile than the cocaine salt.[4,19] The less dangerous method does not involve ether and is used to manufacture "crack."

Properties of free base. The free base thus formed is more stable to heat and more pure because the process removes many of the cutting substances. This free base can then be smoked with a special pipe or sprinkled on a tobacco or marijuana cigarette.[20] Compared to insufflation, free basing is extremely dangerous. When the hydrochloride salt is used intranasally, the local vasoconstrictor action on the nasal mucosa acts to limit absorption. Free base cocaine, when smoked, offers no such protection and actually simulates the immediate effect of intravenous

administration, and the user may inadvertently overdose.[4,17] In addition, the ether used as a solvent can be a fire hazard.

The highly vascularized lung surface facilitates immediate absorption of free base cocaine, and after smoking the onset and progression of effects occur almost immediately. The effect is an intense euphoric experience that is often followed within minutes by a dysphoric "crash," leading to frequently repeated doses and rapid addiction in the susceptible individual.[17] Large doses of cocaine taken by this route have caused death within minutes.

"Crack"

Cocaine has glutted the street market over the last several years, and despite a government crusade against its use it has never been more plentiful, cheaper, purer, or more widely used. Cocaine suppliers have had to resort to new marketing techniques and packaging to stay competitive in the industry. The use of free base has been linked to a shift in cocaine distribution patterns as dealers have switched from selling cocaine powder to free base cocaine in tiny chunks known as "rocks" or "crack."[1] Crack is designed for individuals who wish to try free base cocaine but are unwilling to free base it themselves because they either do not know how or are frightened to try.[16]

Crack is extracted from cocaine powder in a procedure that uses sodium bicarbonate, heat, and water. This eliminates the need for chemicals and glassware. The process is simple and relatively safe compared with the more volatile method of processing cocaine powder into free base.

Free base cocaine is called crack because of the sound made by crystals popping when it is heated[1] and rocks because of its appearance. Dealers prefer to sell crack rather than cocaine powder because of crack's high addiction potential, low unit cost, and ease of handling. Crack is usually in the form of a light brown or beige pellet or a small chunk and is sold in clear plastic or amber vials. There are approximately 300 to 500 mg per vial. One vial usually provides two to three inhalations, and the effects may last approximately 20 minutes.[14]

"Basuco"

Cocaine may also be smoked in the form of coca paste, which is also referred to as "pasta," "bazooka," or "basuco."[21,22] This is a crude extract of the coca leaf that is heated with sulfuric acid, precipitated with sodium carbonate, and then converted to cocaine sulfate.

Oral Administration

As mentioned above, there is a common misconception that cocaine is hydrolyzed in the gastrointestinal tract and rendered inactive. An oral dose of cocaine, however, is at least as effective as the same dose taken intranasally.

"Body Packing"

Because of increased surveillance by narcotics agents, individuals who smuggle drugs must devise schemes of surreptitiously bringing cocaine through customs. "Body packing" is one such scheme, in which extremely large amounts (3 to 6 g) of cocaine are ingested in condoms, toy balloons, or in the fingers of latex gloves with the expectation that these packets will be excreted 1 to 2 days after the smuggler's entry into the country.[2,11,23,24] Some individuals take a substance such as diphenoxylate (Lomotil®) before boarding the plane to slow gastrointestinal motility and prevent passage of the cocaine packets before landing. They then take a laxative once they reach their destination.

Many deaths are associated with body packing because leakage or rupture can occur in one or more of the packets.[2,25] The rupture of even one packet can cause death because of the large dose of pure cocaine that is suddenly absorbed through the intestinal mucosa.[11,23] Often a roentgenogram will show evidence of these condoms, depending on the type of material used, as multiple oval soft tissue densities surrounding a gas halo.[20] Enteric septicemia caused by fecal contamination of subsequently injected cocaine has been reported.

Intravenous Administration

The effects of intravenous administration are similar to those of smoking because both routes of administration demonstrate almost immediate effects. The intravenous injection sites of cocaine users are noted to have prominent ecchymoses, sometimes with a central area of pallor.[26] Multiple ecchymotic areas are probably due to a direct cytotoxic reaction of cocaine coupled with the ischemic vascular injury secondary to vasoconstriction.

Cutting Substances and Contaminants

Various cutting substances may be added to cocaine, some of which may greatly add to its toxicity (Table 31-4). Adulteration of cocaine makes it impossible for cocaine users to know how much cocaine they are taking.[4] The user may only be getting 5% to 40% pure cocaine. Most of the active ingredients used as cutting substances for cocaine come from three major drug categories: xanthine alkaloids, local anesthetics, or decongestants. The use of cutting substances increases the dealer's profit; these particular substances are used because their stimulant effects mimic those of the pure drug to unsophisticated users.

Local anesthetics may be added to simulate the expected anesthetic effect ("freeze") of the cocaine. Procaine is by far the most common local anesthetic cutting agent, followed by lidocaine, benzocaine, and tetracaine. Procaine is also the least toxic; lidocaine is about 2 to 3 times more toxic than procaine.[4] Methidrine,

---

Table 31-4 Cocaine Cutting Substances

Local anesthetics
  Benzocaine
  Lidocaine
  Procaine
Stimulants
  Caffeine
  Amphetamines
  Phencyclidine
Sugars
  Inositol
  Lactose
  Sucrose
Miscellaneous
  Benzene
  Quinine

---

an amphetamine, may be added because it is a cheap alternative to cocaine and has many of the same effects. Phencyclidine, caffeine, and quinine have also been used. The sugars lactose, sucrose, and inositol (an isomer of glucose) may be added as adulterants because they act as fillers and add weight to the cocaine.[17] The disaccharide lactose, which is similar to sucrose, is most commonly used. Quinine is also used for cutting cocaine, just as it is for heroin.

In addition to these substances, the mixture may be contaminated with bacteria, fungi, or viruses.[4]

Toxicity

Clinical Features

The clinical picture of cocaine poisoning can easily be confused with that of amphetamine or phencyclidine poisoning. In most instances, the distinctive clinical feature of cocaine poisoning is the more rapid return of the patient to a normal physical state.

Cocaine overdose is more common than previously thought. Contrary to popular belief, users can overdose by any route of administration, including by insufflation. Serious overdose may occur particularly in those with pseudocholinesterase deficiencies and in body packers, smokers, and intravenous users.

Onset and Duration of Symptoms

Cocaine reaction in the body is of a biphasic nature, with initial sympathetic stimulation followed by abrupt generalized CNS depression (Table 31-5). In cases of acute toxicity, if death occurs it does so usually within 2 to 3 minutes, but sometimes there is a delay of up to 30 minutes. Deaths have been reported after smoking, insufflation, intravenous injection, and oral use.[20,24,27] Nevertheless, cocaine use rarely leads to death.

The predominantly positive feelings that are experienced during the initial phase of cocaine intoxication are of short duration and are commonly followed by dysphoric feelings characterized by anxiety, depression, irritability, fatigue, and a craving for more cocaine.

Table 31-5 Clinical Features of Cocaine Intoxication

CNS
  Excitement
  Euphoria
  Garrulousness
  Headache
  Tremors
  Seizures
  Fever
  Hyperthermia
  Mydriasis
Cardiovascular
  Tachycardia
  Hypertension
  Hypotension
  Dysrhythmias
    Premature ventricular contractions
    Ventricular tachycardia
    Ventricular fibrillation
  Chest pain
  Myocardial infarction
  Angina pectoris
Nonspecific
  Rhabdomyolysis
  Myonecrosis
  Acute tubular necrosis

Central Nervous System Effects

Systematically, cocaine stimulates the CNS from above downward. The first recognizable action is on the cortex and is manifested by excitement, euphoria, garrulousness, and restlessness.[4,12] These are some of the effects sought after by the user. There may also be an increased capacity for muscular work. Nausea, vomiting, and abdominal pain often occur. Other signs and symptoms may include headache, chills, fever, mydriasis, and formication, which is the sensation of insects crawling under the skin (also called Magnan's sign)[12]; these tactile hallucinations may lead to serious degrees of self-excoriation.[11] Cocaine causes mydriasis indirectly by blocking the reuptake of norepinephrine. It usually does not cause cycloplegia.

As the dose is increased lower motor centers are stimulated, causing tremors and seizures. Seizures and death have been associated with a wide range of plasma concentrations. Other effects may include tachypnea and tachycardia. Paradoxical respiratory depression after an initial increase in rate and depth may lead to rapid, shallow respirations or Cheyne-Stokes breathing, and death may occur from central respiratory depression.

Cardiovascular Effects

Small doses of systemically administered cocaine may paradoxically slow the heart either because of central vagal stimulation or as a reflex response to the hypertension; after moderate doses the heart rate increases, probably as a result of cocaine-induced central and peripheral effects on the sympathetic nervous system. Dysrhythmias associated with cocaine use include sinus tachycardia, ventricular premature contractions, ventricular tachycardia and fibrillation, and asystole.[1]

Cocaine may precipitate life-threatening cardiac events.[28] Cocaine represents a potential hazard to individuals with underlying fixed coronary artery disease because it causes predictable increases in heart rate, systolic blood pressure, and myocardial oxygen demand. Angina pectoris and myocardial infarction apparently due to coronary artery constriction have also been reported in young, otherwise healthy individuals who used cocaine.[1]

One proposed mechanism for the cardiac effects of cocaine on these individuals is coronary vasospasm due to sympathetic potentiation or to a direct effect on the vascular smooth muscle.[18] A term for the process, contraction band necrosis, is classically associated with an excessive amount of circulating catecholamines, which increases the local tissue concentration of norepinephrine. In addition, some of the contaminants of cocaine may have cardiovascular effects. The occurrence of an acute myocardial infarction in any young patient should raise the suspicion of coronary artery spasm related to cocaine use.[1] A combination of factors may also lead to dysrhythmias, such as scarring in the conduction system and elevated catecholamine concentrations, both of which develop over the course of time.

Cocaine and Pregnancy

Cocaine has a deleterious influence on the outcome of pregnancy. There is an increased rate of spontaneous abortion, and infants exposed to cocaine in utero have a high risk of congenital malformations, perinatal mortality, and neurobehavioral impairments.[13]

Life-Threatening Effects

With continued high doses of cocaine, irrationality, paranoia, a proneness to violence, and a true toxic psychosis may ensue. With lethal doses, malignant hyperthermia, status epilepticus, ventricular dysrhythmias, and respiratory arrest can occur. Rhabdomyolysis and acute myoglobinuric renal failure have been associated with cocaine abuse.[16] Malignant hyperthermia is due to stimulation of the heat regulatory centers in combination with increased skeletal muscle activity.[3,4] Pneumomediastinum and pneumothorax have been reported as a result of prolonged Valsalva's maneuvers after the inhalation of alkaloidal cocaine (Table 31-6).[19] Sudden death from the recreational use of cocaine may be preceded by delirium, hyperpyrexia, and convulsions.

Cocaine and Dependence

Current data from animal studies suggest that cocaine may be more harmful than heroin because it is a powerful reinforcing drug. Self-administration leading to death has been noted in primates. In one study of laboratory animals, cocaine self-administration was accompanied by a substantially higher incidence of mortality than was heroin self-administration in a 30-day period.[29,30] The number of fatalities occurring after unlimited access to cocaine was more than twice that after unlimited access to heroin. The

Table 31-6 Life-Threatening Effects of Cocaine Intoxication

Angina pectoris
Myocardial infarction
Malignant hyperthermia
Status epilepticus
Ventricular dysrhythmias
Respiratory arrest
Pneumomediastinum
Pneumothorax

mortality rate for 30 days of continuous testing was 36% for the heroin group and 90% for the cocaine group.[29] The attempt to recapture the positive feelings and to relieve the abstinence syndrome appears to be an important factor underlying compulsive cocaine use.[30]

Effects of Chronic Use

In chronic users, septal atrophy, perforation, and ulcerations secondary to intense and repeated vasoconstriction may occur, although these are rare. In addition, reactive hyperemia leading to boggy nasal mucosa and a chronic stuffy nose or "cold" may develop. Atrophy of the nasal mucosa has been reported.[12] These effects may lead individuals to abuse nasal sprays, which cause temporary vasoconstriction but have the same rebound phenomenon as cocaine.

Laboratory Analysis

Patients suspected of cocaine use may undergo a toxicologic screen to confirm the presence of cocaine or its principal metabolite in the urine. Because of the usual acute nature of the overdose and the short half-life of the drug in the body, quantitative laboratory determinations of serum concentrations have no value in assessing the clinical state of the patient. Semiquantitative and qualitative immunoassays are available for detecting the inactive metabolite benzoyl-ecgonine in the urine; such assays may be positive more than 24 hours after cocaine use.[1,12,14] After a single nasal application of cocaine, metabolites may be detected in the urine within 4 hours and for as long as 27 hours.

None of the routine biochemical tests correlate with the clinical severity of cocaine intoxication. Electrocardiograms may be useful in assessing and monitoring cardiac abnormalities, and a chest roentgenogram may help rule out pulmonary edema.

Treatment

The treatment of acute reactions to cocaine is generally unnecessary because the reactions usu-ally run their course before the patient arrives at the emergency department. For example, a patient undergoing a seizure due to cocaine will not usually have a second seizure or need seizure prophylaxis. Generally, when treatment is necessary for cocaine overdose it consists of symptomatic and supportive care (Table 31-7). As usual, ingestion of an unknown substance requires the administration of glucose, thiamine, naloxone, and oxygen. If seizures occur, diazepam or a short-acting barbiturate can be administered.[4] Paranoia can be treated with haloperidol. Lidocaine may be used for ventricular irritability unless the patient is having seizures.[3,4]

β-Adrenergic blocking drugs such as propranolol are rarely needed for hypertension, tachycardias, and dysrhythmias that are hemodynamically significant or for many of the minor symptoms associated with cocaine overdose. Propranolol may result in unopposed α-adrenergic–mediated vasoconstriction, possibly worsening hypertension.[4] For this reason, labetalol, a combined α and β blocker, has been advocated for hypertension rather than the traditional blocker propranolol.[31] Hypertensive crisis may also be treated with a short-acting antihypertensive preparation such as sublingual nifedipine or intravenous nitroprusside.

Active external cooling maneuvers are suggested for hyperpyrexia, and core temperatures should be continuously monitored. Blood pressure should be maintained primarily with intravenous fluids and military antishock trousers, if necessary. Vasopressors should be avoided

---

Table 31-7 Treatment of Cocaine Overdose

Indication	Treatment
Seizures	Diazepam (5 to 15 mg IV)
Hypertension, tachycardia, dysrhythmias	Propranolol (1-mg doses IV up to 10 mg) or labetalol (0.25 mg/kg IV)
Hyperthermia	Active cooling
Hypotension	Fluids or military antishock trousers
Body packing	Surgical removal

because they can be hazardous in a patient who is already sympathetically stimulated.[4]

Any patient, regardless of age, who is complaining of anginal-type symptoms temporally related to the use of cocaine should have an intravenous line in place, have continuous cardiac monitoring, and be admitted to a monitored area to rule out the possibility of an acute myocardial infarction.

Body packing merits serious consideration of surgical removal of the cocaine packages.[2] Some investigators suggested a conservative approach of observation without surgery. If signs of toxicity are present, however, emergency surgery may be lifesaving after pharmacologic intervention. The longer these packages remain in the gastrointestinal tract, the greater the possibility of cocaine leakage. Endoscopic removal of the packages has caused their rupture,[2] so that surgery rather than endoscopy is recommended for removal of all intact packages.[4] Syrup of ipecac-induced emesis has resulted in the successful removal of recently ingested drug packets. In patients who are not body packers but who have recently ingested drug packets to avoid police detection, emesis induced by syrup of ipecac has been successful in expelling the packets because they are still in the stomach.

Withdrawal

Long-term users of cocaine may present to the emergency department as an attempt to abstain from the drug. These patients should be fully evaluated for associated signs of drug abuse and referred to an appropriate facility for detoxification and rehabilitation. There is a strong risk of psychologic dependency from cocaine, and there appears to be a pharmacologic basis for the withdrawal symptoms noted after abrupt cessation of cocaine. Consistent use of cocaine may result in depression when the drug is discontinued. Because the drug affects the dopaminergic neuronal systems, long-term use of cocaine depletes the nerve terminals of dopamine, which contributes to the dysphoria and depression that develops during withdrawal and the subsequent craving for more of the drug.[14]

Bromocriptine (Parlodel®), a dopamine substitute, has shown initial promise in reducing symptoms and cravings in hospitalized cocaine abusers, but controlled outpatient trials are needed to determine whether this treatment can increase abstinence rates.

AMPHETAMINES

Amphetamines became a drug of abuse about 50 years ago when they were available in nasal decongestant inhalers and other over-the-counter preparations. In addition, there were many other nonmedical uses of amphetamines. Subsequent recognition of the limited therapeutic value and high abuse potential of amphetamines led to a marked reduction in their medical use. Current applications include treatment for narcolepsy, for appetite control, and to control hyperkinetic behavior in children. Many authorities believe that less toxic alternatives exist and that, even for these indications, amphetamines should not be employed.

Mechanism of Action

The mechanism of action of amphetamines on peripheral structures is thought to be a combination of an indirect action by a release of norepinephrine from stores in adrenergic nerve terminals and a direct action on both α and β receptor sites.[32] Amphetamines cause a release of catecholamines into the synaptic cleft and decrease the rate of catecholaminergic neuronal firing. The main site of the CNS action appears to be the cerebral cortex. The neurotransmitters in the CNS that are affected are norepinephrine, dopamine, and 5-hydroxytryptamine.[33]

Pharmacokinetics

Amphetamine (phenylisopropylamine) is a noncatechol sympathomimetic adrenergic agent that is structurally related to norepinephrine but that has greater central stimulant activity than norepinephrine and other catecholamines.

The amphetamines (Table 31-8) can be divided into the D-isomer and the L-isomer. The

Table 31-8 Amphetamine Preparations and Their Trade Names

Preparation	Trade Name(s)
Benzphetamine	Didrex
Dextroamphetamine	Dexedrine
	Dexampex
	Ferndex
	Oxydess
Diethylpropion	Tenuate
	Tepanil
Fenfluramine	Pondimin
Methamphetamine	Desoxyn
Methylphenidate	Ritalin
Phendimetrazine	Adipost
	Bontril
	Dyrexan
	Melfiat
	Plegine
	Trimstat
	Wehless
Phenmetrazine	Preludin
Phentermine	Adipex
	Fastin
	Teramine

Source: Adapted from *Topics in Emergency Medicine* (1985; 7[3]:21), Copyright © October 1985, Aspen Publishers, Inc.

D-isomer has 2 to 4 times the potency of the L-isomer for CNS stimulation, and the L-isomer has greater cardiovascular effects. The racemic mixture is marketed as Benzedrine® or "bennies" and the D-isomer as Dexedrine® or "dexies."[34] For all practical purposes, however, the effects of all these products are similar, the differences being relative potency, half-life, CNS activity or peripheral activity, and onset of action. Methamphetamine may be favored by the drug abuser for parenteral use because it is water soluble and can be injected more readily than the other agents. In addition, it is favored because it has more pronounced central effects and less pronounced peripheral effects.

Amphetamines are absorbed rapidly from the gastrointestinal tract. At therapeutic doses, blood concentrations reach their peak 1 to 2 hours after ingestion. The plasma half-life of amphetamines depends on the pH of the urine. With an alkaline urine the plasma half-life is 15 to 30 hours, whereas with an acidic urine the half-life is 8 to 10 hours.

Toxicity

Amphetamines may be taken on a short- or long-term basis by oral, respiratory, intravenous, or vaginal routes.[32] The amount of amphetamine required to produce serious features of overdose (Table 31-9) depends to a large extent on the frequency of previous usage and the size of the doses. There is a relatively large margin of safety between therapeutic and lethal doses. After repeatedly taking amphetamines most users develop a tolerance to the drug, and larger amounts can be taken with each dose.

At average oral doses, amphetamines produce euphoria, a feeling of superabundant energy, extended wakefulness, and decreased appetite.[32] An increase in blood pressure with reflex bradycardia may also be noted, along with a relaxation of bronchial muscles and CNS stimulation. These are the desired effects of the amphetamines that are sought after by the user.

A patient who ingests amphetamine in moderate amounts may become symptomatic within

Table 31-9 Clinical Features of Amphetamine Intoxication

Cardiovascular
  Hypertension
  Bradycardia
  Tachycardia
  Palpitations
  Hypertensive crisis
  Dysrhythmias
Central nervous system
  Delirium
  Euphoria
  Mydriasis
  Coma
  Status epilepticus
  Superabundant energy
  Extended wakefulness
  Hyperpyrexia
  Anxiety
  Seizures
  Cerebrovascular accident
  Psychosis
  Hallucinations
Nonspecific
  Anorexia
  Myoglobinemia
  Rhabdomyolysis
  Sweating

30 minutes. These symptoms may last for several hours and may include tachycardia, flushing, sweating, palpitations, and headache.[10] A significant overdose of amphetamines may cause dilated, reactive pupils, hyperpyrexia, profound anxiety, and seizures. Severe overdosage may be followed by cardiac dysrhythmias, delirium, hypertensive crisis, cerebral vascular accidents,[35] circulatory collapse, coma, and status epilepticus. Hyperthermia and disseminated intravascular coagulation have also been observed.[33] In addition, acute renal failure associated with rhabdomyolysis is a well-recognized entity secondary to amphetamine overdose.[36–38] Evidence of rhabdomyolysis and myoglobinuria usually consists of myalgia, muscle tenderness, myoedema, elevated creatinine phosphokinase concentrations, and myoglobinuria.[38] Ischemic chest pain has occurred and may be secondary to vasospasm.[33]

The intravenous injection of amphetamine produces a sudden "flash" or "rush" that is described as exhilarating; although transient, this experience is often the primary motive for parenteral abuse. The rush is followed by a persistent, invigorating sense of euphoria, clear thinking, gregariousness, self-confidence, excitement, and invulnerability.

Continued high-dose intravenous use induces mental disturbances such as confusion, delirium, and an acute psychosis that may be indistinguishable from schizophrenia. The individual may appear confused with disorganized behavior or may exhibit compulsive repetition of meaningless acts, such as picking at the bed sheets. The patient may become irritable, fearful, or suspicious of his or her surroundings and experience delusions and hallucinations. The hallucinations may be both visual and auditory. In addition to these findings, any of the complications of intravenous use discussed earlier may be noted (see Chapter 28).

Treatment

There is no specific antidote for amphetamine overdose, and most of the treatment is supportive (Table 31-10). Life-threatening overdoses are rare. If the drug has been ingested orally, then emesis or lavage and administration of activated charcoal and a cathartic should be performed. α-Adrenergic blocking agents can be lifesaving in patients with hypertensive crisis or for the hyperpyrexia associated with amphetamine toxicity.

It has been suggested that, because the rate of renal excretion of amphetamines is dependent on the pH of the urine and is more than doubled in the presence of an acid urine, the patient should be given agents that will acidify the urine.[39,40] This is discouraged, however, because if myoglobinuria is present acidifying the urine may favor the development of acute renal failure.[38] Aggressive extracellular volume repletion and attempts to avert acute renal failure, as well as prophylaxis against or treatment of acute hyperkalemia, should be instituted. For treatment of acute psychotic manifestations, haloperidol or phenothiazines are commonly used. Chlorpromazine is believed by some investigators to prolong the half-life of amphetamines, and thus haloperidol (2 to 5 mg intramuscularly) is the preferred drug for treating the acute psychotic reactions. Diazepam can be administered for seizures.

Table 31-10 Treatment of Amphetamine Overdose

Indication	Treatment
Oral ingestion	Emesis or lavage
	Activated charcoal and cathartic
	Sorbitol
Hypertensive crisis, hyperpyrexia	Phentolamine
	Urine acidification (not recommended)
Acute psychosis, agitation	Haloperidol (2 to 5 mg IM)
Seizures	Diazepam (5 to 15 mg IV)

Withdrawal

Although long-term use of amphetamines does not cause a true physiologic withdrawal, serious depression and suicidal ideation may occur and can be quite prolonged. After long-term high-dose use, abusers exhibit a profound depression, apathy, and fatigue. Many have a disturbed, restless, yet prolonged sleep, sometimes up to 20 hours a day.[33] There may also be a lingering impairment of perception and thought processes. This incapacitating tenseness, anxiety, and suicidal tendency may persist for weeks or months. Precautions against suicide should be enacted for patients withdrawing from amphetamines.

THE "LOOK-ALIKE" DRUGS

The "look-alike" drugs and "speed" are included in a recent but growing category of drugs of abuse.[32,41,42] Because many over-the-counter stimulants are inexpensive and less risky to sell than controlled substances, they are often sold singly or more commonly in combinations as speed or cocaine. The most common over-the-counter stimulants sold as look-alikes are phenylpropanolamine, ephedrine, caffeine, and pseudoephedrine. Phenylpropanolamine is also called norephedrine, and pseudoephedrine is an optical isomer of ephedrine.[43] These drugs may be in the form of tablets or capsules that resemble prescription drugs in shape, size, color, and markings, but they do not contain the same ingredients or have the same effectiveness. Phenylpropanolamine is found in more than 75 over-the-counter preparations for relief of colds, in anorectic preparations, in appetite control remedies, and in nasal decongestants.[41] It is the active ingredient in the plant *Catha edulis*, whose leaves are chewed to achieve an amphetamine-like effect. Phenylpropanolamine is a derivative of ephedrine.[43] Both these drugs are noncatecholamines, or indirectly-acting sympathomimetics structurally resembling the amphetamines.[44] Phenylpropanolamine and ephedrine act both peripherally and centrally because, unlike catecholamines, they readily cross the blood-brain barrier. Of the two, ephedrine has a more potent effect on the CNS.[32]

The most common look-alikes are copies of amphetamine compounds, but instead of containing amphetamine they contain 100 to 200 mg of caffeine, 25 to 30 mg of ephedrine, and 25 to 50 g of phenylpropanolamine (Table 31-11). Such preparations are currently considered legal and are available as diet aids or

Table 31-11 Selected Products Containing Phenylpropanolamine

Product Name	Phenylpropanolamine (milligrams)	Caffeine (milligrams)
Anorexin	25–50	100
Codexin	75	100
Dex-a-diet	75	
Dexatrim	50	200
Dietac	25–50	
EZ Trim	75	
PVM Appetite Control	25–75	
Prolamine	37.5	140
Super Odrinex	25	100

Source: Adapted with permission from *Annals of Emergency Medicine* (1982;11:483), Copyright © 1982, American College of Emergency Physicians.

"pick-me-ups" in pharmacies, grocery stores, and drug paraphernalia shops and can even be obtained by mail order.[32]

Uses

The look-alikes are capable of producing mood elevations and an altered state of consciousness, as is seen with amphetamines. Patients have a generalized feeling of well-being and experience anorexia (an effect that is much weaker than that induced by amphetamines and decreases with time), decreased fatigue, enhanced sensory perceptions, and improved motor skills.[32]

One of the problems associated with the look-alike drugs is that the margin of safety between therapeutic and toxic doses of these agents is small. This property exposes patients to potentially toxic amounts at single doses barely exceeding those found in a combination pill. The toxicity of the triple combination of phenylpropanolamine, ephedrine, and caffeine in abuse quantities may even be greater than the toxicity of amphetamines.[34] In addition, an inexperienced drug user may inadvertently overdose because of the mistaken idea that these drugs will not produce a "high" equivalent to that of amphetamines. Such a user may also wrongly assume that the look-alikes are safer, less potent substances and take several pills at a time, causing even greater toxicity.[41]

Mechanism of Action

Phenylpropanolamine has two modes of action: a direct α-adrenergic action and an indirect action by virtue of its ability to release norepinephrine from storage sites at nerve terminals.[44] There is also a weak β-adrenergic stimulatory component that may cause orthostatic hypotension.[43]

Pharmacokinetics

Absorption of oral phenylpropanolamine is rapid, with the maximal clinical effect occurring in 1 to 3 hours.[43] Phenylpropanolamine is a weak base and is eliminated most rapidly in an acid urine. Although the half-life is approximately 2 hours, clinical effects may last for a longer period.[44]

Toxicity

Phenylpropanolamine has a low therapeutic index, which means that there is not a great deal of difference between a therapeutic and a toxic dose. Life-threatening complications may therefore occur at approximately 3 times the over-the-counter dose.[43]

Central Nervous System Effects

Phenylpropanolamine is a less potent CNS stimulant than amphetamine. This can be dangerous if individuals attempt to simulate an amphetamine-like ''high'' and take more than a normal dose of phenylpropanolamine.[44] Intoxication can occur from both central and peripheral adrenergic stimulation. A higher than recommended dose can cause agitation, restlessness, altered sleep patterns, headache, disorientation, and confusion (Table 31-12). Grand mal seizures have also been reported in patients taking phenylpropanolamine together with caffeine.[43] Hemorrhagic and nonhemorrhagic stroke and transient ischemic neurologic deficit have been reported.

Table 31-12 Clinical Features of Intoxication from Look-Alike Drugs

Central nervous system
  Agitation
  Restlessness
  Headache
  Disorientation
  Confusion
  Intracerebral hemorrhage
  Seizures
  Altered sleep patterns
  Mania
  Psychosis
Cardiovascular
  Dysrhythmias
    Premature ventricular contractions
    Premature atrial contractions
    Ventricular tachycardia
    Paroxysmal atrial tachycardia
  Hypertension
  Postural hypotension
  Bradycardia
Miscellaneous
  Rhabdomyolysis
  Myoglobinemia
  Myoglobinuria

Cardiovascular Effects

Because phenylpropanolamine affects the adrenergic receptors and may produce cardiac dysrhythmias, premature ventricular contractions, premature atrial contractions, and atrial and ventricular tachycardia may be noted.[45] Because of the greater peripheral effect, hypertension (both systolic and diastolic) may be more pronounced than with amphetamines and may lead to hypertensive encephalopathy and intracerebral hemorrhage.[32,43] Occasionally, postural hypotension may be observed.[46] Reflex bradycardia has also occurred after phenylpropanolamine ingestion.[43]

Hypertensive crisis can result from even a single therapeutic dose of phenylpropanolamine. Intracerebral hemorrhage has occurred secondary to the severe hypertension. The hypertensive effect may be potentiated by various other drugs, including monoamine oxidase inhibitors, ephedrine, caffeine, anticholinergic drugs, antihistamines, and antihypertensive agents.

Electrocardiographic abnormalities have been reported with phenylpropanolamine and include ventricular dysrhythmias and repolarization abnormalities. Direct myocardial injuries associated with symptoms of chest pain with elevation of the MB fraction of creatine phosphokinase have been described.

Miscellaneous Effects

Renal failure with[41,47] or without[48,49] rhabdomyolysis and hypertension may occur with phenylpropanolamine overdose.

Laboratory Analysis

Qualitative identification of phenylpropanolamine in urine can be accomplished by using thin-layer chromatography or enzyme-modified immunoassay. These techniques may not be readily available, however. Therapeutic doses typically produce serum concentrations between 60 and 200 ng/mL.[43] Qualitative identification in the urine can also be performed.

Treatment

Treatment of patients with a suspected overdose of a look-alike drug (Table 31-13) should comprise immediate and frequent monitoring of the vital signs for possible life-threatening

Table 31-13 Treatment of Overdose Look-Alike Drugs

Indication	Treatment
Oral ingestion	Emesis or lavage
	Activated charcoal and cathartic
Seizures	Diazepam (5 to 15 mg IV)
Severe hypertension	Sodium nitroprusside (3 μg/kg/minute)
Ventricular dysrhythmias	Lidocaine (1 mg/kg followed by 1 to 4 μg/kg/minute)
	β-Adrenergic blocking drugs (use with caution)
Psychosis	Haloperidol (2 to 5 mg IM)

sequelae such as cardiac dysrhythmias and hypertensive crisis. Therapy with emesis or lavage, and activated charcoal and a cathartic should then be instituted.[44] Most episodes of hypertension subside within 3 to 4 hours without treatment or with the addition of a mild sedative such as a benzodiazepine. Hypertension should be treated if accompanied by signs or symptoms of myocardial ischemia or hypertensive encephalopathy[43]; sodium nitroprusside beginning at 3 μg/kg/minute and titrated according to effect is suggested.[43] If serious cardiac dysrhythmias are present, lidocaine should be administered. β-Adrenergic blocking drugs, although potentially useful for the tachydysrhythmias, may be harmful if the hypertension causes a vagal stimulation, which produces a reflex bradycardia that may be potentiated by the β-adrenergic blocking drug.[44] The psychosis, if not responsive to supportive care, can be managed with the use of haloperidol or diazepam. Seizures should be treated with intravenous diazepam.

Acidification of the urine accelerates clearance but entails additional risks such as precipitation of myoglobin in the kidneys with minimal clinical benefit. For this reason, acid diuresis is not suggested.[43] Dialysis and diuresis are not effective because of the large volume of distribution of these drugs.

PROPYLHEXEDRINE

This compound is the active ingredient in Benzedrex® inhalers and is extracted from the wicks of the inhalers by drug abusers for intravenous injection.[50] Compounds of this type are called "crank" or homemade speed. Propylhexedrine is a potent local vasoconstrictor with mild to moderate stimulatory effects on the CNS.[50]

CAFFEINE

Caffeine (1,3,7-trimethylxanthine) belongs to a group of methylated xanthines found in a variety of plants throughout the world. The closely related alkaloids theobromine and theophylline (1,3-dimethylxanthine) are other methylxanthines with similar properties.[51] Although each differs in its potency on a particular organ system, they share many pharmacologic effects. Aqueous extracts of these plants have for centuries formed the basis of a number of popular beverages, from the coffee bean in Arabia, the tea leaf in China, the kola nut in West Africa, to the cocoa bean in Mexico.[52]

Caffeine is widely consumed today in beverages such as coffee, tea, and cocoa. Coffee and tea have been the most popular beverages in Western society for several hundred years. Although the major source of caffeine on a weight-for-weight basis is tea, the highest dose per serving is found in coffee, which has approximately twice the amount of caffeine that is obtained from an equal amount of tea.[53] Caffeine is also an ingredient in chocolate as well as many over-the-counter analgesics, headache remedies, anorectic agents, and stimulants (Table 31-14). Soft drinks represent a major source of dietary caffeine, particularly for children.[53] Ingestion of caffeine, therefore, is common for therapeutic purposes or from consumption of various beverages. Naturopathic therapies such as caffeine enemas have been linked to deaths.[52,54]

Metabolism

Caffeine is absorbed rapidly after oral administration, and serum concentrations reach their peak in 30 to 60 minutes.[43,52,53] The presence or absence of food in the stomach does not influence the absorption of caffeine.[52] It is freely and equally distributed throughout the total body water and has a volume of distribution in adults of 0.5 L/kg.[43] Caffeine has a plasma half-life of 3 to 4 hours in adults.[44,52,54] It is metabolized in the liver to methyluric acid and methylxanthine, both of which are inactive and are excreted in the urine.[52] Caffeine is also metabolized to theophylline.[44]

Actions

Caffeine causes a translocation of intracellular calcium by increasing the permeability of calcium in the sarcoplasmic reticulum, which accounts for its action of increasing the contractility of skeletal and cardiac muscle. It also causes an increased accumulation of cyclic nucleotides, particularly cyclic AMP, by inhibiting the enzyme phosphodiesterase.[43,53,55] This enzyme is necessary for the degradation of cyclic AMP.[44] By inhibiting phosphodiesterase, the metabolic action of endogenous sympathomimetics is enhanced. Additionally, caffeine blocks adenosine receptors.[56,57] Adenosine acts as a neurotransmitter in purinergic neurons, which have diverse functions throughout the body.[53] Some actions of adenosine include dilation of blood vessels, slowing of the rate of cardiac pacemaker cells, and inhibition of the release of norepinephrine from autonomic nerve endings. Because caffeine antagonizes this effect, sympathomimetic effects occur.[53]

Caffeine is a potent releaser of epinephrine and to a lesser extent of norepinephrine from the adrenal medulla.[43,44,53] The cardiac toxic effects as well as the metabolic effects (hyperglycemia, ketosis, and metabolic acidosis) of caffeine are probably due to increasing circulating concentrations of epinephrine and norepinephrine. It has been shown that caffeine can be an effective bronchodilator, although its use is not recommended.

Several of the biochemical effects, such as phosphodiesterase inhibition, calcium mobilization, and prostaglandin antagonism, occur only at relatively high doses. At the doses encountered in foods and beverages, the probable mechanism is that of adenosine receptor antagonism.[43,53]

Table 31-14 Concentrations of Caffeine in Beverages and Pharmaceuticals

Product	Average Caffeine Content per Dose (milligrams)
Coffee	100–150
Tea	40–60
Cocoa	10–40
Carbonated drinks	35–65
Chocolate	25
Headache remedies	50–75
Anorectic agents	100–200
Cold preparations	30–75
Stimulants	75–200

Toxicity

Caffeine is a widely abused drug that is often overlooked as a cause of acute reactions. Caffeine has a wider therapeutic index than theophylline, resulting in a lower incidence of toxicity.[52] The xanthine derivatives stimulate the CNS, produce a mild diuresis, stimulate cardiac muscle, and relax smooth muscle (notably bronchial muscle) (Table 31-15). Considering the widespread consumption of caffeine in drinks and over-the-counter medicines, relatively few cases of acute serious caffeine poisoning have been reported. Nevertheless, death has been reported from oral,[58] rectal, and parenteral administration of caffeine.[59]

Although serious methylxanthine poisoning is much more often the result of theophylline intoxication than caffeine intoxication, the clinical presentation is similar.

Central Nervous System Effects

The primary effect of caffeine is CNS stimulation.[53] The cerebral cortex is particularly sensitive to the effects of caffeine, and small doses result in increased alertness, a more rapid and clear thought flow, decreased drowsiness, and improvement of psychomotor coordination. These effects are milder and of shorter duration than those of amphetamines. Larger doses may produce headache, tremors,[60] nervousness, muscle twitching, insomnia,[61] tachypnea, and irritability, which may be indistinguishable from anxiety neurosis. Transient psychosis and delirium have also been reported.[62]

Cardiovascular Effects

The positive inotropic effect on the myocardium and the positive chronotropic effect at the sinoatrial node may produce palpitations, extrasystoles, sinus or supraventricular tachycardia, and other more major ventricular dysrhythmias such as premature ventricular contractions and bigeminy. Death, although very rare, results from respiratory failure or cardiac arrest. Hypotension and circulatory failure is a late and often terminal complication of massive caffeine overdose. Severe pulmonary edema also appears to be a consistent feature of acute caffeine poisoning.[52]

Recurrent emesis and abdominal pain are characteristic features of caffeine ingested in pill form, which may eliminate a substantial portion of the dose. High doses of caffeine can produce vagal, vasomotor, and respiratory center stimulation causing bradycardia, vasoconstriction, tachypnea, and tonic-clonic seizures.

Laboratory Analysis

Because caffeine and theophylline are both methylxanthines and because caffeine decreases the hepatic clearance of theophylline, serum concentrations of theophylline should be measured when large changes in caffeine intake are to be expected. In addition, theophylline is a known metabolite of caffeine but in typical doses is present in extremely low concentrations.[63,64] Caffeine can be confirmed by either thin-layer or gas chromatography.[52]

Treatment

Treatment of an acute overdose of caffeine usually is limited to support and abstention from the caffeine-containing substance because there is no specific antidote for caffeine. Emesis or

---

Table 31-15 Clinical Features of Caffeine Intoxication

Central nervous system
  Increased alertness
  Decreased drowsiness
  Increased psychomotor coordination
  Headache
  Tremors
  Nervousness
  Muscle twitching
  Transient psychosis
  Delirium
Cardiovascular
  Palpitations
  Extrasystoles
  Supraventricular tachycardia
  Premature ventricular contractions
  Bigeminy
  Pulmonary edema

lavage or administration of activated charcoal and a cathartic should be performed in the acute overdose of caffeine tablets.[44] Seizures should be controlled with a benzodiazepine such as diazepam.[52] Although it may seem to be logical to use a β-adrenergic blocking drug to reverse the manifestations of the hyperadrenergic syndrome, an unopposed α-adrenergic effect may result.[44] For this reason, α-adrenergic blockers may be necessary in the presence of a β-adrenergic blocking drug. Administration of lidocaine or phenytoin is recommended for treatment of cardiac dysrhythmias.[52] In addition, the administration of antacids to neutralize gastrointestinal irritation may be effective.

Withdrawal

Evidence suggests that habituation to caffeine may occur at relatively low dosages that are easily obtained by both children and adults. The withdrawal in some respects may resemble caffeine overdose and consist of headaches, irritation, nervousness, anxiety, nausea, rhinorrhea, dizziness, and mild depression.[53] In addition, there may be an inability to work effectively. The headache is a clinically recognizable syndrome known as caffeine withdrawal headache, which responds to caffeine therapy. Withdrawal may persist for up to 1 week but usually requires no specific treatment.

REFERENCES

1. Cregler L, Mark H: Medical complications of cocaine abuse. *N Engl J Med* 1986;315:1495–1500.

2. Suarez C, Arrango A, Lester L: Cocaine-condom ingestion: Surgical treatment. *JAMA* 1977;238:1391–1392.

3. Dipalma J: Cocaine abuse and toxicity. *Am Fam Physician* 1981;24:236–238.

4. Dargon D: Cocaine. *Top Emerg Med* 1985;7:1–8.

5. Resnick R, Resnick E: Cocaine abuse and its treatment. *Psychiatr Clin North Am* 1984;7:713–728.

6. Cohen S: Cocaine. *JAMA* 1975;231:74–75.

7. Cohen S: Amphetamine abuse. *JAMA* 1975;231:414–415.

8. Gay G: You've come a long way, baby! Coke time for the new American lady of the eighties. *J Psychoactive Drugs* 1981;13:297–318.

9. Gay G, Inaba D, Rappolt R, et al: "An' Ho, Ho, Baby, Take a Whiff on Me": La dama blanca cocaine in current perspective. *Anaesth Analg* 1976;55:582–587.

10. Van Dyke C, Byck R: Cocaine. *Sci Am* 1982;246:128–141.

11. Fairbanks D, Fairbanks G: *Ann Plast Surg* 1983;10:452–457.

12. Gay G: Clinical management of acute and chronic cocaine poisoning. *Ann Emerg Med* 1982;11:562–572.

13. Isenberg S, Spierer A, Inkelis S: Ocular signs of cocaine intoxication in neonates. *Am J Ophthalmol* 1987;103:211–214.

14. Cregler L, Mark H: Relation of acute myocardial infarction to cocaine abuse. *Am J Cardiol* 1985;56:794.

15. Gay G, Inaba D, Sheppard C, et al: Cocaine: History, epidemiology, human pharmacology, and treatment: A perspective on a new debut for an old girl. *Clin Toxicol* 1975;8:149–178.

16. Merigan K, Roberts J: Cocaine intoxication: Hyperpyrexia, rhabdomyolysis and acute renal failure. *Clin Toxicol* 1987;25:135–148.

17. Perez-Reyes M, DiGuiseppi S, Ondrusek G, et al: Free-base cocaine smoking. *Clin Pharmacol Ther* 1982;32:459–465.

18. Mathias D: Cocaine-associated myocardial ischemia. *Am J Med* 1986;81:675–678.

19. Shesser R, Davis C, Edelstein S: Pneumomediastinum and pneumothorax after inhaling alkaloidal cocaine. *Ann Emerg Med* 1981;10:213–315.

20. Allred R, Ewer S: Fatal pulmonary edema after intravenous "freebase" cocaine use. *Ann Emerg Med* 1981;10:441–442.

21. Siegel R: Cocaine hallucinations. *Am J Psychiatr* 1978;135:309–314.

22. Siegel R: Treatment of cocaine abuse: Historical and contemporary perspectives. *J Psychoactive Drugs* 1985;17:1–9.

23. McCarron M, Wood J: The cocaine "Body Packer" syndrome: Diagnosis and treatment. *JAMA* 1983;250:1417–1420.

24. Wetli C, Wright R: Death caused by recreational cocaine use. *JAMA* 1979;241:2519–2522.

25. Bettinger J, Cocaine intoxication: Massive oral overdose. *Ann Emerg Med* 1980;9:429–430.

26. Mittleman R, Weltli C: Death caused by recreational cocaine use. *JAMA* 1984;252:1889–1893.

27. Lundberg G, Garriott J, Reynolds P, et al: Cocaine-related death. *J Forensic Sci* 1977;22:402–408.

28. Isner J, Estes N, Thompson P, et al: Acute cardiac events temporally related to cocaine abuse. *N Engl J Med* 1986;315:1438–1443.

29. Bozarth M, Wise R: Toxicity associated with long-term intravenous heroin and cocaine self-administration in the rat. *JAMA* 1985;254:81–83.

30. Pollin W: The danger of cocaine. *JAMA* 1985;254:98.

31. Dusenberry S, Hicks M, Mariani P: Labetalol treatment of cocaine toxicity. *Ann Emerg Med* 1987;16:142.

32. King P, Coleman J: Stimulants and narcotic drugs. *Pediatr Clin North Am* 1987;34:349–362.

33. Linden C, Kulig K, Rumack B: Amphetamines. *Top Emerg Med* 1985;7:18–32.

34. King J: Hypertension and cerebral hemorrhage after Trimolets ingestion. *Med J Aust* 1979;2:258–259.

35. Goodman S, Becker D: Intracranial hemorrhage associated with amphetamine abuse. *JAMA* 1970;212:480–482.

36. Citron B, Halpern M, McCarron M, et al: Necrotizing angiitis associated with drug abuse. *N Engl J Med* 1970;283:1003–1011.

37. Ginsberg M, Hartzman M, Schmidt-Nowara W: Amphetamine intoxication with coagulopathy, hyperthermia, and reversible renal failure. *Ann Intern Med* 1970;73:81–85.

38. Scanling J, Spital A: Amphetamine-associated myoglobinuric renal failure. *South Med J* 1982;75:237–240.

39. Fann W: Some clinically important interactions of psychotropic drugs. *South Med J* 1973;66:661–665.

40. Lockett S: Poisoning by salicylates, paracetamol, tricyclic antidepressants, and a miscellany of drugs. *Practitioner* 1973;211:105–112.

41. Bernstein E, Diskant B: Phenylpropanolamine: A potentially hazardous drug. *Ann Emerg Med* 1982;11: 311–315.

42. Dietz A: Amphetamine-like reactions to phenylpropanolamine. *JAMA* 1981;245:601–602.

43. Pentel P: Toxicity of over-the-counter stimulants. *JAMA* 1984;252:1898–1903.

44. Bayer M, Maskell L: Abuse and toxicity of over-the-counter stimulants. *Emerg Med Rep* 1983;4:127–132.

45. Peterson R, Vasquez L: Phenylpropanolamine-induced ventricular arrhythmias. *JAMA* 1973;223:324–326.

46. Sawyer D, Conner C, Rumack B: Managing acute toxicity from nonprescription stimulants. *Drug Intell Clin Pharmacol* 1982;1:529–533.

47. Swenson R, Golper T, Bennett W: Acute renal failure and rhabdomyolysis after ingestion of phenylpropanolamine-containing diet pills. *JAMA* 1982;248:1216.

48. Horowitz J, Lang W, Howes L, et al: Hypertensive responses induced by phenylpropanolamine in anorectic and decongestant preparation. *Lancet* 1980;1:60–61.

49. Norvenius G, Widerlov E, Lonnerholm G: Phenylpropanolamine and mental disturbance. *Lancet* 1979;2:1367–1368.

50. Mancusi-Ungaro H, Decker W: Tissue injuries associated with parenteral propylhexedrine abuse. *Clin Toxicol* 1983;21:359–372.

51. Zimmerman P, Pulliam J, Schwengels J, et al: Caffeine intoxication: A near fatality. *Ann Emerg Med* 1985;14:1227–1229.

52. Dalvi R: Acute and chronic toxicity of caffeine: A review. 1986;28:144–150.

53. Abbott P: Caffeine: A toxicological overview. *Med J Aust* 1986;145:518–521.

54. Jarboe C, Hurst H, Rodgers G, et al: Toxicokinetics of caffeine elimination in an infant. *Clin Toxicol* 1986;24: 415–428.

55. Kramer G, Wells J: Effects of phosphodiesterase inhibitors on cyclic nucleotide levels and relaxation of pig coronary arteries. *Molec Pharmacol* 1979;16:813–822.

56. Daly J, Bruns R, Snyder S: Adenosine receptors in the central nervous system: Relationship to the central actions of methylxanthines. *Life Sci* 1981;28:2083–2097.

57. Fredholm B: Are methylxanthine effects due to antagonism of endogenous adenosine? *Trends Pharmacol Sci* 1980;1:29–132.

58. McGee M: Caffeine poisoning in a 19-year-old female. *J Forensic Sci* 1980;25:29–32.

59. Jokela S, Vartianen A: Caffeine poisoning. *Acta Pharmacol Toxicol* 1959;15:331–334.

60. Reimann H: Caffeinism: A cause of long continued low-grade fever. *JAMA* 1967;202:1105–1106.

61. Silver W: Insomnia, tachycardia and cola drinks. *Pediatrics* 1971;47:635.

62. McManamy M, Purcell S: Caffeine intoxication: A report of a case the symptoms of which amounted to a psychosis. *N Engl J Med* 1966;215:616–620.

63. Benowitz N, Osterloh J, Goldschlager N, et al: Massive catecholamine release from caffeine poisoning. *JAMA* 1982;248:1097–1098.

64. Sved S, Hossie R, McGilveray I: The human metabolism of caffeine to theophylline. *Res Commun Chem Pathol Pharmacol* 1976;13:185–192.

ADDITIONAL SELECTED REFERENCES

Alsott R, Miller A, Forney R: Report of a human fatality due to caffeine. *J Forensic Sci* 1973;18:135–137.

Anderson R, Reed W, Hillis L, et al: History, epidemiology, and medical complications of nasal inhaler abuse. *J Toxicol Clin Toxicol* 1982;19:95–107.

Baldessarini RI: Symposium on behavior modification by drugs: pharmacology of the amphetamines. *Pediatrics* 1972;49:694–701.

Becker A, Simons K, Gillespie C, et al: The bronchodilator effects and pharmacokinetics of caffeine in asthma. *N Engl J Med* 1984;310:743–746.

Benchimol A, Bartall H, Desser K: Accelerated ventricular rhythm and cocaine abuse. *Ann Intern Med* 1978;88: 519–520.

Bennett W: Hazards of the appetite suppressant phenylpropanolamine. *Lancet* 1979;2:42–43.

Blum A: Phenylpropanolamine: An over-the-counter amphetamine?, editorial. *JAMA* 1981;245:1346–1347.

Caruana D, Weinbach B, Goerg D, et al: Cocaine-packet ingestion. *Ann Intern Med* 1984;100:73–74.

Chambers H, Morris L, Tauber M, et al: Cocaine use and the risk for endocarditis in intravenous drug users. *Ann Intern Med* 1987;106:833–836.

Curatolo P, Robertson D: The health consequences of caffeine. *Ann Intern Med* 1983;98:641–653.

Duffy W, Senekjian H, Knight T, et al: Acute renal failure due to phenylpropanolamine. *South Med J* 1981;74:1548.

Edison G: Amphetamines: A dangerous illusion. *Ann Intern Med* 1971;74:605–610.

Egan D, Robinson D: Cocaine: Recreational drug of choice? *Rocky Mt Med J* 1978;75:34–36.

Eisele J, Reay D: Deaths related to coffee enemas. *JAMA* 1980;244:1608–1609.

Escobar J, Karno M: Chronic hallucinosis from nasal drops. *JAMA* 1982;247:1859–1862.

Fishbain D, Wetli C: Cocaine intoxication, delirium, and death in a body packer. *Ann Emerg Med* 1981;10: 531–532.

Foley R, Kapatkin K, Verani R, et al: Amphetamine-induced acute renal failure. *South Med J* 1984;77: 258–259.

Gary N, Saidi P: Methamphetamine intoxication. *Am J Med* 1977;64:537–540.

Haddad L: 1978: Cocaine in perspective. *JACEP* 1979;8:374–376.

Harrington H, Heller A, Kawson D, et al: Intracerebral hemorrhage and oral amphetamine. *Arch Neurol* 1983;40:503–507.

Insley B, Grufferman S, Ayliffe E: Thallium poisoning in cocaine abusers. *Am J Emerg Med* 1986;4:545–548.

Jekel J, Podlewski H, Dean-Patterson S, et al: Epidemic free-base cocaine abuse. *Lancet* 1986;1:459–462.

Josephson G, Stine R: Caffeine intoxication: A case of paroxysmal atrial tachycardia. *JACEP* 1976;5:776–778.

Koff R, Widrich W, Robbins A: Necrotizing angiitis in a methamphetamine user with hepatitis B: Angiographic diagnosis, five-month follow-up results and localization of bleeding site. *N Engl J Med* 1973;288:946–947.

Leikin J, Zell M, Hyrhorczuk K: PCP or cocaine intoxication. *Ann Emerg Med* 1987;16:235–236.

Madden J, Payne T, Miller S: Maternal cocaine abuse and effect on the newborn. *Pediatrics* 1986;77:209–211.

May D, Long R, Madden R, et al: Caffeine toxicity secondary to street drug ingestion. *Ann Emerg Med* 1981;10: 549.

Patel R, Dutta D, Schonfeld S: Free-base cocaine use associated with bronchiolitis obliterans organizing pneumonia. *Ann Intern Med* 1987;107:186–188.

Perry D: Heroin and cocaine adulteration, editorial. *Clin Toxicol* 1975;8:239–243.

Post R, Kopanda R: Cocaine, kindling, and psychosis. *Am J Psychiatr* 1976;133:627–640.

Rumack B: Phenylpropanolamine: A potentially hazardous drug, editorial. *Ann Emerg Med* 1982;11:332.

Schatzman M, Sabbadini A, Forti L: Coca and cocaine: A bibliography. *J Psychedelic Drugs* 1976;8:95–128.

Schenck N: The case for cocaine. *Res Staff Physician* 1975;21:67–69.

Scott M, Mullally R: Lithium therapy for cocaine-induced psychosis: A clinical perspective. *South Med J* 1981;74:1475–1477.

Silverstein W, Lewin N, Goldfrank L: Management of the cocaine-intoxicated patient. *Ann Emerg Med* 1987;16:234–235.

Warner A, Pierozynski G: Pseudocatatonia associated with abuse of amphetamine and cannabis. *Postgrad Med* 1977;61:275–276.

Weiss S, Raskind R, Morganstein N, et al: Intracerebral and subarachnoid hemorrhage following use of methamphetamine ("speed"). *Int Surg* 1970;53:123–127.

Wetli C, Mettleman R: The body packer syndrome: Toxicity following ingestion of illicit drugs packaged for transportation. *J Forensic Sci* 1981;26:492–500.

Winek C, Eastly T: Cocaine identification. *Clin Toxicol* 1979;8:205–210.

chapter 32

Phencyclidine

Phencyclidine (phenylcyclohexylpiperidine, PCP) is chemically related to the phenothiazines and consists of a benzene ring, a cyclohexyl ring, and a piperidine ring.[1] Phencyclidine is a synthetic drug and one of a large family of arylcyclohexylamines developed more than 20 years ago as possible anesthetic agents with structures different from those of other psychomimetic drugs and neurotransmitters.[2,3] More than 30 phencyclidine analogs have been developed through minor modifications of the manufacturing process. Many investigators have attempted to classify PCP, and although it is sometimes classified as an atypical hallucinogen it appears to fall into a class of its own. It produces both CNS stimulation and depression, hallucinations, analgesia, and cholinergic-like symptoms along with many other effects.

Phencyclidine was developed for use in humans for general anesthesia and as a short-acting analgesic under the trade name Sernyl®.[4–7] Because of postoperative side effects, however, such as postanesthetic excitement, visual disturbances, and delirium, the drug was withdrawn for human use.[2] Its use continued as a veterinary anesthetic under the trade name Sernylan®, but this was also withdrawn from the market. Since 1978, all legal manufacture and sale has been stopped, and PCP is now classified as a Schedule II controlled substance. Federal reporting of the sale of piperidine, which is necessary for the synthesis of PCP, became mandatory in 1978.

Phencyclidine is structurally similar to ketamine and was first seen as a street drug in San Francisco in 1967, as the *Peace Pill*. It is misrepresented as many other drugs of abuse, such as tetrahydrocannabinol (THC), cannabinol, cocaine, mescaline, psilocybin, peyote, and LSD. It has since replaced other drugs as the most readily available street drug and is difficult to control, probably because it is simple and inexpensive to make. Early in its history PCP developed a negative reputation among the drug-using community, but it no longer carries such a stigma because it is more of an accepted drug of abuse. Today, there are a great many analogues of phencyclidine available on the street.

ACTIONS

Phencyclidine appears to alter the association pathways in the brain, which then interferes with the ability to process and react appropriately to sensory stimuli.[3] PCP is believed to affect multiple neurotransmitter receptors in the brain. Evidence suggests involvement of the noradrenergic, dopaminergic, cholinergic, γ-aminobutyric acid, and serotonergic systems as well as the opiate receptors and the endorphins.[3,8] Because PCP affects so many neurotransmitters, the clinical picture of intoxication can vary greatly.[9]

Phencyclidine is an analgesic with local anesthetic properties that are twice as effective as those of procaine and half as potent as those of cocaine (Table 32-1). In addition, PCP appears to have sympathomimetic activity, causing both CNS stimulation and depression.[10] Although an anticholinergic action may explain many of the manifestations that appear to be adrenergic, there are, in addition, many cholinergic-like effects seen with the drug. PCP also appears both to stimulate and to block the dopaminergic receptors in the brain to cause marked psychomimetic actions.[10]

PHARMACOKINETICS

Absorption

Phencyclidine can be absorbed from most routes. Although it can be ingested orally in the form of tablets, this is rarely seen in the sophisticated drug user. Oral ingestion may be employed, however, in a suicide attempt. Smoking of a ''joint'' is the usual route. The user may sprinkle powdered PCP (''Angel Dust'') on dried parsley, mint, or low-grade marijuana and smoke it, thus allowing maximum control over the dose ingested. Rarely has the intravenous administration of PCP been attempted. In addition, leaf mixtures, rock crystals, and capsules containing the crystalline or granular powder are used, or the user may insufflate the powder.

Phencyclidine enters the bloodstream rapidly by all routes and, because it is highly lipid soluble, quickly distributes to tissues with a high lipid content. Also, because it is a basic compound, it achieves high concentrations in body compartments that have an acidic pH, such as the cerebrospinal fluid and gastric secretions.[3]

Onset of Action

The effects of PCP are noted immediately with parenteral administration. If smoked, effects may begin as early as 2 to 5 minutes. The onset of symptoms with oral administration occurs within 15 minutes. Although the ''high'' may last 4 to 6 hours, the user generally requires 24 to 48 hours to return to a normal state. This is thought to be attributable to some binding of the drug in the CNS[10] as well as to enterohepatic circulation of the drug. In the stomach PCP is in a substantially ionized form because the pKa of the stomach is 8.5.[3] Because it is not very lipid soluble in the stomach, there is little absorption from that area. Most of the drug is absorbed in the alkaline small intestine. The compound undergoes enterogastric reabsorption, whereby it is secreted back into the stomach from the systemic circulation and is then reabsorbed as it proceeds into the more alkaline portions of the intestinal tract. This recirculation may account for the drug's prolonged systemic course and the fact that it continues to be excreted in the urine for several days.

Metabolism

The drug is rapidly metabolized to hydroxylated and glucuronidyl metabolites, which are then excreted in the urine. There is little pharmacologic activity of these metabolites.

TOXICITY

Effects of PCP can be divided into five areas: (1) behavioral, (2) neurologic, (3) cardiovascular, (4) renal, and (5) gastrointestinal. PCP may act as a depressant, a stimulant, or a hallucinogen depending on such variables as route of administration and dosage. Because of this, it is difficult to predict the clinical effects of the drug.[10] Patients may display rapid and unpredictable fluctuations in their clinical state

---

Table 32-1 Actions of Phencyclidine

Analgesic
Local anesthetic
Sympathomimetic
Anticholinergic
Cholinergic
Dopaminergic
Antidopaminergic

of intoxication. Low-dose intoxications may become behavioral emergencies but rarely represent a true medical emergency.

Behavioral Effects

Phencyclidine can cause behavioral changes secondary to either CNS stimulation or depression and may vary markedly depending on individual factors as well as the dose. The risk of dysphoric reactions from PCP may be increased in the presence of previous underlying psychiatric illness (Table 32-2).[9,11]

The behavioral effects at low doses may include euphoria, a pleasurable "high," amnesia, anxiety, agitation, a disordered thought process, and hallucinations. Many times users experience a sense of strength. Although frank hallucinations are not common, illusions or delusions are common. The dissociation of somatic perception, and therefore the lack of experienced pain, leads to illusions of superhuman strength, power, and invulnerability. Most deaths result from aberrant behavior rather from the drug itself.

Phencyclidine is unique in that it may produce a psychosis indistinguishable from schizophrenia. Many similarities exist between the hyperdopaminergic state of schizophrenia and intoxication with PCP. Depersonalization and distortions of body image and perceptions of all sensory modes are the psychological effects most frequently reported. Users describe a sense of distance and estrangement from their surroundings. Time seems to expand, and body movements seem to be slowed. Users report that feelings of immobility, numbness, and detachment are among the desired effects of the drug. Individuals may have fluctuating levels of consciousness, in which at one moment they are mute and at the next propelled into action. This action can take the form of agitated pacing, unprovoked aggression, or loss of impulse control. Other individuals feel paralyzed, off-balance, or restrained. Still others may seem to be catatonic, and although they appear to be awake, with eyes open in a blank stare, they have no response to any external stimuli and may be unable to speak. Catatonic patients characteristically display catalepsy, posturing, mutism, rigidity, staring, and negativism.

Neurologic Effects

The neurological manifestations of PCP intoxication result from cerebellar dysfunction and may include dizziness, ataxia, slurred speech, dysarthria, and nystagmus (Table 32-3). The nystagmus, which is commonly seen, is first horizontal and then vertical or rotatory and can occur at low or moderate doses.[12] It is first noted only with appropriate stimuli but later may occur spontaneously. The nystagmus has irregular burstlike features and can be helpful in establishing a definitive diag-

Table 32-2 Behavioral Effects of Phencyclidine

Euphoria
Amnesia
Body image distortion
Feeling of dissociation
Anxiety
Agitation
Depersonalization
Disordered thought process
Hallucinations
Feeling of superhuman strength
Psychosis
Catatonia
Blank stare

Table 32-3 Neurologic Manifestations of Phencyclidine Intoxication

Dizziness
Ataxia
Slurred speech
Dysarthria
Nystagmus
Miosis
Lack of experienced pain
Decreased proprioception
Tremors
Muscle weakness
Coma
Muscle rigidity
Seizures

nosis.[13,14] Miotic pupils are typically seen, although the pupil size can be variable.[10] In addition, blurred vision, decreased pain perception, decreased proprioception, and unusual temperature response are attributable to the anesthetic action of the drug. Tremors, muscle weakness, slurred speech, drowsiness, salivation, and drooling may also be noted. High-dose intoxication may cause coma or generalized intense muscle rigidity. Intracranial hemorrhage associated with PCP abuse has also been reported.[15] Opisthotonic or decerebrate posturing may be present along with myoclonus and generalized tonic-clonic seizures, which can progress to status epilepticus.[10]

Cardiovascular Effects

The cardiovascular manifestations of PCP intoxication (Table 32-4) may include tachycardia and hypertension. Although the blood pressure elevation can be significant, it usually is mild and transitory and does not lead to serious consequences.[10] Ordinarily, hypertension occurs in the early phases of intoxication (especially when the patient is hypertonic) or as a dopaminergic crisis in the recovery phase. On occasion, accelerated hypertension may result in serious complications, including intracerebral hemorrhage and other cerebrovascular accidents; careful monitoring of the vital signs is therefore essential. Tachyphylaxis to the pressor

---

Table 32-4 Cardiovascular, Renal, and Gastrointestinal Manifestations of Phencyclidine Intoxication

---

Cardiovascular
  Tachycardia
  Hypertension
Renal
  Antidiuresis
  Rhabdomyolysis
Gastrointestinal
  Nausea
  Vomiting
  Salivation
  Drooling
  Abdominal pain
  Hematemesis

---

effects of PCP develops rapidly, and hypertension is not of major consequence in the long-term PCP user.

Renal Effects

One of the major renal consequences of PCP intoxication is myoglobinuria leading to acute tubular necrosis (Table 32-4).[16] The mechanism for muscle injury is thought to be related to a number of factors, including increased and excessive isometric muscle activity and the generalized hypertonicity associated with the severe agitation or as a result of grand mal seizures. There is no evidence that PCP has a direct toxic effect on skeletal muscle.[17] If significant rhabdomyolysis has occurred, myoglobinuria may be present and lead to acute renal failure.

The mechanism of acute renal failure in acute rhabdomyolysis is not clearly understood, and several mechanisms have been suggested.[18,19] Tubular obstruction by myoglobin casts, passive back-diffusion of glomerular filtration through damaged tubular epithelial cells, myoglobin nephrotoxicity, renal ischemia, and a decreased glomerular permeability have all been implicated.[19] Urinary acidification enhances myoglobin and uric acid precipitation in the renal tubules, which could increase the likelihood of acute renal failure.[18] An elevation of the serum uric acid concentration above the normal range and a moderate increase in the serum creatine kinase concentration are indicative of rhabdomyolysis,[19] although these changes may occur without an elevation in serum creatine concentration. A positive urine dipstick test for blood, with no red blood cells on the microscopic examination of the urine, may indicate myoglobinuria secondary to rhabdomyolysis.

Gastrointestinal Effects

Gastrointestinal manifestations of PCP intoxication may include nausea, vomiting, salivation, and drooling (Table 32-4). Abdominal cramps and hematemesis, seen in users of illicit preparations of PCP, may be secondary to the by-products produced during the synthesis of the drug.

Major Complications

Major complications of PCP intoxication include respiratory depression and apnea (which can occur abruptly), seizures and status epilepticus,[20] intracerebral hemorrhage,[21] hypertensive encephalopathy,[10] rhabdomyolysis and myoglobinuria with renal failure, hyperpyrexia, psychosis, adrenergic crisis, laryngospasm, and cardiac arrest (Table 32-5). Trauma injuries are a large part of the major problems associated with PCP abuse. Unrecognized and painless self-injury, automobile accidents, violent behavior, falls, and drowning, sometimes in very shallow water,[9] are associated with PCP overdose. The injuries are due to the anesthetic action of the drug coupled with the user's overconfidence, disorientation, and ataxia and the muscle rigidity, prolonged reaction time, and sensory aberrations induced by the drug.

In the low-dose range, deaths are usually attributable to behavioral disturbances and result from impaired perception or delusional beliefs in addition to the marked tendency that the user has toward violence. In the high-dose range, deaths may be secondary to the physiological changes from sympathetic hyperstimulation.

LABORATORY ANALYSIS

Although a tentative diagnosis of PCP intoxication can be made on clinical grounds, confirmation requires a positive assay of urine, blood, or gastric contents. For the most part, quantitatively measured PCP concentrations do not provide clinically useful information beyond what could be obtained from a qualitative screen. PCP can be rapidly and inexpensively identified by thin-layer chromatography, but gas chromatography with mass spectroscopy and ultraviolet detection have also been used successfully. Gas chromatography with nitrogen detection is a sensitive but time-consuming technique. Gas chromatography with flame ionization is less sensitive and may yield a negative result even when PCP is identified by other means. The enzyme multiplied immunoassay is a rapid and sensitive technique. Analysis of serum for PCP may be misleading, however, because blood concentrations may be unmeasurable several hours after exposure[1] whereas the urine may still be positive.

TREATMENT

In the emergency department various functions should be monitored (Table 32-6), including the respiratory rate and depth (because of acute apnea), blood pressure (because of hypertension or hypotension), muscle tone (because of rhabdomyolysis), renal function (because of acute renal failure secondary to rhabdomyolysis), and temperature (because of hyperthermia).

There is no agent known that is specific in antagonizing the toxic effects of PCP, so that the treatment for intoxicated patients is primarily supportive medical and psychiatric care (Table 32-7).[22] Routine emesis and gastric lavage are not generally necessary because the drug is usually not ingested. Nevertheless if there is any question about the amount taken or, more

---

Table 32-5 Major Complications of Phencyclidine Intoxication

Respiratory depression and apnea
Seizures and status epilepticus
Intracerebral hemorrhage
Hypertensive encephalopathy
Rhabdomyolysis and renal failure
Hyperpyrexia
Psychosis
Adrenergic crisis
Laryngospasm
Cardiac arrest
Trauma

Table 32-6 Physiologic Functions To Monitor in Phencyclidine Overdose

Respiratory rate and depth
Blood pressure
Muscle tone
Renal function
Cardiac monitor
Psychiatric condition

Table 32-7 Treatment of Phencyclidine Overdose

Indication	Treatment
Oral ingestion, multiple drugs	Emesis or lavage
Seizures, muscle spasticity, opisthotonus	Diazepam
Psychosis, severe agitation	Haloperidol (2 to 5 mg IV)

important, about the concomitant ingestion of other drugs, then the stomach should be emptied and activated charcoal and a cathartic administered. Sensory isolation with frequent monitoring and avoidance of unnecessary instrumentation is best for the mildly intoxicated patient.

Control of the Airway

Intubation with ventilatory assistance may be required, possibly for an extended period, because of the prolonged and delayed hypoventilation and apnea that may occur with PCP intoxication. These effects usually occur only at high doses. Intubation, if required, may be difficult because of the increased muscle rigidity. Because laryngeal reflexes are maintained, attempted endotracheal intubation may precipitate laryngospasm. In some cases it has been necessary to use a neuromuscular blocking agent for successful endotracheal intubation.

Nasogastric Suction

Attempts to increase elimination may include intermittent nasogastric suction. As mentioned before, because PCP is a weak base, it is highly ionized in the acid medium of the stomach. Ionized drugs do not pass through biological membranes, so that PCP is not well absorbed in the stomach. If nasogastric suction is used, drug that is secreted back into the stomach from the small intestine is removed before it returns to the small intestine.[10,23] Multiple-dose activated charcoal has also been advocated because it can adsorb any compound secreted into the stomach and be removed by nasogastric suction.

Although these methods may be effective, the potential benefit must be weighed against the risk of the procedure in an uncooperative patient predisposed to rhabdomyolysis. Many investigators hold that the risks of these procedures in this group of patients outweigh the potential benefit.

Control of Seizure Activity

Small doses of diazepam can be administered slowly to control muscle spasticity, opisthotonus, and seizures unless there is an associated closed head injury. Diazepam can be followed by intravenous phenytoin for seizure prophylaxis. The use of barbiturates is not recommended because a synergistic depressant effect may occur. If seizures are persistent, then consideration should be given to the use of a neuromuscular blocking agent and institution of mechanical respiratory support. Although seizures are rare, they should be treated immediately to decrease the risk of rhabdomyolysis.[3]

Acidification of Urine

Urinary elimination of PCP is significantly dependent on urinary pH, and measures aimed at lowering the pH of the urine have been recommended to facilitate excretion of the drug. Although acidification of the urine has been shown to increase excretion,[23] it is not recommended because of the possibility of decreased myoglobin excretion and the development of acute tubular necrosis.[3] Moreover, by reducing uric acid solubility an acid urine may predispose the patient to the development of acute uric acid nephropathy.

Control of Hypertension

Hypertension is not often severe enough to require treatment, but blood pressure monitoring is vital. If treatment is required, nifedipine or nitroprusside is suggested for severe or malignant hypertension. A β blocker may be administered if the adrenergic crisis is severe.

Control of the Violent Patient

Violent and combative patients must be protected from injuring themselves and others. "Talk down" therapy, which may be effective for other drugs, not only is ineffective for PCP but may aggravate the patient's condition.[24] Initially, these patients should be restrained. Physical restraints should be soft in order not to traumatize the patient further. Physical restraints should be used for the shortest possible period of time because they intensify isometric muscle tension, which directly correlates with muscle toxicity and the development of rhabdomyolysis. Pharmacologic therapy may be instituted after the patient has been physically restrained.

Haloperidol, rather than chlorpromazine, should be used and is an excellent agent for sedation of the uncontrollable patient.[11,14,25–27] The phenothiazines should be avoided because they may increase the likelihood of severe hypotension as well as decrease the seizure threshold and thus increase the likelihood of seizures. Neuromuscular blocking agents in a controlled setting may be useful if muscular rigidity remains a problem. Psychiatric intervention is begun only after the patient is clinically stable and no longer profoundly agitated.

Methods To Avoid

The use of sympathomimetics should be avoided because these drugs have the potential to exacerbate tachycardia and hypertension. Dialysis is ineffective in enhancing the removal of PCP.

OTHER PHENCYCLIDINE-LIKE SUBSTANCES

There are many other arylcyclohexylamines that have appeared on the street (Table 32-8) and are similar structurally to PCP. Intoxication with these substances should be considered in a patient having a "bad trip."

Piperidinocyclohexane carbonitrile (PCC) is an intermediary in the synthesis of PCP and is difficult to separate from the final product. PCC appears to be strongly psychoactive and causes unpleasant reactions, including severe psychological side effects, nausea, vomiting, hematemesis, and abdominal cramping.[28] Other by-products of PCP synthesis are of concern in the PCP-intoxicated patient. PCP can be manufactured with piperidine, cyclohexane, and potassium cyanide. The cyano group in PCC is labile, especially with heating, and decomposes to release hydrogen cyanide. The amount of PCC contaminating PCP is probably not sufficient to cause serious complications in moderate to low doses but may worsen the effects of an overdose. On this basis it may be worthwhile to determine blood concentrations of cyanide in patients suspected of having used PCP chronically or in excessive doses.

Phenylcyclohexylpyrrolidine (PHP) is another analog of PCP. It is similar chemically and pharmacologically, has the same effects on ingestion or smoking, and is much easier to synthesize.[10,26] The chemicals for its manufacture are easier to obtain than piperidine, which is now a controlled substance. PHP has also become popular because it is difficult to detect with the thin-layer chromatographic examination that is generally employed by hospital and police toxicology laboratories. The patient may therefore show a negative PCP screen and still be intoxicated with a PCP-like substance.[26,28]

Thienylcyclohexylpiperidine (TCP) is the thiophene analog of PCP and produces similar effects. It was first seen in San Francisco and is considered more potent than PCP but is sold on the same weight basis as PCP.[29,30]

Cyclohexamine (PCE) first appeared in Los Angeles in 1969. This analog is considered somewhat more potent than PCP but has similar effects.

Table 32-8 Selected Phencyclidine Analogs

PCC—Piperidinocyclohexane carbonitrile
PHP—Phenylcyclohexylpyrrolidine
TCP—Thienylcyclohexylpiperidine
PCE—Cyclohexamine
Ketamine

Ketamine (Ketalar®, Ketaject®) is a dissociative anesthetic that has found use in medicine and abuse in the street.[2] Ketamine is considered somewhat less potent than PCP in producing depersonalization and intoxication, and it is considered superior to PCP by some users. It may be administered intranasally, intramuscularly, and intravenously and by inhalation.[2]

REFERENCES

1. Fauman B, Baker F, Coppleson L, et al: Psychosis induced by phencyclidine. *JACEP* 1975;4:223–225.

2. Felser J, Orban D: Dystonic reaction after ketamine abuse. *Ann Emerg Med* 1982;11:673–675.

3. Hartness C, Buchan J, Bayer M: Phencyclidine. *Top Emerg Med* 1985;7:33–38.

4. Owens S, Mayersohn M: Phencyclidine-specific Fab fragments alter phencyclidine disposition in dogs. *Drug Metab Disp* 1986;14:52–58.

5. Burns R, Lerner S: Phencyclidine: An emerging problem. *Clin Toxicol* 1976;9:473–475.

6. Bayer M, Norton R: Solving the clinical problems of phencyclidine intoxication. *ER Rep* 1983;4:7–12.

7. Done A, Aronow R, Miceli J: Pharmacokinetic bases for the diagnosis and treatment of acute PCP intoxication. *J Psychedelic Drugs* 1980;12:253–258.

8. Price W, Giannini A: Management of PCP intoxication. *Am Fam Physician* 1985;32:115–118.

9. Burns R, Lerner S: Perspectives: Acute phencyclidine intoxication. *Clin Toxicol* 1976;9:477–501.

10. Krenzelok E: Phencyclidine: A contemporary drug of abuse. *Crit Care Q* 1982;4:55–63.

11. Balster R, Chait L: The behavioral pharmacology of phencyclidine. *Clin Toxicol* 1976;9:513–528.

12. McCarron M, Schulze B, Thompson G, et al: Acute phencyclidine intoxication: Incidence of clinical findings in 1000 cases. *Ann Emerg Med* 1981;10:237–242.

13. Hershowitz J: More about poisoning by phencyclidine. *N Engl J Med* 1977;297:1405.

14. Showalter C, Thornton W: Clinical pharmacology of phencyclidine toxicity. *Am J Psychiatr* 1977;124:1234–1238.

15. Bessen H: Intracranial hemorrhage associated with phencyclidine abuse. *JAMA* 1982;248:585–586.

16. Hoogwerf B, Kern J, Bullock M, et al: Phencyclidine-induced rhabdomyolysis and acute renal failure. *Clin Toxicol* 1979;14:47–53.

17. Kunel R, Metzler H: Pathologic effect of phencyclidine and restraint on rat skeletal muscle: Prevention by prior denervation. *Exp Neurol* 1974;45:387–402.

18. Patel R, Das M, Palazzolo M, et al: Myoglobinuric acute renal failure in phencyclidine overdose: Report of observations in eight cases. *Ann Emerg Med* 1980;9:549–553.

19. Patel R, Connor G: A review of thirty cases of rhabdomyolysis-associated acute renal failure among phencyclidine users. *Clin Toxicol* 1986;23:547–556.

20. Kessler G, Demus L, Berlin C, et al: Phencyclidine and fatal status epilepticus. *N Engl J Med* 1974;291:979–984.

21. Eastman J, Cohen S: Hypertensive crisis and death associated with phencyclidine poisoning. *JAMA* 1975;231:1270–1272.

22. Owens S, Hardwick W, Blackall D: Phencyclidine pharmacokinetic scaling among species. *J Pharmacol Exp Ther* 1987;242:96–101.

23. Aronow R, Miceli J, Done A: A therapeutic approach to the acutely overdosed PCP patient. *J Psychedelic Drugs* 1980;12:259–267.

24. Stein J: Phencyclidine-induced psychosis: The need to avoid unnecessary influx. *Mil Med* 1973;138:590–591.

25. Fox S: Haloperidol in the treatment of phencyclidine intoxication. *Am J Hosp Pharmacol* 1979;36:448–451.

26. Giannini A, Castellani S: A case of phenylcyclohexylpyrrolidine (PHP) intoxication treated with physostigmine. *J Toxicol Clin Toxicol* 1982;19:505–508.

27. Castellani S, Giannini A, Boeringa J, et al: Phencyclidine intoxication: Assessment of possible antidotes. *J Toxicol Clin Toxicol* 1982;19:313–319.

28. Dulik D, Soine W: Color test for detection of 1-piperidinocyclohexane carbonitrile (PCC) in illicit phencyclidine. *Clin Toxicol* 1981;18:737–742.

29. Shulgin A, MacLean D: Illicit synthesis of phencyclidine (PCP) and several of its analogs. *Clin Toxicol* 1976;9:553–560.

30. Lundberg G, Gupta R, Montgomery H: Phencyclidine: Patterns seen in street drug analysis. *Clin Toxicol* 1976;9:503–511.

ADDITIONAL SELECTED REFERENCES

Aronow R, Done A: Phencyclidine overdose: An emerging concept of management. *JACEP* 1978;7:56–59.

Barton C, Sterling M, Vaziri N: Phencyclidine intoxication: Clinical experience in twenty-seven cases confirmed by urine assay. *Ann Emerg Med* 1981;10:243–246.

Brown J, Malone M: Status of drug quality in the street drug market: An update. *Clin Toxicol* 1976;9:145–168.

Budd R: PHP: A new drug of abuse. *N Engl J Med* 1981;303:588.

Burns R, Lerner S: Phencyclidine deaths. *JACEP* 1978;7:135–141.

Castellani S, Adams P: Effects of dopaminergic and cholinergic agents on phencyclidine-induced behaviors in rats. *Neurosci Abstr* 1980;6:311–314.

Fallis R, Aniline O, Weiner L, et al: Massive phencyclidine intoxication. *Arch Neurol* 1982;39:316.

Fauman B, Aldinger G, Fauman M, et al: Psychiatric sequelae of phencyclidine abuse. *Clin Toxicol* 1976; 9:513–528.

Garey R, McQuitty S, Tootle D, et al: The effects of apomorphine and Haldol on PCP-induced behavioral and motor abnormalities in the rat. *Life Sci* 1980;26:277–284.

Giannini A, Price W, Loiselle R, et al: Treatment of phenylcyclohexylpyrrolidine (PHP) psychosis with haloperidol. *Clin Toxicol* 1985;23:185–189.

Goldfrank L, Osborn H: Phencyclidine (angel dust). *Hosp Physician* 1978;14:18–21.

Gupta R, Lu I, Oei G, et al: Determination of phencyclidine (PCP) in urine and illicit street drug samples. *Clin Toxicol* 1975;8:611–621.

Karp H, Kaufman N, Anand S: Phencyclidine poisoning in young children. *J Pediatr* 1980;97:1006–1009.

Liden C, Lovejoy F, Costello C: Phencyclidine: Nine cases of poisoning. *JAMA* 1975;234:513–516.

Luisada P, Brown B: Clinical management of phencyclidine psychosis. *Clin Toxicol* 1976;9:539–545.

McCann D, Smith C, Winter J: A caution against use of verapamil in phencyclidine intoxication. *Am J Psychiatry* 1986;143:679.

Munch J: Phencyclidine: Pharmacology and toxicology. *Bull Narcotics* 1974;26:9–17.

Nicholas J, Lipshitz J, Schreiber E: Phencyclidine: Its transfer across the placenta as well as into breast milk. *Am J Obstet Gynecol* 1982;143:143–146.

Pearlson G: Psychiatric and medical syndromes associated with phencyclidine (PCP) abuse. *Johns Hopkins Med J* 1981;148:25–33.

Picchioni AL, Consroe P: Activated charcoal: A phencyclidine antidote, in hogs or dogs. *N Engl J Med* 1979; 300:202.

Price W, Giannini A, Krishen A: Management of acute PCP intoxication with verapamil. *Clin Toxicol* 1986;24:85–87.

Rainey J, Criwder M: Prolonged psychosis attributed to phencyclidine: Report of three cases. *Am J Psychiatr* 1975;132:1076–1078.

Rappolt R, Gay G, Farris R: Emergency management of acute phencyclidine intoxication. *JACEP* 1979;8:68–76.

Rappolt R: Phencyclidine (PCP) intoxication: Diagnosis in stages and algorithms of treatment. *Clin Toxicol* 1980; 16:509–529.

Reed A, Kane A: Phencyclidine (PCP): Another illicit psychedelic drug. *J Psychedelic Drugs* 1972;5:8–12.

Reynolds R: Clinical and forensic experiences with phencyclidine. *Clin Toxicol* 1976;9:547–552.

Rumack B: Phencyclidine overdose: An overview, editorial. *Ann Emerg Med* 1980;9:595.

Russ C, Wong D: Diagnosis and treatment of phencyclidine psychosis: Clinical considerations. *J Psychedelic Drugs* 1979;11:277–282.

Sidoff M: Phencyclidine: Syndromes of abuse and modes of treatment. *Top Emerg Med* 1979;1:111–119.

Siegel R: PCP and violent crime: The people vs peace. *J Psychedelic Drugs* 1980;12:317–330.

Smith D, Wesson D: PCP abuse: Diagnostic and psychopharmacological treatment approaches. *J Psychedelic Drugs* 1980;12:293–299.

Soine W, Vincek W, Agee D: Phencyclidine contaminant generates cyanide. *N Engl J Med* 1979;301:438.

Stillman R, Petersen R: The paradox of phencyclidine (PCP) abuse. *Ann Intern Med* 1979;90:428–430.

Thompson T: Malignant hyperthermia from PCP. *J Clin Psychiatr* 1979;40:327.

Tong T, Benowitz N, Becker C, et al: Phencyclidine poisoning. *JAMA* 1975;234:512–513.

Varipapa R: PCP treatment, editorial. *Clin Toxicol* 1977; 10:353–355.

Walker S, Yesavage J, Tinklenberg J: Acute phencyclidine (PCP) intoxication: Quantitative urine levels and clinical management. *Am J Psychiatr* 1981;138:674–675.

Welch M, Correa G: PCP intoxication in young children and infants. *Clin Pediatr* 1980;19:510–514.

chapter 33

Volatile Inhalants

Abuse of volatile inhalants has been practiced since earliest recorded history.[1] The substances inhaled represent a group of diverse chemicals that produce psychoactive vapors and include a wide variety of gases, smokes, powders, and fluids. The abuse of these substances has been slowly but steadily increasing among adolescents. An extremely wide range of volatile fat-soluble compounds is used; in the vapor phase these compounds pass easily through the lungs and into the blood.[2] The efficient pulmonary absorption of the substance bypasses the detoxifying enzymes of the liver, thus avoiding the first-pass metabolism seen with oral administration of some of these compounds.[3] Once within the brain, compounds with a wide variety of chemical structures can cause disturbances of consciousness ranging from mild intoxication through hallucinatory states to coma with cardiorespiratory depression.[4]

Inhaling volatiles is called glue sniffing, solvent sniffing, solvent abuse, and inhalant abuse.[2] Substances that are abused by inhalation can be categorized as aromatic and aliphatic hydrocarbons, alcohols, esters, ketones, aliphatic nitrites, anesthetic agents, halogenated solvents, and propellants (Table 33-1).[5]

All these substances are inhaled for the purpose of achieving a state of altered awareness,[6] and most are easily available at home and in industry. Any volatile substance that has an intoxicating vapor has a potential for abuse, and often the clinical effects are due entirely to the solvent content and not to its other constituents (Tables 33-2 and 33-3).[7]

Solvents constitute a group of lipid-soluble substances widely used in industry. Although solvents make up a heterogeneous group, most are volatile, lipophilic, and have CNS depressant effects (a volatile substance is one that readily vaporizes at ambient temperatures). The selection of a particular intoxicant for abuse seems to follow well-defined trends, with one type of inhalant becoming popular and being widely abused for a time and then giving way to another substance.[8]

There are more than 50 commonly abused solvents of widely different properties cited in the literature.[9] Some of the more popular inhalants include or have included glue, coolants, paint thinner, nail polish remover, petroleum fuels such as gasoline, transmission fluid, and many aerosolized substances such as hair spray, room deodorizers, deodorants, insecticides, glass chillers, and vegetable oil frying pan lubricants.[10,11] Typewriter correction fluid now appears to be a popular item of abuse by inhalation. The volatile nitrites (''poppers'') and nitrous oxide are also popular.

OVERVIEW

Methods of Abuse

Three of the most common methods for inhalation are called ''huffing,'' ''bagging,'' and

Table 33-1 Substances with Abuse Potential by Inhalation

Classification	Examples
Aerosols	Fluorocarbons (see Halogenated hydrocarbons, below)
	Isobutane
Aliphatic hydrocarbons	n-Hexane
	Ethane
	Acetylene
	Butane
	Isopentane
Anesthetic agents	Nitrous oxide
	Ether
	Chloroform
Aromatic hydrocarbons	Benzene
	Toluene
	Xylene
	Styrene
	Naphthalene
Esters	Ethyl acetate
	Isopropyl acetate
Fuels	Gasoline
	Naphtha
Halogenated hydrocarbons	Carbon tetrachloride
	Trichloroethylene
	Trichloroethane
	Perchloroethylene
	Methylene chloride
	Methylchloroform
	Fluorocarbons (dichlorodifluoromethane, trichlorofluoromethane)
Ketones	Acetone
	Methyl-n-butyl ketone
	Methylethyl ketone
Nitrites	Amyl nitrite
	Isobutyl nitrite
	Butyl nitrite

Table 33-2 Solvents Contained in Commercial Products Commonly Abused by Inhalation

Commercial Product	Solvent
Acrylic paints	Toluene
Acrylic spray paints	Toluene
Adhesives	Acetone
	Toluene
	n-Hexane
	Trichloroethylene
Aerosol propellants	Freon
Anesthetic agents	Nitrous oxide
	Ether
	Chloroform
Cleaning fluid	Carbon tetrachloride
	Benzene
	Trichloroethylene
	Trichloroethane

Table 33-2 continued

Commercial Product	Solvent
Coronary vasodilator	Amyl nitrite
Degreasers	Trichloroethylene
Dry cleaning fluid	Trichloroethane
	Trichloroethylene
Nail polish remover	Acetone
Gasoline	Hydrocarbons
	Tetraethyl lead
	Paraffins
	Olefins
Glues and adhesives	Benzene
	Xylene
	Acetone
	Naphtha
	n-Hexane
	Trichloroethylene
	Tetrachloroethylene
	Trichloroethane
	Carbon tetrachloride
Indelible ink	Methylethyl ketone
	Methyl-n-butyl ketone
	Acetone
Lacquer thinner	Toluene
	Aliphatic acetates
	Ethyl alcohol
	Propyl alcohol
Lighter fluid	Naphtha
	Perchloroethylene
	Carbon tetrachloride
	Trichloroethane
Liquid solder	Benzene
Model cement and glue	Acetone
	Toluene
	Naphtha
	Methylisobutyl ketone
Paint thinner	Trichloroethylene
Plastic cement	Acetone
	Toluene
	n-Hexane
	Ethylacetate
Refrigerants	Freon
Room deodorizers	Amyl nitrite
	Isobutyl nitrite
	Butyl nitrite
Rubber cement	Benzene
	n-Hexane
	Trichloroethylene
Shoe polish	Toluene
	Chlorinated hydrocarbons
Spot remover	Trichloroethane
	Trichloroethylene
	Carbon tetrachloride
Tube repair kits	Benzene
Typewriter correction fluid	Trichloroethane
	Trichloroethylene
	Perchloroethylene

Table 33-3 Solvents and Their Commercial Products

Solvent	Commercial Product
Acetone	Plastic cement
	Model cement
	Fingernail polish remover
Carbon tetrachloride	Degreasers
Benzene	Gasoline
Ether	Anesthetic
Freons	Aerosol propellant
	Refrigerant
Gasoline	Motor fuel
Hexane	Plastic cement
	Rubber cement
Hydrocarbons	Gasoline
Naphtha	Lighter fluid
	Model cements
Nitrites	"Room deodorizers"
	Coronary vasodilator
Nitrous oxide	Anesthetics
Perchloroethylene	Typewriter correction fluid
	Degreaser
Styrene	Adhesives
Tetraethyl lead	Gasoline
Toluene	Acrylic sprays and paints
	Plastic cement
	Indelible marking ink
	Lacquer thinner
Trichloroethane	Spot remover
	Dry cleaner
	Typewriter correction fluid
Trichloroethylene	Degreaser
	Dry cleaner
	Anesthetic agent
	Rubber cement
	Paint thinner
	Typewriter correction fluid
Xylene	Indelible inks

"sniffing." In "huffing" a cloth sprayed or soaked with an inhalant is placed in front of the mouth and nose, and the vapors are inhaled.[12] "Bagging" is much more dangerous and involves pouring the material into a plastic bag, shaking the bag so that it is vaporized, inflating the bag by breathing into it, and then inhaling the vapors.[13,14] "Sniffing" describes the simple inhalation of the substance directly from the container. The preferred method is "bagging" because the direct inhalation of the vapor from the air or a bottle may not ensure a high concentration. Because of the potential for abuse of materials containing solvents, many manufacturers add oil of mustard (allyl isothiocyanate), a mucosal irritant, to products in an effort to deter abusers.[15]

Toxicity

General Considerations

Because of the lipid solubility and high vapor pressure of solvents, these materials gain rapid access to the bloodstream across the alveolar-capillary membrane in the lungs when inhaled. Once absorbed, the compounds are distributed to tissues with high lipid content, particularly brain tissue.[3] Excretion occurs primarily through exhalation, with a small fraction metabolized in the liver or excreted through the kidneys.

The early clinical effects of abuse of inhalants, regardless of the substance involved, are similar to those of alcohol consumption or anesthesia and may vary from mild alcohol-like inebriation to frank chemical psychosis and gross behavioral disturbances. With sufficient exposure, drunkenness, dizziness, perceptual changes, and euphoria are seen almost universally.

Users may present to the emergency department with paint around the face or white typewriter correction fluid around the mouth, have a solvent odor on their breath, or with glue on their hands or face.[3] Erythematous spots around the nose and mouth, called "glue sniffer's rash," may be observed when a plastic bag is used for inhalation.[5,14]

When hydrocarbons are inhaled in vapor or fine aerosol form, the effects appear principally to affect the following areas: central and peripheral nervous systems, the cardiovascular system, and the renal system.

Acute Effects

Central nervous system. The clinical effects of solvent inhalation develop rapidly and peak quickly. After several deep inhalations, a state of intoxication is produced that may last from 30 minutes to 3 hours.[4,12,13] As stated above, clinical manifestations resemble those of ethanol intoxication except that the solvents often produce a greater degree of excitation with exhilaration, euphoria, restlessness, incoordination, and delirium (Table 33-4). Mild CNS depression may follow the stage of exhilaration with symptoms of confusion, disorientation, tinnitus, blurred vision, headache, and analgesia. Many patients develop ataxia and nystagmus. Massive exposure can lead to greater degrees of CNS depression, coma, and death.[16] Psychomimetic effects have been reported and include both visual and auditory hallucinations. These effects have been noted with gasoline, lighter fluid, and toluene inhalation.

Cardiovascular. The fluorinated hydrocarbons used as propellants in aerosol sprays and

Table 33-4 Acute Clinical Effects of Volatile Inhalants

Central nervous system
  Confusion
  Euphoria
  Exhilaration
  Hallucinations
  Restlessness
  Incoordination
  Confusion
  Disorientation
  Ataxia
  Nystagmus
  Delirium
  Coma
  Death
Cardiovascular
  Ventricular fibrillation

refrigerants have been implicated in sudden death. Typically the individual looks startled, jumps up and runs for a few hundred feet, and then collapses.[17] Although previous theories suggested suffocation as the cause of death, it is probably attributable to a cardiac dysrhythmia such as ventricular fibrillation, which occurs by sensitization of the patient's myocardium to endogenous circulating epinephrine[8,18–21] as well as by depression of myocardial contractility and consequent reduction in cardiac output. "Sudden sniffing death," as it has been termed in the literature, may occur from any of the volatile inhalants and does not appear to be related to one type of chemical such as the fluorinated hydrocarbons.[22–24] The ability to sensitize myocardial tissue to epinephrine seems to be characteristic of many lipid-soluble chemicals.[23] The most recent reports of sudden sniffing death have occurred after inhalation of trichloroethane, trichloroethene, and gasoline.[20,25,26]

Long-Term Effects

The physical sequelae of prolonged solvent abuse have included aplastic anemia and acute hepatic and renal damage (Table 33-5).[5] Other long-term sequelae include cardiac dysrhythmias, peripheral neuropathies, electrolyte disturbances, and lead poisoning.[12,27]

Neurologic. Neurologic abnormalities attributable to solvent inhalation vary from mild isolated cognitive impairment to severe dementia associated with elemental neurologic signs such as corticospinal tract dysfunction, oculomotor abnormalities, tremor, and deafness.[28] Cognitive dysfunction, optic atrophy, encephalopathy, cerebellar degeneration, and equilibrium disorders have also been reported.

Renal. A characteristic renal lesion of renal tubular acidosis is associated with long-term inhalation of toluene.[29,30] The non–anion gap metabolic acidosis is due to the loss of bicarbonate rather than the addition of any exogenous acid.[31] Patients may exhibit diffuse weakness associated with hypokalemia and hypophosphatemia, often with accompanying rhabdomyolysis.[32] There may also be markedly elevated serum creatine phosphokinase. Deaths from these electrolyte disturbances have been reported.[18]

Lead poisoning. Although lead poisoning is an extremely rare sequela of solvent abuse, repeated intoxication by prolonged, deliberate inhalation of leaded gas may lead to organic lead encephalitis.[16,33–37] Tetraethyl lead is an entity separate and distinct from the inorganic leads that cause lead poisoning and is significantly more toxic than inorganic lead. This is because the molecular species as a whole is involved rather than the metallic constituent alone.[32] Although tetraethyl lead is not by itself toxic, it is converted to the toxic derivative triethyl lead in the liver. Both tetraethyl and triethyl lead are more lipid soluble than inorganic lead and can therefore rapidly accumulate in the CNS, causing early neurologic dysfunction.[12] The most noticeable clinical sign of tetraethyl lead poisoning is encephalopathy.

Laboratory Analysis

In cases of suspected solvent abuse, arterial blood gases and electrolytes may demonstrate either a hyperchloremic metabolic acidosis or an anion gap metabolic acidosis. Tests for renal and liver function may document the status of these organ systems. In the case of a suspected volatile organonitrite, methemoglobin concentrations should be measured.

Table 33-5 Long-Term Sequelae from Inhalation Abuse

Aplastic anemia
Hepatic damage
Renal damage
   Renal tubular acidosis
Neurologic sequelae
   Optic atrophy
   Cognitive impairment
   Corticospinal tract dysfunction
   Deafness
   Dementia
   Encephalopathy
   Oculomotor abnormalities
   Cerebellar degeneration
   Disorders of equilibrium
   Peripheral neuropathies
   Tremor
Electrolyte disturbances
Lead poisoning
Weight loss

Laboratory testing for solvents is required in cases of glue sniffing only when medical complications occur or for medicolegal purposes. These agents are not routinely detected in toxicologic screens, and special precautions should be used to improve the likelihood of recovery, such as the use of volatile analysis containers. Although solvents are relatively inert to biologic degradation, their volatile nature may lead to inaccurate or negative studies if they are not collected properly. Sensitive methods of analysis such as gas chromatography with mass spectrophotometry may be required for the accurate characterization of these compounds. Chromatographic methods are available for the detection of compounds such as acetone, trichloroethene, isopropanol, methylethyl ketone, benzene, trichloroethane, toluene, and many others.[38] Blood concentrations of many of these volatiles may correlate with the depth of narcosis. The blood concentrations may be biphasic, with an initial peak followed by a trough; this reflects lipid binding by the CNS and a subsequent slow release into the blood.

Although blood is the specimen of choice for the detection of the agents abused, the analysis of urine may provide useful additional or corroboratory information in some instances. This applies particularly when abused substances may have cleared the circulation before a blood specimen can be obtained.

Methemoglobinemia should be considered in the cyanotic patient who is unrelieved with oxygen or whose blood appears brown. Methemoglobinemia may be secondary especially to the volatile nitrites.[39,40]

Treatment

Symptomatic, conservative treatment is called for in cases of acute solvent intoxication. Generally, no further intervention is needed except pyschiatric evaluation and followup. Treatment of toluene inhalation includes fluid and electrolyte replacement. Patients presenting with distal renal tubular acidosis and marked metabolic acidosis should be admitted and treated with bicarbonate. Serum electrolyte abnormalities such as hypokalemia, hypophosphatemia, and hypochloremia are common and must be corrected. Treatment for methemoglobinemia secondary to the nitrites should follow the protocol outlined in Chapter 22. In cases of nitrous oxide abuse, vitamin B_{12} and thiamine supplements may correct the mixed neuropathic abnormalities.

AROMATIC HYDROCARBONS

Benzene

The aromatic hydrocarbons most frequently abused are benzene, toluene, and xylene. Benzene is lipophilic and may serve as a vehicle for penetration of other neurotoxic solvents into the nervous system. For example, benzene is a constituent of gasoline and may contribute to the cerebral toxicity noted after chronic inhalation of lead-based gasoline.[4]

Formerly, benzene was the major organic hydrocarbon in paints, lacquers, and thinners (Table 33-6). Because benzene is toxic to bone marrow and liver, however, it has been replaced by toluene (methylbenzene) and aliphatic hydrocarbons, which nevertheless have toxicities of their own.[15]

Table 33-6 Compounds Containing Benzene

Rubber cement, glues, and adhesives
Cleaning fluid
Tube repair kits
Liquid solder
Gasoline

Table 33-7 Compounds Containing Toluene

Plastic cement
Model glue
Lacquer thinner
Shoe polish
Model cement
Acrylic spray paints
Acrylic paints
Indelible ink
Cleaning fluid

Toluene

Toluene is probably the most popular of the solvents abused and is also the best described. It is a common constituent of paints, paint and spot removers, varnishes, lacquers, adhesives (glues and cements), and transmission fluid (Table 33-7).[41]

Toluene is a hydrocarbon that is insoluble in water. On inhalation it is absorbed by the lungs and bound to lipoproteins. Toluene is metabolized in hepatic microsomes by oxidation to benzoic acid, which is conjugated with glycine to form hippuric acid and is eliminated by the kidneys.[29]

The effects of toluene on the CNS may be depression or excitation, with euphoria in the induction phase followed by disorientation, tremulousness, mood lability, tinnitus, dysarthria, diplopia, pleasant hallucinations, and ataxia that may last from 1 to 2 hours.[30] Large doses may produce seizures and coma.[19]

Blood concentrations of toluene may be biphasic. An initial peak is followed by a trough, reflecting lipid binding by the CNS and subsequent slow release into the blood.[41]

Long-term toluene abuse may cause certain symptom complexes such as muscle weakness; gastrointestinal complaints, including abdominal pain and hematemesis; and neuropsychiatric disorders, including an altered mental status, cerebellar abnormalities, and peripheral neuropathy (Table 33-8). Renal tubular damage has been noted in many individuals, with potassium, phosphorus, and bicarbonate wasting.[32] Pyuria, hematuria, proteinuria, and membraneous glomerulonephritis have also been described.[41] Both hyperchloremic metabolic acidosis and an elevated anion gap metabolic acidosis have been noted with toluene sniffing.[30,42] The latter is possibly secondary to accumulation of metabolites of toluene.[29] Long-term exposure may also lead to hepatomegaly with impaired liver function. Aplastic anemia and severe erythroid hypoplasia may occur.

The dose-related neurotoxicity of hydrocarbons, especially toluene, is known.[43] The legally allowed maximum concentration of pure toluene vapor to which an individual may be exposed is 200 parts per million (ppm); at higher concentrations fatigue, headache, paresthesias, and slowed reflexes appear. Exposure to concentrations greater than 600 ppm causes confusion or delirium. Long-term abusers are exposed to concentrations well above 1000 ppm for prolonged periods and often to other compounds as well.

HALOGENATED HYDROCARBONS

Chlorinated or fluorinated hydrocarbons have been used for years as active compounds or inert solvents.[12] The fluorinated hydrocarbons, or freons, have been implicated in many deaths from inhalation, but chlorinated hydrocarbons such as methylene chloride, trichloroethylene, and methylchloroform are also considered dangerous. As mentioned above, the most recent substance of popular abuse appears to be typewriter correction fluid.[7]

The aliphatic fluorinated hydrocarbons are no longer widely used as propellants and refrigerants in over-the-counter preparations; they have been replaced by propane, isobutane, and carbon dioxide.

The halogenated hydrocarbons are potentially toxic to the lungs, bone marrow, liver, kidneys, and heart. Dysrhythmias may be a significant problem after exposure to these agents.

Table 33-8 Clinical Effects of Toluene Intoxication

Gastrointestinal
  Abdominal pain
  Hematemesis
Central nervous system
  Altered mental status
  Cerebellar abnormalities
  Peripheral neuropathy
  Muscle weakness
Renal
  Renal tubular acidosis
  Pyuria
  Hematuria
  Proteinuria
  Membraneous glomerulonephritis
Electrolyte abnormalities
  Hypokalemia
  Hypophosphatemia
  Hyperchloremic metabolic acidosis
  Anion gap metabolic acidosis
Miscellaneous
  Hepatomegaly
  Aplastic anemia

Typewriter Correction Fluid

Typewriter correction fluid (Liquid Paper®, Wite-Out®, Snopake®) is a solvent-containing liquid used to eradicate typing errors. The inhalation of these products is known as getting "whited out."[7,43] Most of these substances contain trichloroethylene, trichloroethane, or perchloroethylene either singly or in combination. These compounds are also used industrially as degreasers and solvents. Typewriter correction fluid is found in offices, schools, and hospitals.[43] It is easily available in many retail outlets and is inexpensive to purchase. All three of the active agents have been associated with seizures, CNS depression, confusion, loss of consciousness, euphoria, and incoordination. In addition, trichloroethylene has been associated with visual disturbances, multiple nerve palsies, and peripheral neuropathies.[25] Trichloroethylene and perchloroethylene have been associated with massive hepatic necrosis.[7] These agents have caused cardiac dysrhythmias as a result of sensitization of myocardial tissue to epinephrine with subsequent ventricular fibrillation.[43]

Many of the new typewriter correction fluids have been reformulated with mustard oil to discourage intentional inhalation.[15]

Other Aliphatic Hydrocarbons

n-Hexane is a principal component of gasoline and naphtha fractions as well as over-the-counter glues and cements. Individuals who inhale the vapors of these products may therefore be exposed to high concentrations of this aliphatic agent. Severe peripheral neuropathy has been attributed to *n*-hexane.[14,15] Other aliphatic hydrocarbons such as ethane, acetylene, propane, propylene, isobutane, butane, and isopentane are toxic to the heart and may produce narcosis.

GASOLINE

Gasoline sniffing was first noted in the 1950s and was most popular among teenagers in remote rural areas, where access to alcohol and other more commonly used drugs was restricted.[32] Gasoline sniffing is more commonly performed by males than females and often begins during childhood; it is done in groups as a social activity along with friends or siblings.[44] Fifteen to twenty breaths of gasoline vapor are sufficient to produce an intoxication that can last for 5 to 6 hours.[15,44]

The toxicity of inhaled gasoline is complex because gasoline is a mixture of alkanes, cycloalkanes, alkenes, and aromatic hydrocarbons. The toxicity of gasoline is related to the composition of the mixture.[4]

Benzene, a known bone marrow depressant, constitutes a small percentage of gasoline. Gasoline may also have organic lead as an ingredient. The most common organolead compound in gasoline is tetraethyl lead. Chronic inhalation of these compounds may lead to organolead intoxication. The symptomatology of organolead poisoning differs from that of inorganic lead poisoning and is discussed in Chapter 41.

KETONES, AND ESTERS

Ketones are largely produced industrially from petrochemicals by dehydrogenation of two alcohols. They are widely used in industrial operations and are components of various household products. They are used as solvents for inks, paints, and resins, as intermediates in organic synthesis, and in some perfumes. Acetone, methyl-*n*-butyl ketone, methylisobutyl ketone, and methylethyl ketone are among the ketones abused by inhalation.

Methylethyl ketone, a highly volatile solvent, is a component in aerosolized paints and coatings, adhesives and cements, sealers, liquid holders, primers, lacquers, varnishes, and brush cleaners. It is abused because of its hypnotic effects, which are considered greater than those of ethanol.[15] The ketones produce sharp irritation that is usually sufficient to prevent acute overexposure. Because of the irritating effects on the nose and mouth, the abuse of these agents is reduced. Both methyl-*n*-butyl ketone and methylethyl ketone may cause peripheral neuropathies.

ANESTHETIC AGENTS

Anesthetics commonly abused by inhalation include ether, chloroform and related gases, and nitrous oxide. Nitrous oxide is the most widely abused member of this class.

Nitrous oxide is produced from ammonium nitrate; extensive commercial purification removes toxic by-products such as ammonia and oxides of nitrogen, principally nitric oxide and nitrogen dioxide.[45] Nitrous oxide is an analgesic-anesthetic gas popularly known as "laughing gas." It has marked analgesic properties in subanesthetic concentrations. Its onset of action is rapid, and its effects disappear in 2 to 3 minutes. The populations at greatest risk for nitrous oxide include health professionals, particularly dentists; medical and dental students; and susceptible members of the general population.[46]

Abuse of nitrous oxide was widespread for many years.[47] It is a commonly used industrial agent, particularly in the food industry, because it is nonflammable and bacteriostatic and has no flavor. For these reasons it has been used as a propellant in whipped cream dispensers. Inhalation of some of these pressurized sources without the use of reducing valves has led to alveolar rupture with dissection of the gas, resulting in pneumomediastinum.[48] Other gases have replaced nitrous oxide as an aerosol propellant in most products.

Inhalation of 50% to 75% nitrous oxide produces an exhilarating "rush" within 15 to 30 seconds that is followed by a sense of euphoria and detachment for 2 to 3 minutes. The most common early symptom reported after inhalation is numbness or tingling of the extremities (Table 33-9). Some long-term abusers present with loss of finger dexterity, ataxia, and leg weakness. Ataxia may also be secondary to sensory loss. Neuropsychiatric symptoms such as depression, impaired memory, or confusion have been noted; these symptoms improve after cessation of abuse.

Polyneuropathies from the inhalation of nitrous oxide have been reported, although some signs suggest a possible cerebellar disorder.[49] The neuropathology has been linked to the inactivation of vitamin B_{12}, which is the coenzyme for methionine synthesis. This neurologic disorder, which may be similar to subacute combined degeneration, includes early sensory complaints, loss of balance, impaired gait, impotence, and sphincter sensorimotor polyneuropathy often combined with signs of involvement of the posterior and lateral columns of the spinal cord. Vitamin B_{12} deficiency may also lead to megaloblastic anemia. In cases of nitrous oxide abuse, vitamin B_{12} and thiamine supplements may correct the mixed neuropathic abnormalities.

VOLATILE ALKYL NITRITES

The volatile alkyl nitrites, predominantly amyl, butyl, and isobutyl nitrite, are formed by combining the corresponding alcohol with sodium nitrite and sulfuric acid. They are powerful oxidizing agents and are also flammable. In the body, the nitrites are hydrolyzed to nitrite ion and the corresponding alcohol.

History of Nitrite Abuse

Amyl Nitrite

Amyl nitrite was introduced into medical practice as a coronary vasodilator more than a

Table 33-9 Signs and Symptoms of Nitrous Oxide Abuse

Neurologic
  Ataxia
  Numbness or tingling of extremities
  Loss of finger dexterity
  Leg weakness
  Impotence
Neuropsychiatric
  Depression
  Impaired memory
  Confusion
Miscellaneous
  Megaloblastic anemia

century ago.[50] It has been abused since at least the 1930s, but recently it has been displaced by the organic nitrites.

Amyl nitrite is a yellowish, volatile, flammable liquid with a fruity odor.[51] It is unstable and decomposes in the presence of air and light. Amyl nitrite has been marketed in fragile glass "perles." The glass is covered with a woven absorbent material, so that the perles can be safely crushed in the hand and the vapors from the liquid inhaled. The term "snappers" or "poppers" is used for these agents because of the sound made by the perles when they are broken. Although amyl nitrite is rapidly absorbed through the lungs, gastric secretions decompose it, and it is thus ineffective when swallowed.[50]

Isobutyl Nitrite

Because amyl nitrite perles are prescription items and somewhat difficult to obtain, new products have appeared and are sold at adult bookshops. These include various isomers of the nitrites.[52] Since the late 1960s, butyl and isobutyl nitrite have been commercially available as "liquid incense" and "room deodorizers." Isobutyl nitrite is marketed in drug paraphernalia stores under such trade names as Rush®, Bolt®, Hardware®, Quick Silver®, and Satan's Scent®.[52,53]

Volatile nitrites are increasingly abused as stimulants, aphrodisiacs, and psychedelic agents. Currently available products are more than 90% nitrites and contain small quantities of the corresponding alcohol and vegetable oil to render them less volatile.[24]

Table 33-10 Clinical Effects of the Alkyl Nitrites

Hypotension
Tachycardia
Nausea
Dizziness
Weakness
Syncope
Slowed perception of time
Headache
Methemoglobinemia

Clinical Effects of Nitrites

Alkyl nitrites produce relaxation of smooth muscle in vessels, including the coronary arteries, thereby producing tachycardia; the meningeal vessels, thereby producing throbbing headache; and the subcutaneous vasculature, thereby producing a cutaneous blush in the upper torso and head.[9] Increased intraocular pressure has also been noted. Hemodynamic effects of the nitrites include a decrease in blood pressure and an increase in heart rate within 10 seconds of inhalation (Table 33-10).[54] Nausea, dizziness, and weakness may also be noted as a result of the

hypotension. Syncope, especially if the patient is standing, can occur. Peak effects occur within 30 seconds, with a return to normal by 90 seconds.

The perceived slowing of time, which is one of the drug's experienced effects, is what gave rise to a modest amount of its nonmedical use. For example, if the vapors are inhaled just before sexual climax, the sensation of orgasm is prolonged and allegedly enhanced.[54]

Methemoglobin concentrations from inhalation of the volatile nitrites average less than 5% in normal individuals and are higher in reductase-deficient individuals.[11,40] Inhaling isobutyl nitrite theoretically can lead to significant methemoglobin accumulation even in normal subjects if the exposure is intense or if inadequate time is allowed between inhalations for methemoglobin reduction. When the alkyl nitrites are ingested, however, they carry the risk of profound and potentially lethal methemoglobinemia.[10,11,54]

Burns can result from hydrolysis of the nitrite to nitrous acid on the skin. The use of the alkyl nitrites can be dangerous in individuals with cerebral hemorrhage, recent head injury, hypotension, or glaucoma.[39]

REFERENCES

1. Novak A: The deliberate inhalation of volatile substances. *J Psychedelic Drugs* 1980;12:105–122.

2. Anderson H, Dick B, Macnair R, et al: An investigation of 140 deaths associated with volatile substance abuse in the United Kingdom (1971–1981). *Hum Toxicol* 1982;1:207–221.

3. Sourindrhin I: Solvent misuse. *Br Med J* 1985; 290:94–95.

4. Polkis A, Burkett C: Gasoline sniffing: A review. *Clin Toxicol* 1977;11:35–41.

5. Davies B, Thorley A, O'Connor D: Progression of addiction careers in young adult solvent misusers. *Br Med J* 1985;290:109–110.

6. Edwards I: Solvent abuse. *N Z Med J* 1982; 95:880–883.

7. Akerman H: The constitution of adhesives, and its relationship to solvent abuse. *Hum Toxicol* 1982;1:223–230.

8. Greer J: Adolescent abuse of typewriter correction fluid. *South Med J* 1984;77:297–298.

9. Garriott J, Petty C: Death from inhalant abuse: Toxicological and pathological evaluation of 34 cases. *Clin Toxicol* 1980;16:305–315.

10. Shesser R, Mitchell J, Edelstein S: Methemoglobinemia from isobutyl nitrite preparations. *Ann Emerg Med* 1981;10:262–264.

11. Shesser R, Dixon D, Allen Y, et al: Fatal methemoglobinemia from isobutyl nitrite ingestion. *Ann Intern Med* 1980;92:131–132.

12. Barnes G: Solvent abuse: A review. *Int J Addict* 1979;14:1–26.

13. Goldfrank L, Kirstein R, Bresnitz E: Gasoline and other hydrocarbons. *Hosp Physician* 1979;15:32–38.

14. Saxena K: Glue sniffing and other deliriants. *Top Emerg Med* 1985;7:55–62.

15. Prockop L: Neurotoxic volatile substances. *Neurology* 1979;29:862–865.

16. Coulehan J, Hirsch W, Brittman J, et al: Gasoline sniffing and lead toxicity in Navajo adolescents. *Pediatrics* 1983;71:113–117.

17. Francis J, Murray V, Ruprah M, et al: Suspected solvent abuse in cases referred to the poisons unit, Guy's hospital, July 1980–June 1981. *Hum Toxicol* 1982; 1:271–280.

18. Kirk L, Anderson R, Martin K: Sudden death from toluene abuse. *Ann Emerg Med* 1984;13:68–69.

19. Taher S, Anderson R, McCartney R, et al: Renal tubular acidosis associated with toluene "sniffing." *N Engl J Med* 1974;290:765–768.

20. Boon N: Solvent abuse and the heart. *Br Med J* 1987;294:722.

21. Reinhardt C, Azor A, Maxfield M, et al: Cardiac arrhythmias and aerosol "sniffing." *Arch Environ Health* 1971;22:265–279.

22. Clark D, Tinston D: Acute inhalation toxicity of some halogenated and non-halogenated hydrocarbons. *Hum Toxicol* 1982;1:239–247.

23. Wason S, Gibler B, Hassan M: Ventricular tachycardia associated with non-freon aerosol propellants. *JAMA* 1986;256:78–80.

24. Wason S, Setsky A, Platt O, et al: Isobutyl nitrite toxicity by ingestion. *Ann Intern Med* 1980;92:637–638.

25. King M, Day R, Oliver J, et al: Solvent encephalopathy. *Br Med J* 1981;283:663–665.

26. King M: Neurological sequelae of toluene abuse. *Hum Toxicol* 1982;1:281–287.

27. Ron M: Volatile substance abuse: A review of possible long-term neurological, intellectual and psychiatric sequelae. *Br J Psychiatr* 1986;148:235–246.

28. Hormes J, Filley C, Rosenberg N: Neurologic sequelae of chronic solvent vapor abuse. *Neurology* 1986;36:698–702.

29. Streicher H, Gabow P, Moss A, et al: Syndromes of toluene sniffing in adults. *Ann Intern Med* 1981;94:758–762.

30. Patel R: Renal disease associated with toluene inhalation. *Clin Toxicol* 1986;24:213–223.

31. O'Brien E, Yeoman W, Hobby J: Hepatorenal damage from toluene in a "glue sniffer." *Br Med J* 1971;2:29–30.

32. Moss M, Cooper P: Gasoline sniffing and lead poisoning. *Acta Pharmacol Toxicol* 1986;59:48–51.

33. Boeckx R, Postl B, Coodin F: Gasoline sniffing tetraethyl lead poisoning in children. *Pediatrics* 1977; 60:140–145.

34. Hanson K, Sharp F: Gasoline sniffing, lead poisoning, and myoclonus. *JAMA* 1978;240:1375–1376.

35. Law W, Nelson E: Gasoline sniffing by an adult: Report of a case with the unusual complication of lead encephalopathy. *JAMA* 1968;204:1002–1004.

36. Seshia S, Rajani K, Boeckx R, et al: The neurological manifestations of chronic inhalation of leaded gasoline. *Dev Med Child Neurol* 1978;2:323–324.

37. Valpey R, Sumi S, Corass M, et al: Acute and chronic progressive encephalopathy due to gasoline sniffing. *Neurology* 1978;28:507–510.

38. Ramsay J, Flanagan R: The role of the laboratory in the investigation of solvent abuse. *Hum Toxicol* 1982;1:299–311.

39. Munjack D: Sex and drugs. *Clin Toxicol* 1979; 15:75–89.

40. Horne M, Waterman M, Simon L, et al: Methemoglobinemia from sniffing butyl nitrite. *Ann Intern Med* 1979;91:417–418.

41. Cohr K, Stokholm J: Toluene: A toxicologic review. *Scand J Work Environ Health* 1979;5:71–90.

42. Fischman C, Oster J: Toxic effects of toluene: A new cause of high anion gap metabolic acidosis. *JAMA* 1979;241:1713–1715.

43. King G, Smialek J, Troutman W: Sudden death in adolescents resulting from inhalation of typewriter correction fluid. *JAMA* 1985;253:1604–1606.

44. Edminster S, Bayer M: Recreational gasoline sniffing: Acute gasoline intoxication and latent organolead poisoning. *J Emerg Med* 1985;3:365–370.

45. Sterman A, Coyle P: Subacute toxic delirium following nitrous oxide abuse. *Arch Neurol* 1983;40:446–447.

46. Rosenberg H, Orkin F, Springhead J: *Anesth Analg* 1979;58:104–106.

47. Layzer R: Myeloneuropathy after prolonged exposure to nitrous oxide. *Lancet* 1978;2:1227–1230.

48. LiPuma J, Wellman J, Stern H: Nitrous oxide abuse: A new cause for pneumomediastinum. *Radiology* 1982;145:602.

49. Layzer R, Fishman R, Schafer J: Neuropathy following abuse of nitrous oxide. *Neurology* 1978;28:504–506.

50. Cohen S: The volatile nitrites. *JAMA* 1979; 241:2077–2078.

51. Haley T: Review of the physiological effects of amyl, butyl, and isobutyl nitrites. *Clin Toxicol* 1980;16:317–329.

52. Fisher A, Brancaccio R, Jelinek J: Facial dermatitis in men due to inhalation of butyl nitrite. *Cutis* 1981; 27:146–153.

53. Smith M, Stair T, Rolnick M: Butyl nitrite and a suicide attempt. *Ann Intern Med* 1980;92:719–720.

54. Dixon D, Reisch R, Santinga P: Fatal methemoglobinemia resulting from ingestion of isobutyl nitrite, a "room odorizer" widely used for recreational purposes. *J Forensic Sci* 1981;26:587–593.

ADDITIONAL SELECTED REFERENCES

Barnes G, Vulcano B: Bibliography of the solvent abuse literature. *Int J Addict* 1979;14:401–421.

Blyth A: Solvent abuse: Summary of a paper presented on behalf of the DHSS. *Hum Toxicol* 1982;1:347–349.

Cherry N, McArthy T, Waldron H: Solvent sniffing in industry. *Hum Toxicol* 1982;1:289–292.

Dossing M, Aren-Soborg P, Petersen L, et al: Liver damage associated with occupational exposure to organic solvents in house painters. *Eur J Clin Invest* 1983;13:151–157.

Evans M: Solvent misuse: Educational implications. *Hum Toxicol* 1982;1:337–343.

Gay M, Meller R, Stanley S: Drug abuse monitoring: A survey of solvent abuse in the county of Avon. *Hum Toxicol* 1982;1:257–263.

Hershey C, Miller S: Solvent abuse: A shift to adults. *Int J Addict* 1982;17:1085–1089.

Jones R, Winter D: Two case reports of deaths on industrial premises attributed to 1,1,1-trichloroethane. *Arch Environ Health* 1983;38:59–61.

Kalf G, Post G, Snyder R: Solvent toxicology: Recent advances in the toxicology of benzene, the glycol ethers, and carbon tetrachloride. *Annu Rev Pharmacol Toxicol* 1987;27:299–427.

Klein B, Simon J: Hydrocarbon poisonings. *Pediatr Clin North Am* 1986;33:411–419.

Lewis J, Moritz D, Mellis L: Long-term toluene abuse. *Am J Psychiatr* 1981;138:368–370.

Lindstrom K: Behavioral effects of long-term exposure to organic solvents. *Acta Neurol Scand* 1982;66:131–141.

Lynn E, Walter R, Harris L, et al: Nitrous oxide: It's a gas. *J Psychedelic Drugs* 1972;5:1–7.

Massengale O, Glaser H, LeLievre R, et al: Physical and psychologic factors in glue sniffing. *N Engl J Med* 1963;269:1340–1344.

McLeod A, Marjot R, Monaghan M, et al: Chronic cardiac toxicity after inhalation of 1,1,1-trichloroethane. *Br Med J* 1987;294:727–729.

Messina F, Wynne J: Homemade nitrous oxide: No laughing matter. *Ann Intern Med* 1982;96:333–334.

O'Conner D: The use of suggestion techniques with adolescents in the treatment of glue sniffing and solvent abuse. *Hum Toxicol* 1982;1:313–320.

Oliver J, Watson J: Abuse of solvents "for kicks." *Lancet* 1977;1:84–86.

Panson R, Winek C: Aspiration toxicity of ketones. *Clin Toxicol* 1980;17:271–317.

Ramsay A: Solvent abuse: An educational perspective. *Hum Toxicol* 1982;1:265–270.

Riihimaki V, Pfaffli P: Percutaneous absorption of solvent vapors in man. *Scand J Work Environ Health* 1978;4:73–85.

Roberts D: Abuse of aerosol products by inhalation. *Hum Toxicol* 1982;1:231–238.

Skuse D, Burrell S: A review of solvent abusers and their management by a child psychiatric out-patient service. *Hum Toxicol* 1982;1:321–329.

Tarsh M: Schizophreniform psychosis caused by sniffing toluene. *J Soc Occup Med* 1979;29:131–133.

Watson J: Morbidity and mortality statistics on solvent abuse. *Med Sci Law* 1979;19:246–252.

Watson J: Solvent abuse: Presentation and clinical diagnosis. *Hum Toxicol* 1982;1:249–256.

Woodcock J: Solvent abuse from a health education perspective. *Hum Toxicol* 1982;1:331–336.

chapter 34

Hallucinogens and Marijuana

Hallucinogens, also known as psychedelic drugs, are chemicals that produce changes in perception, thought, and mood. These drugs are also referred to as psychomimetic agents, psycholytics, or psychotogens and include lysergic acid diethylamide (LSD), mescaline, psylocybin, and some of the "designer drugs."[1] Hallucinogens can be derived from natural products or produced synthetically. Although tetrahydrocannabinol, the psychoactive ingredient in marijuana, may cause hallucinations or illusions, in the typical dosage that is smoked these properties are not noted.

HALLUCINOGENIC SUBSTANCES: GENERAL CONSIDERATIONS

Substances in this group are perhaps more properly called "illusionogenic" because they produce a distortion of an actual stimulus rather than create a new stimulus where none exists.[1]

Mechanism of Action

All the hallucinogenic agents affect the pons, which is the bridge between the higher and lower cortical centers. The mechanism by which the hallucinogens produce psychedelic action is not known, although they appear to interact with serotonin synapses.[1] The emotional response to a hallucinogen can vary from an ecstatic, blissful feeling to a miserable, hopeless dysphoria.

Actions

The hallucinogens produce a flooding of sensation by inhibiting the usual dampening of sensory input. There is a heightened awareness of colors, sounds, and textures, distortion of object contours, a diminished sense of reality, increased suggestibility, and occasionally a sense of anxiety or panic. Distortion of ego functions causes depersonalization. Subjective time appears to be slowed. Illusions are common, but true hallucinations are infrequent. Changes in self-image are substantial. Overflow from one sensory modality to another, or synesthesia, may occur, so that the user may "hear" colors or "feel" sounds.[2] Hallucinations of this type are not typically encountered in any form of functional psychosis.

Toxicity

The uncomplicated hallucinogenic experience rarely comes to the attention of the physician.[3] It is the untoward effects such as acute anxiety, panic, and psychotic episodes that bring the user to the emergency department. Death due directly to an unadulterated hallucinogen is infrequent.

When it has occurred, it is usually accidental and a result of misinterpretation of the environment.

Diagnosis and Treatment

Diagnosis of hallucinogen intoxication is generally based on a history of recent ingestion along with appropriate symptomatology.

An individual under the influence of a hallucinogenic drug is in a state of extreme hypersensitivity, and a hostile environment is harmful. Most cases of hallucinogen intoxication resolve without incident.[3] Panic, acute anxiety, and psychotic episodes may require some form of therapy. Psychological support and reassurance can be helpful for the individual experiencing a "bad trip." A quiet environment is usually sufficient to reduce the dysphoria. The patient should not be left alone but be accompanied by someone familiar or who can provide reassurance. Usually after a period of observation the patient improves.[1] For severe agitation, minor tranquilizers such as diazepam may be used. Major tranquilizers such as haloperidol should be reserved for the most disturbed and agitated patients. Attempts at gastrointestinal decontamination will probably not be useful if the patient is already symptomatic.[1] "Flashbacks" should be managed by support and reassurance.

Withdrawal

A withdrawal syndrome does not occur with hallucinogenic drugs, and physical dependence has not been reported.[1]

TYPES OF HALLUCINOGENS

Indolalkylamines

The indolalkylamines comprise the prototypical drug LSD, psilocybin, and psilocin.

Lysergic Acid Diethylamide

LSD is the most commonly abused drug in the indolalkylamine class. It was first synthesized in the 1930s from the ergot fungus that grows in heads of rye and wheat and from morning glory seeds. This compound was discovered accidentally when a European chemist tasted a small amount of the fungus extract and experienced hallucinogenic effects. It is the most potent psychoactive drug known,[3] producing effects at doses as low as 20 μg.[1]

LSD is a colorless, tasteless substance usually sold in the form of capsules or pills, as a white powder, in thin squares or gelatin ("windowpane"), and in liquid form absorbed onto paper ("blotter acid"), or sugar cubes. The amount of the drug in each dose may vary greatly. The most common route of administration is oral, but it is also absorbed from mucosa. Although LSD can be found in naturally occurring ergot, most of the drug that is currently used is synthetic and derived from ergonovine.

The dose of LSD that produces hallucinogenic effects is 100 to 250 μg (1 to 2 μg/kg), which usually produces an experience lasting 8 to 12 hours. Effects usually begin 20 minutes to 1 hour after ingestion and peak at 2 to 3 hours. LSD is 100 times more potent than psilocybin and 4000 times more potent than mescaline in producing altered states of consciousness.

LSD affects both the sympathetic and parasympathetic nervous system, but sympathetic activities predominate. Initial physical symptoms are sympathomimetic in nature and include mydriasis, hypertension, hyperthermia, tachycardia, and piloerection. Psychological effects soon follow.[1]

Although LSD acts on the auditory, tactile, olfactory, and gustatory senses, the most marked effects are visual. Colors of objects are perceived as more intense than usual, and fixed objects seem to undulate and flow. Because of the disruption of neuronal mechanisms that inhibit sensory input, the user is unable to experience stable, clear sensations. Synesthesia occurs, the attention span is short, and the user may experience poor judgment.[2] Ego dissolution and detachment may occur, and experiences may seem to have increased meaningfulness.

LSD has low toxicity, and deaths due directly to overdose have not been reported.[1] Fatalities are usually secondary to trauma incurred when users attempt unreasonable feats. The greatest danger from the use of LSD and related drugs is to borderline psychotic and depressed patients because suicide and prolonged psychotic behavior have been precipitated in some groups.

A "flashback," or the recurrence of some aspect of the hallucinogenic experience days to months after ingestion of the hallucinogen, is another characteristic of LSD. The phenomenon of flashbacks is not completely understood. Users describe flashbacks as transient, spontaneous recurrences of a previous hallucinogenic experience after a period of apparant normalcy. The effects are usually unpleasant and often involve visual distortions and altered self-perception. Flashbacks appear to occur more frequently in those who previously experienced a "bad trip." There is no set pattern of frequency or intensity of flashbacks. Ordinarily they tend to disappear with time and reassurance if the drug is not taken again.[1,3]

Psilocybin

Psilocybin and psilocin ("magic Mexican mushroom," "silly putty") are derived from several species of mushrooms, notably *Psilocybe mexicana*, which has been used for centuries in Native American ceremonies. Other mushrooms in the genera *Panaeolus* and *Conocybe* also contain these agents. Psilocin and psilocybin are chemically related to LSD.

Psilocybin is the phosphorylated ester of psilocin (4-hydroxydimethyltryptamine).[3] After psilocybin is ingested the phosphoric acid is removed, producing psilocin. Psilocin and psilocybin are 100 to 200 times less potent than LSD. Both substances are found in various hallucinogenic substances.[3]

The hallucinations and distortions of time and space produced by these two drugs are similar to those produced by LSD, but the duration of action is much shorter, between 2 and 4 hours. A dose of 20 to 60 mg produces effects similar to those of LSD. Usually one or two dried mushrooms are ingested to produce the psychedelic effects. CNS effects include an initial anxiety followed by a dreamy state, visual distortions, and feelings of depersonalization.

Phenylisopropylamines

Compounds in this class are more numerous than the indolalkylamines and include hundreds of natural and synthetic compounds.[3]

Mescaline and Peyote

The main representatives of the phenylethylamine group are mescaline (3,4,5-trimethoxyphenylethylamine) and peyote, which are derived from the Mexican peyote cactus (*Lophophora williamsii*) once used in religious ceremonies by the Aztecs. The peyote cactus is common to the Southwestern United States and Mexico; it has a small crown, a long root, and small pink or red flowers. The crown is cut from the cactus and dried to form a hard brown disk; this is frequently referred to as a mescal "button," which is the street name for mescaline. Each button contains from 6 to 45 mg of mescaline.

Mescaline is the least active of the hallucinogens and a close chemical relative of epinephrine. It achieves its effects by stimulating adenylate cyclase activity at central dopaminergic receptors in anterior limbic structures. The effects of mescaline cannot be differentiated from those of LSD, but LSD is approximately 4000 to 5000 times more potent than mescaline.[3]

Mescaline is usually ingested orally in doses of 300 to 500 mg. The drug is completely absorbed from the gastrointestinal tract, and effects appear 1 to 2 hours after ingestion, peak at 5 to 6 hours, and may last 8 to 12 hours. Besides the psychedelic effects, nausea and vomiting occur 30 to 60 minutes after ingestion with subsequent mydriasis, hyperreflexia, ataxia, nystagmus, and tremors. Psychological effects are essentially identical to those of LSD and may include altered sensations of sight, smell, touch, and hearing. There is less mental reorganization with mescaline than with LSD.

"Designer Drugs"

Synthetic derivatives of the peyote cactus include methylenedioxyamphetamine (MDA), 3,4-methylenedioxymethamphetamine (MDMA, or "Adam"), and 3,4-methylenedioxyethamphetamine (MDEA, or "Eve").

MDA, a Schedule I controlled substance, is a potent CNS stimulant.[4] Because MDA is chemically and pharmacologically related to both mescaline and amphetamine,[5] it produces a mixture of psychomotor stimulatory and hallucinogenic effects. Sympathomimetic activity derives from the phenylisopropylamine portion, and the psychoactive properties derive from the methyleneoxy group.[6,7] The sympathomimetic effects of MDA can manifest as hypertension, hyperthermia, mydriasis, salivation, tachycardia, seizures, and death (Table 34-1), and the psychoactive properties give rise to an overwhelming desire to communicate with others, an intensification of feelings, and a facilitation of self-insight.[5,8] MDMA and MDEA also have both stimulant and hallucinogenic effects.[6] MDMA is derived from MDA and is advocated by some psychiatrists as a memory enhancer.[8,9] It was first developed as an appetite suppressant in 1914 but was never marketed. Even though it has had a long history, it is considered one of the new designer drugs. MDMA has recently been widely abused on college campuses for its alleged aphrodisiac effects and is known on the street as "Ecstasy" and "XTC."[6] It has no accepted medical use.

MDMA synthesized clandestinely is sold as a beige powder, a clear unmarked gelatin capsule, or a beige or white unmarked tablet. A typical oral dose may be 75 to 150 mg. Until 1985, MDMA was not a controlled substance and was legally available for use. Since that time, it has been placed on Schedule I on an emergency basis.[6,9] The related drug MDEA has appeared as a nonscheduled substitute for MDMA and has similar but milder effects.

MDMA and MDEA have a rapid onset of action of approximately 30 minutes after oral ingestion. Generally, effects last for 4 to 6 hours and may include CNS stimulation, hypertension, mydriasis, tachycardia, and hyperactivity (Table 34-1). Hallucinations, delusions, and paranoia have also been noted. Seizures, muscle rigidity, and death have also occurred.

MARIJUANA

Marijuana is an ancient drug that was first described as early as 2700 BC.[1,10] It is the most widely abused drug in American society after tobacco, alcohol, and caffeine,[11,12] and it is the most commonly used illegal substance in the United States. Its use has increased dramatically in the United States during the last decade. Marijuana and related drugs are sedative-hypnotics,

Table 34-1 Clinical Effects of MDA, MDMA, and MDEA

CNS stimulation
Hypertension
Tachycardia
Mydriasis
Delusions
Paranoia
Seizures
Muscle rigidity

tranquilizers, hallucinogens, or narcotics. Although they have properties in common with all these classes of drugs, they are in a class by themselves.

The name marijuana is derived from the Mexican Spanish word *maraguana*, which is a general term indicating any substance that can cause intoxication but refers specifically to a mixture of cut, dried, and ground flowers, leaves, and stems of the leafy green hemp plant *Cannabis sativa*.[12,13] Marijuana is the principal drug produced from the hemp plant, although biochemists have identified approximately 400 drug constituents in the plant resin. Approximately 60 are known collectively as the cannabinoids. Of these, δ-9-tetrahydrocannabinol (THC) is by far the most active and is considered the main psychoactive agent in marijuana. Although the concentration of THC in a plant depends on genetic and environmental factors, selective breeding now yields marijuana with a much higher concentration than was previously available.[13] THC is a lipid-soluble, water-insoluble compound. It has been synthesized, but because it is expensive to produce material sold on the street as synthetic THC is likely to be phencyclidine, mescaline, LSD, or other drugs.

Marijuana is frequently classified as a hallucinogen, but at the doses most commonly taken these effects are not noted. The cannabinoids in marijuana have a multitude of effects, including psychotropic, hypnotic, tranquilizing, antiemetic, anticonvulsant, and analgesic effects. They also lower intraocular pressure, increase the appetite, and affect the cardiovascular, respiratory, reproductive, and immune systems.

Marijuana is prepared from all portions of the *Cannabis* plant that are capable of producing psychoactive effects (the stems and seeds are virtually inactive). The most potent type of marijuana is sensemilla, which is prepared from unpollinated female hemp plants.[13] In general the concentration of THC in marijuana is 1% to 2%.

Hashish is a concentrated preparation of the resinous secretions collected from the flowering tops and leaves of high-quality hemp plants. The resin is dried and compressed into balls or cakes.[10] The concentration of THC in hashish is 5% to 15%.

Methods of Administration

Smoking

Marijuana is typically rolled into a cigarette (called a ''joint'') and smoked. The average marijuana cigarette weighs 0.5 to 1 g and may contain 20 to 35 mg of THC. Approximately 25% to 50% of the THC content is delivered to the lungs and brain, and approximately 25% collects in the butt of the cigarette (known as a ''roach''). The remainder is destroyed by pyrolysis. Usual effects after inhalation are noted within 5 to 10 minutes of smoking, reach a peak within 20 minutes, and may last for 2 to 3 hours. The amount of THC per puff varies widely and increases toward the butt of the marijuana cigarette. Water pipes (bongs) or regular pipes may also be used.

Ingestion

Marijuana and hashish may be ingested orally in brownies or other foods. With oral ingestion there is usually a delay in the onset of symptoms from 30 minutes to more than 2 hours. Effects from oral ingestion are more prolonged than those from smoking but are usually not as intense. This is in part due to decreased bioavailability after oral ingestion.

Metabolism

Because THC is lipid soluble, once it enters the bloodstream it is distributed to organs and fatty tissue and readily enters the brain. Inhaled THC is not excreted by the lungs, in contrast to volatile inhalants.

Tetrahydrocannabinol undergoes a complex and extensive transformation in the body, and less than 0.2% of the dose is excreted unchanged. It is stored in body fat, where it has a half-life of 7 to 8 days. Approximately two-thirds of the cannabinoid metabolites are excreted in the feces and the remainder in the urine. Urinary metabolites consist primarily of δ-9-carboxy-THC and 11-hydroxy-δ-9-THC, the latter of which is oxidized to 11-nor-δ-9-carboxylic acid. There are also some 20 other similar acid metabolites, whose concentrations may remain high enough to be detected in some individuals up to 30 days after the last use.

Because of the long half-life of THC and its metabolites, repeated use of marijuana or hashish at intervals shorter than the half-life (7 to 8 days) results in accumulation in body tissues.

Clinical Effects

General Considerations

The quality, intensity, and duration of effects from marijuana and related substances are influenced by many factors, including the route and speed of administration, the experience of the user, the social setting, and the potency of the preparation. Users report feelings of relaxation and well being, mild euphoria, relief of anxiety, heightened sexual arousal, and a keen sense of hearing. The senses of taste, touch, and smell may seem to be enhanced or altered. Ideas may appear to be disconnected, rapid flowing, and altered in emphasis and importance. Time seems to pass slowly, with little activity needed and no sense of boredom. Individuals often spend long periods listening to music or reading. Increased desire to eat, especially sweets, is characteristic of the individual under the influence of marijuana. Short-term memory, learning ability, and psychomotor performance may be impaired after long-term use.

Cardiovascular Effects

The most constant cardiovascular effect of marijuana is sinus tachycardia with increased peripheral blood flow probably mediated by β-adrenergic stimulation. The resting heart rate is elevated in a dose-dependent fashion. Blood pressure is not altered significantly.

Ocular Effects

Conjunctivitis may be noted after the use of marijuana from engorgement of the blood vessels in the eye.[13] This effect appears to be dose related. Pupillary changes tend to be mild and inconsistent. THC has been noted to decrease intraocular pressure.

Miscellaneous Effects

Other physiologic effects of marijuana use include bronchodilation. At the usual doses there are no constant effects on respirations or body temperature. THC has been shown to be an effective antiemetic in patients receiving cancer chemotherapy.

Toxicity

A novice user may experience fearfulness, confusion, and panic attacks. This is especially true if the setting is unfamiliar. Psychologically predisposed individuals are more susceptible to these adverse reactions. High doses may produce such a state even in experienced users.

Although high doses can induce disorientation, delusion, feelings of paranoia, and frank hallucinations, these effects are rarely noted in the United States because the concentrations of THC necessary to induce them are not usually found in marijuana grown in or brought into this country.[14] At the usual doses there is little cognitive or motor dysfunction, but the drug may affect the ability to drive or operate machinery safely.

Effects of Long-Term Use

Heavy smokers of marijuana may experience varying degrees of respiratory tract irritation leading to bronchitis, pharyngitis, sinusitis, and uvular edema. In addition, there may be a reduction in testosterone levels and some degree of suppression of the immune system. Marijuana smoke contains larger amounts of carcinogenic hydrocarbons than tobacco smoke, and this may be a problem in long-term heavy users. Although THC freely crosses the placental barrier and is distributed to the fetus, at present there is no sound evidence to indicate that THC causes genetic abnormalities in humans. Most individuals who use marijuana in moderation for a time are unlikely to suffer any lasting harmful effects. The available evidence suggests strongly that there are no gross structural or neurologic defects attributable to the use of marijuana, and current research does not support the contention that use results in permanent cerebral impairment.

Physical and psychological dependence on marijuana and related substances are suggested but not documented in numerous reports. Although there may not be a true withdrawal syndrome after cessation of smoking, and although physical dependence has not been documented in long-term heavy users, irritability, restlessness, nervousness, and insomnia have been noted in individuals who abruptly discontinue use.[12]

Marijuana and Paraquat

A number of years ago there was some concern that the herbicide paraquat, which was sprayed on marijuana fields in Mexico, would lead to poisoning of marijuana users. Despite the fact that paraquat was detected on marijuana from sprayed fields, lung damage, the major manifestation of paraquat poisoning, has not been reported in human cases.[15] This is probably because paraquat is changed by pyrolysis to bipyridine, a nontoxic by-product.[15,16]

Laboratory Analysis

The most widely used techniques for measuring marijuana in samples include immunoassay, gas chromatography, gas chromatography with mass spectrometry, thin-layer chromatography, and high-performance liquid chromatography.[17] The two most widely used screening procedures are enzyme immunoassay and radioimmunoassay. With few exceptions, the specimen used to test for marijuana is urine.

Plasma concentrations of THC reach a maximum within 1 hour after marijuana is smoked and fall rapidly to about one-tenth the peak plasma concentrations shortly thereafter.[13] The metabolites of THC that account for a positive urine test may remain in the body for up to 21 to 30 days after the last dose in a long-term heavy user.[13] This is because THC is stored in adipose tissues of long-term users and is released back into the circulation.[18] In the occasional user a urine test may be positive for several days up to 1 week after a single exposure, depending on the method of screening.[13]

Treatment

Treatment of effects from the use of marijuana and related substances is usually limited to supportive care. Treatment of panic and paranoid episodes depends on the characteristics and severity of the episode. Reassurance is usually sufficient to calm a distressed patient. Medicating the patient is usually not necessary.

REFERENCES

1. Strassman R: Adverse reactions to psychedelic drugs. *J Nerv Ment Dis* 1984;172:577–595.

2. Baumeister R: Acid rock: A critical reappraisal and psychological commentary. *J Psychoactive Drugs* 1984; 16:339–345.

3. Cohen S: The hallucinogens and the inhalants. *Pediatr Clin North Am* 1984;7:681–688.

4. Lukaszewski T: 3,4-Methylenedioxyamphetamine overdose. *Clin Toxicol* 1979;15:405–409.

5. Simpson D, Rumack B: Methylenedioxyamphetamine: Clinical description of overdose, death, and review of pharmacology. *Arch Intern Med* 1981; 141:1507–1509.

6. Dowling G, McDonough E, Bost R: "Eve" and "Ecstasy": A report of five deaths associated with the use of MDEA and MDMA. *JAMA* 1987;257:1615–1617.

7. Ricaurte G, Bryan G, Strauss L, et al: Hallucinogenic amphetamine selectively destroys brain serotonin nerve terminals. *Science* 1985;229:986–988.

8. Greer G, Strassman R: Information on "Ecstasy." *Am J Psychiatr* 1985;142:1391.

9. Gehlert D, Schmidt C, Wu L, et al: Evidence for specific methylenedioxymethamphetamine (ecstasy) binding sites in the rat brain. *Eur J Pharmacol* 1985;119:135–136.

10. Tashkin D, Soares J, Hepler R, et al: Cannabis, 1977. *Ann Intern Med* 1978;89:539–549.

11. Charles R, Holt S, Kirkham N: Myocardial infarction and marijuana. *Clin Toxicol* 1979;14:433–438.

12. Millman R, Sbriglio R: Patterns of use and psychopathology in chronic marijuana users. *Psychiatr Clin North Am* 1986;9:533–545.

13. Schwartz R: Marijuana: A crude drug with a spectrum of underappreciated toxicity. *Pediatrics* 1984;73:455–458.

14. Beaconsfield P, Ginsburg J, Rainsbury R: Marihuana smoking: Cardiovascular effects in man and possible mechanisms. *N Engl J Med* 1972;287:209–212.

15. Landrigan P, Powell K, James L, et al: Paraquat and marijuana: Epidemiologic risk assessment. *Am J Public Health* 1983;73:784–788.

16. Fairshter R, Wilson A: Paraquat and marihuana. *Chest* 1978;74:357.

17. Moyer T, Palmen M, Johnson P, et al: Marijuana testing—How good is it? *Mayo Clin Proc* 1987;62:413–417.

18. Silber T, Getson P, Ridley S, et al: Adolescent marijuana use: Concordance between questionnaire and immunoassay for cannabinoid metabolites. *J Pediatr* 1987; 111:299–302.

ADDITIONAL SELECTED REFERENCES

Genest K, Farmilo C: The identification and determination of lysergic acid diethylamide in narcotic seizures. *J Pharm Pharmacol* 1964;16:250–257.

Greenland S, Staisch K, Brown N, et al: The effects of marijuana during pregnancy. *Am J Obstet Gynecol* 1982; 143:408–413.

Satinder K, Black A: Cannabis use and sensation-seeking orientation. *J Psychol* 1984;116:101–105.

Schwartz R, Hawks R: Laboratory detection of marijuana use. *JAMA* 1985;254:788–792.

Wert R, Raulin M: The chronic cerebral effects of cannabis use: Part I: Methodological issues and neurological findings. *Int J Addict* 1986;21:605–628.

Wert R, Raulin M: The chronic cerebral effects of cannabis use: Part II: Psychological findings and conclusion. *Int J Addict* 1986;21:629–642.

part IX

ANALGESICS

chapter 35

Acetaminophen

Acetaminophen (*N*-acetyl-*p*-aminophenol; APAP) was first synthesized in the United States in 1877.[1] Its use did not become extensive until 1949, when it was recognized as the principal active metabolite of phenacetin.[2–4] Acetaminophen (paracetamol in the United Kingdom) is one of three para-amino compounds still in use.[5] The other two, acetanalid and phenacetin, owe their analgesic and antipyretic properties to the metabolic generation of acetaminophen.

The status of acetaminophen as a prescription drug is similar to that of the relatively new nonsteroidal anti-inflammatory agent ibuprofen in that acetaminophen was a prescription drug for a short period but since 1960 has been marketed in the United States without a prescription.[6,7] It is now sold under approximately 50 trade names and in 200 proprietary combinations with other drugs (Table 35-1).[5,8] Its use has dramatically increased over the past 20 years,[9,10] and it is one of the most commonly used over-the-counter analgesic and antipyretic agents in the United States, primarily because it is generally considered safer than aspirin and has none of aspirin's undesirable side effects when taken in therapeutic doses.[11–13] In addition to the regular-strength acetaminophen (325 mg) that is available, it is marketed in extra-strength (500-mg) tablets.

Toxic effects of acetaminophen overdose were first noted in 1966. At that time overdose with this substance was one of the most common causes of hepatic necrosis in the United King-

Table 35-1 Selected Preparations of Acetaminophen by Trade Name

Aceta	Halenol
Actamin	Liquiprin
Amphenol	Neopap
Anacin-3	Oraphen-PD
Anuphen	Panex
APAP	Pedric
Bayapap	Phenaphen
Bromo Seltzer	SK-APAP
Conacetol	Sudoprin
Dapa	Tapar
Datril	Tempra
Dolanex	Tenol
Febrigesic	Tylenol
Febrinol	Valadol

dom.[1,6,14] Toxic effects of overdosage were not seen in the United States until 1971.[15–17] Because acetaminophen poisoning is a common toxicological problem that clinicians can expect to encounter even more in the future, a thorough discussion of the pharmacology and toxicology of the compound is warranted.

ACTIONS

Analgesia

Acetaminophen relieves mild to moderate pain. A number of studies comparing acetaminophen with salicylate have shown that both drugs have equal effects on pain when given in equivalent doses if the pain is noninflammatory in origin.[18] For inflammatory pain, salicylates have been shown to be superior to acetaminophen.

The mechanism of action of acetaminophen appears to be related to the inhibition of brain cyclo-oxygenase (prostaglandin synthetase),[5] with much less of an effect on the peripheral enzyme. The peripheral action appears to be blockade of pain impulse generation. In addition to inhibiting cyclo-oxygenase centrally, salicylates also inhibit this enzyme peripherally, which appears to result in anti-inflammatory activity.[19]

Antipyresis

Acetaminophen is also an antipyretic agent, altering the response of the heat-regulating center in the hypothalamus and leading to a lowering of the set point by vasodilation and sweating.[20] This central antipyretic action probably involves inhibition of prostaglandin synthesis in the hypothalamus. Studies comparing acetaminophen and salicylates have shown no significant difference in temperature response, time of onset, time of peak action, or duration of antipyretic action.[21]

ADVANTAGES OF ACETAMINOPHEN

Acetaminophen has several advantages over many of the other analgesic agents. It has relatively few side effects and drug interactions when ingested in therapeutic amounts (Table 35-2). Unlike aspirin, acetaminophen is stable in solution, so that a liquid formulation is available. Hypersensitivity to acetaminophen rarely occurs but when present is manifested by erythema or urticaria. Because acetaminophen and aspirin have completely different chemical structures, there is no cross-sensitivity between the two drugs.[22]

Acetaminophen also has advantages over other analgesics in that it does not share many of their adverse effects.[23] Acetaminophen does not

Table 35-2 Effects Caused by Other Analgesics Not Seen with Acetaminophen

Gastric irritation
Gastric erosion
Platelet function interference
Oral anticoagulant potentiation
Methemoglobinemia
Hemolytic anemia
Mood and mentation changes
Renal damage

cause gastric irritation or erosion, as do the salicylates,[24–26] nor does it interfere with platelet function or platelet aggregation or have any delayed effects on small vessel hemostasis as measured by bleeding time.[5,27,28] Short-term therapy causes no interaction with oral anticoagulants,[29] but there does appear to be some alteration in prothrombin time with doses of acetaminophen administered over a period of weeks.[29] This has not been found to be clinically significant. Occasional or small doses of acetaminophen have little effect on coumarin action. Acetaminophen does not cause methemoglobinemia, hemolytic anemia, or changes in mood, energy, and mentation, as do phenacetin and acetanalid.

PHARMACOKINETICS

Acetaminophen is rapidly absorbed from the gastrointestinal tract, with peak concentrations noted between 60 and 120 minutes after oral administration of tablets and more quickly after ingestion of liquid preparations.[30–32] Therapeutic concentrations occur much earlier; a therapeutic concentration is usually less than 9 μg/mL at 4 hours.[33] The rate of absorption of acetaminophen is even more rapid from an alcoholic solution than from tablets or suspensions.[5] Bezoar formation has not been reported with acetaminophen overdose, as it has with salicylate overdose.

Acetaminophen is a weak acid and therefore is not ionized in the stomach or small intestine; this allows for rapid absorption. Approximately 10% of acetaminophen is bound to plasma proteins. The volume of distribution for both children and adults is approximately 1 to 1.2 L/kg.[34]

The half-life of acetaminophen is 2 to 3 hours and appears to follow first-order, non-cumulative, log-linear kinetics in therapeutic situations. Because its metabolism is largely enzymatic, toxic amounts of acetaminophen are eliminated by zero-order kinetics, and as the concentration increases the half-life also increases. Most investigators believe that the prolonged half-life seen in patients intoxicated with acetaminophen results from impaired metabolism due to ensuing liver damage.[35] It may, however, also be a consequence of the limited capacity of the major biotransformation pathways, namely sulfate and glucuronic acid, because the metabolic conversion of large doses of acetaminophen eventually depletes the free sulfate needed to convert it to acetaminophen sulfate, a nontoxic by-product.[31]

METABOLISM

Acetaminophen is a major metabolite of phenacetin but does not share some of its pharmacologic properties. Phenacetin can cause methemoglobinemia by forming an aniline derivative (*p*-phenitidin) (Fig. 35-1), but acetaminophen lacks the ability to cause methemoglobinemia because of an alternate metabolic pathway in the liver.

A small amount of acetaminophen is excreted unchanged in the urine. Most of a dose is conjugated with either glucuronic acid or sulfate and then excreted by the kidneys. This accounts for 80% to 90% of the metabolic by-product. The toxicity of acetaminophen is not due to either of these pathways.[36,37] The cytochrome P-450 microsomal mixed-function oxidase system metabolizes a small but clinically significant portion of acetaminophen to an active intermediate apparently by first-order kinetics (Fig. 35-2).[32,38,39] Normally this minor metabolite of hydroxylation, which may be an iminodoquinone (*N*-acetyl-*p*-benzoquin-oninine),[40–42] is detoxified by conjugation with hepatic glutathione when it is present, and the end products (mercapturic acid and cysteine) are then excreted.[43–45] When acetaminophen is ingested in pharmacologic doses, 5% to 10% is excreted in the urine as mercapturic acid.[9,10]

When large doses of acetaminophen are ingested, the intermediary formed by this pathway, which is a strong electrophilic and oxidizing agent, depletes the limited supply of glutathione in the liver.[41,46,47] In addition, with an overdose there is saturation of the sulfate- and glucuronide-conjugating systems, shunting even more quantities of acetaminophen through the cytochrome P-450 system and further depleting the supply of glutathione.[44,48] When no more glutathione is available for conjugating the toxic metabolite, the acetaminophen metabolite arylates to proteins of the cytosol and endoplasmic reticulum in the centrilobular zone of the liver and produces cell necrosis and death.[13,33] In other words, the toxic metabolite is neutralized by glutathione, which contains a sulfhydryl group. If all the glutathione is used up other sulfhydryl groups in the liver are attacked, and the cells are damaged or destroyed.[39,49]

TOXICITY

Acute

There are essentially four phases in an acute acetaminophen overdose (Table 35-3).[35] There are no specific early signs or symptoms, and the true gravity of the situation is often not appreciated when the patient is first seen.[33]

Phase 1 occurs within hours after an ingestion and may persist for 24 to 48 hours.[11] Most patients are anorectic, nauseated, and vomiting. This is especially true with children. Diaphoresis may also be noted as a result of the effects of acetaminophen on the heat-regulating center in the hypothalamus. CNS depression is not usually a feature during this phase unless the patient has also ingested other depressant-type drugs,[10] such as codeine, propoxyphene, alcohol, antihistamines, and decongestants. The early symptoms are due to the local action of acetaminophen; the more severe the overdose, the more likely these symptoms are to be present. An important feature of this phase is that there are no specific symptoms to indicate how serious the intoxication may eventually become. Some patients may be completely asymptomatic during the initial phase of intoxication, even after ingest-

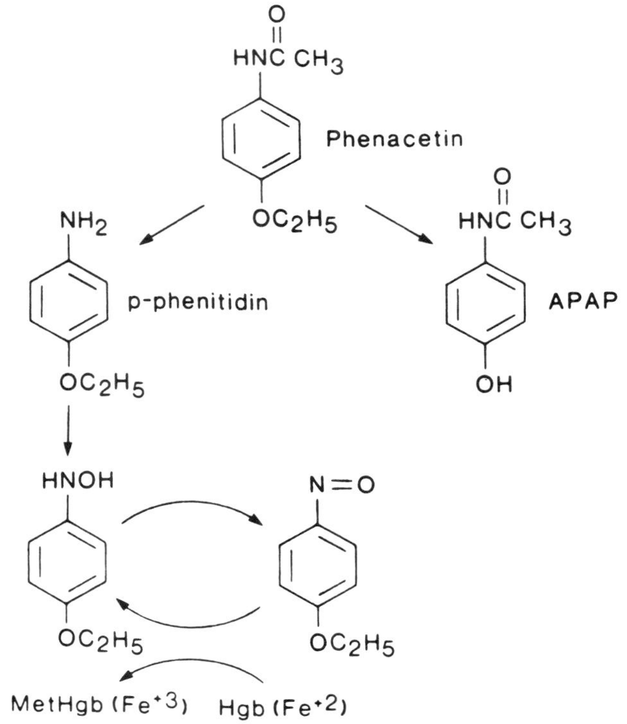

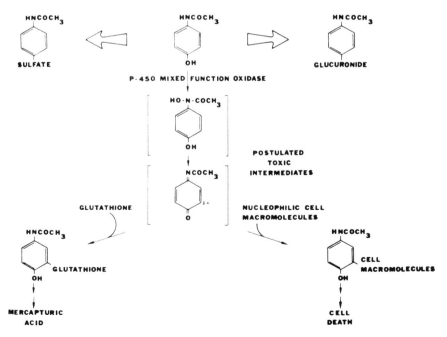

Figure 35-1 Metabolic pathway of phenacetin. *Source:* Reproduced by permission from *Pediatrics* (1978;62:877), Copyright © 1978, American Academy of Pediatrics.

Figure 35-2 Metabolic pathway of acetaminophen. *Source:* Reprinted with permission from *Clinical Pharmacology and Therapeutics* (1974;16:677), Copyright © 1974, CV Mosby Company.

Table 35-3 Phases of Acute Acetaminophen Intoxication

Phase 1 (30 minutes to 4 hours)
Anorexia
Nausea
Vomiting
Diaphoresis

Phase 2 (24 to 72 hours)
Abatement but continuation of phase 1 symptoms
Liver function abnormalities
Right upper quadrant pain

Phase 3 (3 to 5 days)
Jaundice
Coagulopathy
Hypoglycemia
Encephalopathy
Renal failure
Myocardiopathy

Phase 4 (7 to 8 days)
Abnormalities return to normal, OR
Condition continues to deteriorate

ing large doses. As a rule, liver enzyme abnormalities do not occur during this period.[9,10]

Phase 2 occurs between 24 and 72 hours after ingestion, and although the previously described symptoms may lessen in severity they may continue for up to 48 hours. Laboratory evidence of abnormal liver function (bilirubin, alkaline phosphatase, serum glutamic-oxaloacetic transaminase, serum glutamic-pyruvic transaminase, and lactic acid dehydrogenase) may now appear. In general, the elevations of serum transaminase concentrations do not correlate well with the clinical outcome. The patient may complain of right upper quadrant pain at this time.

Phase 3 occurs 3 to 5 days after an ingestion; there may be evidence of hepatic necrosis in patients who have ingested a significant overdose.[50] Symptoms consist of jaundice, hypoglycemia, and encephalopathy. In acute hepatic necrosis, coagulation disorders may be severe and may include disseminated intravascular coagulation and bleeding diathesis.[17,51] Liver enzyme abnormalities may peak during this phase; a concentration of serum glutamic-oxaloacetic transaminase greater than 1000 IU/L is taken to define hepatotoxicity (see Fig. 35-3).[9,10] Although renal failure and myocardiopathy have been reported in association with liver disease, they appear to occur only as secondary events if the overdose results in severe hepatic failure[52]; it has not been definitively determined whether they are primary events.[53] Acetaminophen metabolites accumulate in the

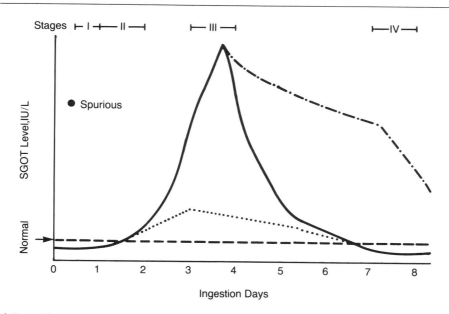

Figure 35-3 Dotted line is course of those who received acetylcysteine; solid line, those with natural course; and dotted-and-dashed line, those with severe course. *Source:* Reprinted with permission from *Archives of Internal Medicine* (1981;141:385), Copyright © 1981, American Medical Association.

renal medulla, where reactive free radicals may cause direct nephrotoxicity. Acute renal failure secondary to severe hepatic failure manifests itself as the hepatorenal syndrome. The renal lesion is acute tubular necrosis and is usually associated with death.[2,13,52]

Phase 4 occurs 7 to 8 days after an ingestion. In most patients this is usually the period in which the abnormal laboratory values return to normal. In a small number of patients liver abnormalities continue, leading to liver failure and death.

Chronic

On the basis of the kinetics of acetaminophen as well as other factors, intoxication from long-term accumulation of acetaminophen does not appear to occur.[5,54,55] There are sporadic reports that imply complications from long-term use in select individuals, but these reports are anecdotal.[12,56–58] More investigation is needed before a clear statement regarding long-term intoxication can be made.[57]

PREDICTING HEPATOTOXICITY

A number of factors should be taken into account in predicting whether liver disease may occur (Table 35-4). One factor is the total quantity of drug ingested. It has been shown in laboratory animals that liver necrosis occurs after an ingested dose of acetaminophen sufficient to deplete more than 70% of the glutathione in the liver.[11,46] Because approximately 4% of the acetaminophen ingested is metabolized by this pathway, it has been estimated that approximately 15 g of acetaminophen is required to cause liver toxicity in a 70-kg person.[5,59,60] Many clinicians accept 7.5 g as the toxic dose to take into account those individuals with liver disease from any cause or those individuals with decreased glutathione stores. The minimum toxic dose in children is considered 150 mg/kg.

Correlating the ingested dose with degree of liver damage is problematic because information obtained regarding the amount of drug ingested or eliminated by vomiting may be inexact, or there may be a lack of information regarding

Table 35-4 Factors Involved in Predicting Hepatotoxicity from Acetaminophen

Total quantity of ingested material
History of spontaneous emesis
Time from ingestion to medical attention
Activity of the cytochrome P-450 system
Age of the patient
Serum concentration in relation to nomogram
  (see Fig. 35-3)

whether other drugs were taken that could affect the metabolic disposition of the acetaminophen. A history, then, should only be used as a rough guide. It has been suggested that the 4-hour plasma acetaminophen concentration (C_p) in a patient seen at any point between 2 to 16 hours after ingestion may be predicted from the following formula:

$$C_p = 0.59 \times \text{dose (in milligrams per kilogram)}$$

Although there are many factors that are not taken into account by this formula (such as degree of emesis), it may enable an early assessment to be made of the relative severity of the overdose until laboratory results are available. It should not be used as an indication for treatment.

Whether the patient has undergone a spontaneous emesis before arriving in the emergency department influences the course of the intoxication. Vomiting is an early effect of acetaminophen, and its occurrence lessens the likelihood of a severe toxic reaction.

The metabolic activity of the cytochrome P-450 pathway is a factor in the extent of toxicity of an overdose. Certain drugs, such as phenobarbital and ethyl alcohol, stimulate the cytochrome P-450 pathway when chronically administered. A patient taking such drugs on a long-term basis may have an increased likelihood of intoxication because that pathway is metabolizing a greater percentage of the acetaminophen to the potentially toxic intermediate.[46]

On the other hand, use of cimetidine may afford protection against a toxic dose of acetaminophen.[61,62] Most of a dose of cimetidine is excreted unchanged in the urine, but a small portion is metabolized by the cytochrome P-450 system. It has been shown that standard therapeutic doses of cimetidine can reduce cytochrome P-450 metabolism of some drugs, including acetaminophen, because they appear to have a lower affinity for cytochrome P-450 than cimetidine. Metabolism of these drugs through this pathway is therefore inhibited, and in the case of acetaminophen a smaller amount of the toxic intermediary is formed.[61,63] The acute ingestion of ethyl alcohol appears to decrease the toxicity of acetaminophen in the same manner. Although positive findings associated with cimetidine have been seen in laboratory animals, studies concerning the use of cimetidine in humans have not shown promising results, and it is still too early to know whether cimetidine offers significant protection.[64]

Other known inhibitors of the cytochrome P-450 system, such as piperonylbutoxide,[46] cobaltous chloride, and metyrapone, either have not been clinically effective or have shown undesirable side effects. Although in animals prior administration of inhibitors of oxidative metabolism such as cimetidine can reduce the formation of *N*-acetyl-*p*-benzoquinonamine, research has concentrated on the use of other sulfur-containing compounds with the aim of detoxifying this metabolite.

Children appear to be less vulnerable than adults to the toxic effects of acetaminophen. Although there are a few reports, it is extremely rare for clinical intoxication or death to occur in the pediatric age group even when toxic blood concentrations are found.[11,65-67] The reasons for this phenomenon are still unclear. The plasma half-life of acetaminophen in adults and children is nearly identical, and the volume of distribution is similar.[68-70] The only difference appears to be the major pathway for conjugation in adults and children.[71] In adults glucuronide conjugation is the major pathway, and in children between 3 and 9 years of age the sulfate conjugate is the major pathway.[69] This factor should not, however, account for the difference in toxicity because the conjugated pathways do not have an effect on toxicity, the intermediary formed from the cytochrome P-450 pathway being the entity that leads to liver toxicity. Other proposed mechanisms suggest that decreased toxicity in young children may be due to smaller amounts of the drug being metabolized through the cytochrome P-450 system.[66] Children older than 6 years of age can be considered similar to adults with regard to elimination of acetamino-

phen as well as the proportion of sulfate and glucuronide metabolites excreted.[66]

The single most important prognostic indicator of acetaminophen hepatotoxicity is obtained from a serum concentration, which is placed on the acetaminophen nomogram (Fig. 35-4).[72] Serum concentration has been shown to be a more accurate indicator of the possibility of liver toxicity than the amount of drug ingested. The nomogram that was first described in 1976 is based on the correlation between liver toxicity and plasma concentration of acetaminophen measured between 4 and 24 hours after ingestion.[73] This nomogram is accurate to a high confidence level. The nomogram has been modified to include a second elimination curve 25% lower than the standard curve, which allows for errors in the history of the time of ingestion. Those patients whose plasma acetaminophen concentrations fall between 150 and 200 μg/mL at 4 hours after ingestion, or between the two lines at any later time, are considered at "possible" risk for toxicity. Concentrations higher than those indicated by the standard nomogram line are considered at "probable" risk.[10,34,63] (To avoid confusion, values should always be reported in micrograms per milliliter. Serious illness and death have resulted from the withholding of treatment because of confusion as to the units used to report plasma concentrations.[41,42])

To interpret properly the serum acetaminophen concentration, the time of ingestion must be established as accurately as possible. As an example, a concentration greater than 150 μg/mL at 4 hours is considered potentially toxic, and concentrations greater than this indicate antidotal therapy.[36] The nomogram begins 4 hours after ingestion, which is considered the time when peak concentration is attained. Before 4 hours concentrations may be falsely low[63] but can be used if they are high because they may indicate that a significant amount was ingested earlier than suspected.

Serum half-life, although used in the past, is not as reliable in predicting toxicity as a laboratory determination of serum concentration.[13,63,73] If the estimated time of ingestion cannot be obtained, making prognosis from the nomogram impossible, then the half-life may be helpful.[10] The half-life of acetaminophen at

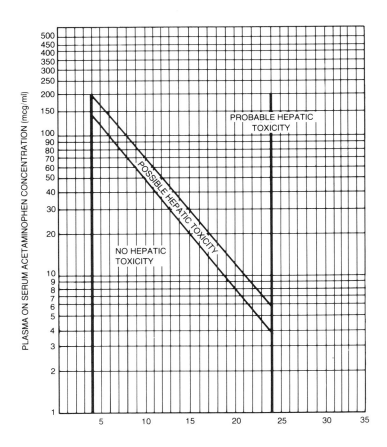

Figure 35-4 Acetaminophen nomogram. *Source:* Adapted with permission from *Pediatrics* (1975; 55:871), Copyright © 1975, American Academy of Pediatrics.

---

therapeutic plasma concentrations is 2 to 3 hours.[73] Because its metabolism is largely enzymatic, elimination is according to zero-order kinetics as concentrations increase. It has been shown that, if the half-life is greater than 4 hours, liver damage is likely and appropriate treatment should be instituted.[63] The half-life has been observed to increase to 8 hours in individuals who have ingested hepatotoxic quantities of acetaminophen.[10]

Histologic Findings

The histologic abnormalities associated with acetaminophen overdose include centrilobular hemorrhagic hepatic necrosis.[40] The sinusoids are often congested and dilated centrally. This location coincides with the centrilobular location of the enzymes responsible for the main metabolism of the drug. Tissue regeneration and repair are normally rapid and complete.[40]

LABORATORY DETERMINATIONS

Venous blood samples should be drawn for a complete blood cell count and for evaluation of platelets, prothrombin time, electrolytes, blood urea nitrogen, glucose, and liver function such as serum glutamic-oxaloacetic transaminase, serum glutamic-pyruvic transaminase, bilirubin, and alkaline phosphatase. A toxicology screen should also be performed.[10] If the acetaminophen concentration is found to be within the toxic range, then evaluation of liver function

Table 35-5 Laboratory Determinations in Acetaminophen Overdose

Toxicology screen with acetaminophen level
If toxic then serial;
Complete blood count
Platelet count
Prothrombin time
Liver function tests
   Serum glutamic-oxaloacetic transaminase
   Serum glutamic-pyruvic transaminase
   Alkaline phosphatase
   Bilirubin

Table 35-6 Treatment of Acetaminophen Overdose

Emesis or lavage
Activated charcoal and cathartic
N-Acetylcysteine (within 24 hours)
   Loading dose: 140 mg/kg orally
   Maintenance dosage: 70 mg/kg every 4 hours for 17 doses
Supportive measures (after 24 hours)
   Neomycin enema
   Fresh frozen plasma
   Glucose

should be performed at 24-hour intervals for at least 4 days (Table 35-5).

Prompt determination of serum acetaminophen concentrations can have a significant impact on the patient's treatment and prognosis. Therefore, rapid and reliable techniques for measuring the drug are required. Laboratory methods may include colorimetric techniques, radioimmunoassay, high-performance liquid chromatography, and gas chromatography.[74] The preferred method of analysis for acetaminophen is high-performance liquid chromatography, but this has a high initial cost and requires a trained technician for operation.[75] Another successful method is enzyme-modification immunoassay, but this may also be expensive and is not feasible for use by a small laboratory because of reagent instability.[74] Spectrophotometric methods, such as those involving nitration and ferric reduction, may be unreliable because of the presence of interfering substances.[75]

TREATMENT

Ineffective Methods

Several studies seem to have demonstrated that hemoperfusion removes acetaminophen.[51,76–78] Nevertheless, because the toxic metabolite is formed relatively rapidly, and because the drug has such a short half-life, there appears to be little point in trying to remove the drug by this method.[76,79] Hemodialysis reduces the half-life of acetaminophen and readily removes it from circulation, but because hepatic injury is an early event there is no strong evidence that this procedure will alter the clinical course.[80,81] Peritoneal dialysis is also ineffective because of the strong protein-binding properties of acetaminophen.[82] Forced diuresis is not indicated because only 5% of the unaltered drug is excreted in the urine.[40]

Effective Methods

Effective treatment and management of the acetaminophen-intoxicated patient consists of the following measures (Table 35-6).

Nonspecific

Emesis should be induced with the appropriate dose of syrup of ipecac and then water. As an alternate approach, gastric lavage should be performed with the proper-sized tube and an adequate amount of lavage fluid.[73] These methods should be performed in a timely fashion.

Activated charcoal is an effective adsorbent for acetaminophen,[24] and its use is suggested to adsorb the remaining acetaminophen or to adsorb any other compound ingested in conjunction with the acetaminophen.[83] There is controversy concerning its role, however, because an orally administered antidote may be also absorbed by the activated charcoal.[24] If oral *N*-acetylcysteine as an antidote (see below) is deemed necessary, an attempt could be made to remove the charcoal by gastric lavage before its administration. Even so, coadministration of activated charcoal and oral *N*-acetylcysteine has not been shown to affect peak *N*-acetylcysteine concentrations, absorption rate, time to peak concentration, or half-life.[84]

A cathartic should be administered in conjunction with the activated charcoal to decrease the transit time in the gastrointestinal tract.

Specific

A protocol for treatment of acetaminophen intoxication based on the drug's metabolism was tested in 1973. It was demonstrated that hepatotoxicity could be decreased by the administration of cysteine, which is a sulfhydryl precurser of glutathione. The protocol was based on the observation that when glutathione is present in sufficient quantity there is no toxic effect of acetaminophen on the liver, but when glutathione is depleted because of an overwhelming amount of acetaminophen metabolized through the cytochrome P-450 pathway liver toxicity may occur. Attempts have been made to find a glutathione substitute that offers protection to the liver by virtue of supplying sulfhydryl groups for use in the detoxification of acetaminophen's metabolic intermediary. Glutathione, the obvious choice, is synthesized intracellularly and is not readily taken into cells when administered orally; it is also expensive and so has not met with success.[63] A number of smaller sulfhydryl substances, however, can be taken into hepatocytes and have been found to be effective. Methionine, a precurser of glutathione, had been tried in the past but was abandoned because of some of the adverse reactions associated with its use.[53,63,83,85] For the same reason cysteamine, a glutathione substitute, was tried and abandoned.[86,87]

N-Acetylcysteine

The antidote of choice for acetaminophen overdose in the last few years has been N-acetylcysteine (Mucomyst®, N-acetyl-3-mercaptoalanine), an N-acetyl derivative of the naturally occurring amino acid L-cysteine.[10,33,88,89] N-Acetylcysteine has been in clinical use as a mucolytic agent since the mid-1950s. There is a relatively wide margin of safety between therapeutic and toxic doses. This compound has been shown to offer protection against liver toxicity when administered within the first 24 hours after an acute acetaminophen overdose.[70,90] Statistically significant differences in severity of hepatotoxicity have been observed between patients treated within 16 hours after ingestion and those treated between 16 and 24 hours after ingestion.[10] Because of this, it is suggested that treatment begin within the first 16 hours after an acute ingestion.[36,66] Initiating therapy after 24 hours appears not to be effective.

Mechanism of action. N-Acetylcysteine is metabolized to cysteine and is taken up by cells, where it acts as a glutathione substitute, combining directly with the hepatotoxic metabolite to detoxify it. There may be other mechanisms by which N-acetylcysteine is effective, as evidenced by studies showing an increase in the rate of elimination of acetaminophen after administration of N-acetylcysteine. This finding suggests that it may also serve as a biologic source of inorganic sulfate, enhancing the formation of acetaminophen sulfate and thereby allowing metabolism through nontoxic routes.[38,73,89,91] Another proposed mechanism for this compound is that it may stabilize cellular constituents against the possible deleterious effects of the covalent binding of the reactive metabolite.[40,92]

Route of administration. N-Acetylcysteine may be administered orally or intravenously. It has been approved for intravenous use in Canada and Europe[66] and is the therapy of choice in the United Kingdom, where it has been shown to be well tolerated and effective.[86,87] In the United States, a special pyrogen-free preparation is available for investigational use.

The intravenous protocol under investigation in the United States differs considerably from that used in Europe and Canada. The rationale for intravenous administration is that, because vomiting is a frequent effect in most patients receiving oral N-acetylcysteine, administering it parenterally would ensure complete absorption.[85,86] Nevertheless, activated charcoal can be administered as long as it is retrieved before administration of the antidote. Some investigators believe that there are theoretical advantages to the oral administration of N-acetylcysteine because of a significant first-pass effect, which would cause a significant portion of the drug to be extracted by the liver (the organ requiring protection) because of direct entry through the portal vein.[41,66,84]

Dosage. The current recommended dosage regimen for *N*-acetylcysteine is to administer a loading dose of 140 mg/kg and then a maintenance dose of 70 mg/kg every 4 hours for 17 additional doses or for a total of 72 hours. This is given as a 10% or 20% solution diluted to 5% with a soft drink or juice to disguise the unpleasant taste. If the patient refuses to ingest the material, it can be administered down a nasogastric tube. If the drug is administered orally and the patient has an emesis within 1 hour, the dose should be repeated.[10,66] If emesis persists, insertion of a weighted tube such as a Miller-Abbott or Cantor tube and administration directly into the duodenum are suggested.

The intravenous protocol used in the United States consists of the same loading and maintenance doses as are used in the oral route. The preparation for intravenous use is administered for only 2 days.[66] *N*-Acetylcysteine is administered on the basis of a potentially toxic plasma concentration of acetaminophen obtained from the nomogram. Once treatment has begun, subsequent measurements of plasma concentration should be of interest only and should not be used to determine whether treatment should continue. Even if a second concentration shows a decrease below the nomogram line, treatment should continue for the entire course. If treatment is started before a measurement of plasma acetaminophen concentration is available, it should be terminated in patients subsequently found not to be at risk.

Even though children less than 6 years of age with confirmed toxic blood concentrations of acetaminophen are unlikely to develop significant toxic effects, the recommendation is that any child with a plasma acetaminophen concentration in the toxic range on the nomogram should be offered the same treatment as adults.[34,66]

In a patient being treated with *N*-acetylcysteine, serial liver function tests should be performed. These should include the tests described in Table 35-5 as well as serum blood urea nitrogen and serum creatinine determinations.

Side effects. *N*-Acetylcysteine does not have some of the adverse effects seen with other antidotes, such as increasing the likelihood of liver failure if administered too late in the course of an ingestion. It is relatively free from major adverse reactions when administered orally. When given parenterally, allergy and anaphylaxis have been reported 15 to 60 minutes after the onset of infusion; symptoms include angioedema, bronchospasm, flushing, hypotension, nausea, vomiting, rash, pruritus, and tachycardia.[93] These reactions are rare and are not associated with oral use.[34] The safety of *N*-acetylcysteine in pregnancy is not established.

Other Methods

As stated above, in patients who are treated more than 24 hours after an overdose of acetaminophen *N*-acetylcysteine appears not to be effective. Such patients should be treated by supportive measures such as reduction of protein intake and neomycin enemas to reduce the degree of liver toxicity.[9,10] In addition, fresh frozen plasma, vitamin K, and glucose may be administered if the patient shows signs of hypoprothrombinemia or hypoglycemia.

Despite the known potential for toxicity in massive overdose of acetaminophen, the great majority of cases do not result in fatalities, serious liver toxicity, or long-term complications. Mortality rates in patients with toxic plasma concentrations who do not receive antidotal therapy have been in the range of 2% to 4%.

SUMMARY

In summary, an overdose of acetaminophen may overwhelm the liver stores of glutathione and cause a rise in liver enzymes, which reflects the hepatic toxicity that may ensue. The patient can be protected from this by the timely administration of *N*-acetylcysteine, which supplies sulfhydryl groups to the toxic intermediary. Therapy should ideally be instituted as soon as possible, but significant protection is achieved if the antidote is administered within the first 24 hours.[10]

REFERENCES

1. Black M, Raucy J: Acetaminophen, alcohol, and cytochrome P-450. *Ann Intern Med* 1986;104:427–428.

2. Prescott L, Matthew J: Cysteamine for paracetamol overdosage. *Lancet* 1974;1:998.

3. Proudfoot A, Wright N: Acute paracetamol poisoning. *Br Med J* 1970;3:557–558.

4. Hinson J: Reactive metabolites of phenacetin and acetaminophen: A review. *Environ Health Perspect* 1983; 49:71–79.

5. Ameer B, Greenblatt D: Acetaminophen. *Ann Intern Med* 1977;87:202–209.

6. Spooner J, Harvey J: The history and usage of paracetamol. *J Int Med Res* 1976;4:1–6.

7. Levy G, Khanna N, Soda D, et al: Pharmacokinetics of acetaminophen in the human neonate. *Pediatrics* 1975;55:818–824.

8. Beaver W: Aspirin and acetaminophen as constituents of analgesic combinations. *Arch Intern Med* 1981; 141:293–300.

9. Rumack B, Matthew H: Acetaminophen poisoning. *Pediatrics* 1975;55:871–876.

10. Rumack B, Meredith T, Peterson R, et al: Panel discussion: Management of acetaminophen overdose. *Arch Intern Med* 1981;141:401–403.

11. Temple A: Emergency treatment of acetaminophen overdose. *Curr Top Emerg Med* 1981;3:1–5.

12. Gerber J, MacDonald J, Harbison R, et al: Effect of *N*-acetylcysteine on hepatic covalent binding of paracetamol (acetaminophen). *Lancet* 1977;1:657–658.

13. Prescott L, Sutherland G, Park J, et al: Cysteamine, methionine, and penicillamine in the treatment of paracetamol poisoning. *Lancet* 1976;2:109–113.

14. Clark R, Thompson R, Borirakchanyavat V, et al: Hepatic damage and death from overdose of paracetamol. *Lancet* 1973;1:66–69.

15. Goldfrank L, Kerstein R, Weisman R: Acute acetaminophen overdose. *Hosp Physician* 1980;16:52–60.

16. McJunkin B, Barwick K, Little W, et al: Fatal massive hepatic necrosis from acetaminophen overdose. *JAMA* 1976;236:1874–1875.

17. Gazzard B, Davis M, Spooner J, et al: Why do people use paracetamol for suicide? *Br Med J* 1976;1:212–213.

18. Cooper S: Comparative analgesic efficacies of aspirin and acetaminophen. *Arch Intern Med* 1981;141:282–285.

19. Levy G: Comparative pharmacokinetics of aspirin and acetaminophen. *Arch Intern Med* 1981;141:279–281.

20. Manoguerra A: Acetaminophen intoxication. *Clin Toxicol* 1979;14:151–155.

21. Yaffe S: Comparative efficacy of aspirin and acetaminophen in the reduction of fever in children. *Arch Intern Med* 1981;141:286–292.

22. Hansten P: Acetaminophen interactions. *Drug Interact Newslett* 1983;3:55–59.

23. Hayes A: Therapeutic implications of drug interactions with acetaminophen and aspirin. *Arch Intern Med* 1981;141:301–304.

24. Levy G, Houston B: Effect of activated charcoal on acetaminophen absorption. *Pediatrics* 1976;58:432–435.

25. Goulston K, Shyring A: Effect of paracetamol (*N*-acetyl-*p*-aminophenol) on gastrointestinal bleeding. *Gut* 1964; 5:463–466.

26. Jick H: Effects of aspirin and acetaminophen on gastrointestinal hemorrhage. *Arch Intern Med* 1981; 141:316–321.

27. Mielke C: Comparative effects of aspirin and acetaminophen on hemostasis. *Arch Intern Med* 1981; 141:305–310.

28. Mielke C, Herden D, Britten A, et al: Hemostasis, antipyretics and mild analgesics. *JAMA* 1976;235:613–616.

29. Antlitz A, Awalt L: A double-blind study of acetaminophen used in conjunction with oral anticoagulant therapy. *Curr Ther Res* 1969;11:360–361.

30. Clements J, Heading R, Nimmo W, et al: Kinetics of acetaminophen absorption and gastric emptying in man. *Clin Pharmacol Ther* 1978;24:420–431.

31. Slattery J, Koup J, Levy G: Acetaminophen pharmacokinetics after overdose. *Clin Toxicol* 1981;18:111–117.

32. Slattery J, Levy G: Acetaminophen kinetics in acutely poisoned patients. *Clin Pharmacol Ther* 1979;25:184–185.

33. Prescott L, Roscoe P, Wright N, et al: Plasma paracetamol half-life with hepatic necrosis in patients with paracetamol overdosage. *Lancet* 1971;1:519–522.

34. Rumack B, Peterson R: Acetaminophen overdose: Incidence, diagnosis and management in 416 patients. *Pediatrics* 1978;62(suppl):901.

35. Ferguson D, Snyder S, Cameron A: Hepatotoxicity in acetaminophen poisoning. *Mayo Clin Proc* 1977;52: 246–248.

36. Rumack B, Peterson R, Koch G, et al: Acetaminophen overdose: 662 cases with evaluation of oral acetylcysteine treatment. *Arch Intern Med* 1981;141:380–385.

37. Gillette J: An integrated approach to the study of chemically reactive metabolites of acetaminophen. *Arch Intern Med* 1981;141:375–379.

38. Mitchell J, Thorgeirsson S, Potter W, et al: Acetaminophen-induced hepatic injury: Protective role of glutathione in man and rationale for therapy. *Clin Pharmacol Ther* 1974;16:676–684.

39. Mitchell J, Jollow D, Potter W, et al: Acetaminophen-induced hepatic necrosis: Part I: Role of drug metabolism. *J Pharmacol Exp Ther* 1973;187:185–201.

40. Prescott L: Paracetamol overdose: Pharmacological considerations and clinical management. *Drugs* 1983; 25:290–314.

41. Flanagan R: The role of acetylcysteine in clinical toxicology. *Med Toxicol* 1987;2:93–104.

42. Flanagan R, Mant T: Coma and metabolic acidosis early in severe acute paracetamol poisoning. *Hum Toxicol* 1986;5:179–182.

43. Hinson J, Nelson S, Mitchell J: Studies on the microsomal formation of arylating metabolites of acetaminophen and phenacetin. *Mol Pharmacol* 1977;13:625–633.

44. Gemborys M, Gribble G, Mudge G: Synthesis of *N*-hydroxyacetaminophen, a postulated toxic metabolite of acetaminophen, and its phenolic sulfate conjugate. *J Med Chem* 1978;21:649–652.

45. Mitchell J, Jollow D: Metabolic activation of drugs to toxic substances. *Gastroenterology* 1975;68:392–410.

46. Mitchell J, Lauterburg B: Drug-induced liver injury. *Hosp Pract* 1978;13:95–106.

47. Potter W, Thorgeirsson S, Jollow D: Acetaminophen-induced hepatic necrosis: Part V: Correlation of hepatic necrosis, covalent binding and glutathione depletion in hamsters. *Pharmacology* 1974;12:129–143.

48. Abramowicz M: Acetaminophen hepatotoxicity. *Med Lett Drug Ther* 1978;20:61–63.

49. Jollow D, Thorgeirsson S, Potter W, et al: Acetaminophen-induced hepatic necrosis: Part VI: Metabolic disposition of toxic and nontoxic doses of acetaminophen. *Pharmacology* 1974;12:251–271.

50. Black M: Acetaminophen hepatotoxicity. *Annu Rev Med* 1984;35:577–593.

51. Gazzard B, Willson R, Weston M, et al: Charcoal hemoperfusion for paracetamol overdose. *Br J Clin Pharmacol* 1974;1:271–274.

52. Boyer T, Rouff S: Acetaminophen-induced hepatic necrosis and renal failure. *JAMA* 1971;218:440–441.

53. Maxwell L, Cotty V, Marcus A, et al: Prevention of acetaminophen poisoning. *Lancet* 1975;2:610–611.

54. Forrest J, Aldrienssens P, Finlayson N, et al: Paracetamol metabolism in chronic liver disease. *Eur J Clin Pharmacol* 1979;15:427–431.

55. Benson G: Acetaminophen in chronic liver disease. *Clin Pharmacol Ther* 1983;33:95–101.

56. Barker J, Carle D, Anuras S: Chronic excessive acetaminophen use and liver damage. *Ann Intern Med* 1977;87:299–301.

57. Johnson G, Tolman K: Chronic liver disease and acetaminophen. *Ann Intern Med* 1977;83:302–304.

58. Lesser P, Vielti M, Clark W: Lethal enhancement of therapeutic doses of acetaminophen by alcohol. *Dig Dis Sci* 1986;31:103–105.

59. Clark P, Clark J, Wheatley J: Urine discoloration after acetaminophen overdose. *Clin Chem* 1986;32:1777–1778.

60. Prescott L: Treatment of severe acetaminophen poisoning with intravenous acetylcysteine. *Arch Intern Med* 1981;141:386–389.

61. Jackson J: Cimetidine protects against acetaminophen hepatotoxicity. *Vet Hum Toxicol* 1981;23:7–9.

62. Ruffalo R, Thompson J: Cimetidine and acetylcysteine as antidotes for acetaminophen overdose. *South Med J* 1982;75:954–958.

63. Prescott L, Newton R, Swainson C, et al: Successful treatment of severe paracetamol overdosage with cysteamine. *Lancet* 1974;1:588–592.

64. Critchley J, Scott A, Dyson E, et al: Is there a place for cimetidine or ethanol in the treatment of paracetamol poisoning? *Lancet* 1983;1:1375–1376.

65. Nogen A, Bremme J: Fatal acetaminophen overdosage in a young child. *J Pediatr* 1978;95:832–833.

66. Rumack B: Acetaminophen overdose in children and adolescents. *Pediatr Clin North Am* 1986;33:691–701.

67. Miller R, Roberts R, Fisher L: Acetaminophen elimination kinetics in neonates, children and adults. *Clin Pharmacol Ther* 1976;19:284–294.

68. Peterson R, Rumack B: Toxicity of acetaminophen overdose. *JACEP* 1978;7:202–205.

69. Peterson R, Rumack B: Pharmacokinetics of acetaminophen in children. *Pediatrics* 1978;62 (suppl):877–879.

70. Peterson R, Rumack B: Age as a variable in acetaminophen overdose. *Arch Intern Med* 1981;141:390–393.

71. Spyker D: Expediting accurate assessment and specific therapy in acetaminophen poisoning. *Emerg Med Rep* 1987;8:1–8.

72. Atwood S: The laboratory in the diagnosis and management of acetaminophen and salicylate intoxications. *Pediatr Clin North Am* 1980;27:871–879.

73. Prescott L, Park J, Proudfoot A: Cysteamine for paracetamol poisoning. *Lancet* 1976;1:357.

74. Bridges R, Kinneburgh D, Keehn B, et al: An evaluation of common methods for acetaminophen quantitation for small hospitals. *J Toxicol Clin Toxicol* 1983;20:1–17.

75. Osterloh J: Limitations of acetaminophen assays. *J Toxicol Clin Toxicol* 1983;20:19–22.

76. Gazzard B, Clark R, Borirakchavyavat V, et al: A controlled trial of heparin therapy in the coagulation defect of paracetamol-induced hepatic necrosis. *Gut* 1974;15:89–93.

77. Widdop B, Medd R, Braithwaite R, et al: Experimental drug intoxication: Treatment with charcoal hemoperfusion. *Arch Toxicol* 1975;34:27–32.

78. Willson R, Winch J, Thompson R, et al: Rapid removal of paracetamol by hemoperfusion through coated charcoal. *Lancet* 1973;1:77–82.

79. Helliwell M, Essex E: Hemoperfusion in ''late'' paracetamol poisoning. *Clin Toxicol* 1981;18:1225–1233.

80. Farid N, Glynn J, Kerr D: Hemodialysis in paracetamol self-poisoning. *Lancet* 1972;2:396–398.

81. Winchester J, Gelfand M, Helliwell M, et al: Extracorporeal treatment of salicylate or acetaminophen poisoning—Is there a role? *Arch Intern Med* 1981;141:370–374.

82. Maclean D, Peters T, Brown P, et al: Treatment of acute paracetamol poisoning. *Lancet* 1968;2:849–852.

83. Klein-Schwartz W, Oderda G: Adsorption of oral antidotes for acetaminophen poisoning (methionine and *N*-acetylcysteine) by activated charcoal. *Clin Toxicol* 1981;18:283–290.

84. Renzi F, Donovan J, Marten T, et al: Concomitant use of activated charcoal and N-acetylcysteine. *Ann Emerg Med* 1985;14:568–572.

85. Vale J, Meredith T, Crome P, et al: Intravenous N-acetylcysteine: The treatment of choice in paracetamol poisoning?, editorial. *Br Med J* 1979;2:1435–1436.

86. Prescott L, Illingworth R, Critchley J, et al: Intravenous N-acetylcysteine: Still the treatment of choice for paracetamol poisoning, editorial. *Br Med J* 1980;1:46–47.

87. Prescott L, Illingworth R, Critchley J, et al: Intravenous N-acetylcysteine: The treatment of choice for paracetamol poisoning. *Br Med J* 1979;2:1097–1100.

88. Peterson R, Rumack B: Treating acute acetaminophen poisoning with acetylcysteine. *JAMA* 1977; 237:2406–2407.

89. Galinsky R, Levy G: Effect of N-acetylcysteine on the pharmacokinetics of acetaminophen in rats. *Life Sci* 1979;5:693–700.

90. Piperno E, Berssenbruegge D: Reversal of experimental paracetamol toxicosis with N-acetylcysteine. *Lancet* 1976;2:738–739.

91. Pond S, Tong T, Kaysen G, et al: Massive intoxication with acetaminophen and propoxyphene: Unexpected survival and unusual pharmacokinetics of acetaminophen. *J Toxicol Clin Toxicol* 1982;19:1–16.

92. Labadarios D, Davis M, Portmann B, et al: Paracetamol-induced hepatic necrosis in the mouse: Relationship between covalent binding, hepatic glutathione depletion and the protective effect of α-mercaptopropionylglycine. *Biochem Pharmacol* 1977;26:31–35.

93. Walton N, Mann T, Shaw K: Anaphylactoid reaction to N-acetylcysteine. *Lancet* 1979;2:1298.

ADDITIONAL SELECTED REFERENCES

Gilligan J, Kemp R, Pain R, et al: Paracetamol concentrations, hepatotoxicity, and antidotes. *Br Med J* 1980; 280:114.

Hamlyn A, James O, Douglas A: Treatment of paracetamol overdose. *Lancet* 1976;2:362.

Heading R, Nimmo J, Prescott L, et al: The dependence of paracetamol absorption on the rate of gastric emptying. *Br J Pharmacol* 1973;47:415–421.

Hinson J, Pohl L, Monks T, et al: Acetaminophen-induced hepatotoxicity. *Life Sci* 1981;29:107–116.

James O, Lesna M, Roberts S: Liver damage after paracetamol overdosage. *Lancet* 1975;2:579–581.

Koch-Weser J: Acetaminophen. *N Engl J Med* 1976; 295:1297–1300.

Manor E, Marmor A, Kaufman S, et al: Massive hemolysis caused by acetaminophen. *JAMA* 1976;236:2777–2778.

Meredith T, Vale J, Goulding R: The epidemiology of acute acetaminophen poisoning in England and Wales. *Arch Intern Med* 1981;141:397–400.

Mitchell M, Schenker S, Avant G, et al: Cimetidine protects against acetaminophen hepatotoxicity in rats. *Gastroenterology* 1981;81:1052–1060.

Pearson H: Comparative effects of aspirin and acetaminophen on hemostasis. *Pediatrics* 1978;62 (suppl): 926–929.

Plotz P, Kimberly R: Acute effects of aspirin and acetaminophen on renal function. *Arch Intern Med* 1981;141:343–348.

Schreiner G, McAnally J, Winchester J: Clinical analgesic nephropathy. *Arch Intern Med* 1981;141:349–357.

Seeff L, Cuccherini B, Zimmerman H, et al: Acetaminophen hepatotoxicity in alcoholics. *Ann Intern Med* 1986; 104:399–404.

Stewart M, Barclay J: Emergency estimation of plasma paracetamol. *Lancet* 1976;1:362–363.

Vale J, Meredith T, Goulding R, et al: Treatment of acetaminophen poisoning: The use of oral methionine. *Arch Intern Med* 1981;141:394–396.

Wilson J, Kasantikul V, Harbison R, et al: Death in an adolescent following an overdose of acetaminophen and phenobarbital. *Am J Dis Child* 1978;132:466–473.

Zimmerman H: Effects of aspirin and acetaminophen on the liver. *Arch Intern Med* 1981;141:333–342.

chapter 36

Salicylates

Salicylates in rudimentary form have been known since ancient times and were first described by Hippocrates. Toxicity was described much later, after aspirin (acetylsalicylic acid) was synthesized by the Bayer company in the 1850s. For many decades salicylate intoxication was the leading cause of accidental poisonings and deaths among children.[1-3] Although recently there has been a substantial reduction in these accidental poisonings and deaths,[4-6] salicylate poisoning continues to be relatively common because of accidental ingestion in children, intentional overdose in adults, and therapeutic intoxication in persons of all ages.[7-9] The great decrease in the number of accidental pediatric salicylate ingestions and deaths over the last few years is due primarily to the introduction of safety lids on containers, the restriction on the number of flavored aspirin to 45 grains or 36 1.25-grain tablets per container, and the decreased use of salicylates in children.[4-6,9] More than 20 billion tablets of salicylate are consumed per year,[10] and more than 200 aspirin-containing products are available. Salicylates probably exist in more different formulations than any other drug.[11]

Salicylates are nonsteroidal, anti-inflammatory, synthetic derivatives of salicylic acid.[6,12] Salicylic acid is not used systemically because of its severe irritating effect on gastrointestinal mucosa and other tissues. Because of these side effects, better tolerated chemical derivatives have been prepared for systemic use (Table 36-1). Acetylsalicylic acid (ASA, aspirin) is the prototypical salicylate found in most compound analgesics. Aspirin is metabolized by hy-

Table 36-1 Commonly Used Salicylates by Trade Name

Type of Salicylate	Trade Name(s)
Aspirin	Anacin
	Alka-Seltzer
	ASA
	Ascriptin
	Bufferin
	Easprin
	Measurin
	Ecotrin
	Zorprin
Choline magnesium trisalicylate	Arthropan
	Trilisate
Magnesium salicylate	Durasal
	Magan
	Mobidin
	Trilisate
Methyl salicylate	Oil of wintergreen
Salsalate	Disalcid
	Arcylate
Salicylic acid	Calicylic
	Fomac
	Keralyt
	Mediplast
	Debucare

drolysis into the active salicylate and acetate. Sodium, choline, and magnesium salts of salicylate are also used as antipyretics and are hydrolyzed into salicylic acid. Salsalate is the salicylate ester of salicylic acid and hydrolyzes to two molecules of salicylate. All these drugs distribute rapidly throughout all tissues and are bound to serum proteins, especially to albumin. A topical preparation, methyl salicylate (also known as oil of wintergreen), is the most toxic salicylate compound because of the high content of salicylate (7 g per 5 mL). This is equivalent to 21 325-mg tablets of aspirin and can be rapidly lethal in young children.[12] Methyl salicylate is also an ingredient in Ben-Gay®. Salicylic acid ointment, a topical preparation used for removing scales of psoriasis and corns, can also cause salicylate intoxication. Aspercreme® and kerolytic agents[12] are examples of this salicylic compound.

Although related to the salicylates structurally and pharmacologically, salicylamide and sodium thiosalicylate are not hydrolyzed to salicylate. Diflunisal is a salicylic acid derivative that is not metabolized to salicylic acid and has less of an effect than aspirin on platelet function.[13] For this reason these compounds are not considered true salicylates. Salicylamide is a weak analgesic and is a substance in some over-the-counter preparations. It was once commonly used for the pediatric population. Salicylamide has a different toxicity than aspirin and is relatively ineffective and unreliable as an antipyretic.

ACTIONS

All the salicylates have analgesic, anti-inflammatory, and antipyretic actions. The salicylates act as antipyretics by altering the response of the hypothalamus to pyrogens, which then causes vasodilation and sweating.[14] These effects are due to the actions of both the acetyl and the salicylate portions of the molecule as well as the active salicylate metabolite.

The irreversible inhibition of platelet aggregation that is one of aspirin's effects specifically involves its ability to act as an acetyl donor to the platelet membrane; the nonacetylated salicylates have no clinically significant effect on platelet

aggregation. Salicylates other than aspirin may therefore be particularly useful in patients with gastrointestinal intolerance to aspirin or in patients in whom interference of normal platelet function by aspirin or other nonsteroidal anti-inflammatory agents is undesirable. The anti-inflammatory and toxic effects of the drug are produced by the hydrolysis product, salicylic acid.

Peripherally, salicylates inhibit the synthesis of prostaglandins in inflamed tissues and thus prevent the sensitization of pain receptors to mechanical stimulation or to chemicals such as bradykinin that appear to mediate the pain response.

PHARMACOKINETICS

Salicylic acid is a weak acid with a pKa of 3 and thus tends to ionize to a greater degree at an alkaline pH and to a lesser degree at an acidic pH.[15,16] Although the volume of distribution of salicylates increases with increasing plasma concentration, in the therapeutic range it is usually between 0.15 and 0.2 L/kg. In toxic states the volume of distribution can increase to more than 0.6 L/kg; this is due to decreased binding of salicylate to plasma proteins.[9] The practical implication of this phenomenon is that high serum concentrations result in disproportionately high tissue concentrations.

The biologic half-life of aspirin in the therapeutic situation is about 15 minutes, and the half-life of salicylic acid is 2 to 4 hours except in an overdose situation, when it can be more than 20 hours. In therapeutic situations, plasma concentrations of salicylate greater than 30 mg/dL are often associated with adverse systemic effects.[16]

Absorption

The absorption of salicylate is quite rapid under normal circumstances, and serum concentrations are measurable in 15 to 30 minutes.[1] The oral absorption of salicylate is limited by the rate of dissolution of the particular preparation. When antacid is added to the salicylate, absorption is increased.[16]

Aspirin is not stable in solution and must be dissolved just before use. This usually requires the addition of a base, typically sodium bicarbonate, because the weakly acidic aspirin is not readily water soluble.

The absorption of enteric-coated tablets is erratic, delayed, and sometimes incomplete; such tablets may be found many hours later still undissolved in the gastrointestinal tract.[15,17] Clinical toxicity and peak plasma salicylate levels may not appear for as long as 12 hours or even longer.[12] Patients who retain these enteric-coated preparations in the stomach are at risk for multiple gastric perforations and rapid death. Rectal suppositories are also absorbed very slowly and incompletely. The viscous preparation of methyl salicylate may take as long as 6 to 8 hours to be absorbed in significant amounts.[12]

Even though therapeutic amounts of aspirin are absorbed rapidly, large doses of aspirin may be absorbed slowly partly because of the inhibitory effect of aspirin on gastric emptying and the impaired dispersion of the salicylate in gastrointestinal fluids. It has been shown that large doses of salicylates can result in delayed absorption from salicylate-induced pylorospasm. Because of these factors, in the acutely overdosed patient the plasma salicylate concentration may rise continually for as long as 24 hours after an ingestion. In addition, the formation of concretions (or bezoar) has been reported with aspirin overdose and may result in continued absorption for several days even after charcoal and cathartics have been administered.

There are many causes of intoxication by salicylates (salicylism), such as the administration of aspirin in too large a dose,[9,18] the administration of adult aspirin or adult rectal suppositories to a child,[8,9] and concomitant administration of salicylate with other salicylate-containing medicines.[9,19] This last is common because many over-the-counter preparations contain aspirin and may be taken for various reasons. In addition to these causes of acute salicylism, chronic salicylate intoxication can occur after the prolonged routine administration of aspirin to a dehydrated patient or to one with other alterations in body homeostasis.[17] Chronic salicylism may also occur in young children with an acute illness who are receiving salicylate too frequently or in elderly patients who, because of the chronicity of their problems, may be taking salicylate over a long period of time and become intoxicated in an insidious manner.[19] Serious salicylate poisonings now seem to be most commonly associated with long-term or therapeutic administration of aspirin because of the peculiar metabolism of the salicylates, which change kinetics and begin to accumulate even with therapeutic doses.[20,21]

Metabolism

Salicylate is metabolized principally in the liver by the microsomal enzyme system and is predominately conjugated with glycine to form salicyluric acid.[6,20] Salicylate is also conjugated with glucuronic acid to form salicylphenolic glucuronide and salicylacyl glucuronide.[22] In addition, small amounts of salicylate are hydrolyzed to form gentisic acid, which is an active metabolite and a potent inhibitor of prostaglandin synthesis. Renal excretion of the unmetabolized drug also occurs.

Two of these pathways, those involved in the formation of salicyluric acid and salicylphenolic glucuronide, are of limited capacity and are rapidly saturated even at therapeutic plasma salicylate concentrations.[6,17] This is an example of Michaelis-Menten kinetics, which leads to possible accumulation and intoxication at therapeutic doses.[9,22] Therefore, a 50% increase in the daily dose of aspirin may produce a 300% increase in the concentration of salicylate in the serum.[16]

As a consequence of the saturation of the salicylurate and salicylphenolic glucuronide pathways, the renal excretory pathway contributes even more to the elimination of salicylate as the dose increases, giving urinary pH a much greater role in either enhancing or retarding excretion.[16,22] For example, renal excretion of unmetabolized drug is usually less than 19% at low doses, but it could account for 50% or more at high doses or in an overdose if the pH of the urine is properly adjusted. Renal excretion of salicylate and formation of salicylic acid glucuronides become relatively more important elimination pathways for large single doses and for multiple doses that produce high plasma salicylate concentrations.[17]

At some therapeutic plasma concentrations salicylate follows first-order kinetics, so that as more is ingested more is excreted in a linear fashion. At high therapeutic doses and for toxic concentrations, excretion changes to zero-order kinetics, allowing only a certain quantity to be excreted hourly regardless of the amount present in the plasma.[23] When a steady state from repeated doses occurs, as in the long-term administration of salicylates, then saturation kinetics may take effect, and relatively small increases in dose result in large increases in plasma concentration.[15] Chronic salicylism, therefore, occurs because of the early saturation of these enzymes and a switch in the kinetics from first-order to zero-order elimination.[16]

TOXICITY

Clinical Features

The pathophysiology of salicylate overdose is complex because of the range of toxic effects produced and their manifestations (Table 36-2). The principal toxic effects are extensions of the drug's pharmacologic actions and include direct CNS stimulation of respiration, uncoupling of oxidative phosphorylation leading to hyperpyrexia, electrolyte disturbances and dehydration, altered glucose metabolism through inhibition of Krebs cycle enzymes, interference with hemostatic mechanisms leading to clotting disorders, and local gastrointestinal irritation leading to gastrointestinal bleeding.[3,5,9] Acute renal failure, CNS dysfunction, and pulmonary edema are the more serious consequences of salicylism.[6,24]

Respiratory Alkalosis

Early acid-base disturbances occur because aspirin increases medullary sensitivity to carbon dioxide, directly stimulating the CNS respiratory center in the medulla oblongata and resulting in hyperpnea and tachypnea.[6] This leads to a decreased Pco_2, an increased pH, and respiratory alkalosis (Table 36-3).[9,25,26] Because of the excretion of the acidic carbon dioxide through the lungs a compensatory increase in the renal excretion of bicarbonate occurs, which then causes loss of potassium and sodium in the

Table 36-2 Disorders Associated with Salicylate Overdose

Acid-base disturbance
Hyperpyrexia
Electrolyte disorder
Dehydration
Clotting disorder
Gastrointestinal bleeding
Acute renal failure
CNS depression
Pulmonary edema

Table 36-3 Pathophysiology of Respiratory Alkalosis

Stimulation of respiratory center
Increased respirations
Increased carbon dioxide excretion
Decreased Pco_2
Increased plasma pH
Increased renal excretion of bicarbonate

urine.[27] Many intoxicated adults and older children present with respiratory alkalosis with early bicarbonate excretion.[17] This alkalosis fortuitously slows the entrance of salicylate into tissues and organs, including the brain.

It has been shown that the effects of CNS depressants may blunt the hypocapneic effect of salicylates, thereby reducing the incidence of respiratory alkalosis.[27] Ingestion of CNS depressant drugs with aspirin, however, may not only diminish salicylate-induced hyperventilation in some patients but may also cause hypoventilation and respiratory acidosis, thus worsening the patient's condition.[25]

Metabolic Acidosis

A metabolic acidosis (Table 36-4) may follow the physiologic compensation of respiratory alkalosis for a number of reasons. Acidosis develops principally from accumulation of organic acids. Salicylate and its metabolic byproducts represent a large acid load but do not fully account for the metabolic acidosis.[26] Pyruvic and lactic acids accumulate from the inhibition of α-ketoglutaric and succinic acid dehydrogenases of the Krebs cycle. In addition, inhibition of amino transferases causes an increase in the amount of amino acids, and increased lipid metabolism leads to increased

Table 36-4 Pathophysiology of Metabolic Acidosis

Inhibition of Krebs cycle
Increased amounts of pyruvic and lactic acids
Increased peripheral demand for glucose
Stimulation of lipid metabolism
Increased formation of ketones

amounts of ketones such as acetoacetic acid, β-hydroxybutryic acid, and acetone.[9,27] Inorganic phosphoric and sulfuric acids accumulate secondary to salicylate-induced renal impairment.[25] Depletion of buffer capacity as a result of the initial compensatory increase in renal excretion of bicarbonate also contributes to the development of metabolic acidosis. Together these changes produce a decrease in plasma *p*H and a metabolic acidosis.[26,27]

Metabolic acidosis, however, may not occur until 12 to 24 hours after an acute ingestion of salicylate in an adult.[28,29] The severity of the metabolic acidosis increases with decreasing age, and thus infants and children younger than 5 years of age are more susceptible to the development of ketosis with subsequent acidosis.[12] A more rapid metabolic acidosis occurs in children because their ability to increase alveolar ventilation is quickly overcome by the accumulated acids.[17] As a result, children quickly pass through the respiratory alkalosis stage to metabolic acidosis.

The likelihood of metabolic acidosis increases with the severity of salicylate intoxication.[9] Chronic salicylism, too, may present with a compensated metabolic acidosis. The acutely salicylate-intoxicated adult usually exhibits a simple or compensated respiratory alkalosis and seldom proceeds to acidosis unless the poisoning is severe or salicylate was taken together with a respiratory depressant.

Uncoupling of Oxidative Phosphorylation

Salicylates have been shown to uncouple oxidative phosphorylation,[3,30] resulting in failure to produce high-energy phosphates such as adenosine triphosphate while at the same time increasing oxygen utilization and carbon dioxide production, which increases heat production.[12] In other words, because of the uncoupling energy normally conserved as a nucleotide tri-phosphate (adenosine triphosphate) is dissipated as heat. In addition, salicylates in toxic doses decrease the efficiency of the normal cooling mechanisms. Hyperthermia may be striking, resulting in temperatures as high as 41° to 42°C (105.8° to 107.6°F).[30,31]

Hyperglycemia and Hypoglycemia

Uncoupling of oxidative phosphorylation increases tissue glycolysis and peripheral demand for glucose. The altered glucose metabolism may result in hyperglycemia or hypoglycemia. Hyperglycemia usually occurs early in the course of intoxication as a result of interference with tissue utilization of glucose.[9] Hypoglycemia, which can be severe, may occur late in the course of an acute intoxication after sufficient time has passed for glycogen stores to be depleted.[7] Hypoglycemia may be life threatening and is most likely to occur in infants.

Uncoupling of oxidative phosphorylation also leads to increased cerebral glycolysis.[32] CNS glucose may be depleted even when the rest of the body is maintaining normal glucose concentrations[32] because the rate of glucose utilization from cerebrospinal fluid may exceed the rate of supply by the blood.[9] Hypoglycemia should therefore be considered in a salicylate-intoxicated patient with seizures, coma, or altered mental status, and appropriate treatment should be initiated.[32] Concurrent administration of glucose with salicylate overdose has been associated with striking improvement.

Fluid and Electrolyte Disorders

Dehydration and electrolyte loss occur early in salicylate intoxication as a result of a number of factors (Table 36-5). Because salicylates cause diaphoresis, water and sodium are lost. Further, because of the hyperventilation that occurs directly from salicylate ingestion, there is greater than normal insensible water loss from the lungs, which contributes to dehydration.[7] Salicylates are an irritant to the gastrointestinal tract, causing vomiting and resultant fluid and electrolyte losses. Sodium and potassium are lost through the kidneys during respiratory alkalosis because the kidneys attempt to excrete bicarbonate and to conserve hydrogen ion.[3] Dehydration may also be enhanced by decreased intake of fluids.

Table 36-5 Pathophysiology of Fluid and Electrolyte Disturbances

---

Increased metabolism and heat production
Increased cutaneous insensible water loss through sweating
Organic aciduria and increased solute excretion
Increased renal output of water
Loss of gastric contents by emesis
Increased respiratory rate
Increased pulmonary insensible water loss
Increased renal excretion of bicarbonate
Increased excretion of sodium and potassium

Hypokalemia is caused by both renal and extrarenal factors. The renal factor is excretion of bicarbonate, sodium, and potassium to compensate for the respiratory alkalosis. The extrarenal factor is loss of potassium from cells and an accumulation of sodium and water in cells due to the inhibition of the active cellular system for sodium-potassium transport caused by the uncoupling of oxidative phosphorylation. Hypokalemia may be a significant clinical finding, so that special attention may be required to normalize potassium during treatment. Patients can be assumed to have total body potassium depletion even though normal serum potassium concentrations are present.

Clotting Disorders

Salicylates have important long-lasting effects on hemostasis. Clotting disorders occur because salicylates decrease the production of factor VIII, which results in a warfarin-like action of increasing prothrombin time; this can be treated by the administration of vitamin K.[9] Other disorders include decreased prothrombin formation, decreased platelet adhesiveness, increased capillary fragility, and even decreased platelet amounts.[25] The last effect is thought to be an autoimmune response. The effects of interference with platelet function remain for the life span of the platelets, which is 7 to 10 days. The result of this defect in platelet function is increased bleeding time[33] and is due to irreversible acetylation of platelet prostaglandin cyclo-oxygenase. It has been shown that aspirin doses as low as 5 grains interfere with platelet aggregation.[33] This effect is of possible therapeutic benefit in the prophylaxis of ischemic heart disease

and cerebral transient ischemic attacks.[34] Hypoprothrombinemia is considered secondary to inhibition of the vitamin K–dependent synthesis of factor VIII and, as stated above, can be reversed by administration of vitamin K.[33]

Although bleeding can occur for many reasons, it is rarely secondary to the inhibition of clotting mechanisms in acute salicylate overdose. If bleeding does occur, it is usually from the gastrointestinal tract because salicylates exert a local effect on the mucosal lining: particulate aspirin in contact with the gastric mucosa dissolves the protective mucous lining, resulting in superficial erosions.[35,36]

Signs and Symptoms of Intoxication

The possibility of salicylate poisoning should be considered in any patient who presents with unexplained hyperpnea in association with vomiting, confusion, lethargy, fever, coma, or convulsions (Table 36-6).[6,37] Nausea and vomiting commonly occur after salicylate overdose from the direct irritative effect on the gastric mucosa and the direct central effect, which is independent of the route of absorption. Tinnitus is also common in a significant overdose. As discussed, hyperpyrexia is a result of the uncoupling of oxidative phosphorylation. Hyperpnea is a reflection of the direct effect of salicylate on the respiratory center, causing a respiratory alkalosis (Table 36-7). Disorientation, coma, and seizures are ominous findings that suggest a serious overdose.[6]

Morbidity

The causes of morbidity from salicylate overdose are CNS dysfunction, cardiac dysfunction, and noncardiogenic pulmonary edema.[31]

Central Nervous System Dysfunction

Many of the deaths from salicylate poisoning are attributable to CNS dysfunction.[9,37] There appears to be a critical concentration of salicylate in brain tissue at which death occurs that is achieved over a wide range of serum salicylate concentrations.[38]

Table 36-6 Features of Acute Salicylate Intoxication

Gastrointestinal
  Nausea
  Vomiting
Neurologic
  Dizziness
  Confusion
  Vertigo
  Tinnitus
  Disorientation
  Hallucinations
  Coma
  Seizures
  Hearing loss
Miscellaneous
  Acid-base disorder
  Electrolyte disorder
  Hyperpnea
  Hyperpyrexia
  Diaphoresis
  Dehydration
  Oliguria
  Pulmonary edema

Table 36-7 Metabolic Abnormalities Associated with Salicylate Overdose

Hypoglycemia and hyperglycemia
Respiratory alkalosis
Metabolic acidosis
Hypokalemia
Hyponatremia and hypernatremia
Hypoprothrombinemia
Increased bleeding time
Ketosis
Altered renal function

Table 36-8 Central Nervous System Effects of Salicylate Overdose

Seizures
Coma
Cerebral edema
Disorientation
Irritability
Hallucinations

Symptoms of CNS dysfunction may include disorientation, hallucinations, and irritability or the more serious symptoms of coma, seizures, and cerebral edema (Table 36-8).[39] The severity of CNS symptoms is directly related to the concentration of salicylate in the brain.

Acidosis increases the permeability of brain tissue to salicylate from the intravascular space because a low *p*H shifts the ratio of ionized to nonionized salicylate in favor of the nonionized form.[9] Because the blood-brain barrier is more permeable to this nonionized salicylate, more of it will enter the brain if the *p*H is lowered.[38,40] As an example, a decrease in blood *p*H from 7.4 to 7.2 will double the amount of nonionized salicylate acid crossing the blood-brain barrier into the CNS.[41] Therefore, one of the major therapeutic goals is to correct or avoid an acidosis.

Seizures may be a result of hypoglycemia or hypocalcemia, both of which can occur secondary to alkalosis or may be due to a direct effect of salicylate on the brain.[38] Because seizures lead to a metabolic acidosis, their presence indicates a grave prognosis.

Another factor altering the distribution of salicylate is plasma protein binding. With high serum concentrations of salicylate, proportionately more is unbound and free to cross the blood-brain barrier.

Cardiac Dysfunction

Cardiac dysfunction may manifest as congestive heart failure, dysrhythmias, or sudden cardiac arrest. There are many factors contributing to cardiac abnormalities. The patient may be acidotic, hypokalemic, and hyperpyrexic, all of which may exacerbate any potential cardiac dysfunction and lead to decreased cardiac output and cardiac dysrhythmias.

Noncardiogenic Pulmonary Edema

Noncardiogenic pulmonary edema due to salicylate overdose is more common than has generally been realized.[5,24,28,42–47] Pulmonary edema, although rare in children, appears to be a significant complication of salicylate intoxication in adults older than 30 years of age.[5,48] Although pulmonary edema may occur from an acute overdose of salicylates, an increased risk for its development appears to be associated with chronic aspirin ingestion.[49] In addition, pulmonary edema may be precipitated or aggravated by forced alkaline diuresis, but volume overload is not necessary for its occurrence.[24,45]

The exact mechanism of salicylate-induced pulmonary edema remains unclear. Salicylates may cause pulmonary edema by increasing alveolar capillary membrane permeability.[50] Most experimental evidence indicates that salicylates induce pulmonary edema by damaging the pulmonary vascular endothelium, thereby increasing permeability to fluid and protein in the pulmonary vascular bed,[48,49] possibly mediated by inhibition of prostaglandin synthesis.[9,51] Inappropriate secretion of antidiuretic hormone resulting in fluid retention has also been implicated as a possible mechanism triggering pulmonary edema.[43] Some investigators have suggested that the edema may be centrally mediated and related to brain salicylate concentrations, secondary to hypoxia or myocardial failure, or due to a direct toxic effect of salicylate on the lungs or lung vasculature.[9,46]

Salicylate-induced noncardiogenic pulmonary edema is usually manifested by tachypnea or dyspnea and hypoxemia.[5] Physical examination usually reveals diffuse rales without signs of congestive heart failure such as gallop rhythm, cardiomegaly, peripheral edema, or jugular venous distension.[43] Diffuse, bilateral alveolar infiltrates may be seen on the chest roentgenogram. Because the edema is noncardiogenic, the cardiac silhouette is not enlarged unless coincidental cardiac dysfunction is present.[50] Proteinuria and adverse neurologic effects such as lethargy or confusion, profound respiratory failure, and the adult respiratory distress syndrome are often associated with pulmonary edema. Typically, patients with pulmonary edema may have a normal pulmonary capillary wedge pressure and are normotensive with normal cardiac output.[5] Pulmonary edema appears to occur more frequently when the serum salicylate concentration exceeds 40 mg/dL, but in general serum salicylate concentration correlates poorly with the subsequent development of pulmonary edema. With early diagnosis and prompt therapy most patients survive, and there is clearing of the chest roentgenogram in 1 to 7 days.

Chronic Salicylism

Although chronic salicylate poisoning frequently occurs, it may be occult and difficult to

Table 36-9 Signs and Symptoms of Chronic Salicylism

Gastrointestinal
  Gastrointestinal hemorrhage
  Gastric ulcer
  Nausea
  Vomiting
Neurologic
  Tinnitus
  Mental deterioration
  Personality changes
  Seizures
  Coma
  Hallucinations
  Confusion
  Disorientation
  Slurred speech
  Stupor
  Hyperpyrexia
Miscellaneous
  Pulmonary edema
  Hypotension
  Diaphoresis
  Tachypnea
  Abnormal bleeding diathesis

diagnose unless there is a high degree of suspicion.[12,17] Chronic salicylism usually occurs accidentally and unknowingly from ingestion of moderate doses of aspirin prescribed for coexisting medical conditions. Chronic salicylism is usually associated with significant mortality.[37] A 25% mortality has been reported in chronic salicylate intoxication when the diagnosis was delayed.[41] Many times the patient is elderly and on various medications containing salicylates and may present with atypical clinical features.[12] Because of the cumulative kinetics of salicylate intoxication, these symptoms may include tinnitus, gastric ulcer with a gastrointestinal hemorrhage, abnormal bleeding parameters, weight loss, and mental deterioration or signs of "senility" (Table 36-9). The possibility of salicylate intoxication should always be kept in mind when attempting to diagnose the cause of these abnormalities.[12]

Although serum salicylate concentrations are not reliable for an estimation of severity of intoxication or prognosis, they should be determined in all patients suspected of having chronic salicylism. A serum concentration in the therapeutic range does not rule out salicylate toxicity because the metabolic acidosis results in redistribution of salicylate from serum to tissue.[37]

Assessment of Severity of Salicylate Overdose

In acute salicylate ingestions, the severity of intoxication can be roughly estimated by obtaining a history of the amount ingested (Table 36-10), evaluating the clinical condition of the patient, and measuring serum salicylate concentration in relation to the time since ingestion.[20] As determined from the history, if the patient has ingested less than 150 mg/kg of salicylate the likelihood of any serious symptoms developing is negligible. Patients who ingest 150 to 300 mg/kg may experience mild to mod-

Table 36-10 Assessing Severity of Salicylate Overdose by History

Ingested Dose (milligrams per kilogram)	Estimated Severity
<150	Asymptomatic
150–300	Mild to moderate
300–500	Serious
>500	Potentially lethal

Source: Adapted with permission from *Archives of Internal Medicine* (1981;141:364–369), Copyright © 1981, American Medical Association.

erate toxic reactions. At doses in excess of 300 mg/kg patients may show prolonged and severe effects (Table 36-10).

Even though there may be an accurate history of the quantity ingested, laboratory evidence of

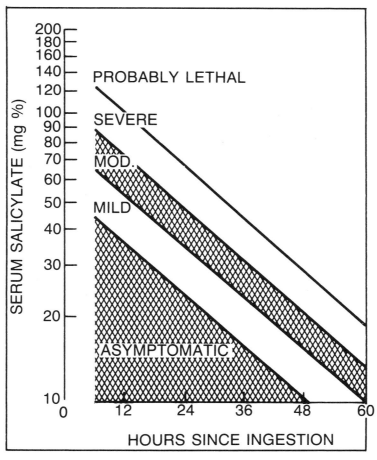

Figure 36-1 Salicylate nomogram for acute salicylate toxicity. *Source:* Reproduced by permission from *Pediatrics* (1960; 26:800), Copyright © 1960, American Academy of Pediatrics.

the drug in the blood should be relied on to make a prognosis and therapeutic decision. In the past, laboratory determinations were problematic because of the poor correlation between serum salicylate concentration and clinical severity. Efforts to resolve this problem gave rise to the salicylate nomogram (Fig. 36-1), which is based on the stronger correlation between serum salicylate concentrations and the severity of symptoms when the time of ingestion is used as a point of reference.[20,21] Severity is determined on the basis of the magnitude of the peak concentration, whenever it may have occurred.[52]

The nomogram may be helpful in deciding the need for hospitalization and the type of therapy that may be required. Nevertheless, it can only be used with single, acute ingestions and has no relevance to chronic or multiple ingestions.[39] It is also not applicable to overdoses with liquid salicylate preparations or enteric-coated tablets, for which peak concentrations may occur earlier (liquids) or later (enteric preparations) than for uncoated tablets.[20] Other factors that may delay salicylate absorption must be considered when using the nomogram, including concomitant use of narcotics or anticholinergic agents or pre-existing peptic ulcer disease.

The nomogram can be used for the acute ingestion of salicylates beginning at 6 hours after ingestion. Because absorption and distribution of salicylate may continue during the first 6 hours, blood concentrations measured before 6 hours should not be used to predict toxicity, although they may be useful in confirming an overdose.[20] More than one measurement should always be made to ensure that a peak concentration is obtained,[6] and a patient should never be released from the hospital on the basis of a single measurement. A concentration measured before 6 hours can be used if more than one measurement is made to establish that the concentration is declining.

For the patient who is within the asymptomatic range on the nomogram there are usually no objective signs of salicylate poisoning. The patient who falls within the mild range may experience some hyperpnea, lethargy, vomiting, and a small degree of hyperthermia. Acidosis is not usually noted. The patient in the moderate range has a greater degree of hyperpnea and may develop prominent neurologic disturbances, such as marked lethargy or perhaps excitability. More severe neurologic disturbances such as seizures or coma usually do not occur. Hypoglycemia may develop, and later in the course a compensated metabolic acidosis may ensue. The patient in the severe range may present in coma or become comatose, undergo seizures, and eventually develop a partially compensated metabolic acidosis. Usually patients with readings of moderate or severe on the salicylate nomogram require hospitalization.

In massive overdoses, plasma salicylate concentrations may continue to rise up to 24 hours after ingestion. Bezoar formation should be considered in a patient who does not respond to therapy as predicted or in whom serum salicylate concentrations continue to rise after therapy has been instituted.

LABORATORY ANALYSIS

A number of laboratory tests are recommended for the patient intoxicated with salicylate (Table 36-11). As discussed above, the plasma salicylate concentration is the single most important prognostic indicator for the salicylate-intoxicated patient. Arterial blood gases should be measured to confirm the patient's acid-base status, especially if bicarbonate therapy is to be instituted. A urine specimen should be obtained for pH measurement, and a complete blood cell count and prothrombin time studies should be performed for baseline analysis. Electrolyte studies should be performed because of the potential for acid-base and fluid and electrolyte imbalances.

Bedside tests may aid in the detection of salicylism in a qualitative manner.[17] The ferric chloride test can be performed on urine. This test is positive in the presence of any amount of salicylic acid, acetoacetic acid, or phenylpyruvic acid. Ferric chloride (10%) is added to a small amount of boiled urine, which removes any interfering substances such as ketones. A purple color indicates the presence of salicylates. A false-positive result may be produced by some phenothiazines.[20,53]

Phenistix® can be used in a semiquantitative manner[12]; this test is used in the diagnosis of

Table 36-11 Suggested Laboratory Tests for Salicylate Overdose

Plasma salicylate concentration
Arterial blood gases
Complete blood cell count
Urinalysis
Electrolytes
Prothrombin time

Table 36-12 Treatment of Salicylate Intoxication

Indication	Treatment
Acute overdose	Emesis or lavage
	Activated charcoal and cathartic
Dehydration	Correction of fluid losses with normal saline and potassium chloride
Acidosis	Alkali therapy with sodium
Coagulopathies	Vitamin K
Hyperthermia	Sponge baths
Hypoglycemia	Glucose (25 g IV)
Seizures	Antiseizure medicines (diazepam or short-acting barbiturates)
Pulmonary edema	Oxygen or positive end-expiratory pressure

phenylketonuria. Development of a color when a stick is dipped into serum or urine indicates that salicylate or phenothiazines are present. The addition of one drop of sulfuric acid bleaches out the color from phenothiazines but not from salicylate. If a tan color develops, the salicylate concentration is considered less than 40 mg/dL. A deeper brown indicates a concentration in the range of 40 to 90 mg/dL, and a purple color indicates a concentration greater than 90 mg/dL. A gray-green to blue color develops if the test is positive for phenylketonuria.[20,21]

TREATMENT

A specific antidote for salicylate is not available; consequently, treatment of intoxication is limited to symptomatic, supportive care (Table 36-12), which is not always adequate.[12] The emphasis should be on removing and adsorbing or decontaminating the remaining drug, control of hyperthermia, correction of the metabolic dis-

turbances and dehydration, and hastening of excretion of the drug.[9,12] Avoidance of systemic acidosis is a primary therapeutic goal in salicylate intoxication because acidemia has been shown to be associated with increased neurologic abnormalities and a grave prognosis. Care must be taken that there is no interference with carbon dioxide excretion through the lungs, so that adequate ventilation must be maintained.

Decontamination should be attempted if the intoxicant is a topically absorbed preparation such as salicylic acid or oil of wintergreen. Emesis or lavage and administration of activated charcoal and a cathartic should be performed for orally ingested salicylate even late after ingestion because there may be decreased absorption of salicylate when it is taken in large amounts in addition to the concretions that sometimes form.[12,54] Salicylates have a small volume of distribution and are dialyzable, so that multiple-dose activated charcoal has been suggested as a noninvasive approach to increasing clearance by an intestinal dialysis.[55]

Intravenous fluids may be administered for correction of fluid loss and diuresis. Correction of fluid loss should be vigorous, with fluid administered in volume to compensate for the great amounts that may have been lost. Repletion may be performed at a rate of as much as 10 to 15 mL/kg/hour for the first 1 to 2 hours and then 4 to 8 mL/kg/hour. Potassium chloride (20 to 40 mEq/L) should be added.[9]

There is controversy concerning the role of forced diuresis in the treatment of salicylate overdose. Proponents of forced diuresis have argued that it provides a safe and effective method of enhancing salicylate elimination, with clearance rates comparable to those achieved by hemodialysis.[56–58] Opponents have questioned its efficacy and emphasized possible side effects, including hypernatremia and fluid overload.[6] Large amounts of crystalloid solutions have the potential to increase lung microvasculature pressure and the transfer of fluid across the injured pulmonary vascular bed and to decrease colloid oncotic pressure, which is a factor that may be important in the pathogenesis of noncardiogenic pulmonary edema.[5]

Another concern is whether diuresis is effective in producing an alkaline urine in the severely intoxicated patient with electrolyte abnormalities.[6] Recently, sodium bicarbonate without a diuresis was shown to be at least as effective as bicarbonate diuresis in enhancing elimination of salicylate but, unlike the diuresis regimens, did not cause fluid retention or any noticeable biochemical abnormalities.[17,58] Until further work is done a conservative approach, with the use of bicarbonate and administration of fluids for the massive fluid losses and without the use of diuresis, is recommended.[5,58,59]

As a rule of thumb, a concentration of 30 mg/dL in adults indicates that renal excretion of salicylate should be enhanced by alkalinization.[17] Because acidemia carries such an ominous prognosis, it should be corrected as rapidly as possible to minimize the entry of salicylate into CNS and other tissues.[9,60] Furthermore, the acidotic state promotes retention of the drug because it reduces the effectiveness of the salicylate excretory mechanism of the kidney. Parenteral alkalinization with sodium bicarbonate, which is almost solely an extracellular alkalinizer, should be attempted for plasma ion trapping effects and to raise the pH of the urine for enhancement of excretion. The rate at which salicylate is removed from the body is augmented by making the urine alkaline, and a change in urine pH from 6.5 to 7.5 will enhance urinary excretion tenfold.[56]

Oral alkalinization enhances gastrointestinal salicylate absorption and should not be used in therapy. Also, attempts to reduce hyperventilation through the use of CNS depressant drugs should never be made because they may depress the respiratory center and induce or exacerbate a potentially fatal metabolic acidosis.[58]

Acetazolamide (Diamox®), a carbonic anhydrase inhibitor, causes a loss of bicarbonate in the urine and so may be considered a logical choice for increasing salicylate excretion[61]; it should not be used alone, however, because it also causes retention of hydrogen ions and thereby a metabolic acidosis and because salicylate becomes trapped in brain and other tissues as a result of its use.[62] There are reports of severe intoxication resulting from the combined therapeutic use of aspirin and a carbonic anhydrase inhibitor.[61,62] This is probably due to the acidemia induced by the carbonic anhydrase inhibitor, which increases the concentration of freely diffusable nonionized salicylic acid and thereby enhances the ability of salicylate to penetrate into the CNS.

Alkalinization should be attempted only in patients who require this therapy, and because salicylate can cause an alkalosis care must be taken not to overalkalinize these patients, which may exacerbate hypokalemia or cause tetany or cardiac dysrhythmias.[5] In severely intoxicated patients, however, it may be important to administer bicarbonate to replace that lost in the urine; loss of bicarbonate can lead to a metabolic acidosis and ultimately worsen the patient's condition.[63] This is especially true for children who go through a transient stage of respiratory alkalosis. Vigorous potassium repletion may be required to ensure adequate alkalinization of the urine.

An alkaline urine may not be possible to achieve in the patient who needs it most.[58] Such a situation is most probably due to marked metabolic acidosis, potassium depletion, and consequent aciduria. The potassium deficit may be severe because of the pre-existing acidosis, which leads to intracellular penetration of hydrogen ion and displacement of potassium ion. Potassium is thereby lost in the urine. These underlying disorders may require correction before an alkaline urine can be obtained.[12]

Sponge baths and cooling blankets can be used for hyperthermia, and the use of salicylates should be avoided if the patient is hyperthermic for an unknown reason.

When measured, pulmonary capillary wedge pressure has been found to be normal during acute manifestations of salicylate-induced pulmonary edema.[50] Treatment of pulmonary edema therefore is generally supportive and includes adequate oxygenation.[24] Early hemodynamic monitoring, including arterial and pulmonary artery catheter placement, may be highly desirable.[5,6] Ventilation management for these patients is similar to that recommended for patients with other forms of adult respiratory distress syndrome.[24] Positive end-expiratory pressure may be necessary if oxygenation is not adequate, but diuretics have not been shown to be helpful. Resolution of roentgenographic abnormalities is frequent in 3 to 8 days, but fatal outcome has also been reported.[50]

The intravenous administration of vitamin K (10 to 50 mg) is suggested only if hemorrhagic complications occur or if bleeding parameters are markedly abnormal.

The possibility of hypoglycemia should be considered in any patient with salicylate poisoning who deteriorates unexpectedly. Therefore, glucose should be administered if coma, seizures, or an altered mental status occurs.[7,9] If seizures continue, short-acting barbiturates or diazepam can be administered.

Although hemodialysis and hemoperfusion are effective in removing salicylate from the body, their role in the acute salicylate overdose is limited. Hemodialysis is preferred over hemoperfusion because acid-base and electrolyte disturbances are corrected more rapidly with the former (Table 36-13). For the most part, however, neither dialysis nor hemoperfusion is necessary in the care of the overdosed patient. Hemodialysis may be particularly useful in chronically intoxicated patients with high serum salicylate concentrations.[17] Regardless of serum

Table 36-13 Indications for Hemodialysis in Salicylate Overdose

---

Renal failure
Clinical findings
   Persistent CNS manifestations
   Seizures
   Coma
   Pulmonary edema
Failure to respond to other therapy
Worsening acid-base disorder
Worsening electrolyte disorder

---

salicylate concentrations, hemodialysis may be especially useful in patients with an unresponsive acidosis, impaired renal function, pulmonary edema, persistent CNS manifestations, or progressive deterioration despite appropriate therapy or for patients who have a pre-existing disease that prohibits usual theapeutic measures.[9,17] If the drug is present in a significant amount and if renal failure occurs, dialysis is necessary to remove the drug.

REFERENCES

1. Andrews H: Salicylate poisoning. *Am Fam Physician* 1973;8:102–106.

2. Temple A: Pathophysiology of aspirin overdosage toxicity, with implications for management. *Pediatrics* 1978;62(suppl):873–876.

3. Temple A: Acute and chronic effects of aspirin toxicity and their treatment. *Arch Intern Med* 1981;141:364–369.

4. Sherz R: Safety packaging impact on childhood poisoning in the United States. *Vet Hum Toxicol* 1979;21(suppl):127–129.

5. Fisher C, Albertson T, Foulke G: Salicylate-induced pulmonary edema. *Am J Emerg Med* 1985;3:33–37.

6. Henry J, Volans G: ABC of poisoning: Analgesic poisoning: Part I: Salicylates. *Br Med J* 1984;289:820–823.

7. Hill H: Current concepts: Salicylate intoxication. *N Engl J Med* 1973;288:1110–1112.

8. Griffith R, Decker W, Wright C: Iatrogenic salicylate poisoning of an infant by adult rectal aspirin suppositories. *J Fam Pract* 1981;12:757–760.

9. Snodgrass W, Rumack B, Peterson R, et al: Salicylate toxicity following therapeutic doses in young children. *Clin Toxicol* 1981;18:247–259.

10. Hammond A: Aspirin: New perspectives on everyman's medicine. *Science* 1971;174:48–51.

11. Leist E, Banwell J: Products containing aspirin. *N Engl J Med* 1974;291:710–712.

12. Sullivan J, Lander D: Planning an effective therapeutic strategy in salicylate poisoning. *Emerg Med* 1986;7:89–96.

13. Brogden R, Heel P, Pakes G, et al: Diflunisal: A review of its pharmacological properties and therapeutic use in pain and musculoskeletal strains and sprains and pain in osteoarthritis. *Drugs* 1980;19:84–106.

14. Lovejoy F: Aspirin and acetaminophen: A comparative view of their antipyretic and analgesic activity. *Pediatrics* 1978;62(suppl): 904–909.

15. Levy G: Clinical pharmacokinetics of aspirin. *Pediatrics* 1978;69(suppl):867–872.

16. Levy G, Tsuchiya T: Salicylate accumulation kinetics in man. *N Engl J Med* 1972;287:430–432.

17. Skiendzielewski J, Parrish G, Harrington T: Mental confusion in an elderly chronically ill patient. *Ann Emerg Med* 1986;15:571–575.

18. Mitchell I: ''Therapeutic'' salicylate poisoning in children. *Br Med J* 1979;1:1081.

19. Cline M, Williams H: The clinical pharmacology of salicylates: Medical staff conference. *Calif Med* 1969;110:410–422.

20. Done A, Temple A: Treatment of salicylate poisoning. *Mod Treat* 1971;8:528–551.

21. Done A: Aspirin overdosage: Incidence, diagnosis, and management. *Pediatrics* 1978;62(suppl):890–897.

22. Netter P, Faure G, Regent M, et al: Salicylate kinetics in old age. *Clin Pharmacol Ther* 1985;38:6–11.

23. Beveridge G, Forshall W, Munro J, et al: Acute salicylate poisoning in adults. *Lancet* 1964;1:1406–1412.

24. Davis P, Burch R: Pulmonary edema and salicylate intoxication. *Ann Intern Med* 1974;80:553–554.

25. Smith M: The metabolic basis of the major symptoms in acute salicylate intoxication. *Clin Toxicol* 1968; 1:387–392.

26. Bartels P, Lund-Jacobsen H: Blood lactate and ketone body concentrations in salicylate intoxication. *Hum Toxicol* 1986;5:363–366.

27. Gabow P, Anderson R, Potts D, et al: Acid-base disturbances in the salicylate-intoxicated adult. *Arch Intern Med* 1978;138:1481–1484.

28. Tashima C, Rose M: Pulmonary edema and salicylates. *Ann Intern Med* 1974;81:274–279.

29. Goldfrank L, Bresnitz X: Salicylism. *Hosp Physician* 1979;15(3):50–60.

30. Miyahara J, Karlei R: Effect of salicylate on oxidative phosphorylation of mitochondrial fragments. *Biochem J* 1965;97:194–198.

31. Segar W, Holliday M: Physiologic abnormalities of salicylate intoxication. *N Engl J Med* 1958;259:1191–1194.

32. Thurston J, Pollack P, Warren S, et al: Reduced brain glucose with normal plasma glucose in salicylate poisoning. *J Clin Invest* 1970;49:2139–2142.

33. Pearson H: Comparative effects of aspirin and acetaminophen on hemostasis. *Pediatrics* 1978;62 (suppl):926–929.

34. Krasnoff S, Bernstein M: Acetylsalicylic acid poisoning. *JAMA* 1947;135:712–714.

35. Robins J, Turnbull J, Robertson C: Gastric perforation after acute aspirin overdose. *Hum Toxicol* 1985; 4:527–528.

36. Ashworth C, McKemie J: Hemorrhagic complications, with death probably from salicylate therapy. *JAMA* 1944;126:806–810.

37. Anderson R, Potts D, Rumack B, et al: Unrecognized adult salicylate intoxication. *Ann Int Med* 1976;85:745–748.

38. Fink M, Irwin P: Central nervous system effects of aspirin. *Clin Pharmacol Ther* 1982;32:362–365.

39. Wortzman D, Grunfeld A: Delayed absorption following enteric-coated aspirin overdose. *Ann Emerg Med* 1987;16:434–436.

40. Reed J, Palmisano P: Central nervous system salicylate. *Clin Toxicol* 1975;8:623–631.

41. Paul B: Salicylate poisoning in the elderly: Diagnostic pitfalls. *J Am Geriatr Soc* 1972;20:387–390.

42. Granville-Grossman K, Sergeant H: Pulmonary edema due to salicylate intoxication. *Lancet* 1960; 1:575–577.

43. Greenstein S: Pulmonary edema due to salicylate intoxication: Report of a case. *Dis Chest* 1963;44:552–553.

44. Hrnicek G, Skelton J, Miller W: Pulmonary edema and salicylate intoxication. *JAMA* 1974;230:866–867.

45. Hefner J: Noncardiogenic pulmonary edema: A complication of salicylate toxicity. *Respir Care* 1982; 27:1215–1218.

46. Karliner J: Noncardiogenic forms of pulmonary edema. *Circulation* 1972;46:212–216.

47. Sorensen S: Adult respiratory-distress syndrome in salicylate intoxication. *Lancet* 1979;1:1025–1028.

48. Greenbaum D, Togba J, Blecker M, et al: Salicylate intoxication: An unusual presentation. *Chest* 1974; 66:575–576.

49. Bowers R, Brigham K, Owen P: Salicylate pulmonary edema: The mechanism in sheep and review of the current literature. *Am Rev Respir Dis* 1977;115:261–268.

50. Shanies H: Noncardiac pulmonary edema. *Med Clin North Am* 1977;61:1319–1337.

51. Hyman A, Spannhoke E, Kadowitz P: Prostaglandins and the lung. *Ann Rev Respir Dis* 1978;117:111–136.

52. Brown S, Cameron J, Matthew H: Plasma salicylate levels in acute poisoning in adults. *Br Med J* 1967; 2:738–739.

53. Trinder P: Rapid determination of salicylate in biological fluids. *Biochem J* 1954;57:301–303.

54. Boxer L, Anderson F, Rowe D: Comparison of ipecac-induced emesis with gastric lavage in the treatment of acute salicylate ingestion. *J Pediatr* 1970;74:800–803.

55. Hillman R, Prescott L: Treatment of salicylate poisoning with repeated oral charcoal. *Br Med J* 1985; 291:1472.

56. Cumming G, Dukes D, Widdowson G: Alkaline diuresis in treatment of aspirin poisoning. *Br Med J* 1964; 4:1033–1036.

57. Lawson A, Proudfoot A, Brown S, et al: Forced diuresis in the treatment of acute salicylate poisoning in adults. *Q J Med* 1969;38:31–48.

58. Elenbaas R: Critical review of forced alkaline diuresis in acute salicylism. *Crit Care Q* 1982;4:89–95.

59. Prescott L, Balali-Mood M, Critchley J, et al: Diuresis or urinary alkalinization for salicylate poisoning? *Br Med J* 1982;285:1383–1386.

60. Prowse K, Pain M, Marston A, et al: The treatment of salicylate poisoning using mannitol and forced alkaline diuresis. *Clin Sci* 1970;38:327–337.

61. Morgan A, Polak A: Acetazolamide and sodium bicarbonate in treatment of salicylate poisoning in adults. *Br Med J* 1969;1:16–19.

62. Sweeney K, Chapron D, Brandt L, et al: Toxic interaction between acetazolamide and salicylate: Case reports and a pharmacokinetic explanation. *Clin Pharmacol Ther* 1986;40:518–524.

63. McCain H, Teague R: Metabolic complications of salicylate overload. *Drug Ther* 1979;xx:70–80.

ADDITIONAL SELECTED REFERENCES

Cabooter M, Elewaut A, Barbier F: Salicylate-induced pancreatitis. *Gastroenterology* 1981;80:214–215.

Cooper S, Needle S, Kruger G: Comparative analgesic potency of aspirin and ibuprofen. *J Oral Surg* 1977; 35:898–903.

Hefner J, Sahn S: Salicylate-induced pulmonary edema: Clinical features and prognosis. *Ann Int Med* 1981; 95:405–409.

Kahn A, Blum D: Fatal respiratory-distress syndrome and salicylate intoxication in a two-year-old. *Lancet* 1979; 2:1131–1132.

McGuigan M: A two-year review of salicylate deaths in Ontario. *Arch Intern Med* 1987;147:510–512.

Miller R, Jick H: Acute toxicity of aspirin in hospitalized medical patients. *Am J Med Sci* 1977;274:271–279.

Paynter A, Alexander F: Salicylate intoxication caused by teething ointment. *Lancet* 1979;2:1132.

Proudfoot A, Brown S: Acidemia and salicylate poisoning in adults. *Br Med J* 1969;2:547–550.

Walters J, Woodring J, Stelling C, et al: Salicylate-induced pulmonary edema. *Radiology* 1983;146:289–293.

Zimmerman G, Clemmer T: Acute respiratory failure during therapy for salicylate intoxication. *Ann Emerg Med* 1981; 10:104–106.

chapter 37

Nonsteroidal Anti-inflammatory Agents

Nonsteroidal anti-inflammatory drugs (NSAIDs) have become the most frequently prescribed drugs, and within the last 10 years there has been a proliferation in the number of new NSAIDs.[1,2] These drugs make up a heterogenous group of compounds that share certain therapeutic actions and side effects but that may be structurally dissimilar (Table 37-1).[3]

CLINICAL USES

The NSAIDs are used extensively as antiarthritics, analgesics, and antigout and pseudogout agents as well as for pain and inflammation associated with bursitis, tendonitis, costochondritis, pericarditis, and dysmenorrhea (Table 37-2).[2,3] NSAIDs have also been used to treat venous thrombosis, cerebrovascular disease, patent ductus arteriosus in premature infants, and hypercalcemia associated with certain malignancies.

The NSAIDs produce their antipyretic effects by acting on the hypothalamus, with heat dissipation being increased as a result of vasodilation and increased peripheral blood flow.

PHARMACOKINETICS

All the NSAIDs are highly protein bound, and only the unbound drug is biologically active. In

Table 37-1 Nonsteroidal Anti-inflammatory Drugs (NSAIDs)

Acetic acid derivatives
  Indomethacin (Indocin®)
  Sulindac (Clinoril®)
  Tolmetin (Tolectin®)
Fenamate derivatives
  Flufenamic acid
  Meclofenamate (Meclomen®)
  Mefenamic acid (Ponstel®)
Oxicam derivatives
  Piroxicam (Feldene®)
Propionic acid derivatives
  Fenbufen
  Fenoprofen (Nalfon®)
  Ibuprofen (Motrin®, Rufen®, Advil®, Nuprin®, Mediprin®)
  Indoprofen
  Ketoprofen
  Naproxen (Naprosyn®, Anaprox®)
Pyrazole derivatives
  Oxyphenbutazone (Tandearil®)
  Phenylbutazone (Azolid®, Butazolidin®)

general, less than 10% of a dose is excreted unchanged by the kidney; the drug is metabolized predominately by the liver.[2] Most of the NSAIDs bind only to albumin. Once the albumin binding sites are saturated, the concentration of free drug rapidly increases. This accounts for the relatively speedy efficacy of most NSAIDs as well as for their self-prophylaxis: the free drug is rapidly excreted by the kidney, so that drug

Table 37-2 Indications for NSAIDs

Analgesia and anti-inflammation
  Arthritis
  Gout
  Pseudogout
  Bursitis
  Tendonitis
  Costochondritis
  Sprain or strain
  Pericarditis
  Dysmenorrhea
Antipyresis
Patent ductus arteriosus
Venous thrombosis
Hypercalcemia

Table 37-4 Characteristics of the Prostaglandins

Composed of unsaturated fatty acids
Synthesized from linoleic, linolenic, and arachidonic
  acids
Physiologic stimulation of synthesis
  Infection
  Trauma
  Fever
  Platelet aggregation
Properties
  Short half-life
  Located in tissue membranes
  Not stored in the body
  "Local hormones"
  Distributed throughout body

Table 37-3 Protein-Bound Drugs Whose Concentrations May Increase with Concomitant NSAID Therapy

β-Adrenergic blocking agents
Oral anticoagulants
Phenytoin
Salicylates
Sulfonamides
Sulfonylurea agents

accumulation is prevented. For many NSAIDs an increase in dose does not bring about a linear increase in blood concentration; rather, with an increased dose more drug is free and thus rapidly excreted.[4] This is not the case with benoxaprofen (Oraflex®), for which blood concentrations rise steadily with repeated dosing.[2] This drug is dangerous and was removed from the market after several cases of fatal cholestatic jaundice were reported.[5]

Because the NSAIDs are so strongly protein bound, they can be displaced from binding sites or can displace other protein-bound drugs, including sulfonylurea agents, some β blockers, oral anticoagulants, hydantoins, salicylates, and sulfonamides (Table 37-3). This can potentiate the effects of the other agent.[2]

Mechanism of Action

The generation of inflammatory reactions appears to require the action of a number of mediators, but the class of mediators most

directly linked to the action of anti-inflammatory drugs is the prostaglandins.[6] This group of biologically active molecules is now known to be a part of a broad class of lipids referred to as the eicosanoids.[7]

The prostaglandins are unsaturated fatty acid compounds derived from 20-carbon essential fatty acids.[1] They are found in tissue membranes, primarily phospholipids.[2] These are synthesized from the dietary essential fatty acids linoleic acid and linolenic acid (Table 37-4). The most important of the precursors to prostaglandin synthesis is arachidonic acid.[7,8]

Prostaglandin synthesis is initiated within the cell by cleavage of arachidonic acid from membrane phospholipids through the action of a phospholipase. Synthesis is initiated by a stimulus that damages or distorts the cell membrane, such as infection, trauma, fever, or platelet aggregation.[9] Because the prostaglandins have an effect on target cells in the immediate vicinity of their site of biosynthesis, they are called "local hormones."[1] The prostaglandins appear in minute quantities, have a short half-life (seconds to minutes), are not stored in appreciable quantities in either cells or tissues, and are ubiquitous in their distribution throughout the body. In this respect the prostaglandins differ from circulating hormones.[8]

NSAIDs block prostaglandin production, and hence their actions, by inhibition of the enzyme cyclo-oxygenase (prostaglandin synthetase).[1,10] Through the blockade of prostaglandin-derived mediators, NSAIDs reduce inflammation.[9] Because NSAIDs bind reversibly to cyclo-oxygenase, both the beneficial and the toxic effects of the prostaglandins recede when the drug is stopped.

Corticosteroids, which are the most potent of the anti-inflammatory drugs, are also potent inhibitors of prostaglandin synthesis.[8] The mechanisms of other anti-inflammatory drugs such as gold salts, penicillamine, and antimalarials are unknown at present, but they differ from NSAIDs and seem to have no important effects on prostaglandin synthesis.

The inhibition of prostaglandin biosynthesis may only partly explain the therapeutic effects of NSAIDs.[9] Another postulated mechanism is interaction with the adenylate cyclase system. Some NSAIDs inhibit phosphodiesterase, thereby elevating the intracellular concentration of cyclic AMP. Cyclic AMP has been shown to stabilize membranes, including lysosomal membranes in polymorphonuclear leukocytes, thus preventing the release of enzymes that appear to play a major role in the inflammatory response.[9]

Side Effects

Although the NSAIDs are among the most widely used drugs in medicine and are generally well tolerated, toxic effects have been noted, some of which may be quite severe.[3] In rare instances, these drugs can cause allergic reactions, peptic ulcer disease, elevation of liver enzymes, and kidney failure (Table 37-5). Problems with zomepiric (Zomax®) and benoxaprofen (Oraflex®) are extreme examples of known side effects[10,11]; zomepiric has also been removed from the market.[1] The voluntary withdrawal of these drugs by their manufacturers as well as recent reports of hepatic and renal toxicity have drawn attention to the potential toxicities of NSAIDs.[5]

Gastrointestinal

The most common side effects of NSAIDs occur in the upper gastrointestinal tract.[1,12] NSAIDs may cause dyspepsia, epigastric pain, erosive gastritis, peptic ulceration, and gastrointestinal bleeding. Because prostaglandins decrease gastric acid secretion and help to maintain the gastric mucosal barrier, inhibition of

Table 37-5 Side Effects of NSAIDs

Gastrointestinal
  Dyspepsia
  Epigastric pain
  Gastritis
  Peptic ulceration
  Gastrointestinal bleeding
Hematologic
  Impairment of platelet function
  Mild bleeding diathesis
Renal
  Acute renal failure
  Chronic renal failure
  Nephrotic syndrome
  Interstitial nephritis
Hepatic
  Heptatoxicity (rare)

prostaglandin synthesis may account for many of the upper gastrointestinal symptoms caused by these drugs.[2] The prodrugs, such as fenbufen and sulindac, are not active until they are absorbed and metabolized by the liver and consequently are of low ulcerogenicity.

Hematologic

NSAIDs impair platelet aggregation through inhibition of platelet cyclo-oxygenase–induced synthesis of thromboxane. Although this effect produces at most a mild bleeding diathesis in hematologically normal patients, in patients with coagulation defects caused by anticoagulants or hereditary clotting factor deficiencies bleeding may be severe.

Renal

The NSAIDs have been known to produce a wide array of untoward renal effects, including acute interstitial nephritis, acute papillary necrosis, nephrotic syndrome, and acute and chronic renal failure.[1]

Prostaglandins are potent vasodilators in the kidney, and it appears that renal disease occurs by the inhibition of renal prostaglandin. This phenomenon occurs rarely with virtually all the NSAIDs that are primary prostaglandin inhibitors. The reaction is reversible if the drug is discontinued and appropriate supportive measures are taken. In addition, abnormalities of water metabolism and of sodium and potassium homeostasis have been noted.

Hepatic

Because the liver plays a central role in metabolism of NSAIDs, it is not surprising that there has been associated hepatotoxicity.[2] Liver toxicity is rare with most NSAIDs but has been noted with phenylbutazone and oxyphenbutazone, which are the most hepatotoxic of the NSAIDs.

CHARACTERISTICS OF THE NSAIDs

The NSAIDs can be divided into several chemical groups (see Table 37-1). Some of the NSAIDs are considered prodrugs, which are precursor drugs requiring metabolism to an active metabolite.

Acetic Acid Derivatives

Indomethacin

Indomethacin (Indocin®) is rapidly absorbed from the upper gastrointestinal tract and may be absorbed even more quickly when given as a rectal suppository.[9] Indomethacin is highly (more than 90%) protein bound, and its apparent volume of distribution ranges from 0.39 to 1.5 L/kg.[6] The elimination half-life of a therapeutic dose varies from 2.6 to 11.2 hours and is similar in duration to the half-life reported in the overdosed patient.[13] Biotransformation is the major elimination pathway.[3]

Acute intoxication with indomethacin may cause nausea, vomiting, anorexia, abdominal pain, headache, tinnitus, dizziness, lethargy, drowsiness, confusion, paresthesia, aggressive behavior, disorientation, restlessness, gastrointestinal bleeding, electrolyte imbalance, coma, and seizures (Table 37-6).[3] Although blood dyscrasias such as leukopenia, thrombocytopenia, and agranulocytosis have occurred, they are usually a consequence of chronic administration.[9]

Sulindac

Sulindac (Clinoril®) is a prodrug that is converted to active sulfide and sulfone metabolites by the cytochrome P-450 enzyme system.[6] Sulindac and its metabolites undergo extensive

Table 37-6 Clinical Features of Acute Indomethacin Overdose

Gastrointestinal
Nausea
Vomiting
Anorexia
Abdominal pain
Hematemesis
Neurologic
Headache
Tinnitus
Dizziness
Lethargy
Drowsiness
Confusion
Paresthesia
Disorientation
Restlessness
Coma
Seizures

enterohepatic circulation.[3] Sulindac bears a chemical resemblance to indomethacin but is a substituted indene rather than an indole. It was synthesized as the result of a search for a compound as effective as indomethacin but with less ulcerogenic potential.[9]

The elimination half-lives of sulindac and its active metabolites are 7 and 16 hours, respectively. Because it is metabolized slowly, it can be given in twice-daily doses. The plasma protein binding of sulindac is approximately 95%.[3]

Tolmetin

Tolmetin (Tolectin®) has a structural resemblance to indomethacin and sulindac but an action and toxicity similar to those of the propionic acid derivatives.[6] It is well absorbed from the gastrointestinal tract and is highly (99%) protein bound.[3] The plasma half-life of tolmetin is approximately 1 hour, and the drug has an apparent volume of distribution of 0.10 to 0.14 L/kg.[9]

The side effects that may be seen after long-term administration of tolmetin may also be noted in the acute overdose and may consist of nausea, vomiting, epigastric pain, headache, dizziness, and tinnitus (Table 37-7). Central nervous system manifestations such as anxiety, nervousness, insomnia, drowsiness, and visual disturbances have also been reported.[9]

Table 37-7 Clinical Features of Acute Tolmetin Overdose

Gastrointestinal
  Nausea
  Vomiting
  Epigastric pain
Neurologic
  Headache
  Dizziness
  Tinnitus
  Anxiety
  Nervousness
  Insomnia
  Drowsiness
  Visual disturbances

Fenamate Derivatives

Meclofenamate

Meclofenamate (Meclomen®) is highly protein bound and undergoes significant enterohepatic circulation. The half-life is approximately 3 hours.[3,6] After acute massive overdose, CNS stimulation manifested as irrational behavior, marked agitation, and generalized seizure may occur. This initial phase may be followed by renal toxicity, including decreased urine output and increased serum creatinine concentration, and may be accompanied by oliguria or anuria and azotemia.[3]

Mefenamic Acid

Mefenamic acid (Ponstel®) is rapidly absorbed from the gastrointestinal tract. The plasma half-life of this highly protein-bound drug is 2 to 4 hours. Although it is eliminated by biotransformation, enterohepatic recirculation of metabolites also appears to occur.[6]

The major side effect of mefenamic acid is diarrhea.[3] This is a special problem in the elderly, and renal insufficiency has been reported in patients who became dehydrated as a result of the diarrhea.[9] In addition, dyspepsia, upper gastrointestinal tract discomfort, and occasional ulceration with hemorrhage have been reported.[14] Other findings in the acute overdose include coma, hypoprothrombinemia, and acute renal failure. Unlike overdosage with other NSAIDs, overdosage with mefenamic acid appears to be characterized by a relatively high incidence of seizures.[3] Patients who have taken overdoses of mefenamic acid must be closely observed, particularly during the first few hours, when seizures are most likely to occur.[14] The drug is usually eliminated very quickly, with rapid recovery noted.[3]

Oxicam Derivatives

Piroxicam

Piroxicam (Feldene®) is structurally distinct from other NSAIDs. It is a potent anti-inflammatory agent that is extensively bound to plasma protein. At therapeutic doses piroxicam has an elimination half-life of 45 hours.[3] Piroxicam is one of the most widely used NSAIDs in the world because of its long half-life.[15] Pharmacokinetic studies in the elderly and patients with renal impairment show no evidence of drug accumulation.[3]

Acute overdose may cause nausea, vomiting, diarrhea, abdominal pain, gastrointestinal bleeding, dizziness, blurred vision, excitability, coma, seizures, hematuria, proteinuria, and acute renal failure.[16]

Propionic Acid Derivatives

Fenbufen

Fenbufen is a prodrug with no anti-inflammatory activity of its own.[3] Thus there is a low incidence of gastrointestinal side effects associated with its use. After absorption, it is converted in the liver to its active metabolite.[6] Fenbufen is highly protein bound, and plasma concentrations reach their peak 1 to 2 hours after ingestion of therapeutic doses. The elimination half-life of the parent drug and that of its two principal metabolites after administration of therapeutic doses are approximately 10 hours.

Fenoprofen

Fenoprofen (Nalfon®), as either the sodium or the calcium salt, is rapidly and completely absorbed from the gastrointestinal tract. Plasma concentrations reach a peak 2 hours after a single oral dose. Fenoprofen has a plasma half-life of 2 to 3 hours.[9] It is bound extensively to human serum albumin and has a low apparent volume of distribution of 0.08 to 0.10 L/kg.[3] It is metabolized extensively, and less than 5% of a dose is excreted unchanged in the urine. When substantial quantities of fenoprofen are ingested in acute overdose, hematuria and acute renal failure may occur.

Ibuprofen

Ibuprofen (Motrin®, Rufen®, Advil®, Nuprin®, Mediprin®) was the first phenylpropionate to be marketed in the United States.[17] Although ibuprofen has shown anti-inflammatory, antipyretic, and analgesic activity, higher doses are required for anti-inflammatory effects than for analgesia. Ibuprofen is now available in several over-the-counter preparations.[6,18] The drug is well (80%) absorbed from the gastrointestinal tract, and plasma concentrations reach their peak about 1 to 2 hours after a single oral dose.[19] Ibuprofen is highly bound to plasma proteins and is eliminated chiefly by biotransformation. The half-life is about 2 to 4 hours.[9] There is no evidence of accumulation after multiple doses, and in the overdose setting the elimination half-life does not appear to be prolonged.[20]

Since its introduction to the United States in 1974, ibuprofen has been shown to be relatively safe and effective for the treatment of inflammatory disorders. It is generally well tolerated, although mild and transient gastrointestinal discomfort may occasionally occur.[15] Central nervous system complaints such as headache and giddiness may also occasionally occur. Diarrhea, vomiting, stomatitis, erythematous or urticarial skin rashes, constipation, deafness, and edema have been reported less frequently.

As with other propionic acid derivatives, acute overdose with ibuprofen causes nausea, vomiting, abdominal pain, drowsiness, nystagmus, diplopia, headache, tinnitus, impaired renal function, coma, and hypotension (Table 37-8). In addition, serious effects associated with a single large ingestion have included profound metabolic acidosis, hypotension, acute renal failure, acute liver cell injury, and acute cholestasis.[18,20]

Ibuprofen is known to be extensively metabolized by oxidation of the isobutyl group and

Table 37-8 Clinical Features of Acute Ibuprofen Overdose

Gastrointestinal
  Nausea
  Vomiting
  Abdominal pain
Neurologic
  Tinnitus
  Coma
  Nystagmus
  Diplopia
  Headache
Miscellaneous
  Metabolic acidosis
  Hypotension
  Acute renal failure
  Acute liver cell injury
  Acute cholestasis

eliminated primarily by the kidney. Because ibuprofen and its metabolites are acidic compounds, their accumulation in the blood could be responsible for a metabolic acidosis.[18] The ability of ibuprofen to inhibit renal prostaglandin synthesis may explain the renal toxic effects noted.

If measurements of ibuprofen plasma concentrations are available, the ibuprofen nomogram (Fig. 37-1) may aid in predicting which patients are at risk for developing symptoms at a later time.[20]

Naproxen

Naproxen (Naprosyn®, Anaprox®) is a propionic acid derivative with a long half-life (12 to 15 hours).[9] It is well absorbed from the upper gastrointestinal tract, and plasma concentrations reach a peak in 2 to 4 hours.[21] Naproxen is highly (99%) bound to plasma albumin.[3] Because of the long half-life, it is suitable for twice-daily administration; approximately 3 days are required to reach equilibrium. The apparent volume of distribution of naproxen is 0.1 L/kg. Large doses result in a disproportionate increase in renal excretion without evidence of saturation of the excretory mechanism. It therefore is a safer drug when taken in large amounts than, for example, aspirin.

Side effects after therapeutic dosing or overdosage may include stomatitis, headache, vertigo, drowsiness, lightheadedness, dyspepsia,

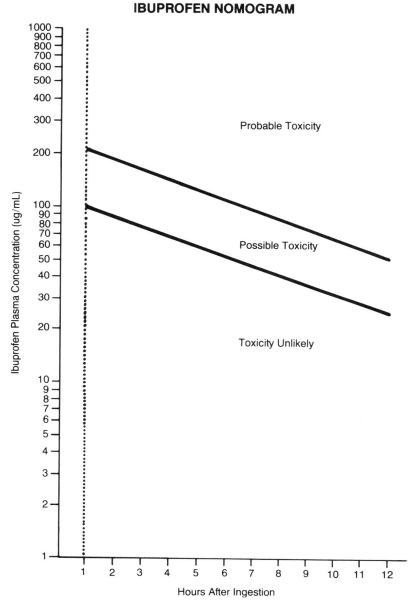

Figure 37-1 Ibuprofen nomogram. *Source:* Adapted with permission from *Annals of Emergency Medicine* (1986;15:1309), Copyright © 1986, American College of Emergency Physicians.

nausea, and vomiting. Severe effects are rare.[3,9,22]

Pyrazalone Derivatives

Phenylbutazone and Oxyphenbutazone

Phenylbutazone (Butazolidin®, Azolid®) and oxyphenbutazone (Tandearil®), which is a major

metabolite of phenylbutazone, are two of the oldest and most potent NSAIDs but are also two of the most toxic.[6] Phenylbutazone and oxyphenbutazone are both highly (98%) protein bound. The apparent volume of distribution of phenylbutazone is 0.17 L/kg and that of oxyphenbutazone is 0.14 L/kg. Phenylbutazone is extensively metabolized; the major metabolites are formed by oxidation and conjugation with glucuronic acid. The elimination half-life of phenylbutazone is approximately 75 hours.[3]

Both compounds have a high incidence of unpleasant side effects associated with long-term therapy (Table 37-9), which has limited their use in this setting. A serum-sickness reaction can be alarming but is usually self-limiting. Ulcerative stomatitis, hepatitis, and blood dyscrasias such as agranulocytosis and aplastic anemia occasionally occur during prolonged therapy. These hematologic effects are dose related and are more likely to occur in the elderly. Although they are very uncommon, mortality due to aplastic anemia is significant.

Acute poisoning from phenylbutazone and oxyphenbutazone may produce myriad abnormalities (Table 37-10). Because the margin of safety between therapeutic and toxic doses is narrow acute overdose is quite common, and the toxic effects may be severe. Toxicity is most frequently associated with serum phenylbutazone concentrations exceeding 100 μg/mL.

Gastrointestinal symptoms include nausea, vomiting, diarrhea, abdominal pain, peptic ulceration, and hematemesis.[3] Neurological findings may include euphoria, restlessness, psychosis, disorientation, nystagmus, tinnitus, trismus, hallucinations, ataxia, drowsiness, coma, and tonic-clonic seizures.

Metabolic disturbances reported with overdose of pyrazalone derivatives resemble those of salicylate overdose and may include a respiratory alkalosis due to hyperventilation and metabolic acidosis, which may occur either alone or after the respiratory alkalosis.

Hepatic dysfunction usually results in elevated liver enzymes and occasionally in jaundice and hepatomegaly. Acute renal failure together with sodium and water retention have also been

described. This may be substantial and may lead to hypertension and peripheral edema. Hematuria has been noted as well as red discoloration of the urine due to a phenylbutazone metabolite. In addition, proteinuria, oliguria, and, rarely, nephritis may be noted. Cardiovascular collapse with subsequent cardiac arrest has occurred.[3]

TOXICITY

Despite the widespread availability of NSAIDs, relatively few cases of acute poisoning have been reported. Unless a substantial overdose is ingested, clinical features of acute NSAID poisoning are usually confined to the gastrointestinal tract and CNS and are mild. Nevertheless, serious complications such as seizures, cardiovascular collapse, acute renal failure, coma, and respiratory distress may com-

Table 37-10 Clinical Features of Pyrazole Overdose

Gastrointestinal
  Nausea
  Vomiting
  Abdominal pain
  Hematemesis
  Peptic ulcer
Neurologic
  Euphoria
  Restlessness
  Psychosis
  Disorientation
  Tinnitus
  Trismus
  Hallucinations
  Ataxia
  Drowsiness
  Seizures
  Coma
Miscellaneous
  Respiratory alkalosis
  Metabolic acidosis
  Acute renal failure
  Hepatotoxicity
  Sodium retention
  Peripheral edema
  Cardiovascular collapse

Table 37-9 Side Effects of Pyrazalone Derivatives

Serum-sickness reaction
Ulcerative stomatitis
Hepatitis
Blood dyscrasias
  Agranulocytosis
  Aplastic anemia

plicate a major overdose. Acid-base disturbances have been described with ibuprofen and phenylbutazone.

TREATMENT OF NSAID OVERDOSE

Other than for confirming a diagnosis of acute NSAID overdose, the routine determination of plasma concentrations of these agents is neither clinically useful nor easily performed.[3] The exception to this may be ibuprofen, for which a nomogram has been formulated that may be of prognostic value (see Fig. 37-1).[20]

Management of acute NSAID poisoning is essentially supportive and symptomatic. Gastric emptying procedures may be of benefit if instituted soon after the ingestion. Emptying should be followed by the administration of activated charcoal and a cathartic.[20]

It is essential to maintain adequate respirations, so that an artificial airway may be required. Rarely, mechanical ventilation is necessary in severely poisoned patients who develop respiratory depression. If marked hypotension occurs, for example after phenylbutazone poisoning or after gastrointestinal bleeding, fluid therapy (including blood) may be necessary.[3]

Seizures induced by NSAIDs tend to occur only once and are short lived. In adults, intravenous diazepam (5 to 10 mg or 0.1 to 0.3 mg/kg), if necessary, may be an effective treatment.

H_2-Receptor antagonists such as cimetidine and ranitidine have been employed to minimize or prevent gastrointestinal irritation, ulceration, and hemorrhage. Although this treatment is expensive and its efficacy has not been shown, it is unlikely to be harmful.

The acid-base disturbances seen with phenylbutazone and ibuprofen overdose are rare and usually transient. Except in the case of renal failure they do not usually require active treatment, but the patient should be closely monitored and appropriate treatment begun if deemed necessary.[3]

Most NSAIDs are highly protein bound and extensively metabolized, so that it is both pharmacologically inappropriate and clinically unnecessary to undertake forced diuresis, dialysis, or hemoperfusion because such methods are unlikely to enhance elimination significantly.

As in salicylate poisoning, the rate of excretion of some of the NSAIDs is increased if the urine is alkaline, but the difficulty of alkalinizing urine in a seriously poisoned patient may militate against the value of the procedure.

Many of the NSAIDs undergo enterohepatic circulation, so that repeated doses of activated charcoal may be useful in reducing their elimination half-life. Although this remains to be shown, it is not a harmful procedure.[20]

REFERENCES

1. Clive D, Stoff J: Renal syndromes associated with nonsteroidal antiinflammatory drugs. *N Engl J Med* 1984; 310:563–572.

2. Corre K: Nonsteroidal antiinflammatory drugs. *Top Emerg Med* 1986;8:12–25.

3. Vale J, Meredith T: Acute poisoning due to nonsteroidal anti-inflammatory drugs. *Med Toxicol* 1986; 1:12–31.

4. O'Brien W: Pharmacology of nonsteroidal anti-inflammatory drugs: Practical review for clinicians. *Am J Med* 1983;73:32–39.

5. Patmas M, Wilborn S, Shankel S: Acute multisystem toxicity associated with the use of nonsteroidal anti-inflammatory drugs. *Arch Intern Med* 1984;144:519–521.

6. Kantor T: Control of pain by nonsteroidal anti-inflammatory drugs. *Med Clin North Am* 1982;66:1053–1059.

7. Metz S: Anti-inflammatory agents as inhibitors of prostaglandin synthesis in man. *Med Clin North Am* 1981; 67:713–757.

8. Robinson D: Prostaglandins and the mechanism of action of anti-inflammatory drugs. *Am J Med* 1983; 73:26–31.

9. Simon L, Mills J: Nonsteroidal antiinflammatory drugs. *N Engl J Med* 1980;302:1179–1243.

10. Panush R, Yonker P: Practical points on nonsteroidal antiinflammatory drugs. *Am Fam Physician* 1984; 29:258–262.

11. Warren S, Mosley C: Renal failure and tubular dysfunction due to zomepirac therapy. *JAMA* 1983;396–397.

12. Bartle W, Gupta A, Lazor J: Nonsteroidal antiinflammatory drugs and gastrointestinal bleeding. *Arch Intern Med* 1986;146:2365–2367.

13. Sheehan T, Boldy D, Vale J: Indomethacin poisoning. *Clin Toxicol* 1986;24:151–158.

14. Balali-Mood M, Proudfoot A, Critchley J, et al: Mefenamic acid overdosage. *Lancet* 1981;1:1354–1356.

15. Nuki G: Non-steroidal analgesic and anti-inflammatory agents. *Br Med J* 1983;287:39–43.

16. MacDougall L, Taylor-Smith A, Rothberg A: Piroxicam poisoning in a 2-year-old child. *South Am Med J* 1984; 66:31–33.

17. Davies E, Avery G: Ibuprofen: A review of its pharmacological properties and therapeutic efficacy in rheumatic disorders. *Drugs* 1971;2:416–446.

18. Lee C, Finkler A: Acute intoxication due to ibuprofen overdose. *Arch Pathol Lab Med* 1986;220:747–749.

19. Steinmetz J, Lee C, Wu A, et al: Tissue levels of ibuprofen after fatal overdosage of ibuprofen and acetaminophen. *Vet Hum Toxicol* 1987;29:381–383.

20. Hall A, Smolinske S, Conrad F, et al: Ibuprofen overdose: 126 cases. *Ann Emerg Med* 1986;15:1308–1313.

21. Alun-Jones E, Williams J, Clwyd G: Hyponatremia and fluid retention in a neonate associated with maternal naproxen overdose. *Clin Toxicol* 1986;24:257–260.

22. Fredell E, Strand L: Naproxen overdose. *JAMA* 1977;238:938.

ADDITIONAL SELECTED REFERENCES

Goodwin J: Toxicity of nonsteroidal anti-inflammatory drugs. *Arch Intern Med* 1987;147:34–35.

Roth S: Nonsteroidal anti-inflammatory drug gastropathy. *Arch Intern Med* 1986;146:1075–1076.

part X

METALS

chapter 38

Introduction to Metals and Chelating Agents

There are 72 elements on the periodic table that are classified as metals; of these, iron, mercury, lead, and arsenic are of interest in toxicology and are discussed in this section. Metals may exist in the elemental, inorganic, and organic forms. Some are essential for life, being vital parts of life processes, and significant disease results when they are deficient from body systems; others have no known biologic function.[1] Many are potent toxins. Metals that are essential nutrients can also exert toxic actions if the homeostatic mechanism maintaining them within physiologic limits is unbalanced.[2]

Although metals were once important therapeutic agents, their use in this area has declined. This is particularly true with the advent of more effective organic drugs in the treatment of infectious diseases.[1] Present interest in the metals lies primarily in the toxic reactions they are capable of producing. The problems created by food contamination, water and air pollution from industrial and exhaust fumes, and the widespread use of agricultural chemicals are largely attributable to these toxins.[3]

All organic poisons are eventually destroyed in the body through various metabolic processes, but no organism is capable of transforming toxic metals into harmless compounds. They therefore persist in the body and exert their toxic effects by combining with one or more reactive groups essential for normal physiological function.

Most metals can be divided into two classes. Those in the first class bind preferentially to oxygen and nitrogen atoms; these include calcium, barium, and strontium.[1] Those in the second class bind preferentially to sulfur and phosphorus atoms; these include mercury, arsenic, and gold. Most toxic metals fall into the second class. Lead is in a separate class because it binds to all four atoms.[1]

It is generally recognized that the absorption of inorganic compounds depends heavily on the compound's water solubility. Metals coming in contact with the body in elemental form are usually poorly absorbed. In compound form they vary considerably in the ease with which they cross biologic membranes. Soluble salts of metals dissociate readily in the aqueous environment of biologic membranes, which facilitates their transport as metal ions.

Table 38-1 Organs Affected by Metal Intoxication

Skin
Gastrointestinal tract
Liver
Kidney
Hematologic organs
Central and peripheral nervous systems

Some metals occur in the environment as alkyl (organometallic) compounds, in which the metal is firmly bonded to carbon. These alkyl compounds remain largely intact in the biologic environment. They are lipid soluble and pass readily across biologic membranes unaltered by the surrounding medium. The most notable examples of organometallic compounds of interest in toxicology are methyl mercury and tetraethyl lead.

MECHANISM OF ACTION

Once absorbed into the body, inorganic metals are capable of being taken up at various binding sites. Metals exert their toxic effects by combining with one or more reactive groups of enzymes that are essential for normal physiologic functions. An example of this is the binding of many metals to sulfhydryl groups, which are essential for the activity of certain enzymes. Other complexes are to amino, phosphate, carboxylate, imidazole, and hydroxyl radicals of enzymes and other essential biological proteins. The sensitivity of the particular system attacked by the metal and the degree of interference with cellular activity caused by the metal-protein complex determine the clinical effects and course of an intoxication.

Whenever the clinical picture indicates involvement of several organ systems, metal poisoning should be considered in the differential diagnosis.[1] The clinical picture can also vary depending on whether exposure is acute or chronic. The skin, gastrointestinal tract, liver, kidney, blood-forming organs, and peripheral and central nervous systems may be involved (Table 38-1). The digestive tract is involved because of its part in absorption; the liver is affected by virtue of its role as blood filter and detoxifier; and the kidney glomeruli and tubular cells are damaged through their function in excretion.

ROUTES OF EXCRETION

The main routes by which the human body rids itself of small amounts of toxic metals are the excretory routes. The sloughing off of the skin, the growth of the hair, and, for volatile poisons, the breath can also be minor routes for elimination of toxic metals.

LABORATORY ANALYSIS

In suspected metal poisoning both blood and urine should be obtained. Quantitative 24-hour urine collections are preferred because concentrations in random samples of urine may sometimes be misleading.[1]

METAL FUME FEVER

Metal fume fever is an occupational syndrome that develops on exposure to fresh metal oxide fumes.[4,5] This occurs when fumes from metals heated above their melting point are inhaled.[6] Many metal oxides can cause metal fume fever, such as copper, zinc, manganese, silver, tin, aluminum, magnesium, iron, selenium, cadmium, antimony, and nickel.[4,5] Exposure is most common in the metal (steel and iron) industry, metal grinding and welding, zinc foundries, galvanizing, and chrome plating. Although the symptoms of metal fume fever are recognized by welders and metal workers and are well known to physicians in occupational medicine, most primary care physicians are unaware of this disorder.[7]

The syndrome occurs mainly in nonatopic individuals who inhale an organometallic dust of particle size less than 1.5 μm, which can penetrate the alveoli of the lungs.[7] The pulmonary and subsequent systemic reactions occur when this material is retained and absorbed after exposure.[5]

Clinical Features

The initial symptoms of metal fume fever are of sudden onset (usually within 4 to 8 hours of exposure) and begin with mild upper airway irritation that later resembles the onset of a viral or bacterial infection.[5] Individuals experience malaise, high fever, chills, frontal headache, nausea, myalgia, and thirst. This may be followed by diaphoresis, cough, and chest tightness.[6]

Physical findings noted may be moist rales at the bases of the lungs with or without wheezing. The chest film is usually normal.[5] In addition, the precipitating antibodies and pulmonary infiltrates present in the occupational and vocational hypersensitivity pneumonitides are absent in metal fume fever.[7]

Mechanism of Intoxication

The pathogenesis of metal fume fever is unknown, and there are various theories as to the mechanism of intoxication including anaphylaxis, endotoxic mechanisms, protein denaturative mechanisms, and immunological mechanisms.[4] None of these theories has been proved.

Diagnosis

Diagnosis of metal fume fever is usually based on an occupational history of exposure to metal fumes. There is no specific test for confirming this condition.[5] Arterial blood gases may show hypoxemia if pulmonary involvement is extensive. In addition, the complete resolution of symptoms and functional abnormalities by 24 to 48 hours favors the diagnosis of metal fume fever.[6]

Treatment

Metal fume fever usually resolves completely in 24 to 48 hours without the need for treatment and without causing permanent lung damage.[7] Patients who present in a toxic state require immediate care in the emergency department.[6] Oxygen should be administered to correct hypoxemia, and bronchospasm can be treated with xanthine bronchodilators.[4]

HEAVY METAL ANTAGONISTS

Because metals persist in the body, a major therapeutic objective in poisoning is the administration of drugs that enhance their excretion. This is done with the aid of chelating agents,[8] which take up and firmly bind metallic ions.[2,9] Chelation is a common chemical reaction that takes place in a large number of compounds. Among the familiar and important endogenous chelating agents are vitamin B_{12} (for cobalt), hemoglobin (for iron), chlorophyll (for magnesium), and cytochrome oxidase (for iron and copper).

Chelating agents are generally nonspecific with regard to their affinity for metals. To varying degrees they mobilize and enhance the excretion of a wide range of metals, including essential metals such as calcium and zinc. Some chelating agents may not be useful because they are rapidly metabolized to inactive forms in the body. Others bind tightly to a toxic metal but at the same time remain immobilized.

Because chelating agents have the common property of reacting with metals to form tightly bound complexes, they can prevent or reverse the binding of toxic metals in biological substrates.[2] This can only be achieved when the chemical affinity of the complexing agent for the metal ions is higher than the affinity of the metal for the sensitive biological molecules.[10] When two or more ligands (such as sulfhydryl groups) in a molecule simultaneously form bonds with a metal atom by giving up protons or electrons, the donor molecule is properly referred to as a chelating agent. The resultant compound is more stable than others with just one binding site.[2] The product of such a reaction is a heterocyclic ring, which can be excreted in urine, feces, or both. Chelators are generally less stable at low pH, so that control of the pH of body fluids may be an important consideration during treatment.

Drugs that function as chelating agents include dimercaprol (British anti-lewisite; BAL), calcium ethylene diamine tetra-acetate (calcium EDTA), penicillamine (Cuprimine®, Depen®), and deferoxamine (Desferal®). Some of the newer agents not yet approved by the FDA are 2,3-dimercaptosuccinic acid (DMSA),[2] dimercaptopropanesulfonic acid (DMPS), and *N*-acetyl-D,L-penicillamine.[8] Calcium EDTA is used in acute lead poisoning; dimercaprol is widely used in poisoning with mercuric, arsenic, and occasionally lead salts; penicillamine is used in copper, lead, and mercury poisoning; and deferoxamine is used for acute iron poisoning.[10]

Dimercaprol

Dimercaprol is a dithiol compound that was developed as an antidote for the organoarsenic war gas lewisite,[2,10] which is a deadly gas that acts on the lungs and skin.[3] Because arsenic is known to be poisonous by inhibiting sulfhydryl groups in essential enzymes, an effort was made to find sulfhydryl substances that had a stronger attraction for arsenic than endogenous body constituents.[2,8]

Indications

Dimercaprol forms a poorly dissociable chelate with a number of metals and is effective for arsenicals, mercurials, and gold salts; it reduces the toxicity of chromium and nickel more than that of other metals (Table 38-2). It is of little value in alkyl lead and cadmium poisonings. In general, with the exception of copper, less depletion of trace metals is observed during therapy with dimercaprol than with calcium EDTA and penicillamine.[3]

Dimercaprol is the antidote of choice in the treatment of acute mercury, arsenic (except arsine), and gold poisoning.[2] When treating acute poisoning by mercury salts, dimercaprol is more effective if administered within 2 hours of ingestion because renal damage caused by mercury cannot be reversed. Dimercaprol is ineffective for alkyl mercury compounds, and the drug is only minimally effective in long-term mercury poisoning.

Even though dimercaprol chelates lead, other chelators such as calcium EDTA or penicillamine are preferred in treating lead poisoning. Dimercaprol, however, is useful as an adjunct to calcium EDTA in the treatment of acute lead encephalopathy or when blood lead concentration is greater than 70 µg per deciliter of whole blood. Dimercaprol is not useful in acute poisoning with alkyl lead compounds (tetraethyl lead), antimony, and bismuth. It should not be used in iron, cadmium, or selenium poisoning because the resulting dimercaprol-metal complexes are more toxic than the metal alone, especially to the kidneys.[8]

Dimercaprol not only protects sulfhydryl enzymes from inactivation by metals but reactivates enzyme systems. The degree to which the

Table 38-2 Characteristics and Effects of Dimercaprol

Metals well chelated
 Arsenic
 Mercury (except alkyl mercury)
 Gold
 Lead (encephalopathy, as adjunct to calcium EDTA)
 Chromium
 Nickel

Metals poorly chelated
 Alkyl lead
 Alkyl mercury
 Antimony
 Iron
 Cadmium
 Selenium

Dosage
 2.5 mg/kg IM every 4 hours for 2 days, then
 2.5 mg/kg IM twice daily for 1 day, then
 2.5 mg/kg IM once or twice daily for 5 to 10 days

Side effects
 Vomiting
 Tremors
 Hypertension
 Tachycardia
 Local pain
 Sterile abscess
 Burning sensation (lips, mouth, throat, penis)
 Abdominal pain
 Seizures
 Rhinorrhea
 Coma
 Death

enzyme can be reactivated is inversely proportional to the length of time it has been inactivated. Therefore, in the treatment of metal poisoning, especially of the acute type, therapy with dimercaprol is most effective if provided early in the course of poisoning.[2]

If the affinity of the metal for dimercaprol is greater than that for enzymes, a mercaptide is formed and can be excreted from the body. The dimercaprol-metal complex can dissociate or be oxidized, however, thus releasing the metal to exert its toxic effects again.

Pharmacokinetics

Because of the instability of dimercaprol in aqueous solutions, peanut oil is the solvent employed in pharmaceutical preparations.[2] Dimercaprol is administered by deep intramuscular injection. After injection of therapeutic doses, blood concentrations reach their peak in 30 to 60 minutes. On absorption, dimercaprol is distributed to all tissues including brain, with highest concentrations in liver and kidney. Elimination is complete within 4 hours. Dimercaprol can be administered in the presence of renal impairment because it is predominantly excreted in bile.[3]

Dosage

Dimercaprol is available as a 10% preparation in peanut oil. The recommended dosage for mercury, arsenic, and gold poisoning is approximately 2.5 mg/kg administered at 4-hour intervals during the first 2 days, twice on the third day, and once or twice daily thereafter for 5 to 10 days or until the patient has recovered. In acute mercury poisoning, an initial dose of 5 mg/kg is given and then is followed by the above regimen. For acute lead encephalopathy, 4 to 5 mg/kg is given alone in the first dose and is followed by the same regimen in combination with calcium EDTA.

Adverse Effects

Reactions to dimercaprol are common but not cumulative and may occur in approximately 50% of patients.[2] Dimercaprol has a strong mercaptan-like odor, which may be noted on the patient's breath. The outstanding side effects are on the CNS and the cardiovascular system. Toxic doses may cause vomiting, tremors, seizures, hypertension, and tachycardia beginning 15 to 30 minutes after injection.[8] In addition, frequent pain and occasional sterile abscesses occur at the injection site, particularly if the drug is not administered deeply enough. A burning sensation around the lips, mouth, throat, and penis, tingling in the hands, abdominal pain, blepharal spasm, rhinorrhea, fever, transient elevation of hepatic transaminase, coma, and death may also occur. Most side effects are transient and rapidly subside as the drug is metabolized and excreted.[2]

Dimercaprol should not be given concurrently with iron therapy because intensification of vomiting and reduction of lead excretion may occur. Renal damage is not a contraindication to its use. On the other hand, dimercaprol is potentially nephrotoxic. Because the chelate dissoci-

ates and breaks down in an acid medium, the urine should be kept alkaline during dimercaprol therapy to protect the kidneys. In patients with G-6-PD deficiency, dimercaprol would be used only in life-threatening situations because it may induce hemolysis.

Calcium EDTA

Calcium EDTA (edathamil calcium disodium, calcium disodium versenate), a polyaminocarboxylic acid, can chelate any divalent or trivalent metal that has a higher binding affinity for it than calcium.[8] It forms a stable soluble complex with the metal by displacement of the calcium on the molecule. This complex can then be excreted in the urine. In the past, the rapid intravenous administration of various sodium salts of EDTA produced precipitous decreases in the serum concentration of ionized calcium and symptoms of hypocalcemia.[2] Unlike sodium EDTA, calcium EDTA is saturated with calcium and therefore can be administered intravenously in relatively large quantities without causing any substantial changes in serum or total body calcium. The drug is usually administered to adults by intravenous infusion, and intramuscular administration is also suggested for children and in patients with incipient or overt lead encephalopathy.

Indications

Calcium EDTA is the treatment of choice for lead poisoning (Table 38-3).[8] It may also be useful in acute cadmium poisoning. Calcium EDTA may also be beneficial in the treatment of poisoning from other metals such as chromium, manganese, nickel, zinc, and possibly vanadium.[2] It may also be useful in the treatment of poisoning by radioactive and nuclear fission products such as plutonium, thorium, uranium, and yttrium.[11] The drug is not effective in the treatment of mercury, gold, or arsenic poisoning.[2] Although calcium EDTA was once administered orally to increase the excretion of lead, this route of administration is no longer recommended because the drug enhances absorption of lead in the gastrointestinal tract. In addition, orally administered calcium EDTA is poorly ab-

Table 38-3 Characteristics and Effects of Calcium EDTA

Metals well chelated
  Lead
  Cadmium
Metals somewhat chelated
  Chromium
  Manganese
  Nickel
  Zinc
  Vanadium
  Plutonium
  Thorium
  Uranium
  Yttrium
Metals poorly chelated
  Mercury
  Gold
  Arsenic
Dosage
  50 mg/kg/day in 6 doses for 5 days
Side effects
  Lacrimation
  Nasal congestion
  Sneezing
  Muscular pain
  Hypotension
  Hypercalcemia
  Renal tubular necrosis

---

sorbed from the gastrointestinal tract and is therefore considered ineffective.[8]

Pharmacokinetics

Calcium EDTA has a plasma half-life of 20 to 60 minutes with intravenous administration and 1.5 hours with intramuscular administration.[11] Fifty percent of a dose is excreted in the urine in 1 hour and 95% in 6 hours. When calcium EDTA is administered intravenously in the treatment of lead poisoning urinary excretion of chelated lead begins within about 1 hour, and peak excretion occurs within 24 to 48 hours.

Calcium EDTA is not metabolized. After parenteral administration it is rapidly excreted by glomerular filtration in urine either unchanged or as the metal chelate.[8] Calcium EDTA does not enter the cells, and thus it removes metals such as lead from the extracellular compartment; indirectly, the remainder of the metal is reduced in soft tissues, CNS tissue, and red blood cells.[11] When EDTA is used for lead poisoning, the amount of metal eliminated after an initial max-

imum in urine tends to decline and then again increases. This is because lead that is weakly bound to body constituents is eliminated initially and lead from intracellular locations is removed after a fairly long interval.[2]

Dosage

Calcium EDTA is available commercially as a 20% solution that is diluted before injection. For intravenous use, calcium EDTA should be diluted with 5% dextrose or normal saline to a concentration of less than 0.5%. This solution should be infused over a matter of hours. In mildly and moderately ill patients, a dosage of 50 mg/kg per 24 hours should not be exceeded. Administration takes place over a 5-day period, after which treatment is stopped for 2 to 5 days before a second dose, if necessary, is administered. Adequate urine flow must be established before the drug is given, and renal failure is a contraindication to its use. For acute lead intoxication, calcium EDTA used alone without concomitant dimercaprol therapy may aggravate symptoms. Combined chelation therapy with dimercaprol is therefore warranted in patients with acute encephalopathy or high blood lead concentrations. After the course of therapy, penicillamine can be administered orally.

During chelation with EDTA, urinalysis, blood urea nitrogen, serum creatinine, and liver function tests should be carefully monitored.

Adverse Effects

In general, calcium EDTA is an agent of relatively low toxicity. Hypocalcemia has occurred with disodium EDTA injected in too rapid a fashion. Because calcium EDTA has produced electrocardiographic changes, such as inversion of the T wave, patients should be monitored for cardiac rhythm irregularities during parenteral therapy.[2,8]

Mild side effects are common and include histamine-like reactions such as lacrimation, nasal congestion, and sneezing. Muscular pains, hypotension, and hypercalcemia may also occur. Calcium EDTA is potentially nephrotoxic, the principal lesion being renal tubular necrosis. Nephrotoxicity can usually be prevented by careful dosage regulation and use of intermittent therapy.

Penicillamine

Penicillamine (Cuprimine®, Depen®, dimethylcysteine), a monothiol agent, is a hydrolysis product of penicillin.[12] It has no antibacterial activity. It is an effective chelating agent for copper, mercury, iron, zinc, lead, and gold (Table 38-4).[13] The primary use of this drug as a chelating agent is to remove copper from individuals suffering from Wilson's hepatolenticular degeneration. Penicillamine is also effective in the treatment of rheumatoid arthritis and cystinuria.[12]

Penicillamine is well absorbed from the gastrointestinal tract; therefore, one of its advantages is that it can be administered orally.[8] Blood concentrations reach a peak approximately 1 hour after ingestion. Penicillamine is rapidly excreted in the urine. The drug is currently available in capsules of 125 and 250 mg. The usual dosage is 30 mg/kg/day or 250 mg 4 times a day in adults.

Penicillamine is relatively nontoxic. Adverse effects include hypersensitivity reactions, rash, fever, nausea, vomiting, nephrotic syndrome, optic neuritis, drug-induced systemic lupus erythematosus, leukopenia, neutropenia, and coagulation deficits.[13] Reactions are usually mild. Rarely, severe and even life-threatening reactions such as autoimmune hemolytic anemia and Stevens-Johnson syndrome have been observed. In addition, penicillamine is a pyridoxine antagonist because pyridoxal-dependent enzyme systems are inhibited. Dietary supplementation of pyridoxine is therefore recommended.[13] Penicillin allergy is not usually a problem, but the possibility of an allergic reaction exists.

Chelating Agents Not Approved by the FDA

Dimercaptopropanesulfonic Acid and Dimercaptosuccinic Acid

DMSA and DMPS are water-soluble chemical analogs of dimercaprol. In contrast to dimercaprol, they have less toxicity, greater water solubility, and limited lipid solubility and are effective when given orally.[10,14,15]

Table 38-4 Characteristics and Effects of Penicillamine

Metals well chelated
  Copper
  Mercury
  Iron
  Zinc
  Lead
  Gold
Dosage
  250 mg 4 times a day, or 30 mg/kg/day
Side effects
  Hypersensitivity
  Nausea
  Vomiting
  Nephrotic syndrome
  Optic neuritis
  Systemic lupus erythematosus
  Leukopenia
  Neutropenia
  Pyridoxine deficiency
  Autoimmune hemolytic anemia
  Stevens-Johnson syndrome

DMSA has recently been shown to be highly effective for the treatment of occupational plumbism as well as childhood lead intoxication, occupational mercurialism, and possibly methyl mercury poisoning.[16–18] DMSA also appears to be highly effective in the treatment of arsenic poisoning.[19]

Both DMPS and DMSA have been studied for more than 25 years in countries other than the United States and have been found to lack serious adverse effects at clinically effective doses.[10,15,20] Of the two drugs, DMSA appears to be more promising in treating heavy metal poisoning, primarily because of its lower median lethal dose and wider therapeutic index.[21] At present, DMSA remains an investigational drug in the United States and has recently been classified as an orphan drug by the FDA.[22] Studies appear to indicate that DMSA is more specific and less toxic than parenteral calcium EDTA and dimercaprol[9] and far more effective than penicillamine in reducing the body lead burden. For this reason, DMSA may soon become the drug of choice for the treatment of lead poisoning.[10,15]

DMSA has no effect on the elimination of iron, calcium, or magnesium.[22] When used in therapeutic doses, neither DMSA nor DMPS appears to have any marked effect on trace metals in the body except for a small increase in urinary excretion of zinc and copper.[20]

The acute toxicity of DMSA is less than that of DMPS, which is much less than that of dimercaprol.[21] Side effects of DMPS include nausea, weakness, vertigo, and pruritus. Nephrotoxicity has not been noted.[15,20]

N-Acetyl-D,L-Penicillamine

N-Acetyl-D,L-penicillamine is formed by the acetylation of the amine group of penicillamine. It is not active as a substrate for the amino acid oxidases and cysteine desulfhydrase, which allows for metal binding by its sulfhydryl groups.[9]

Thus far, experience with N-acetyl-D,L-penicillamine has been encouraging. Toxicity is low and therapeutic effectiveness relatively high. Nevertheless, it is still classified as a "chemical" and not as an experimental drug; this classification impairs its use. Although a number of investigators have advocated the use of this agent, it is not currently available in North America.

Most patients treated with N-acetyl-D,L-penicillamine experienced urinary excretion of mercury, and those with neurologic impairment improved.

REFERENCES

1. Chisolm J: Poisoning due to heavy metals. *Pediatr Clin North Am* 1970;17:591–615.

2. Greenhouse A: Heavy metals and the nervous system. *Clin Neuropharmacol* 1982;5:45–92.

3. Oehme F: Mechanism of heavy metal toxicities. *Clin Toxicol* 1972;5:151–167.

4. Mueller E, Seger D: Metal fume fever—A review. *J Emerg Med* 1985;2:271–274.

5. Johnson J, Kilburn K: Cadmium-induced metal fume fever: Results of inhalation challenge. *Am J Industr Med* 1983;4:533–540.

6. Dula D: Metal fume fever. *JACEP* 1978;7:448–450.

7. Hopper W: Metal fume fever. *Postgrad Med* 1978; 63:123–127.

8. Chenoweth M: Clinical uses of metal-binding drugs. *Clin Pharmacol Ther* 1968;9:365–387.

9. Kostyniak P, Clarkson T: Role of chelating agents in metal toxicity. *Fundam Appl Toxicol* 1981;1:376–380.

10. Aaseth J: Recent advances in the therapy of metal poisoning with chelating agents. *Hum Toxicol* 1983; 2:257–272.

11. Craven P, Morelli H: Chelation therapy. *West J Med* 1975;122:277–278.

12. Silva A, Fleshman D, Shore B: The effects of penicillamine on the body burdens of several heavy metals. *Health Phy* 1973;24:535–539.

13. Halverson P, Kozin F, Bernhard C, et al: Toxicity of penicillamine. *JAMA* 1978;240:1870–1871.

14. Graziano J, Cuccia D, Friedheim E: The pharmacology of 2,3-dimercaptosuccinic acid and its potential use in arsenic poisoning. *J Pharmacol Exp Ther* 1978; 20:1051–1055.

15. Lenz K, Hruby K, Druml W, et al: 2,3-Dimercaptosuccinic acid in human arsenic poisoning. *Arch Toxicol* 1981;47:241–243.

16. Graziano J, Leong J, Friedheim E: 2,3-Dimercaptosuccinic acid: A new agent for the treatment of lead poisoning. *J Pharmacol Exp Ther* 1978;206:696–700.

17. Friedheim E, Corvi C: Meso-dimercaptosuccinic acid: A chelating agent for the treatment of mercury poisoning. *J Pharm Pharmacol* 1975;27:624–626.

18. Bentur Y, Brook G: Meso-2,3-dimercaptosuccinic acid in the diagnosis and treatment of lead poisoning. *Clin Toxicol* 1987;25:39–51.

19. Graziano J, Siris E, LoIacono N, et al: 2,3-Dimercaptosuccinic acid as an antidote for lead intoxication. *Clin Pharmacol Ther* 1985;37:431–438.

20. Aposhian H: DMSA and DMPS—Water-soluble antidotes for heavy metal poisoning. *Annu Rev Pharmacol Toxicol* 1983;23:193–215.

21. Friedheim E, Graziano J, Popovac D, et al: Treatment of lead poisoning by 2,3-dimercaptosuccinic acid. *Lancet* 1978;2:1234–1235.

22. Graziano J: Role of 2,3-dimercaptosuccinic acid in the treatment of heavy metal poisoning. *Med Toxicol* 1986; 1:155–162.

ADDITIONAL SELECTED REFERENCES

Anseline P: Zinc-fume fever. *Med J Aust* 1972;2:316–318.

Day A, Golding J, Lee P, et al: Penicillamine in rheumatoid disease: A long-term study. *Br Med J* 1974;1:180–183.

Hughes R, Gazzard B, Murray-Lyon I, et al: The use of cysteamine and dimercaprol. *J Int Med Res* 1976; 4(suppl):123–129.

Oehme F: British anti-lewisite (BAL): The classic heavy metal antidote. *Clin Toxicol* 1972;5:215–222.

chapter 39

Iron

Iron is distributed throughout all life forms and is one of the most abundant and important of the biological trace metals. Although written reports of the toxic effects of iron have been known for more than 100 years,[1] iron has been used medicinally for several centuries.[2,3] Iron and its compounds were once widely regarded as relatively harmless, and most adults and some medical personnel still may not be fully aware of iron's serious potential as a poison.[3] Iron poisonings still occur each year in the United States. Although the mortality rate today is less than 5%,[4,5] at one time it was as high as 50% in serious poisonings.[3,6–8] The decline in mortality rate is due in part to the use of the chelating agent deferoxamine (Desferal®), but in addition better supportive medical care has become available.[8]

Ferrous sulfate and ferrous gluconate are two of the most common preparations of iron. The accidental ingestion of preparations containing iron is still relatively common in children because of the multitude of such preparations (Table 39-1)[9]; intentional overdose from iron is occasionally seen in adults.[6,10] Many iron preparations are sugar-coated and brightly colored, which increases their attractiveness to children.[2] Iron tablets may also be confused with similar-appearing sugar-coated candies.[11] In addition, in homes with young children containers may be kept on the dining room table or the kitchen counter rather than in the medicine cabinet.[12–14] The failure to dispense iron in child-resistant containers also may contribute to the problem.[15] Because of such factors, the incidence of iron

Table 39-1 Selected Iron Preparations by Trade Name

Ferrous Sulfate	Ferrous Gluconate	Ferrous Fumarate
Feosol	Fergon	Feco-T
Fer-In-Sol	Ferralet	Femiron
Fero-Gradumet	Ferrous-G	Feostat
Ferralyn		Fumasorb
Mol-Iron		Fumerin
		Ircon
		Laud-Iron
		Maniron
		Toleron

poisonings in children younger than 5 years of age appears to be greater than in adults.

Iron is capable of producing chronic poisoning as a result of dietary or medicinal overload, from various types of iron storage diseases, or secondary to occupational exposure. The emergency department physician, however, is most commonly confronted with the acute ingestion of iron.

ABSORPTION

Iron crosses cell membranes only in the ferrous state; ferric ions in food are liberated in the stomach by acid digestion, reduced to the ferrous state, and absorbed. Typical daily intake of iron is approximately 15 to 40 mg,[16] but because of an intestinal mucosal block only 10% of ingested iron is absorbed.[12,17] In the routine daily absorption of dietary iron, the transport of ferrous compounds is energy dependent. This saturable, carrier-mediated uptake process is dependent on binding of iron in the lumen of the gastrointestinal tract and is the rate-limiting step for iron absorption. Absorption occurs mostly in the duodenum and upper jejunum, although the entire intestinal tract, including the colon, is able to absorb iron.[11,18] The divalent (ferrous) iron is absorbed into the gastrointestinal mucosa and converted to the trivalent (ferric) form, which attaches to ferritin in the intestinal mucosal cell wall.[2] The ferritin-ferric complex then passes into the bloodstream and is attached to transferrin.[12] Iron is then carried to the reticuloendothelial cells of the bone marrow for hemoglobin synthesis or to the liver or spleen for storage as ferritin or hemosiderin (Fig. 39-1).[17]

Toxic amounts of iron in solution are rapidly absorbed in the large and small bowel in a concentration-dependent fashion. With toxic amounts the capacity of the normal mechanisms of absorption is exceeded, and absorption becomes a passive, first-order process.[12]

DISTRIBUTION

The body contains approximately 4 to 5 g of iron, of which approximately 60% is contained in hemoglobin, 25% is stored as ferritin and hemosiderin (mainly in the liver), 3% is in myoglobin, and 1% is distributed among various heme-containing enzymes such as cytochrome oxidase, xanthine oxidase, and catalase.[16,18]

EXCRETION

Once iron is absorbed, its removal from the body is difficult. Although iron is lost through sweat, bile, and the desquamation of skin and mucosal surfaces, this loss only totals roughly 1.5 mg/day. In women an additional 0.5 mg/day may be lost in the menses.[12] There is no effective physiologic mechanism for iron excretion,[16,18] which is a fact of great importance in iron intoxication.

TOXICITY

When estimating toxicity of an acute ingestion of iron, the amount of elemental iron should be used in the calculation rather than the milligrams of a particular iron preparation.[2] Ferrous sulfate contains approximately 20% elemental iron, ferrous gluconate 12%, ferrous fumarate 33%, and ferrocholinate 13%.[2,19] Conversion factors for calculating the amount of elemental iron in an iron preparation are given in Table 39-2. For example, there is 60 mg of elemental iron in

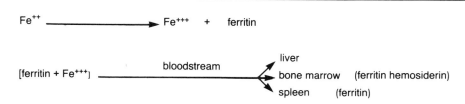

Figure 39-1 Absorption of Iron

Table 39-2 Amounts of Elemental Iron in Various Iron Preparations

Preparation	Percentage of Iron	Conversion Factor*
Ferrous Sulfate	20	5
Ferrous Gluconate	12	8.7
Ferrous Fumarate	33	3
Ferrocholinate	13	7.7

* Conversion factor to calculate amount of elemental iron from milligrams of prepared iron.

300 mg of ferrous sulfate (the total milligrams of prepared iron [300] divided by 5).

Reduced or metallic iron in powder form is nontoxic unless it is oxidized and enters the metabolic cycles.[20] A dose of 20 to 60 mg/kg of elemental iron is considered toxic, and a lethal dose is within the range of 60 to 180 mg/kg.[5,18,21]

The basic pathophysiologic effects of iron in toxic doses are of five types: (1) metabolic disorders, (2) hepatic dysfunctions, (3) CNS dysfunctions, (4) cardiovascular system dysfunctions, and (5) gastrointestinal tract disturbances.[12]

The symptoms of iron poisoning are due to both local and systemic effects and may be influenced by factors such as the chemical and physical forms of the iron, dose, route of administration, and duration of exposure.[22] In general, the ferrous salts are more toxic than the ferric salts. Although a mucosal block or barrier to the absorption of iron exists with normal intake of iron, in overdose situations the mucosal barrier ceases to exist and great amounts of iron may be absorbed.[14] In this event, absorbed iron exceeds the binding capacity of transferrin and passes into various tissues, causing toxicity.

There are five phases of intoxication associated with the acute significant ingestion of iron (Table 39-3). These phases represent a rough guideline for the evolution of various toxic effects.

Phase 1

Phase 1 may begin 30 minutes to 2 hours after an acute ingestion. The first obvious signs of toxicity are gastrointestinal; this symp-

Table 39-3 Phases of Iron Intoxication

Phase 1: gastrointestinal (30 minutes to 2 hours)
Vomiting
Hematemesis
Abdominal pain
Diarrhea
Lethargy
Shock
Hypotension
Metabolic acidosis
Phase 2: "recovery" (2 to 24 hours)
Apparent response to therapy
Phase 3: metabolic acidosis (12 to 48 hours)
Shock
Coma
Phase 4: hepatic (2 to 4 days)
Hepatic necrosis
Bleeding diathesis
Phase 5: gastrointestinal (2 to 4 weeks)
Gastric scarring
Pyloric stenosis
Achlorhydria
Hepatic cirrhosis
CNS abnormalities

tomatology not only is predominant but is considered the *sine qua non* of iron poisoning. Vomiting is invariably the first manifestation of toxicity and usually occurs in the first hour after ingestion.[5] This may possibly proceed to hematemesis as a result of acute hemorrhagic gastritis, which may occasionally be life threatening.[1] Other symptoms include colicky abdominal pain and diarrhea (which sometimes may be bloody and explosive). Lethargy (a common early symptom), coma, hypotension, and metabolic acidosis may ensue during this early phase.[23]

Iron is a corrosive agent and, on direct contact, may produce lesions similar to those caused by acids, although generally they are more superficial in nature.[24] Because iron is a solid, it spares the mouth, pharynx, and upper esophagus. Liquid preparations and tablets primarily affect the pyloric region of the stomach and the duodenum. Enteric-coated tablets may also involve the lower small intestine.[14] Chewable tablets are associated with more proximal lesions.

Phase 2

Phase 2 may occur 2 to 24 hours after an ingestion; at this time the patient appears to recover. This phase may be quite deceptive because the patient may seem to have responded to therapy or the condition may continue to go undiagnosed.[24] The course of the intoxication proceeds directly to the next phase, however.

Phase 3

Phase 3 usually begins 12 to 48 hours after ingestion. A metabolic acidosis that may be particularly resistant to bicarbonate therapy, as well as shock and coma, may ensue. Metabolic acidosis from iron may be due to the hydrogen ion produced during conversion of ferrous to ferric iron in the blood, with the formation of ferric hydroxide complexes in the circulatory system.[6,16,25] In addition, however, there is an interference with the Krebs cycle enzymes in the liver and other tissues, which causes a block in organic acid metabolism and a buildup of lactic and citric acids.

Shock is a cardinal feature of fatal acute iron poisoning in children. It may be diphasic, occurring within the first 6 to 8 hours and again approximately 36 hours after ingestion.[26] The shock is thought to be due to peripheral circulatory failure induced by absorbed iron as well as to other factors such as ferritin, which may be acting as a vasodepressant. In addition, serotonin or histamine release may act to cause hypotension. The most likely explanation for shock is a combination of these factors in addition to the direct vasodilation effect of iron on blood vessels, which leads to shock. After acute ingestion of a large dose of iron there is a dramatic decrease in circulating plasma volume, as reflected in increases in the hematocrit. Cardiac output is lowered on the basis of a decreased filling pressure.

Phase 4

Phase 4 may begin 2 to 4 days after an ingestion. The liver may rarely be a target organ for damage by direct uptake of iron, leading to hepatic necrosis. This may be evidenced by elevation of bilirubin, serum glutamic-oxaloacetic transaminase, and alkaline phosphatase concentrations and possibly manifested clinically by jaundice.[27] In severe cases, hepatic coma with behavioral changes and elevated blood ammonia values have been reported. Damage is thought to be due to cellular injury from the direct action of iron on the mitochondrial cells of the liver. Another theory suggests that hepatic necrosis may be caused by depletion of sulfhydryl enzymes secondary to iron, which then allows another unknown toxin to produce necrotic changes.[27,28]

A bleeding diathesis may also be noted during this phase.[5] These changes, if present, are due to a direct effect of iron on the various proteins involved in blood coagulation and are not a consequence of acidosis, shock, or liver damage.[20] Interference with these clotting mechanisms may contribute to severe hemorrhagic manifestations, which may include prolongation of the prothrombin time, reduction in thromboplastin generation, poor to absent clot retraction, and thrombocytopenia.[5] All three stages of clotting may be involved: the generation of thromboplastin becomes impaired (first stage), the prothrombin time is prolonged (second stage), and the conversion of fibrinogen to fibrin becomes defective (third stage).

Phase 5

Phase 5 may occur 2 to 4 weeks after ingestion as a result of the early corrosive effect of iron on the gastrointestinal tract. It may be manifested by intractable nausea and vomiting secondary to gastric scarring as well as fibrosis leading to pyloric obstruction or stenosis.[24] One report described a severe corrosive gastroduodenitis with subsequent fibrosis and scarring of the stomach and duodenum, necessitating abdominal surgery.[29] Also, perforation and stricture formation are not uncommon. These lesions can be demonstrated by barium contrast studies. Because of this destruction, achlorhydria may supervene together with other nutritional problems caused by the destruction of the mucosa.[18]

DIAGNOSIS AND LABORATORY ANALYSIS

History and Physical Examination

The diagnosis of acute iron poisoning in a young child is frequently complicated by an unreliable history and by the diphasic nature of the symptoms. Patients may present without a definite history of iron ingestion, but it should be suspected in any patient who is vomiting, has bloody diarrhea, or is lethargic, comatose, or in shock. If iron poisoning is suspected an examination of the patient's emesis may reveal iron tablets, and the stool should then be examined for a black color secondary to iron ingestion (Table 39-4).[30]

Plain Roentgenography

Plain roentgenography of the abdomen can be a useful diagnostic procedure in the management of iron overdose (Fig. 39-2).[13,31] Depending on the time after ingestion of iron-containing tablets, the preparation's solubility, and the degree of prior emesis or gastric lavage, the film can be a guide to the number of tablets taken and can indicate whether removal is necessary. A normal roentgenogram, however, does not rule out an ingestion because iron in solution is no longer radiopaque[29] and because iron-containing vitamins can be imaged for only a brief period and appear with low density. Ferrous sulfate, gluconate, and fumarate all have a high content of elemental iron, which results in a slower dissolution of the tablets and thereby renders the preparations radiopaque for a longer period of time.

Table 39-4 Diagnostic Workup of Iron Poisoning

Unknown poisoning
Historical clues
Lethargy
Vomiting
Hematemesis
Shock
Bloody diarrhea

(*If positive, proceed to suspected or confirmed poisoning*)

Suspected poisoning
Plain roentgenogram of abdomen
Examination of emesis for iron
Examination of stool for black color
Provocative deferoxamine test of gastric aspirate

(*If positive, proceed to confirmed poisoning*)

Confirmed poisoning
Plain roentgenogram of abdomen
Iron and total iron-binding capacity
Fischer test (unreliable)
Clotting studies
Complete blood cell count
Blood type and crossmatch
Electrolyte studies
Arterial blood gas analysis

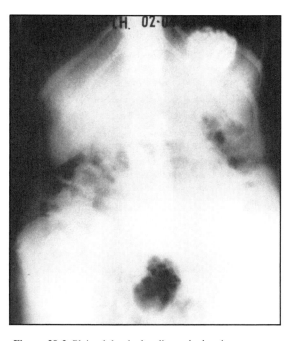

Figure 39-2 Plain abdominal radiograph showing concretion of iron tablets in the stomach. *Source*: Reprinted with permission from *Medical Toxicology* (1986;1:89), Copyright © 1986, Adis Press International Inc.

Colorimetric Tests

Colormetric testing has serious limitations, and the results should not be relied on to make a diagnosis or to determine extent of injury.[32] Two tests that have been employed in a suspected iron overdose involve the chelating agent deferoxamine. One test involves the oral administration of deferoxamine and is an attempt at diagnosis. The other involves intravenous administration of deferoxamine and is an attempt at determining whether free iron is in the blood, which is an indication for chelation therapy.

In the first test, a small amount of deferoxamine is mixed with gastric aspirate. If a red color is produced, the presence of iron in the gastrointestinal tract is confirmed.[32] The major limitation of this test is that gastrointestinal bleeding is usually associated with a moderate to severe iron intoxication.[31]

The second test is provocative and is not suggested for routine use; however, it may be helpful in the occasional situation where no laboratory analysis is available. This test involves the administration of deferoxamine intravenously (10 to 15 mg/kg). Production of a reddish-brown urine indicates that there is free iron circulating in the body that has been chelated with the deferoxamine. The value of this test may be limited because the characteristic color may not always develop despite the presence of chelated iron in the urine.[31]

Serum Iron and Total Iron-Binding Capacity

Further workup for suspected iron overdose should include a definitive test of the serum iron and iron-binding capacity, the results of which are crucial when deciding whether chelation treatment is to be instituted. As mentioned earlier, iron is considered toxic when the plasma concentration exceeds the total iron-binding capacity of transferrin because, once plasma transferrin has been saturated, the iron is distributed into cells and causes damage. Many hospitals do not perform serum iron and total iron-binding capacity tests as a "stat" procedure, but the importance of this test requires that there be some backup facility that can do so.

Emergency serum iron measurements should be available around the clock to obviate the use of indirect methods.[31]

The serum iron concentration must be measured after absorption is complete and before distribution and protein binding in the tissues have contributed to a significant decrease in the initial peak concentration.[14] Although the kinetics of iron after overdose have not been thoroughly investigated, the limited evidence available indicates that serum iron concentration usually peaks 3 to 5 hours after ingestion and decreases rapidly thereafter[22,33,35]; it is therefore advisable to obtain measurements during that time.[31] Because of the rapid clearance of free iron, severely toxic conditions may be associated with only minimally elevated plasma iron concentrations if values are obtained after the peak period.[35] Once the initial serum iron concentration has been determined to be in the toxic range, there is little value to continued measurements of the serum iron or total iron-binding capacity.

The normal serum iron concentration is 50 to 150 µg/dL in adults and children older than 5 years of age and 40 to 100 µg/dL for children younger than 5 years of age (Table 39-5). Total iron-binding capacity or plasma transferrin is roughly one-third saturated under normal conditions, with the total iron-binding capacity ranging from 300 to 450 µg/dL.[18] Serum iron concentrations less than 350 µg/dL have rarely been associated with significant illness.

Most commonly used methods for the measurement of serum iron concentrations involve the liberation of ferric iron bound to transferrin by weak reducing agents followed by the formation of a colored complex with ferrous iron and a chromogenic agent such as ferrozine. If chelation therapy is instituted these methods may reveal spuriously low serum iron concentrations because of the chelation of some of the iron liberated from transferrin.[31]

Miscellaneous Laboratory Procedures

The Fischer test[34] or variations of the colorimetric test[21] that attempt to determine free iron are unreliable, and their results should not be substituted for serum iron and total iron-binding

Table 39-5 Serum Iron Concentrations and Toxicity

Iron Concentration (micrograms per deciliter)	Degree of Toxicity
100	Nontoxic (normal value)
100-300	Minimal
350-500	Moderate
500-1000	Serious
1000	Potentially lethal

capacity.[31,32] Clotting studies as well as a complete blood cell count, electrolyte studies, arterial blood gas analysis, and liver function tests should be obtained for baseline values. A blood type and hold should be performed because patients sometimes need blood transfusions. There is little value in obtaining indicators of hepatic function early in the course of iron intoxication other than for baseline values.[36] It is reasonable to obtain transaminase values after the first 24 hours to assess baseline hepatic function. Prognosis is correlated with the presence of severe symptoms (shock, coma, or vasomotor instability) as well as the serum iron concentration in relation to the total iron-binding capacity within the first 3 to 5 hours after ingestion.[31,37]

TREATMENT

Treatment must be vigorous and prompt and must consist of supportive measures, prevention of absorption of iron in the gastrointestinal tract, and chelation therapy (Table 39-6). Diuresis and dialysis have been shown to be ineffective. Although phlebotomy has been tried, the use of chelating agents is the preferred method of increasing excretion of iron.

Prevention of Absorption

Iron is notorious for its resistance to traditional stomach-emptying procedures probably because of its ability to clump together and form large aggregates. Initial treatment, however, should still consist of emesis or lavage. Gastric lavage in this instance may be preferable because agents can be administered down the lavage tube that form a poorly soluble complex with iron and so limit its absorption.

Table 39-6 Treatment of Iron Poisoning

Indication	Treatment
Acute ingestion	Emesis or lavage
Fluid loss	Normal saline
Metabolic acidosis	Bicarbonate instillation
Shock	Sodium bicarbonate
	Military antishock trousers
	Parenteral fluids
	Vasopressors
Severe overdose	Deferoxamine
	IV: 1 g not to exceed 10 to 15 mg/kg/hour (or 6 g per 24 hours or 80 mg/kg per 24 hours)
	IM: 40 to 90 mg/kg every 8 hours

Intragastric Complexation

The use of intragastric complexation in iron intoxication is controversial,[37] but phosphates, deferoxamine, bicarbonate, and magnesium hydroxide have been suggested as complexing agents to decrease absorption of iron remaining in the gastrointestinal tract.

Phosphates. Sodium biphosphate (Fleet® enema) solution combines with the ingested iron to form ferrous phosphate and ferric phosphate. Because maximum phosphate absorption occurs in the midgut, even if a small amount of the lavage solution is not retrieved it could present a significant phosphate load for absorption.[14,31] In addition, the absorption of phosphate may be enhanced across an intestinal mucosal barrier that is disrupted by the direct irritant action of ingested iron. Because of reports of toxicity after the administration of phosphate in children, with ensuing hyperphosphatemia, hypocalcemia, and other disturbances (including dysrhythmias), this therapy is not recommended.[38,39]

Deferoxamine. The oral administration of deferoxamine has been suggested to reduce the absorption of iron, but there is evidence that this complex is absorbed and may lead to further iron toxicity. Because deferoxamine is only effective in chelating ferric iron and all medicinal preparations contain ferrous salts, intragastric deferoxamine would seem to be of little value.[31] In addition, deferoxamine is poorly absorbed from the gut when the mucosa is intact. Thus its use is not recommended.

Bicarbonate. An alternative lavage solution is sodium bicarbonate, which when administered down the lavage tube forms an insoluble complex of ferrous and ferric carbonate that is not absorbed from the gastrointestinal tract. Because sodium bicarbonate appears to be less dangerous than other intragastric complexing agents, its use is recommended. In addition, absorption of sodium bicarbonate could reduce the metabolic acidosis that occurs in iron intoxication.[38] After gastric emptying, 100 mL of a 5% solution of sodium bicarbonate or sodium bicarbonate ampules can be instilled through the gastric lavage tube and then retrieved. Although the efficacy of this treatment has recently been questioned,[37] there does not appear to be great potential for toxicity from this regimen.

Whole Gut Lavage

Whole gut emptying has been suggested if a slow-release iron formulation was ingested or if an abdominal radiograph after gastric lavage shows persistence of tablets in the stomach or small intestine.[31,40] When a large number of opacities are identified in a single location, it may be reasonable to consider surgical intervention. The clinician must consider the stability of the patient, the number of tablets seen on the radiograph, and the potential for other procedures such as lavage and emesis successfully to remove these tablets.

Other Therapeutic Measures

An important part of therapy consists of adequately correcting any third-space fluid losses with appropriate crystalloid. Military antishock trousers may also be applied in an effort to increase venous return. An indwelling urinary catheter should be placed to measure the urine output and to observe the color of the urine for determining whether the chelating agent should be continued. Sodium bicarbonate should be administered for metabolic acidosis, and vasopressors may be necessary for shock if fluid administration and military antishock trousers are ineffective.

Chelation Therapy with Deferoxamine

Deferoxamine mesylate is a chelating agent that was originally obtained from a species of *Streptomyces*, one of the organisms that produces low–molecular weight chelators as part of its iron-transport system. It was discovered as a result of the investigation of the antibiotic properties of the siderochromes, a class of naturally occurring compounds.[25] Clinical use of deferoxamine mesylate for cases of acute iron poisoning was first reported in the early 1960s.

When deferoxamine chelates with iron, it forms a brownish-red complex with iron bound in the center.[41] This stable ring, unlike free iron, is soluble in water and readily excreted by the kidneys. Theoretically, 100 mg of deferoxamine can bind 8 to 9 mg of elemental iron.[20,35] Deferoxamine has an affinity for iron that is 10 times greater than that of any other known chelator and thus combines more firmly than other chelators, with resultant greater urinary excretion of iron.[23] Deferoxamine also has the advantage of being specific for iron, with virtually no attraction to other metals. It therefore does not cause excretion of calcium, copper, magnesium, or zinc.[14,20,35] Deferoxamine has a volume of distribution of about 60% body weight and a plasma half-life of 10 to 30 minutes. It is metabolized to inactive products by plasma and other tissues.

Indication for Chelation Therapy

Chelation therapy is indicated when iron concentrations exceed the total iron-binding capacity or if the serum iron concentration is greater than 350 μg/dL,[1,33] or in any patient who exhibits serious systemic toxicity when no measurements can be obtained.[31] Chelation is not indicated if the patient is asymptomatic or has minor symptoms with no evidence of gastrointestinal bleeding or if the total iron-binding capacity is greater than the serum iron concentration and the patient has ingested approximately 150 to 300 mg/kg of elemental iron.

Method of Action

It is believed that the efficacy of deferoxamine involves the enhancement of iron elimination through the formation of water-soluble, renally excreted ferrioxamine.[42] Several reports suggest that deferoxamine also exerts a protective effect at the cellular level by chelation of iron in the extracellular space.[23] Another possibility is that deferoxamine enters cells and chelates extra-mitochondrial iron.[31]

Route of Administration and Dosage

Various regimens and routes of administration of deferoxamine have been recommended. Deferoxamine is poorly absorbed from the gut if the mucosa is intact and therefore should be administered parenterally. Intravenous administration is preferred,[1,35] but intramuscular administration was at one time suggested because of reports of hypotension from intravenous administration. It has been shown, however, that hypotension is a consequence of too rapid an intravenous administration. As long as deferoxamine is administered properly, there should be no significant side effects noted.

It has been shown that a dose of deferoxamine given by slow infusion results in more effective chelation and iron excretion than when the same dose is given as a single injection.[25,43] In addition, maximal iron mobilization may require constant exposure of labile iron pools to deferoxamine.[35] The pharmacodynamics of deferoxamine appear to support its use as a continuous infusion in acute iron overdosage to maximize net iron excretions. One gram should be administered in normal saline, with infusion rates not to exceed 10 to 15 mg/kg/hour.[31] This rate can then be reduced to 5 mg/kg/hour after 4 to 6 hours. In severe cases this therapy may be required for 48 to 72 hours.[44] In view of the possible intracellular action of deferoxamine, it appears reasonable to continue treatment until after the pink color of the urine has disappeared and the patient is without signs and symptoms of iron poisoning for at least 24 hours.[4] The total amount of deferoxamine should not exceed 6 g in any 24-hour period in an adult or 80 mg/kg in a child, whichever is lower.[35] In the absence of toxicity, larger doses may be administered.[31,42]

Although deferoxamine may be administered intramuscularly, the quantities required may cause pain at the site of injection, sterile necrosis, and local discoloration.[41] The dose for intramuscular administration in a child ranges from 40 to 90 mg/kg, not to exceed 1 g every 8 hours.[14,18,44] In an adult, 1 g is administered initially and is followed by 500 mg every 4 hours.[33]

Toxicity

The toxicity of deferoxamine is minimal, but symptoms may include gastrointestinal discomfort after oral administration and hypotension after excessively rapid intravenous administration of a large dose, which is probably a result of venous dilation.[24,35] If hypotension develops, the infusion should be temporarily stopped and begun again at a lower infusion rate.[31] In addition, tachycardia as a result of the hypotension and urticaria as an allergic response may occur. Lens opacification has been reported in animals after long-term administration of deferoxamine, but this is not a problem in the acute overdose situation.[25]

Dialysis

Although dialysis can be effective in removing the ferrioxamine complex or chelated iron, it is not as effective as renal excretion in iron removal. Dialysis is indicated only if renal shutdown occurs after chelation therapy has been instituted.[31]

Miscellaneous Methods

Exchange transfusion has been employed, but in view of the rapid intracellular movement of iron it is not an efficient therapeutic modality.[45] Surgical intervention may be necessary for the patient who develops signs of perforation and peritonitis in the early stages of intoxication or subsequent stricture formation,[24,46] and some investigators have recommended early laparotomy in patients with massive iron ingestion to resect potentially gangrenous bowel.[29] Individuals who recover from significant iron overdose should have adequate followup for potential long-term complications.

REFERENCES

1. Greengard J: Iron poisoning in children. *Clin Toxicol* 1975;8:575–597.

2. Crotty J: Acute iron poisoning in children. *Clin Toxicol* 1971;4:615–619.

3. Aldrich R: *Iron in Clinical Medicine*. Berkeley, University of California Press, 1958, pp 58–65.

4. Leiken S, Vassough P, Mocher-Faterni F: Chelation therapy in acute iron poisoning. *J Pediatr* 1967;71:425–428.

5. Wasserman G, Martens V: Early aggressive treatment of iron poisoning. *Am Fam Physician* 1977;15:125–127.

6. Eriksson F, Johansson S, Mellstedt H, et al: Iron intoxication in two adult patients. *Acta Med Scand* 1974;196:231–236.

7. Ross F: Pyloric stenosis and fibrosis stricture of the stomach due to ferrous sulfate poisoning. *Br Med J* 1953;2:1200–1202.

8. Greenblatt D, Allen M, Koch-Weser J: Accidental iron poisoning in childhood: Six cases including one fatality. *Clin Pediatr* 1976;15:835–838.

9. Angle C: Symposium on iron poisoning. *Clin Toxicol* 1971;4:525–527.

10. Wallack M, Winkelstein A: Acute iron intoxication in an adult. *JAMA* 1974;229:1333–1335.

11. Murphy B: Hazards of children's vitamin preparations containing iron. *JAMA* 1974;229:324.

12. Oderda G: Iron and vitamin toxicities. *Ear Nose Throat* 1983;62:40–44.

13. Ng R, Perry K, Martin D: Iron poisoning: Assessment of radiography in diagnosis and management. *Clin Pediatr* 1979;18(10):614–616.

14. Robertson W: Treatment of acute iron poisoning. *Med Treat* 1970;8:552–560.

15. Krenzelok E, Hoff J: Accidental childhood iron poisoning: A problem of marketing and labeling. *Pediatrics* 1979;63:591–596.

16. Harrison P: Biochemistry of iron. *Clin Toxicol* 1971;4:529–544.

17. Murray M: Iron absorption. *Clin Toxicol* 1971;4:545–558.

18. Haddad L: Iron poisoning. *JACEP* 1976;5:691–694.

19. Erler M: Iron poisoning. *JEN* 1980;6:40–42.

20. Robertson W: Iron poisoning: A problem of childhood. *Top Emerg Med* 1979;1:57–63.

21. Cheng C, Sullivan T, Li P, et al: Iron toxicity screening. *JACEP* 1979;8:238–240.

22. Whitten C, Chen Y, Gibson G: Studies in acute iron poisoning: Part II: Further observations on desferrioxamine in the treatment of acute experimental iron poisoning. *Pediatr Res* 1978;2:479–485.

23. Whitten C, Brough A: The pathophysiology of acute iron poisoning. *Clin Toxicol* 1971;4:585–595.

24. Whitten C, Chen Y, Gibson G: Studies in acute iron poisoning: Further observations on desferrioxamine in the treatment of acute experimental iron poisoning. *Pediatrics* 1966;38:102–110.

25. Jacobs A: Iron chelation therapy for iron loaded patients. *Br J Haematol* 1979;43:1–5.

26. Jacobs J, Greene H, Gendel B: Acute iron intoxication. *N Engl J Med* 1965;273:1124–1127.

27. Gleason W, Demello D, Decastor F, et al: Acute hepatic failure in severe iron poisoning. *J Pediatr* 1979;95:138–140.

28. Witzleben C, Buck B: Iron overload hepatotoxicity: A postulated pathogenesis. *Clin Toxicol* 1971;4:579–583.

29. Knott L, Miller R: Acute iron intoxication with intestinal infarction. *J Pediatr Surg* 1978;13:720–721.

30. Lacouture P, Wason S, Temple A, et al: Emergency assessment of severity in iron overdose by clinical and laboratory methods. *J Pediatr* 1981;99:89–91.

31. Proudfoot A, Simpson D, Dyson E: Management of acute iron poisoning. *Med Toxicol* 1986;1:83–100.

32. McGuigan M, Lovejoy F, Marino S, et al: Qualitative deferoxamine color test for iron ingestion. *J Pediatr* 1979;94:940–942.

33. James J: Acute iron poisoning: Assessment of severity and prognosis. *J Pediatr* 1970;77:117–119.

34. Fischer DS: A method for the rapid detection of acute iron toxicity. *Clin Chem* 1967;13:6–11.

35. Robotham J, Lietman P: Acute iron poisoning—A review. *Am J Dis Child* 1980;134:875–879.

36. McEnery J: Hospital management of acute iron ingestion. *Clin Toxicol* 1971;4:603–613.

37. Dean B, Krenzelok E: In vivo effectiveness of oral complexation agents in the management of iron poisoning. *Clin Toxicol* 1987;25:221–230.

38. Bachrach L, Correa A, Levin R, et al: Iron poisoning: Complications of hypertonic phosphate lavage therapy. *J Pediatr* 1979;94:147–149.

39. Geffner M, Opas L: Phosphate poisoning complicating treatment for iron ingestion. *Am J Dis Child* 1980;134:509–510.

40. Fischer DS, Parkman R, Finch S: Acute iron poisoning in children: The problem of appropriate therapy. *JAMA* 1971;218:1179–1184.

41. Westlin W: Deferoxamine as a chelating agent. *Clin Toxicol* 1971;4:597–602.

42. Peck M, Rogers J, Rivenbark J: Use of high doses of deferoxamine (Desferal) in an adult patient with acute iron overdosage. *J Toxicol Clin Toxicol* 1982;19:865–869.

43. Hussain M, Flynn D, Green N, et al: Effect of dose, time and ascorbate on iron excretion after subcutaneous desferrioxamine. *Lancet* 1977;1:977–979.

44. Chisholm J: Poisoning due to heavy metals. *Pediatr Clin North Am* 1970;17:591–615.

45. Movassaghi N, Purugganan G, Leikin S: Comparison of exchange transfusion and deferoxamine in the treatment of acute iron poisoning. *J Pediatr* 1969;75:604–608.

46. Peterson C, Fifield G: Emergency gastrotomy for acute iron poisoning. *Ann Emerg Med* 1980;9:262–264.

ADDITIONAL SELECTED REFERENCES

Gezernik W, Schmaman A, Chappell J: Corrosive gastritis as a result of ferrous sulphate ingestion. *S Afr Med J* 1980;57:151–153.

Henretig F, Karl S, Weintraub W: Severe iron poisoning treated with enteral and intravenous deferoxamine. *Ann Emerg Med* 1983;12:306–309.

Kleinman M, Linn W, Bailey R, et al: Human exposure to ferric sulfate aerosol: Effects on pulmonary function and respiratory symptoms. *Am Ind Hyg Assoc J* 1981; 42:298–304.

Snyder R, Mofenson H, Greensher J: Acute iron poisoning in infancy: Guide to treatment. *N Y State J Med* 1974; 74:2215–2217.

Tenenbein M: Whole bowel irrigation in iron poisoning. *J Pediatr* 1987;111:142–145.

chapter 40

Mercury

Mercury is a highly toxic metal that is slightly volatile at ordinary temperatures. Because every known compound of mercury is potentially dangerous, the opportunity for accidental intoxication is widespread. Mercury is one of the oldest industrial poisons; reports of intoxications date back several hundred years. Mercury nitrate was used by the felt hat industry in France, and the resulting poisoning gave rise to the term "mad as a hatter."[1-3] As with many other pollutants, mercury contamination of the environment has paralleled increasing industrial activity. The largest contribution to atmospheric mercury contamination is the burning of coal and other fossil fuels.

SOURCES OF MERCURY EXPOSURE

Throughout the years mercury has been used in medicine, agriculture, and industry.[4] The main industrial sources of inorganic mercury pollutants are the paint, chemical, and paper manufacturing industries (Table 40-1).[5,6] The chemical industry requires organic mercury compounds for the production of vinyl chloride, which is important in the synthesis of many plastics.[7,8] Mercury is employed in dental laboratories in amalgam fillings, and the continual handling of amalgam by technicians may be a cause of chronic mercury poisoning (mercurialism) that may go unrecognized.[9-12]

Mercury is used in thermometers, barometers, mercury electrical switches, direct current meters, and in the vapor lamps that illuminate traffic arterials (Table 40-2).[13] Polyvinyl alcohol preservative used in hospitals as a mounting medium for ova and parasites contains mercuric

Table 40-1 Sources of Mercury Exposure

Industrial
   Paper production
   Chlorine manufacturing
   Vinyl production
   Fungicides
   Fingerprinting procedures
Medical laboratories
Dental laboratories
Mine ore reduction

Table 40-2 Uses of Mercury

Thermometers
Barometers
Small batteries
Electrical switches
Vapor lamps
Photoengraving chemicals
Medicinals
   Contraceptives
   Bacteriostatic agents
   Diuretics

chloride in various concentrations.[14] Mercuric oxide is used for making dry batteries for hearing aids, small flashlights, and a number of electronic products.[15,16] Mercury is also used in photoengraving. Contraceptives, bacteriostatic agents, and diuretics make use of both inorganic and organic mercury salts.[17,18] Mercury has been popular in agricultural use because of its ability to counteract fungi and mold, and therefore it has been widely used to prevent grain spoilage.

TYPES OF MERCURY COMPOUNDS

Mercury compounds are divided into three chemical classes: elemental mercury, inorganic mercury compounds, and organic mercury compounds (Table 40-3). The inorganic mercury salts also exist either in the mercurous or mercuric state; mercuric salts are more toxic than mercurous salts. Within each class there are also subgroups with significantly different toxicological properties. (Table 40-4).

Elemental Mercury (Quicksilver)

Effects of Ingestion

Elemental mercury (free or metallic mercury) exists in the un-ionized form and is the most volatile of all forms of mercury.[10] It is a liquid at room temperature and is the only metal known that remains in liquid form at 0°C.

Typically, elemental mercury has no toxic effects when swallowed because it is poorly absorbed from the gastrointestinal tract (see Table 40-4). Patients who swallow mercury

---

Table 40-3 Types of Mercury Compounds

Elemental mercury
Inorganic mercury compounds
  Mercurous salts
  Mercuric salts
Organic mercury compounds
  Alkoxyalkyl mercury compounds
  Aryl mercury compounds
  Alkyl mercury compounds

---

from a thermometer or from rupture of a Cantor or Miller-Abbott tube do not experience toxicity from absorption of mercury. To effect systemic absorption of mercury requires the conversion of metallic mercury to the divalent form. If the integrity of the intestinal mucosa is preserved, metallic mercury normally passes through the gastrointestinal tract rapidly enough to preclude significant conversion to the divalent state. If a site for mercury stasis exists oxidation-reduction may occur slowly in the presence of water and chloride at body temperature, ultimately transforming metallic mercury into divalent mercuric compounds.[19,20]

Effects of Inhalation

Elemental mercury has a high vapor pressure, and significant poisoning occurs when the substance is inhaled because it is almost completely absorbed through the alveolar membranes.[17] As a result of its high lipid solubility and lack of charge, elemental mercury easily crosses the blood-brain barrier and accumulates in the cerebral and cerebellar cortex.[10] There it is quickly oxidized to the divalent or mercuric ion, which forms a highly undissociated bond to sulfhydryl radicals on various protein molecules and leads to neurologic and behavioral abnormalities.[21]

Table 40-4 Characteristics of Mercury Compounds

Type	Absorption	Excretion	Systems Affected
Elemental	Inhalation	Kidney	Pulmonary and central nervous systems
Inorganic	Gastrointestinal absorption	Kidney	Gastrointestinal and renal systems
Organic	Dermal and gastrointestinal absorption	Kidney	Gastrointestinal and renal systems
Alkyl	Inhalation, dermal and gastrointestinal absorption	Bile	CNS

Inorganic Mercury Compounds

Inorganic mercury compounds contain mercury in the oxidized or ionized form and readily form salts and complexes with sulfhydryl groups.[22] The monovalent (mercurous) form is highly insoluble, and the divalent (mercuric) form is highly soluble.[10,23] Partly because of the divalent form's high degree of solubility, one of the most common and most toxic salts of mercury is mercuric chloride, which is also known as bichloride of mercury or corrosive sublimate.[24]

Inorganic mercury compounds are absorbed through the gastrointestinal tract or, if aerosolized, through inhalation. Little inorganic mercury is absorbed by skin contact.[25] Oral ingestion of inorganic mercury can cause severe inflammation of the mouth, esophagus, stomach, and small intestine. Inorganic mercury is distributed preferentially to the kidney; secondarily, it accumulates in the liver. It is excreted mainly through the urine.[10]

Although the mercuric salts can be extremely toxic, the mercurous salts, because of their low solubility, represent a minimal hazard. Nevertheless, children who ingested mercurous chloride (calomel) in teething powder developed a syndrome known as acrodynia (painful extremities) or pink disease.[5,23]

Organic Mercury Compounds

Organic mercury compounds, in contrast to elemental and inorganic mercury, are environmental contaminants and pollutants.[10] These compounds contain mercury bound covalently to at least one carbon atom; examples are, dimethylmercury or phenylmercuric acetate.

For toxicologic purposes, organic mercury compounds are divided into two classes on the basis of their toxic clinical effects.[23] Differences in toxicity among the organic mercurials are due to the ease of dissociation of the organic moiety from the anion.[21] Compounds in the first class break down readily in the body to yield inorganic mercury; these are primarily the alkoxyalkyl mercurials and the aryl compounds. Phenylmercuric salts such as methoxyethylmercuric chloride are examples of the alkoxyalkyl salts. In the aryl mercurials, mercury is bound to a carbon on an aromatic ring such as benzene, toluene, phenol, cresol, or nitrophenol. Compounds in the second class are short-chain alkyl mercury compounds in which the integrity of the carbon-mercury bond is maintained. These compounds demonstrate greater toxicity than those in the first class.

In view of these features, it is a mistake to differentiate inorganic from organic mercury, at least from a toxicologic point of view, because the mammalian body handles aromatic mercury compounds and some long-chain alkyl mercury compounds by breaking the mercury-carbon bond, thus rendering the mercury inorganic. In the methyl and ethyl forms of mercury the mercury-carbon bonds are extremely stable; the attachment of the alkyl radical makes the compound more lipid soluble, enabling it to cross the blood-brain barrier more easily.

Alkoxyalkyl Mercury Compounds

Alkoxyalkyl mercury compounds are salts of phenyl and methoxyethyl mercury. The physical properties of these compounds render them more easily absorbable than inorganic salts.[21] Hence their distribution throughout the body may be more widespread initially, but as they undergo biotransformation with splitting of the carbon-mercury bond and release of inorganic mercury their distribution pattern becomes similar to that of the inorganic mercury compounds. These compounds therefore act as inorganic mercury in the body.[26]

Aryl Mercury Compounds

The aryl compounds have distributional patterns different from those of the short-chain alkyl derivatives. The aryl compounds are not well absorbed, and being relatively unstable they are excreted mainly as mercuric ion through the kidneys.[5] Phenylmercuric salts therefore are much safer than alkyl compounds because they are less volatile, much less able to enter the brain, much more readily metabolized, and more rapidly excreted.[26]

Alkyl Mercury Compounds

The short-chain alkyl mercury compounds behave differently from the other organic mercurials. Chemically, these are organic compounds in which the mercury has at least one strong covalent bond with a carbon atom.[27] This bond does not dissociate readily either within or outside the body, and toxic effects are attributed to the action of the intact molecule.[21]

Methyl mercury compounds are biologically the most significant of the short-chain alkyl compounds because of their potential to enter the food chain. They become concentrated as they move up the phylogenetic chain and thus become considerably toxic pollutants.[10] These compounds are soluble in organic solvents and lipids, pass readily through biological membranes, and in the body bind to sulfhydryl groups of proteins. Methyl mercury poisoning is usually accidental and unrecognized until 4 to 6 weeks after which time neurologic symptoms appear.

Alkyl mercury compounds are absorbed through the gastrointestinal tract, respiratory system, and skin.[28] On ingestion approximately 90% of a dose is absorbed directly from the intestine, in contrast to the considerably lower absorption shown by inorganic or phenyl mercury compounds. Alkyl mercury compounds distribute themselves more uniformly in the body than the inorganic compounds, concentrating in the liver, blood, brain, hair, and epidermis.[28] The biologic half-life is 70 to 90 days, and the major clinical effects occur in the CNS.

The main excretion route of methyl mercury is through the bile to the intestine, where it is almost immediately reabsorbed into the blood; this internal recycling process partially accounts for the long half-life of methyl mercury in the body. Less than 10% is excreted in the urine.[21]

MECHANISM OF ACTION

In general, mercury can be described as a potent, nonspecific enzyme poison. It produces its detrimental actions by releasing mercuric ions, which readily form covalent bonds with sulfhydryl groups.[2,29] This results in the inactivation of metabolic enzymes, denaturation and precipitation of structural proteins, and disruption of cell membranes in the cells of the target organs.[22] The inhibition of sulfhydryl enzymes is reversible after removal of mercury. Although this is a major mechanism of toxicity, it is proba-

bly not the only means by which mercury may interfere with metabolic processes.[17] There are other ligands such as amine, phosphoryl, and carboxyl groups, also present in any living cell, with which mercury can form strong bonds. Mercury may also act by a local corrosive action on the gastrointestinal tract.

SYMPTOMS AND SIGNS OF INTOXICATION

Depending on the compound, mercury can be locally irritating or corrosive and damage the skin and mucous membranes, or it may cause systemic toxicity, or both. In addition, toxicity can result from acute or chronic exposure to agents that release the mercuric ion or to the alkyl mercuric compounds, which have different toxicities. The diagnosis is difficult during the earliest phases of mercury intoxication because the manifestations are nonspecific and could arise from causes other than mercury exposure.

Acute

Inhalation

Respiratory absorption of mercury vapor is rapid because of the vapor's excellent diffusion through alveolar membranes.[10] Whereas the CNS is the target organ after chronic exposure to mercury vapor, the lung is the critical organ in acute inhalational exposure.[10,30] The mercury is oxidized in vivo to mercurous and mercuric ions, which are toxic. The kidney then becomes the elimination site, and buildup of mercury concentrations in this organ eventually causes renal damage.[21]

Symptoms of acute mercury poisoning by inhalational exposure include an immediate salivation, a burning sensation in the mouth and throat, a paroxysmal dry cough, dysphagia, nausea, vomiting, substernal chest pain with subsequent shallow respiration, tachypnea, a necrotizing bronchiolitis, bronchitis, and interstitial pneumonitis (Table 40-5).[17] Chronic bronchiolitis may ensue and is suggested by the persistence of severe dyspnea despite negative radiographic findings and by the advent of air-

Table 40-5 Signs and Symptoms of Mercury Vapor Inhalation

Salivation
Burning
  Mouth
  Throat
Cough
Dysphagia
Nausea
Vomiting
Abdominal pain
Chest pain
Tachypnea
Dyspnea
Neurologic
Pulmonary
  Bronchiolitis
  Bronchitis
  Pneumonitis
  Interstitial fibrosis
  Pneumomediastinum
  Pneumothorax

Table 40-6 Clinical Features of Acute Ingestion of Inorganic and Aryl Mercuric Compounds

Early
  Necrosis of mucosa
  Gastrointestinal
    Local pain
    Nausea
    Vomiting
    Hematemesis
    Abdominal pain
    Hematochezia
    Metallic taste in the mouth
  Shock
  Vascular collapse
Subsequent
  Stomatitis
  Salivation (ptyalism)
  Membranous colitis
  Renal abnormalities
    Tubular necrosis
    Albuminuria
    Hematuria
    Anuria

way obstruction in pulmonary function testing. Diffuse interstitial pulmonary fibrosis has also been reported in patients with acute mercury poisoning who survived for several weeks. Complications such as interstitial emphysema, pneumomediastinum, and pneumothorax can occur.[17] In addition to the severe lung damage that may occur as a result of mercury vapor inhalation, the lung also serves as a site from which mercury is absorbed. It is widely distributed throughout the body and passes across the blood-brain barrier, with subsequent neurologic and behavioral abnormalities noted. Fine muscle tremors are among the early signs of mercurialism. Tremors usually begin in the fingers, eyes, or tongue. Mercury is largely ionized to mercuric ion in erythrocytes and other tissues.[17]

Ingestion

When ingested, inorganic mercury is rapidly absorbed by the gastrointestinal tract; this should be considered an emergency of the highest priority. Ingestion is rarely encountered in industry but in other settings may be accidental or purposeful.[2]

Ionizable mercuric salts are corrosive. Necrosis begins immediately in the mucosa of the mouth, throat, esophagus, and stomach. Gas-

trointestinal symptoms consist of local pain, nausea, profuse vomiting with hematemesis, violent abdominal pain, and hematochezia (Table 40-6). The patient may note a metallic taste in the mouth. Volume loss may lead to shock and vascular collapse, which can result in death within a few hours.[26] The alimentary effects of many mercury compounds are so rapid that the course and prognosis are determined largely by events within the first 10 to 15 minutes, particularly by the intervention of vomiting or a therapeutic lavage. Albuminuria and skin lesions may also be noted, although these lesions are more commonly associated with organic than with inorganic mercury exposure. Renal tubular injury occurs with an initial diuresis and subsequent renal shutdown. CNS symptoms may also be noted.[2]

If death does not intervene, subsequent effects noted with both corrosive and noncorrosive mercurials develop within 1 to 3 days after the exposure and may include mercurial stomatitis, marked salivation (ptyalism), membranous colitis, and necrosis of the renal tubules with resultant polyuria, albuminuria, hematuria, and anuria. Death is usually the result of complete and irreversible renal failure. Psychological and

CNS symptoms are uncommon in acute mercury poisoning, in contrast to chronic mercury poisoning.[26]

Chronic

Inorganic, Elemental, and Aryl Compounds

Long-term, low-level exposure to mercury vapor is a common hazard in various industries. With the exception of alkyl mercury poisoning, the signs and symptoms of inorganic and aryl mercury poisonings are identical because of the rapid metabolic breakdown of these mercurials to mercuric ion.[21] The CNS is affected more than any other system in chronic mercury poisoning, and the predominant manifestations are neurologic.[21] The violent gastrointestinal reactions elicited in acute poisonings are absent, but excessive salivation, anorexia, digestive disturbances, vague abdominal distress, and mild diarrhea are common.

Initial symptoms of inorganic, elemental, or aryl mercury poisoning may be insidious in onset and appear after only a few weeks, or they may not be evident for several years despite continuing exposure (Table 40-7). A triad of manifestations has become associated with the diagnosis of chronic mercurialism: (1) oral cavity disorders, such as gingivitis, stomatitis, or excessive salivation; (2) a fine involuntary tremor of the hands, feet, and tongue that is aggravated by voluntary movements[31] (this ''intention'' or ataxic tremor occurs only when there is purposeful movement of a limb, especially when the limb approaches its intended object); and (3) psychological disturbances, called ''erethism,'' manifested as anxiety, irritability, depression, regressive behavior, timidity, or nervousness[1,21] (the term erethism refers to the blushing and sweating that also occurs[25]). Renal involvement is well documented and may be evidenced by proteinuria and edema. Additionally, nonspecific symptoms such as weakness, fatigue, pallor, anorexia, weight loss, and gastrointestinal disturbances have also been reported.[31]

Alkyl Compounds

Methyl, ethyl, propyl, and butyl mercury derivatives are potent neurotoxins on either

Table 40-7 Signs and Symptoms of Chronic Exposure to Inorganic, Elemental, and Aryl Mercury Compounds

Oral cavity disorders
Gingivitis
Stomatitis
Salivation
Tremor
Hands
Feet
Tongue
Psychological disturbances ("erethism")
Anxiety
Irritability
Depression
Regressive behavior
Timidity
Nervousness
Renal
Proteinuria
Edema
Miscellaneous
Weakness
Fatigue
Pallor
Anorexia
Weight loss
Gastrointestinal disturbances

acute or chronic exposure.[27] They are especially hazardous because of their volatility, their ability to penetrate epithelial cells and the blood-brain barrier, and their persistence in the body.

Chronic exposure to organic mercurials primarily affects the CNS (Table 40-8). Whereas the effects of elemental mercury are neuropsychiatric, those of short-chain organic mercury compounds are sensorimotor.[10,30] These compounds produce no biochemical or physiologic disturbances, such as proteinuria, that are clearly associated with exposure. At present, reliance on the neurologic examination or on subjective complaints by the patient is necessary.

The clinical picture may be gradual and delayed, with a latent period of as much as 2 months or more from exposure to the development of symptoms. Loss of sensation and paresthesias of the mouth, lips, tongue, hands, and feet may occur.[28] Dysarthria, inability to concentrate, extreme fatigue, difficulty in swallowing, ataxia, and concentric constriction of the visual fields or ''tunnel vision'' may be noted.[27]

Table 40-8 Signs and Symptoms of Intoxication with Alkyl Mercury Compounds

Central nervous system
  Neurasthenia
  Headache
  Paresthesia
  Ataxia
  Intention tremor
  Hearing loss
  Visual field loss
  Paralysis
  Coma
Nonspecific
  Weakness
  Fatigue
  Apathy
  Dysphagia

Table 40-9 Laboratory Determinations in Mercury Exposure

Inhalation
  Chest roentgenogram
  Arterial blood gas values
  Blood mercury concentrations
  24-Hour urinary sampling
  Urinalysis
Ingestion
  Serum electrolytes
  Blood mercury concentrations
  24-Hour urinary sampling
  Urinalysis

Tremors occur, but motor effects such as incoordination, paralysis, and abnormal reflexes are a result of defects in sensory input. Hearing impairment, coma, and death have also been noted in severe poisonings.[28] Fetuses and neonates are most sensitive to methylmercury, which can produce severe derangement of the developing CNS.

Epidemic methylmercury poisoning has occurred among populations where fish or shellfish is the major dietary staple. This was described in the 1960s in Minamata Bay, Japan, and was due to contamination by nearby industrial wastes discharged into public waters.[2,27] Although inorganic mercurials may have been discharged into the water, methylation of the mercury by microorganisms subsequently consumed by fish may have occurred. Other contaminations have been reported in Iraq, Pakistan, and Guatemala as a result of the ingestion of flour and wheat seed treated with methyl and ethyl mercury fungicide compounds.[27,28,32]

LABORATORY DETERMINATIONS

Because of the often vague clinical picture, confirmatory laboratory tests are desirable (Table 40-9). Unlike the situation for lead poisoning, there are no specific biochemical tests that can be used to determine whether mercury exposure has occurred. The only indicator available is the concentration of mercury in the blood, urine, or hair. Determinations of mercury concentrations in blood or urine are most commonly used, although both are subject to wide variation. Urinary or blood concentrations may be nondiagnostic in many cases because they may vary among symptomatic patients and in individual patients on a daily basis. Findings of higher than normal concentrations of mercury in blood or urine may confirm exposure to mercury, but they correlate poorly with the appearance of clinical symptoms.

Because the mercuric ion is excreted by the kidney, poisoning from elemental, aryl, or long-chain organic mercury or mercuric salts can be best assessed by measuring the 24-hour urinary excretion of mercury. Although monitoring urinary concentration of mercury is the most common method for determining acute exposure and is helpful after chelation therapy,[21] it is not useful after a chronic mercury exposure. The range of 10 to 50 μg/L is considered within the upper limits of normal. If a 24-hour collection shows mercury in the range of 100 to 300 μg/L, either before or after therapy, then significant exposure has occurred. Symptoms may appear when the 24-hour collection contains more than 300 μg/L.

There is a considerably larger variability of the mercury concentrations in urine than in blood. Possible explanations may be difficulty in adequately controlling urine sampling, variations in renal mercury excretion during the day, and the influence of variations in kidney function on mercury excretion. Blood sampling is easier to control, and blood mercury concentrations are not affected in a misleading way by disturbed renal function.

In contrast to the other mercury compounds, the short-chain alkyl organic mercury compounds are mainly excreted in bile. Although they form a tight carbon bond, preferentially to red blood cells, they are uniformly distributed throughout the body. Because urinary excretion accounts for only 10% of total excretion, urinary measurements are not reliable in the assessment of poisoning by these compounds. There is excellent correlation between the average mercury concentration in 1 cm of hair and the blood concentration at the time of formation of the hair sample. Measurement of concentrations in either red blood cells or hair correlates accurately with symptoms. The normal blood mercury concentration is 10 μg/dL in persons with no history of mercury ingestion. A blood concentration of 20 to 50 μg/dL or a hair concentration of 50 to 125 μg/g may be associated with early clinical symptoms.

As a rough guideline, a mercury concentration of 3.5 μg/dL in blood is approximately equivalent to 150 μg/L in a 24-hour urine collection. The concentration in hair is approximately 250 to 300 times the concentration in blood.

TREATMENT

Inorganic and Organic Compounds (Excluding Alkyl Compounds)

The treatment of acute mercury poisoning aims at removal of mercury from the gastrointestinal tract, the inactivation of absorbed mercuric ions, and general supportive measures to maintain electrolyte and fluid balance (Table 40-10). To be successful, treatment must be prompt and intensive. Emesis or gastric lavage should be performed, with subsequent administration of charcoal and a cathartic. Shock due to peripheral vascular collapse is treated with volume repletion.

Patients exposed to high concentrations of mercury vapor should be removed from the contaminated environment. If pulmonary toxicity is suspected, careful monitoring of chest roentgenograms and arterial blood gas values is indicated. Positive end-expiratory pressure may be required to assist ventilation.[26]

Table 40-10 Treatment of Mercury Poisoning

Emesis or lavage
Activated charcoal and cathartic
Volume repletion
Chelation therapy
  Dimercaprol (acute inorganic mercury)
    3 to 5 mg/kg IM every 4 hours for 2 days, then
    3 to 5 mg/kg IM every 6 hours for 1 day, then
    3 to 5 mg/kg IM once or twice a day for 10 days
  Penicillamine (chronic intoxication and mercury
  vapor)
    250 mg 4 times a day for 3 to 10 days, or 30 mg/
    kg per 24 hours not to exceed 1 g/day

Elimination of the toxic mercuric ion is the specific objective in therapy for mercury poisoning. This is done with the use of chelating agents. A chelating agent is indicated in all mercury poisonings except those due to short-chain alkyl compounds. Treatment of mercury poisoning is limited to two commercially available agents, dimercaprol and penicillamine.[23]

Dimercaprol

Extensive clinical experience with dimercaprol has established it as the antidote of choice in acute poisonings due to inorganic mercuric salts, in which the critical target organ is usually the kidney. Dimercaprol is maximally effective when given early in the course of an acute episode and can often be lifesaving under those circumstances. If dimercaprol is given within 3 hours after ingestion, severe renal damage may be prevented. Dimercaprol enhances the renal excretion of mercury, so that caution is indicated in cases of acute renal insufficiency, in which the drug may aggravate the renal damage or manifest its own toxicity.

Dimercaprol is much less effective in chronic mercurialism, in which the brain is the critically diseased organ. Although it often provokes an increase in urinary mercury the rise is usually small in terms of estimated body burden, and the clinical improvement is typically marginal.

The currently suggested treatment schedule for dimercaprol is intramuscular administration as a 10% solution in oil. Dosage is 3 to 5 mg/kg injected every 4 hours for 2 days, the same dose every 6 hours on the third day, and then daily or twice daily for 10 days. The dimercaprol-mercury complex is excreted in both the feces and urine.[23]

Some hazard is attendant on the use of dimercaprol. The mobilization of large quantities of mercury from the body after its administration may impose an overwhelming mercury load on the kidneys with some risk of damage. Redistribution of body stores of mercury after injection of dimercaprol may also result in excessive deposition in the brain.[21]

Penicillamine

Penicillamine appears to be preferable to dimercaprol in treating acute poisoning by mercury vapor and chronic mercurialism of almost any form.[17] Penicillamine is preferable for mercury inhalation because of the tendency for absorbed mercury vapor to enter the brain and for dimercaprol therapy to increase mercury concentration in the brain.

Penicillamine is marketed as 125-mg and 250-mg capsules and is orally administered on an empty stomach in a dose of 250 mg 4 times a day for 3 to 10 days. A dosage of 30 mg/kg/day divided every 6 hours up to 1 g/day should be given for 5 to 10 days. A repeated 5-day course of treatment with a 2-day rest period between courses is indicated until the 24-hour urine mercury excretion is less than 50 μg/L. Although *N*-acetyl-D,L-penicillamine appears to be more effective and less toxic than penicillamine, it is not approved for use in the United States. Doses suggested have been equal to those of penicillamine.

Dimercaprol is preferable to oral penicillamine for acute mercury ingestion because vomiting may prevent retention of penicillamine and because penicillamine may enhance the gastrointestinal absorption of mercury.

Alkyl Compounds

Methyl and other alkyl derivatives of mercury pose more formidable problems in therapy than other mercurials because they are rapidly absorbed and penetrate quickly into the brain, where they are bound to plasma and cellular proteins. There is no specific therapy for alkyl mercury poisoning, and treatment is symptomatic.[21] The use of chelating agents has been of limited value in aiding the elimination of short-chain organic mercury, probably because little of the organic mercury compounds dissociate to yield inorganic mercury ions. Dimercaprol is contraindicated for methyl mercury poisoning because it increases mercury accumulation in the brain.[33] Several newer agents have been clinically evaluated, including *N*-acetylcysteine,[34] *N*-acetyl-D,L-penicillamine,[1] dimercaptopropanesulfonic acid (DMPS), and dimercaptosuccinic acid (DMSA).[35–37] Results have been promising with these water-soluble, orally active agents.

Hemodialysis and peritoneal dialysis may be helpful in renal insufficiency, but they have little or no value for removing mercury because it is bound tightly to plasma and tissue proteins.[38]

REFERENCES

1. Kark R, Poskanzer D, Bullock J, et al: Mercury poisoning and its treatment with *N*-acetyl-D,L-penicillamine. *N Eng J Med* 1971;285:10–16.

2. Winek C, Fochtman F, Bricker J, et al: Fatal mercuric chloride ingestion. *Clin Toxicol* 1981;18:261–266.

3. Markowitz L, Schaumburg H: Successful treatment of inorganic mercury neurotoxicity with *N*-acetyl-penicillamine despite an adverse reaction. *Neurology* 1980;30:1000–1001.

4. Baruch A, Haas A: Injury to the hand with metallic mercury. *J Hand Surg* 1984;9:446–448.

5. Aronow R, Fleischmann L: Mercury poisoning in children. *Clin Pediatr* 1976;15:936–945.

6. Duffield D, Paddle G, Woolhead G: A mortality study of non-malignant genitourinary tract disease in electrolyte mercury cell room employees. *J Soc Occup Med* 1983; 33:137–140.

7. Janus C, Klein B: Aspiration of metallic mercury: Clinical significance. *Br J Radiol* 1982;55:675–676.

8. Snodgrass W, Sullivan J, Rumack B, et al: Mercury poisoning from home gold ore processing. *JAMA* 1981; 246:1929–1931.

9. Brodsky J, Cohen E, Whitcher C, et al: Occupational exposure to mercury in dentistry and pregnancy outcome. 1985;111:779–780.

10. Bauer J: Action of mercury in dental exposures to mercury. *Oper Dent* 1985;10:104–113.

11. Mackert J: Hypersensitivity to mercury from dental amalgams. *J Am Acad Dermatol* 1985;12:877–879.

12. Abraham J, Svare C, Frank C: The effect of dental amalgam restorations on blood mercury levels. *J Dent Res* 1984;63:71–73.

13. Hudson P, Vogt R, Brondum J, et al: Elemental mercury exposure among children of thermometer plant workers. *Pediatrics* 1987;79:935–938.

14. Siedel J: Acute mercury poisoning after polyvinyl alcohol preservative ingestion. *Pediatrics* 1980;66:132–134.

15. Mant T, Lewis J, Mattoo T, et al: Mercury poisoning after disc-battery ingestion. *Hum Toxicol* 1987;6:179–181.

16. Adams C, Ziegler D, Lin J: Mercury intoxication simulating amyotrophic lateral sclerosis. *JAMA* 1983; 250:642–643.

17. Lien D, Todoruk D, Rajani H, et al: Accidental inhalation of mercury vapor: Respiratory and toxicologic consequences. *Can Med Assoc J* 1983;129:591–595.

18. Giunta F, DiLandro D, Chiaranda M, et al: Severe acute poisoning from ingestion of a permanent wave solution of mercuric chloride. *Hum Toxicol* 1983;2:243–246.

19. Bredfeldt J, Moeller D: Systemic mercury intoxication following rupture of a Miller-Abbott tube. *Am J Gastroenterol* 1978;69:478–480.

20. Geffner M, Sandler A: Oral metallic mercury. *Clin Pediatr* 1980;19:435–437.

21. Joselow M, Louria D, Browder A: Mercurialism: Environmental and occupational aspects. *Ann Intern Med* 1972;76:119–130.

22. Felton J, Kahn E, Salick B, et al: Heavy metal poisoning: Mercury and lead. *Ann Intern Med* 1972;76:779–792.

23. Goldfrank L, Bresnitz E: Mercury poisoning. *Hosp Physician* 1980;6:36–46.

24. Laundy T, Adam A, Kershaw J, et al: Deaths after peritoneal lavage with mercuric chloride solutions. *Br Med J* 1984;289:96–98.

25. Rosenman K, Valciukas J, Meyers B, et al: Sensitive indicator of inorganic mercury toxicity. *Arch Environ Health* 1986;41:208–215.

26. Greenhouse A: Heavy metals and the nervous system. *Clin Neuropharmacol* 1982;5:45–92.

27. Eyl T: Organic-mercury food poisoning. *N Engl J Med* 1971;284:706–709.

28. Bakir F, Damluji S, Amin-Zaki L, et al: Methylmercury poisoning in Iraq. *Science* 1973;181:230–241.

29. Oehme F: Mechanisms of heavy metal toxicities. *Clin Toxicol* 1972;5:151–167.

30. Levine S, Cavender G, Langolf G, et al: Elemental mercury exposure: Peripheral neurotoxicity. *Br J Ind Med* 1982;39:136–139.

31. Lilis R, Miller A, Lerman Y: Acute mercury poisoning with severe chronic pulmonary manifestations. *Chest* 1985;88:306–308.

32. Mahaffey K: Toxicity of lead, cadmium, and mercury: Considerations for total parenteral nutritional support. *Bull N Y Acad Med* 1984;60:196–209.

33. Canty A: British anti-lewisite and organomercury poisoning. *Nature (London)* 1975;253:123–125.

34. Lund M, Clarkson T, Berlin M: Treatment of acute methylmercury ingestion by hemodialysis with *N*-acetylcysteine (Mucomyst) infusion and 2,3-dimercaptopropane sulfonate. *Clin Toxicol* 1984;22:31–49.

35. Graziano J: Role of 2,3-dimercaptosuccinic acid in the treatment of heavy metal poisoning. *Med Toxicol* 1986;1:155–162.

36. Aaseth J, Alexander J: Treatment of mercuric chloride poisoning with demercaptosuccinic acid and diuretics: Preliminary studies. *J Toxicol Clin Toxicol* 1982;19: 173–186.

37. Aaseth J: Recent advances in the therapy of metal poisoning with chelating agents. *Hum Toxicol* 1983; 2:257–272.

38. Pellinen T, Karjalainen K, Haapanen E: Hemoperfusion in mercury poisoning. *J Toxicol Clin Toxicol* 1983; 20:187–189.

ADDITIONAL SELECTED REFERENCES

Aposhian H: DMSA and DMPS—Water soluble antidotes for heavy metal poisoning. *Annu Rev Pharmacol* 1983; 23:193–215.

Cassar-Pullicino V, Taylor D, Fitzpatrick J: Multiple metallic mercury emboli. 1985;58:470–474.

Chisolm J: Poisoning due to heavy metals. *Pediatr Clin North Am* 1970;17:591–615.

Clarkson T, Cox L, Greenwood M, et al: Tests of efficacy of antidotes for removal of methylmercury in human poisoning during the Iraq outbreak. *J Pharmacol Exp Ther* 1981;218:74–83.

Dale I: An unusual case of mercury contamination. *J Soc Occup Med* 1985;35:95–97.

Gothe C, Langworth S, Carleson R, et al: Biological monitoring of exposure to metallic mercury. *Clin Toxicol* 1985;23:381–389.

Robillard J, Rames L, Jensen R, et al: Peritoneal dialysis in mercurial diuretic intoxication. *J Pediatr* 1976;88:79–81.

Smith P, Langold G, Goldberg J: Effects of occupational exposure to elemental mercury on short-term memory. *Br J Ind Med* 1983;40:413–419.

Vermeiden I, Oranje A, Vuzevski V, et al: Mercury exanthem as occupational dermatitis. *Contact Dermatitis* 1980;6:88–90.

chapter 41

Lead

Lead, one of the earliest metals used by humans, is poisonous in all forms. It is one of the most hazardous of the toxic metals because the poison is cumulative and because the toxic effects are many and severe.[1] Lead occurs naturally in the earth's crust, atmosphere, and hydrosphere, and it is also a ubiquitous environmental pollutant.

In the body lead is a trace element that has no known essential biological role.[2] Because it occurs widely the environment exposure to it is almost inevitable, even for fetuses, infants, and children.[3] Lead poisoning (plumbism) usually results from cumulative absorption of small amounts of lead until toxic concentrations are reached in the body.[4,5] Months or even years may go by before symptoms appear. Although there have been recent advances in the recognition and management of lead poisoning, it continues to be a significant problem.[6,7]

SOURCES OF LEAD POISONING

Usually, lead compounds are emitted into the atmosphere from three sources: gasoline-powered vehicles, industrial processes, and incineration.[1,8,9] Exposure may occur from air, water, food, and dusts (Table 41-1). Besides the elemental form, lead may exist in both an inorganic and organic form. More than 95% of lead is inorganic and occurs as a lead salt; for practical purposes, all the inorganic forms of lead have the same action in the body.[10] The carbonate and chromate salts and various oxides are found in paints and pottery glazes; the carbonate salt is known as "white lead." Organic lead (lead bound to carbon atoms in an organic molecule) is prevalent only in areas where leaded gasoline is combusted.[11,12]

Table 41-1 Sources of Lead Poisoning

Industrial
  Ammunition manufacture
  Battery manufacture
  Lead refineries
  Pigment manufacture
  Printing
  Shipbuilding
  Smelting plants
  Welding
Miscellaneous
  Automobile exhaust
  Contaminated alcohol
  Firing ranges
  Health foods
  Intravenous drugs of abuse
  Lead bullets
  Lead-based paints
  Leaded gasoline
  Oriental herbal medicines
  Pica
  Pottery glaze

Occupational Exposure

Lead toxicity continues to be a major health problem in many occupations because lead and its salts are used in a wide variety of processes. Most occupational exposures occur in the manufacturing or use of ammunition, brass, bronze pipes, storage batteries, lead shielding, pigments, chemicals, or processed metals.[1,7] Most current exposures occur primarily through inhalation of lead dust during sanding, grinding, scraping, or powder mixing or of lead fumes from burning, refining, pouring, or smelting.[13,14] Studies have shown workers to be at risk in lead refineries, smelting plants, battery manufacturing plants, pigment manufacturing plants, shipyards, and other industries.[8] These workers may also bring dust into their homes on their work clothes and expose their families to high ambient concentrations of lead.[15] In addition, lead is used in printer's type, in welding or soldering of lead-coated steel, electric cable covering, and bearing alloys.[7,16,17]

Household Exposure

Contaminated drinking water from lead-containing pipes, the ingestion of lead-containing health foods, and Chinese herbal medicines are domestic sources of lead poisoning.[8,16] In addition, cases of lead poisoning have been traced to illicit alcoholic beverages such as "moonshine," from the burning of color magazines that contain leaded ink, and from paints and pottery glaze.[1,18,19]

Environmental Exposure

The alkyl lead compounds (Table 41-2) are used primarily in gasoline, and combustion of leaded gasoline accounts for most of the ambient air lead.[9] Organolead compounds are added to motor fuel to eliminate the "knock" or detonation in the internal combustion engine.[8,16] After combustion, these compounds are oxidized and emitted in exhaust as a mixture of lead salts.[7] Although local "fallout" from industrial plants processing lead can be severe, this is a minor contribution to regional pollution compared to

Table 41-2 Alkyl Lead Compounds

Tetraethyl lead
Tetramethyl lead
Tetraethylmethyl lead
Diethyldimethyl lead
Ethyltrimethyl lead

automobile exhausts. Dust and soil may be contaminated principally by automobile exhaust and by the weathering and deterioration of old lead paint.[13,15]

Sniffing of gasoline, both leaded and unleaded, is a problem of some magnitude in the young age group and in areas where there is local legal prohibition against alcohol because of the pleasurable effects of acute inhalation and the availability and low cost of gasoline (see Chapter 33).[12]

Miscellaneous Exposures

Although cases of lead poisoning due to retained bullets are reported only rarely, they may represent potentially life-threatening reactions. Certain ammunition such as lead shot and .22-caliber bullets may provide a large surface area of lead dissolution and absorption.[8,18,20,21] Inadequately ventilated firing ranges may also result in lead toxicity.

Illicit methamphetamine has been reported to contain substantial amounts of lead, and acute lead toxicity has been reported in intravenous amphetamine users.[22]

Age-Related Exposure

In general, lead poisoning in children is a different health problem from that in adults.[7,23] In children it occurs as accidental poisoning, whereas in adults it is usually a result of occupational exposure.[24,25] Young children are exposed to lead in soil, air, house dust, food, and water.

In general, the main routes of entry of lead in children are inhalation and ingestion.[17] Lead-based paint on both the interior and exterior surfaces of housing remains the most common high-dose source of lead for preschool-aged children.[4,16] A lead chip weighing only 2 g and containing 10% lead can deliver a potential dose of 100 mg; for comparison, the safe upper limit for daily intake of lead by children is 5 μg/kg.[3,26] Pica, or the abnormal craving for and indiscriminate eating of nonfood substances, is a frequent exposure factor in children in the development of chronic plumbism.[13,23] This occurs most commonly in preschool children and is most prevalent among those 18 to 24 months old.[8] Developing fetuses are also at risk from the exposure of the mother.[10]

ABSORPTION

Lead enters the bloodstream through the gastrointestinal tract, respiratory tract, and, to a lesser extent, mucous membranes.[7,16] Although lead is not well absorbed through the skin, skin abrasions may allow significant absorption.[27] Absorption from the respiratory tract is rapid because of prompt phagocytosis and because lead enters directly into the general circulation instead of passing through the liver, as in gastrointestinal absorption.

Adults consume approximately 300 μg of lead per day, of which only 10% is absorbed.[1,27] A larger percentage of ingested lead is absorbed by children.[1,7] Deficiencies of other metals, such as iron, calcium, and zinc, all result in increased gastrointestinal absorption of lead.

In contrast to inorganic lead salts, which do not penetrate the skin, alkyl derivatives are capable of rapidly penetrating the intact skin.

DISTRIBUTION

Inorganic lead is distributed into three compartments: blood, soft tissues, and bone.[7] Lead is first distributed as lead diphosphate to the soft tissues, especially kidney, lung, liver, and spleen.[1,4] In time, lead is redistributed and deposited in teeth, hair, and bone, where it is stored as insoluble lead triphosphate.[16] Bone is the largest compartment of body lead, comprising about 95% of the body burden of the metal and acting as a reservoir for endogenous intoxication; lead stored in bone is available for diag-

nosis by EDTA mobilization. Only a small quantity of inorganic lead accumulates in the brain, with most of that in gray matter and the basal ganglia.[11]

TOXICITY OF ELEMENTAL AND INORGANIC LEADS

Lead has diverse biologic effects manifested at the subcellular level. None are beneficial.[17] The basis of lead's toxicity is its ability, as a metallic cation, to bind with specific ligands such as sulfhydryl, amino, and carboxyl groups present in biomolecular substances that are crucial to various physiologic functions.[4] These lead-containing complexes then interfere with normal function by competing with essential metals for binding sites, inhibiting enzyme activity, and inhibiting or altering energy metabolism and essential ion transport.[14]

The critical target organelle for lead toxicity is the mitochondrion, with resultant structural changes and marked functional disturbance noted.[27] Uptake of lead by mitochondria causes swelling, loss of cristae, and interference with oxidative phosphorylation and ion transport.[7] Inhibition of mitochondrial respiration exerts obvious deleterious effects on cell function in various systems.[4] In addition, intracellular lead metabolism overlaps considerably with that of calcium, which gives rise to a potential site of interaction between the elements and a plausible means by which lead impairs intracellular ion transport.[16]

Lead may cause multisystem dysfunction in the gastrointestinal system (lead colic), the hematopoietic system (anemia), the CNS (lead encephalopathy), joints and ligaments (arthralgia and lead gout), the endocrine system (thyroid, adrenocortical, and testicular dysfunctions), and the kidneys.[16]

Two clinically discrete syndromes of lead intoxication have been identified. In relatively acute intoxication, caused by brief exposure to high lead concentrations, the classic symptoms of colic, anemia, and encephalopathy are often seen.[11] Chronic forms of intoxication, which occur after long-term exposure, may have few of the findings typical of classic lead intoxication. Both acute and chronic intoxications may be associated with organic brain disturbances and depression.[4,16]

Acute Intoxication

Intoxication from a single exposure is unusual but has resulted from both accidental and intentional ingestion of solutions of soluble lead salts (Table 41-3).[1] Initial clinical features of acute ingestion of a large amount of any soluble lead salt, especially acetate, carbonate, or chromate, are largely due to local irritation of the alimentary tract.[3,28] The stool may be black if lead sulfide is ingested. Radiopaque flakes may be seen in the gastrointestinal tract after recent ingestion of lead-containing compounds.[1,17] If sufficient lead is retained after a single exposure, a syndrome identical to that of chronic intoxication may develop, with symptoms of leg cramps, muscle weakness, paresthesias, CNS depression, coma, and death within 1 or 2 days.[2]

Chronic Intoxication

Long-term exposure to lead causes a wide range of systemic disorders (Table 41-4).

Gastrointestinal Tract

The most common form of plumbism is gastrointestinal. After a prodromal stage of variable duration and associated with vague symptoms of anorexia, dyspepsia, constipation, and a metallic taste in the mouth, severe abdominal cramps or colic may occur.[1] This is due to the intense spasm that is sometimes associated with rigidity of the abdominal wall. This colic is characteristically severe and paroxysmal.[4]

Table 41-3 Signs and Symptoms of Acute Lead Intoxication

Gastrointestinal toxicity
Leg cramps
Muscle weakness
Paresthesia
CNS depression
Coma
Death

Table 41-4 Signs and Symptoms of Chronic Inorganic Lead Intoxication

Gastrointestinal
Anorexia
Dyspepsia
Constipation
Metallic taste in the mouth
Abdominal pain
Hematopoietic
Anemia (hypochromic, normocytic)
Basophilic stippling
Neurologic
Peripheral neuropathy
"Wrist drop" or "foot drop"
Lead encephalopathy
Vomiting
Apathy
Drowsiness
Stupor
Seizures
Death
Renal
Albuminuria
Hematuria
Pyuria
Oral cavity
Ulcerative stomatitis
"Lead line"
Reproductive
Female
Abnormal ovarian cycle
Infertility
Spontaneous abortion
Stillbirth
Male
Chromosomal alterations
Decreased sperm count
Altered sperm morphology
Decreased sexual drive
Impotence
Sterility
Fetal
Macrocephaly
Low birth weight
Nervous system disorders
Increased death rate during first year

Hematopoietic System

The lead in blood is mostly bound to the erythrocytes, and the earliest demonstrated effect of lead poisoning is inhibition of heme formation. Lead at low blood concentrations can inhibit at least three enzymes that are important for heme synthesis (Fig. 41-1).[17] These enzymes are δ-aminolevulinic acid dehydratase

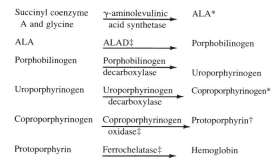

Succinyl coenzyme A and glycine	γ-aminolevulinic acid synthetase	ALA*
ALA	ALAD‡	Porphobilinogen
Porphobilinogen	Porphobilinogen decarboxylase	Uroporphyrinogen
Uroporphyrinogen	Uroporphyrinogen decarboxylase	Coproporphyrinogen*
Coproporphyrinogen	Coproporphyrinogen oxidase‡	Protoporphyrin†
Protoporphyrin	Ferrochelatase‡	Hemoglobin

Figure 41-1 Synthesis of hemoglobin and the effect of lead (symbols: *elevated in urine; †elevated in blood; ‡blocked by lead). *Source*: Adapted with permission from *Medical Toxicology* (1986;1:387–410), Copyright © 1986, Adis Press International Inc.

(ALAD), coproporphyrinogen oxidase, and ferrochelatase.[1,29] The erythrocyte ALAD activity is inhibited at blood lead concentrations of no more than 10 μg/dL in adults and therefore can act as a sensitive marker of lead intoxication.[30] Lead prevents the conversion of δ-aminolevulinic acid (ALA) to porphobilinogen and the conversion of coproporphyrinogen to protoporphyrin by blocking the action of ALAD and coproporphyrinogen oxidase, respectively. This in turn causes ALA and corproporphyrin to accumulate in the urine, where they can be used as markers for lead poisoning.[16]

Two effects are often seen in the human body when an enzyme is inhibited: first, the molecule on which the enzyme acts accumulates because it cannot undergo chemical reaction to produce the desired product; and second, the amount of desired product decreases.[11] With interference with heme synthesis, there is an increase in concentration of free erythrocyte protoporphyrin, erythrocyte zinc protoporphyrin, urinary ALA, and urinary coproporphyrin while erythrocyte ALAD activity and hemoglobin values are decreased (see Table 41-7).[29] Urinary ALA concentration may be elevated by other means, so that it is not specific for lead exposure.[17]

The hematologic effects are seen more commonly in children than in adults and may be helpful in arousing suspicion of lead poisoning.[23]

Anemia. Clinical anemia is an important finding in inorganic lead poisoning but not in organic lead poisoning.[1,16] This is the most clear-cut functional defect caused by lead. The anemia is usually hypochromic and normocytic[7] because of a combination of decreased hemoglobin production and increased red blood cell destruction.[16,31] To compensate the marrow increases red blood cell production, releasing immature red blood cells. Reticulocytes and basophilic stippled cells also may appear in the blood.[19,32] Macrocytosis may develop if anemia persists for any length of time. These symptoms of anemia may be nonspecific but are characteristic of the increased load on the cardiac system.[16,28] They may include weakness; fatigue; pallor; waxy, sallow complexion; headache; irritability; and others.

Basophilic Stippling. Because of the retardation of RNA catabolism in maturing cells from lead poisoning, an accumulation of aggregates of incompletely degraded ribosomal fragments results in the phenomenon known as basophilic stippling.[7,31] This is a nonspecific finding in many other conditions as well, such as hemolytic anemia, malaria, thalassemia, leukemia, and exposure to other toxins,[1] and should be regarded as an unreliable index of lead intoxication (Table 41-5).

Central Nervous System

The neurologic manifestations of acute or chronic lead intoxication are quite variable. Peripheral neuropathy is usually painless and limited to the extensor muscle groups. This may result in the classic picture of "wrist drop" or "foot drop."[7,16]

Table 41-5 Conditions Demonstrating Basophilic Stippling

Hemolytic anemia
Malaria
Thalassemia
Leukemia
Exposure to toxins
 Lead
 Aniline dyes
 Benzene
 Carbon monoxide
 Copper

The cerebral manifestations of lead poisoning have been called lead encephalopathy; this condition is less common in adults than in children.[9] Lead encephalopathy constitutes the most severe consequence of lead intoxication.[3] The most severe, often fatal form of encephalopathy may be preceded by lethargy, intermittent vomiting, apathy, drowsiness, irritability, stupor, poor memory, muscle tremors progressing to seizures, coma, and eventually death.[7]

Renal System

Kidney disease due to exposure to lead is far more prevalent than was previously believed.[33] The hazard is compounded by the fact that, unlike the situation for the hematopoietic system, routine screening is ineffective in early diagnosis.[7,34,35] In the adult, lead nephropathy is an insidious and progressive disease characterized by albuminuria, hematuria, pyuria, or a concentrating defect (in the early phases).[34,36] When less than two-thirds of kidney function is lost, blood urea nitrogen and serum creatinine may still be normal.[37]

Oral Cavity

Oral manifestations include ulcerative stomatitis, a blue gingival "lead line," gray spots on the buccal mucosa, and a heavy coating on the tongue.[1] A lead line is a great help in establishing exposure, but its presence does not mean that lead is being absorbed at that time. This blue line along the margin of the gums is caused by the action of hydrogen sulfide on the lead compound; hydrogen sulfide is a product of bacterial degradation in the gingival sulcus. This line is usually absent in edentulous patients or in patients who take care of their teeth.[1]

Reproductive System

Exposure to lead has profoundly adverse effects on reproduction functions in both men and women, and lead is considered a potential human teratogen.[38]

Exposure of women to lead is associated with abnormal ovarian cycles and menstrual disorders. An increased incidence of infertility, spontaneous abortion, stillbirth, and fetal macrocephaly has been associated with industrial lead exposure.[39] Lead crosses the placenta and appears to be mobilized from maternal stores during pregnancy. Infants of mothers with lead poisoning have lowered birth weights, slow growth, and nervous system disorders, and death is more likely in the first year of life.

Lead also affects the male gamete, and increased numbers of chromosomal alterations as well as abnormalities in sperm number, vigor, and morphologic features have been reported in lead workers. There may also be decreased sexual drive, impotence, and sterility.[40]

TOXICITY OF ORGANOLEAD COMPOUNDS

The signs and symptoms of organolead poisoning differ significantly from those of inorganic and elemental lead poisoning (Table 41-6). Like the organomercurials, tetraethyl and tetramethyl lead are lipid-soluble, highly volatile liquids that are absorbed quickly. The major effects of intoxication occur in the CNS.

The symptomatology of organic lead encephalopathy may be early in onset and correlate poorly with blood lead concentrations. Massive doses have caused death from cerebral and pul-

---

Table 41-6 Signs and Symptoms of Organolead Intoxication

Neurologic
  Tinnitus
  Headache
  Weakness
  Ataxia
  Gait abnormalities
  Tremors
  Seizures
  Coma
  Cerebral edema
Psychiatric
  Insomnia
  Fatigue
  Nightmares
  Restlessness
  Irritability
  Psychosis
  Delusions
  Depression
  Mania

---

monary edema.[8] Small amounts of alkyl lead may cause sleep disturbances, including insomnia and nightmares; fatigue; headache; tinnitus; restlessness; irritability; weakness; ataxia; tremors; psychosis; delusions; suicidal tendencies; mania; and seizures.[9] The most consistently observed neurologic manifestations are an abnormal jaw jerk, hyperactive deep tendon reflexes, stance and gait abnormalities, and an intention tremor.[12] There may be a latent period, which is variable in duration but usually ranges from 5 to 7 days; the more severe the exposure, the shorter the latent period.

Organolead poisoning is not associated with metaphyseal lead lines in the long bones, gingival lead lines, or nailbed changes. Hemoglobin synthesis does not appear to be greatly inhibited by organoleads, and anemia and basophilic stippling generally do not occur.[8]

DIAGNOSIS

Lead poisoning should be suspected in patients with nonspecific aches, pains, gastrointestinal symptoms, and subtle personality or CNS complaints who are employed in a susceptible occupation. Lead encephalopathy should be suspected in patients with unexplained seizures that do not respond to conventional therapy and in patients with evidence of diffuse encephalopathy with or without focal signs in whom more common causes of encephalopathy have been excluded.[41]

Childhood lead poisoning is an important differential diagnosis to keep in mind when a child presents with vomiting, abdominal pain, history of irritability, mood changes, or seizures.

The examination of a patient with a potential exposure to lead should include a work and medical history, a thorough physical examination, and appropriate laboratory studies. Once a diagnosis of increased lead absorption has been confirmed, the most important act of intervention is the prompt and complete termination of any further exposure to lead.

LABORATORY DETERMINATIONS

Laboratory determinations in suspected lead intoxication should include measurement of blood lead concentration, complete blood cell count with peripheral smear morphology and red cell indexes, a reticulocyte count, and, if indicated and available, assays for serum iron and total iron-binding capacity and serum ferritin (Tables 41-7 and 41-8).[29] Because chelating agents that may be used in treatment are potentially nephrotoxic, a routine urinalysis for specific gravity and glucose and protein content should be performed first, together with microscopic examination and measurements of blood urea nitrogen and serum creatinine, to rule out occult renal disease.[4] Long bone roentgenograms may be helpful in assessing chronic lead toxicity, and the diagnosis of acute lead intoxication may be aided by an abdominal roentgenogram.[16]

Many screening tests for lead poisoning are based on the inhibition of heme synthesis, which as discussed above results in the buildup of heme precursors.[11] A lead mobilization test may also

Table 41-7 Laboratory Tests in Elemental and Inorganic Lead Poisoning

Test	Finding
ALAD	Decreased
Urinary ALA	Increased
Blood ALA	Increased
Free erythrocyte protoporphyrin	Elevated
Zinc protoporphyrin	Elevated
Whole blood lead concentration	Elevated
Complete blood cell count	Anemia
Urinalysis	Abnormal
Blood urea nitrogen	Elevated
Serum creatinine	Elevated
Long bone roentgenograms	Lead line

Table 41-8 Laboratory Tests in Organolead Poisoning

Test	Finding
ALAD	Decreased
Urinary ALA	Increased or decreased
Blood ALA	Decreased
Free erythrocyte protoporphyrin	Increased or decreased
Whole blood lead concentration	Elevated
Urine lead concentration	Elevated

be helpful in making the diagnosis in some patients.[29]

In the early stages of lead intoxication, heme synthesis derangements may not be evident; the only abnormality may be an elevated blood lead concentration.[42] Conversely, in chronic lead poisoning the various biochemical abnormalities may be noted but the circulating lead concentrations may often appear to be normal.

Blood Lead Concentrations

Blood lead concentration index is the most popular measure of recent exposure to lead because of its convenience and its accurate reflection of circulating lead concentration (Table 41-9).[42] In general, blood lead determination, even with its limitations, is accepted as the most valid and reliable indicator of recent excessive lead absorption.[29] Because the half-life of circulating lead in blood is short, however, this measurement does not provide a realistic estimate of body burden.[22] Unless exposure is constant and continuous, blood lead concentrations may not reflect previous uptake, absorption, or extent of biochemical injury.[1] In other words, blood lead concentrations have no value in predicting excessive body stores of lead.[1] In addition, the relationship between blood concentration and clinical effects varies. In general, adults tolerate high concentrations better than children.[3]

Because 90% of the lead in circulating blood is fixed to red blood cell surfaces, it is critical that the assay for lead be done on whole blood.[17] The value may fluctuate depending on current ingestion and metabolic shifts.[5] A blood lead concentration greater than 25 μg/dL of whole blood and an erythrocyte protoporphyrin concentration greater than 35 μg/dL indicate undue absorption of lead.[3] Especially in pregnant patients blood lead should be well below this concentration. These clinical standards have been lowered over the last 20 years with the growing awareness of the health risks associated with prolonged blood lead concentrations equal to or greater than 25 μg/dL; these include impaired heme synthesis, red blood cell nucleotide metabolism, and vitamin D and cortisol metabolism; decreased intelligence; and signs of subclinical

Table 41-9 Correlation between Blood Lead Concentration and Symptoms of Intoxication

Lead Concentration (micrograms per deciliter)	Symptoms
25–30	Subclinical (greater risk if pregnant)
40–50	Mild behavioral changes
50–70	Mild to moderate clinical symptoms
70–80	Severe symptoms
>80	Encephalopathy

alterations. A lead concentration of 40 μg/dL of whole blood is considered the threshold for behavioral changes and mild CNS symptoms in adults.[1] Patients whose blood lead concentrations are 50 to 70 μg/dL may have mild to moderate clinical symptoms. Concentrations of 70 to 80 μg/dL may indicate severe lead intoxication, and those in excess of 80 μg/dL are often associated with encephalopathy (see Table 41-8).[3]

Blood lead concentration should thus be interpreted with caution.[32] A single elevated value may not indicate current excessive absorption, and a low value does not necessarily exclude a high bone burden of lead.[29] A false impression of severity may be created by reliance on blood lead concentrations for the diagnosis of lead poisoning in adults.[1] Serial determinations are needed to determine trends. Samples should be drawn by venipuncture rather than by fingerstick because of the possibility of skin contamination.[30]

Normal Urinary Lead Excretion

Measurement of urinary lead excretion without chelation is unreliable in assessing lead stores because the lead concentration in urine depends on diuresis and specific gravity.[1] Lead may also be in the soft tissues and not available for excretion until mobilized by a chelating agent.

Calcium EDTA Mobilization Test

For blood lead concentrations in the borderline toxic range, calcium EDTA mobilization should be performed to assess lead stores and the necessity for subsequent treatment.[5,22] An abnormal or increased lead concentration in urine after administration of calcium EDTA is the best predictor of a significant risk of toxicity.

Calcium EDTA acts as an exchange medium for lead; chelation results in a water-soluble complex that is readily measurable in the urine. Approximately 40% of the body burden of chelatable lead is mobilized and excreted in the urine in the 24 hours after calcium EDTA therapy.[3]

There has not been agreement as to what is considered the upper limit of normal urinary lead excretion after chelation therapy. The range extends from 300 to 600 μg per 24 hours, and more than 500 μg in 24 hours is generally considered abnormal. Some investigators, especially those dealing with the pediatric age group, prefer to use a lead excretion ratio to identify intoxicated patients (see discussion below).[3]

In performing a mobilization test, urine and blood lead concentrations should be measured before chelator therapy begins. Urine is then collected from 8 to 24 hours in lead-free equipment. The concentration is measured every 24 hours with reference to the pretreatment concentration, or a ratio can be calculated from the total amount of lead excreted divided by the amount of calcium EDTA given (in milligrams). A mobilization test is considered positive if the lead excretion ratio exceeds 0.60.[3]

Tests for Biochemical Abnormalities

Most objective tests available for evaluating the adverse consequences of *inorganic* lead exposure depend on the disruption of the pathways of heme synthesis. As discussed above, increased amounts of ALA in urine, decreased ALAD activity in red blood cells, and increased amounts of free erythrocyte protoporphyrin and zinc protoporphyrin are used as early warning signs of biochemical derangement produced by lead.

Concentrations of ALAD are consistently low in *organolead* poisoning, providing the most sensitive screening test; other markers of hemoglobin synthesis are not consistently altered.[12]

Because the amount of ALAD remaining is sufficient to synthesize hemoglobin[4] hemoglobin synthesis is not significantly inhibited by organolead compounds. There may, however, be a measurable increase in concentrations of ALA and, to a lesser extent, free erythrocyte protoporphyrin because of reduced activity of both ALAD and hemoglobin synthetase enzymes. Blood and urine concentrations of lead may also be moderately elevated.

Free Erythrocyte Protoporphyrin

The production of free erythrocyte protoporphyrin is not altered by environmental lead and is stable from day to day, but its concentration is nonspecific, being elevated in iron deficiency, sickle cell anemia, and chronic infection (Table 41-10).[6,30] Concentrations greater than 50 μg/dL of whole blood are abnormal in children.[7]

The amount of free erythrocyte protoporphyrin is a more sensitive indicator than the amount of lead in blood, of metabolically active lead in soft tissue, and of lead loosely bound to bone.[43] It is a direct measurement of the toxic effects of lead on heme synthesis and thus correlates better with lead toxicity than these other values. Elevations in free erythrocyte protoporphyrin become evident at blood lead concentrations greater than 15 μg/dL because ferrochelatase, the enzyme that converts protoporphyrin to hemoglobin, is inhibited.

Zinc Protoporphyrin

The measurement of zinc protoporphyrin concentrations has recently become a rapid method of screening for lead toxicity.[16] An increase in zinc protoporphyrin is a sign of deficient incorporation of iron into the heme system, the deficiency depending on a direct effect of lead on the

Table 41-10 Conditions that Elevate Blood Concentrations of Free Erythrocyte Protoporphyrin

Chronic infection
Iron deficiency
Lead poisoning
Sickle cell anemia

enzyme ferrochelatase or on a dysfunction of the intramitochondrial transport of iron in the blood-forming tissues. Under normal circumstances about 95% of the protoporphyrin in circulating human erythrocytes is in the form of iron proto-porphyrin. In lead poisoning the porphyrin acquires a zinc ion instead of iron. This zinc protoporphyrin is fluorescent[13] and constitutes the basis for a portable field device (the hema-tofluorometer) that has become useful in screen-ing for lead poisoning.

Zinc protoporphyrin is tightly bound in the available heme slots for the life of the erythro-cyte, which is approximately 120 days. Meas-urements therefore reflect the absorption of lead over the preceding 3 to 4 months. Because zinc protoporphyrin accumulates only in erythrocytes formed when lead is present in erythropoietic tissue,[13] there is a lag of several weeks before the concentration of new erythrocytes rich in zinc protoporphyrin is large enough to influence the total zinc protoporphyrin concentration.[44] Conversely, the presence of increased amounts of zinc protoporphyrin in erythrocytes long after lead exposure has ceased appears to be a better indicator of total body burden of lead than other measurements.

Elevations of zinc protoporphyrin concentra-tions correlate exponentially with blood lead concentrations in children beginning at 15 μg/dL. Once the blood lead concentration reaches 40 μg/dL, there is a precipitous rise in the amount of zinc protoporphyrin from its normal range of less than 100 μg/dL of whole blood. This test therefore appears to be one of the most reliable means of monitoring chronic lead absorption in its early stages.

Hair Analysis

Lead concentration in hair has been used to estimate body burden, but sample contamination from exogenous lead is difficult to control. Thus hair analysis has found little use.[13]

Roentgenograms

Roentgenograms of the abdomen may reveal radiopaque material in the bowel if lead has been ingested during the preceeding 72 hours.[1] Lead lines at the metaphyses of long bones reflect prolonged previous lead absorption but do not indicate current exposure.[6] Lead lines may also be noted at the ends of the metacarpals, ribs, tips of the scapulae, or over the iliac crests.

TREATMENT

Treatment of lead intoxication is aimed pri-marily at alleviating the acute symptoms and then at reducing the body lead stores (Ta-ble 41-11).[1] In the acute ingestion of lead, attempts at decreasing absorption should include ipecac syrup or gastric lavage and subsequent administration of activated charcoal and a cathartic.

In acute lead encephalopathy the management of intracranial hypertension is essential and may prove lifesaving if carried out rapidly and effec-tively.[45] Reducing cerebral edema must be con-sidered an urgent first step, especially because chelators do not work immediately. Volume replacement is restricted to basal requirements, and continuing losses must be carefully moni-tored. An adequate flow of urine must be estab-lished before intravenous chelation therapy is begun.[30]

For initial control of seizures, diazepam is the preferred drug. Barbiturates and phenytoin are reserved for the long-term management of recur-ring seizures after the acute episode is managed and consciousness has been fully recovered.[3]

There is no specific therapy for organolead poisoning. The efficacy of the therapeutic reg-imen for lead encephalopathy has not been ade-quately established for this type of intoxication.[8]

Table 41-11 Treatment of Lead Intoxication

Acute
Ipecac syrup or lavage
Charcoal and cathartic
Supportive care
Chelation therapy (see Table 41-12)
Chronic
Calcium EDTA mobilization test
Chelation therapy (see Table 41-12)

Although the therapeutic use of chelating agents in organolead poisoning has been somewhat disappointing compared with their effects on elemental and inorganic lead poisoning, these agents are not entirely without value.[12]

Chelation Therapy

Chelating agents are the main modality of therapy in chronic inorganic lead poisoning (Table 42-12). Lead binds to all four sites on the

Table 41-12 Indications for Chelation Therapy

Clinically Asymptomatic Patients	
Blood lead, 40 to 70 μg/dL Negative calcium EDTA mobilization No encephalopathy Normal free erythrocyte protoporphyrin	No chelation
Blood lead, 40 to 70 μg/dL Positive calcium EDTA mobilization No encephalopathy	Calcium EDTA, 3 to 5 days
Blood lead, 25 to 50 μg/dL Metabolic evidence of poisoning Positive calcium EDTA mobilization	Calcium EDTA, 3 to 5 days, or penicillamine
Clinically Symptomatic Patients	
Blood lead, >70 μg/dL No encephalopathy Clinical evidence of poisoning	Calcium EDTA (50 mg/kg/day in six divided doses) and dimercaprol (4 mg/kg, then 16 mg/kg/day in six divided doses)
Blood lead, 56 to 69 μg/dL No encephalopathy Clinical evidence of poisoning	Calcium EDTA and penicillamine
Lead encephalopathy	Dimercaprol (24 mg/kg/day in six divided doses) and calcium EDTA (75 mg/kg/day in six divided doses)
Long-term therapy	Penicillamine (250 mg orally 4 times daily)

chelator (oxygen, nitrogen, sulfur, and phosphorus).[16] The three drugs approved for use as chelating agents are dimercaprol, calcium EDTA, and penicillamine.[8] Lead forms a complex with each of the chelating agents, and except for penicillamine all are excreted in the urine. Penicillamine-lead complex is excreted in both urine and feces.

Calcium EDTA is the drug of choice for acute and chronic lead poisoning and lead encephalopathy.[45] This compound forms a stable, soluble, nontoxic, nonionic complex with lead ions. Dimercaprol also forms a complex with lead, but for reasons that are not fully understood dimercaprol by itself has seldom been useful in the treatment of clinical lead poisoning.[16]

The lead-mobilizing patterns of dimercaprol and calcium EDTA differ and complement each other.[8] Dimercaprol acts to chelate lead both intracellularly and extracellularly. Two molecules of dimercaprol combine with one atom of lead to form a complex that is excreted in the urine. Calcium EDTA removes lead from the extracellular compartment in soft tissues, CNS tissue, and red blood cells[8] and increases its urinary excretion.

Calcium EDTA should be diluted to a concentration of less than 0.5% in dextrose and water or in a 0.9% saline solution. When administered intravenously as a single dose, it should be diluted similarly and administered by slow infusion over 15 to 20 minutes.[3] Treatment with calcium EDTA should continue for no more than 5 days and should be followed by a rest period, usually of 5 to 7 days depending on patient response, to allow recovery from zinc depletion.[1]

In the management of acute lead encephalopathy or when blood lead concentration is greater than 70 μg/dL, co-administration of dimercaprol and calcium EDTA is preferred.[45] This therapy increases the rate of excretion of lead, lowers mortality, and may lower the incidence of brain damage compared with the use of calcium EDTA alone.[3] The clinical deterioration seen with the use of calcium EDTA as the sole agent is thought to be due to partial dissociation of lead from the chelate, with release of lead into the brain. Dimercaprol, which penetrates the CNS, seems to protect against this effect.[45] Treatment is therefore begun with a priming dose of dimercaprol only. Once urine flow is established, administration of calcium EDTA may begin.[3]

High-dosage therapy for lead encephalopathy consists of dimercaprol administered intramuscularly at 24 mg/kg/day in six divided doses and calcium EDTA administered intravenously at 75 mg/kg/day in six divided doses not to exceed 1.5 g/day.[12] After the initial 5-day course of combined parenteral therapy, oral treatment should commence with 40 mg/kg/day of penicillamine 2 to 4 times per day until two consecutive measurements of blood lead concentration are less than 40 μg/dL and the 24-hour urine lead concentration is less than 100 μg per 24 hours.[7,12]

Asymptomatic patients without encephalopathy and with blood lead concentrations greater than 70 μg/dL may receive low-dose therapy with calcium EDTA and dimercaprol or with calcium EDTA alone. Calcium EDTA is administered intravenously at 50 mg/kg/day in six divided doses, and dimercaprol is administered intramuscularly at an initial dose of 4 mg/kg and then 16 mg/kg/day in six divided doses. Symptomatic patients without encephalopathy and with blood lead concentrations between 56 and 69 μg/dL can be treated with low-dose calcium EDTA. Penicillamine may be used after completion of parenteral chelation therapy.[1]

Use of the Calcium EDTA Mobilization Test

As discussed earlier, the calcium EDTA mobilization test is useful when blood lead concentration is elevated but there is uncertainty about the need for chelation, as in patients with blood lead concentrations of 25 to 50 μg/dL accompanied by erythrocyte protoporphyrin concentrations persistently greater than 35 μg/dL or in patients with free erythrocyte protoporphyrin concentration out of proportion to blood lead concentrations.[42] This test provides an index of the mobile fraction of body lead and directly demonstrates whether a significant diuresis of lead will result from chelation.[22] Patients with moderately elevated blood lead concentrations (25 to 50 μg/dL), no encephalopathy, and a positive mobilization test may be

treated with penicillamine alone. Patients with blood lead concentrations less than 40 μg/dL, and those with moderately elevated blood concentrations (40 to 59 μg/dL) but negative mobilization tests and no encephalopathy, require no chelation therapy.

Chelation Therapy in Renal Disease

Adults with lead nephropathy who have serum creatinine concentrations of 2 mg/dL or less may receive 1 g of calcium EDTA daily for 5 days.[36] In patients with serum creatinine concentrations of 2 to 3 mg/dL, 500 mg every 24 hours for 5 days should be administered. In children, the dosage is 50 to 75 mg/kg daily with the total amount divided into two daily doses and each part dissolved in 500 mL of normal saline or 5% dextrose and water.[36]

Role of Penicillamine

Penicillamine chelates lead but not to the same degree as dimercaprol or calcium EDTA.[16] For this reason, it is not recommended for acute therapy but may be employed for long-term therapy.[7] Because it can be given by mouth, penicillamine has found particular utility in mild and uncomplicated plumbism and for supplemental therapy.[16]

Role of Dimercaptosuccinic Acid

Dimercaptosuccinic acid appears to have great promise as an effective chelating agent for lead, but it has not been approved for clinical use by the FDA. This agent has the advantage of dramatically inducing lead excretion. It also reduces blood lead concentrations and has no apparent side effects.[46–49] Its other advantage is that it has no effect on calcium, magnesium, iron, or zinc excretion.[50] Effective doses have been reported as 3 to 5 mg/kg ingested orally at 6-hour intervals.[51]

REFERENCES

1. Ibels L, Pollock C: Lead intoxication. *Med Toxicol* 1986;1:387–410.

2. Lin-Fu J: Undue absorption of lead among children—A new look at an old problem. *N Engl J Med* 1972;286:702–710.

3. Piomelli S, Rosen J, Chisolm J, et al: Management of childhood lead poisoning. *J Pediatr* 1984;105:523–532.

4. Chisolm J: Treatment of acute lead intoxication—Choice of chelating agents and supportive therapeutic measures. *Clin Toxicol* 1970;3:527–540.

5. Sachs H, Blanksma L, Murray E, et al: Ambulatory treatment of lead poisoning: Report of 1155 cases. *Pediatrics* 1970;46:389–396.

6. Nelson M, Chisolm J: Lead toxicity masquerading as sickle cell crisis. *Ann Emerg Med* 1986;15:748–750.

7. Pincus D, Saccar C: Lead poisoning. *Clin Pharmacol* 1979;19:120–124.

8. Greenhouse A: Heavy metals and the nervous system. *Clin Neuropharmacol* 1982;5:45–92.

9. Schottenfeld R, Cullen M: Organic affective illness associated with lead intoxication. *Am J Psychiatry* 1984;141:1423–1426.

10. Lin-Fu J: Vulnerability of children to lead exposure and toxicity. *N Engl J Med* 1973;289:1229–1233.

11. Chisolm J: Management of increased lead absorption and lead poisoning in children. *N Engl J Med* 1973;289:1016–1017.

12. Edminster S, Bayer M: Recreational gasoline sniffing: Acute gasoline intoxication and latent organolead poisoning. *J Emerg Med* 1985;3:365–370.

13. Bushnell P, Jaeger R: Hazards to health from environmental lead exposure: A review of recent literature. *Vet Hum Toxicol* 1986;28:255–261.

14. Chisolm J: The use of chelating agents in the treatment of acute and chronic lead intoxication in childhood. *J Pediatr* 1968;73:1–38.

15. Rose D, Cummings C, Molinaro J, et al: Screening for lead toxicity among autobody repair workers. *Am J Ind Med* 1982;3:405–412.

16. Gordon N, Brown S, Khosla V, et al: Lead poisoning. *Oral Surg* 1979;47:500–512.

17. Chisolm J, Mellits E, Keil J: A simple protoporphyrin assay microhematocrit procedure as a screening technique for increased lead absorption in young children. *J Pediatr* 1974;84:490–495.

18. Selbst S, Henretig F, Fee M, et al: Lead poisoning in a child with a gunshot wound. *Pediatrics* 1986;77:413–416.

19. Cohen G, Ahrens W: Chronic lead poisoning. *J Pediatr* 1959;54:271–284.

20. Dillman R, Crumb C, Lidsky M: Lead poisoning from a gunshot wound. *Am J Med* 1979;66:509–514.

21. Machle W: Lead absorption from bullets lodged in tissues. *JAMA* 1940;115:1536–1541.

22. Allcott J, Barnhart R, Mooney L: Acute lead poisoning in two users of illicit methamphetamine. *JAMA* 1987;258:510–511.

23. Cohen N, Modai D, Golik A, et al: An esoteric occupational hazard for lead poisoning. *Clin Toxicol* 1986;24:59–67.

24. Lin-Fu J: Vulnerability of children to lead exposure and toxicity. *N Engl J Med* 1973;289:1289–1293.

25. Hammer L, Ludwig S, Henretig F: Increased lead absorption in children with accidental ingestions. *Am J Emerg Med* 1985;3:301–304.

26. Charney E, Kessler B, Farfel M, et al: Childhood lead poisoning. *N Engl J Med* 1983;309:1089–1093.

27. Oehme F: Mechanisms of heavy metal toxicities. *Clin Toxicol* 1972;5:151–162.

28. Green V, Wise G, Callenbach J: Lead poisoning. *Clin Toxicol* 1976;9:33–51.

29. Keate R, DiPietrantonio P, Randleman M: Occupational lead exposure. *Ann Emerg Med* 1983;12:786–788.

30. Piomelli S, Davidow B, Guinee V, et al: The FEP test: A screening micromethod for lead poisoning. *Pediatrics* 1973;51:254–259.

31. Cohen G: Lead poisoning. *Clin Pediatr* 1980;19:245–250.

32. Alessio L, Castoldi M, Odone P, et al: Behavior of indicators of exposure and effect after cessation of occupational exposure to lead. *Br J Ind Med* 1981;38:262–267.

33. Wedeen R, Mallik D, Batuman V: Detection and treatment of occupational lead nephropathy. *Arch Intern Med* 1979;139:53–57.

34. Batuman V, Landy E, Maesaka J, et al: Contribution of lead to hypertension with renal impairment. *N Engl J Med* 1983;309:17–21.

35. Campbell B, Beattie A, Elliott H, et al: Occupational lead exposure and renin release. *Arch Environ Health* 1979;34:439–443.

36. Khan A, Patel U, Rafeeq M, et al: Reversible acute renal failure in lead poisoning. *J Pediatr* 1983;102:147–149.

37. Wedeen R: Lead and the gouty kidney. *Am J Kid Dis* 1983;2:559–563.

38. Needleman H, Gunnoe C, Leviton A, et al: Deficits in psychologic and classroom performance of children with elevated dentine lead levels. *N Engl J Med* 1979;300:689–695.

39. Needleman H, Rabinowitz M, Leviton A, et al: The relationship between prenatal exposure to lead and congenital anomalies. *JAMA* 1984;251:2956–2959.

40. Needleman H, Landrigan P: The health effects of low-level exposure to lead. *Annu Rev Public Health* 1981;2:277–298.

41. Smith M: Recent work on low-level lead exposure and its impact on behavior, intelligence, and learning: A review. *J Am Acad Child Psychiatry* 1985;24:24–32.

42. Carton J, Maradona J, Arribas J: Acute-subacute lead poisoning: Clinical findings and comparative study of diagnostic tests. *Arch Intern Med* 1987;147:697–703.

43. Berwick D, Komaroff A: Cost effectiveness of lead screening. *N Engl J Med* 1982;306:1392–1398.

44. Rosen I, Wildt K, Gullberg B, et al: Neurophysiological effects of lead exposure. *Scand J Work Environ Health* 1983;9:431–441.

45. Coffin R, Phillips J, Staples W, et al: Treatment of lead encephalopathy in children. *J Pediatr* 1966;69:198–206.

46. Aposhian H: DMSA and DMPS—Water-soluble antidotes for heavy metal poisoning. *Annu Rev Pharmacol Toxicol* 1983;23:193–215.

47. Aaseth J: Recent advances in the therapy of metal poisonings with chelating agents. *Hum Toxicol* 1983;2:257–272.

48. Friedheim E, Graziano J, Kaul B: Treatment of lead poisoning by 2,3-dimercaptosuccinic acid. *Lancet* 1978;2:1234–1236.

49. Graziano J: Role of 2,3-dimercaptosuccinic acid in the treatment of heavy metal poisoning. *Med Toxicol* 1986;1:155–162.

50. Graziano J, Leong J, Friedheim E: 2,3-Dimercaptosuccinic acid: A new agent for the treatment of lead poisoning. *J Pharmacol Exp Ther* 1978;206:696–700.

51. Graziano J, Siris E, LoIacono N, et al: 2,3-Dimercaptosuccinic acid as an antidote for lead intoxication. *Clin Pharmacol Ther* 1985;37:431–438.

ADDITIONAL SELECTED REFERENCES

Cohen A, Trotzky M, Pincus D: Reassessment of the microcytic anemia of lead poisoning. *Pediatrics* 1981;67:904–906.

Edwards E, Edwards E: Allergic contact dermatitis to lead acetate in a hair dye. *Cutis* 1982;30:629–630.

Ernhart C, Landa B, Schell N: Lead levels and intelligence. *Pediatrics* 1981;68:903–905.

Fischbein A, Cohn J, Ackerman G: Asbestos, lead, and the family: Household risks. *J Fam Pract* 1980;10:989–992.

Glickman L, Valciukas J, Lilis R, et al: Occupational lead exposure. *Int Arch Occup Environ Health* 1984;54:115–125.

Gloag D: Sources of lead pollution. *Br Med J* 1981;282:41–44.

Mahaffey K, Annest J, Roberts J, et al: National estimates of blood lead levels: United States, 1976–1980. *N Engl J Med* 1982;307:573–579.

Miwa S, Ishida Y, Takegawa S, et al: A case of lead intoxication. *Am J Hematol* 1981;11:99–105.

Nathanson B, Nudelman H: Ambient lead concentrations in New York City and their health implications. *Bull N Y Acad Med* 1980;56:866–875.

Sixel-Dietrich F, Doss M, Pfeil C, et al: Acute lead intoxication due to intravenous injection. *Hum Toxicol* 1985;4:301–309.

Triebig G, Weltle D, Valentin H: Investigations on neurotoxicity of chemical substances at the workplace. *Int Arch Occup Environ Health* 1984;53:189–204.

Valciukas J, Lilis R: A composite index of lead effects. *Int Arch Occup Environ Health* 1982;51:1–14.

chapter 42

Arsenic

Arsenic was first recorded as a medicinal agent in ancient Greece by Hippocrates. Although it is rarely part of the modern pharmacopeia, it is widely used in other applications.

Because arsenic is nearly tasteless and odorless it was used extensively as a means of criminal poisoning, and, although not as common, homicidal, suicidal, and accidental arsenic poisoning occur even today.[1] Self-administration of arsenic by accident in children and as a suicide attempt in adults represent the most common types of ingestion. Purposeful self-administration of arsenic for the purpose of creating and maintaining a state of chronic invalidism has also been reported.[2]

USES

Arsenic is a common ingredient in insecticides, rodenticides, weed killers, wallpaper, paint, ceramics, and glass (Table 42-1). It is also used in wood preservation and as an additive to metal alloys to increase hardening and heat resistance.[3] Organic arsenicals such as dimethylarsenic acid and monosodium methylarsenate are used in forestry as herbicides.[4] Lead, calcium, and magnesium arsenate are the most common arsenicals; these are used primarily as pesticides in sprays of various kinds.[5] Inorganic arsenic poisoning was fairly common in the United States before the Second World War[6]

mainly because of the widespread use of medicinal arsenic and contamination of fruits and vegetables by arsenical sprays.[7]

In some areas organic arsenicals are still used in the treatment of certain protozoan diseases. Arsenic is also an ingredient in numerous homeopathic medicines. The use of penicillin for the treatment of syphilis drastically curtailed the medicinal importance of arsenicals, but they continue to have major agricultural and industrial importance, thereby affording innumerable opportunities for exposure. Arsenic-containing compounds are widely used in feed for poultry, cattle, and swine, purportedly to improve the nutritional status of the animals. Contamination of well water and of illicitly manufactured alcohol have been causes of arsenic poisoning.

TYPES OF ARSENIC COMPOUNDS

From the toxicological standpoint, the important compounds of arsenic fall into three major groups: (1) inorganic arsenicals, such as white arsenic, and the arsenate and arsenite salts; (2) organic arsenicals, which differ in the valence state of the arsenic atom (trivalent and pentavalent); and (3) arsine gas.

Pentavalent arsenate, which is the naturally occurring environmental form of arsenic, is less toxic than trivalent arsenite. Pentavalent compounds are relatively physiologically inactive;

Table 42-1 Uses of Arsenic

Insecticides
Rodenticides
Weed killers
Wallpaper
Paint
Ceramics
Glass
Livestock feed

they are water soluble and therefore rapidly absorbed through mucous membranes. This leads to rapid penetration into all body tissues, most of which are capable of reducing arsenate to toxic arsenite. This mechanism has not been completely determined, however.[7]

Although arsenic trioxide is less toxic than some of the more soluble herbicidal arsenicals, the dust can cause poisoning through ingestion, inhalation, or skin contact. Trivalent arsenic compounds are less readily absorbed through mucous membranes because of their lipid solubility but are better absorbed through the skin.[7] Trivalent arsenicals such as phenylarsenoxide are more potent inhibitors of certain sulfhydryl enzymes than inorganic arsenites.

ABSORPTION, DISTRIBUTION, AND EXCRETION OF ARSENICALS

Under usual circumstances approximately 1 mg of arsenic is ingested daily.[8] After absorption, arsenic combines with the globin portion of the hemoglobin in erythrocytes. After a period of 24 hours, arsenic leaves the bloodstream and is distributed to organs such as the liver, spleen, lung, and kidney. A smaller amount accumulates in muscle and nerve tissue because penetration of the blood-brain barrier is minimal. Arsenic that remains in the bloodstream is bound to proteins. Two to four weeks after ingestion, incorporation into hair, nails, and skin occurs as arsenic binds to sulfhydryl groups of keratin.[7]

After oral ingestion of inorganic arsenic, two metabolites predominate: methylarsinic acid and dimethylarsinic acid. The major route of excretion is through the kidney, but feces, skin, and

hair may also contain appreciable amounts of arsenic.[9]

MECHANISM OF TOXICITY OF ARSENICALS

There are several mechanisms by which arsenic exerts its toxic effects (Table 42-2). The most clinically significant is reversible combination with sulfhydryl groups. Because sulfhydryl groups are present in many enzyme systems, it is not surprising that many enzyme systems are vulnerable; the pyruvate and succinate oxidation pathways are especially sensitive to disruption by arsenic. The Krebs cycle, where oxidative phosphorylation takes place, is also interrupted. This blockade may eventually result in cell death from marked depletion of cellular energy stores and disruption of multiple metabolic systems.

In another major form of toxicity from arsenic, termed arsenolysis, arsenic acts as an anion and can substitute for phosphate in many reactions. This also disrupts oxidative phosphorylation by replacing the stable phosphoryl group with the less stable arsenyl group.[8] The arsenyl decomposes, resulting in a loss of high-energy phosphate bonds and eventual stimulation of cellular respiration to restore lost energy.

Arsenic poisoning results in a clinical picture similar to that of thiamine deficiency because of prevention of the transformation of acetyl and succinyl coenzyme A.[7] Many other enzymes are susceptible to deactivation by arsenic, including monoamine oxidase, lipase, acid phosphatase, liver arginase, cholinesterase, and adenylcyclase, but these are less important clinically.[5]

Table 42-2 Biochemical Effects of Arsenicals

Blockade of oxidative phosphorylation
Inhibition of acetyl and succinyl coenzyme A
  transformation
Inhibition of other enzymes
  Monoamine oxidase
  Lipase
  Acid phosphatase
  Liver arginase
  Cholinesterase
  Adenylcyclase

Systemic poisoning is the principal concern with all arsenic compounds, but arsenic trichloride and some organic derivatives such as lewisite are also strong local irritants that may penetrate the skin and act as vesicants.[9]

TOXICITY OF ARSENICALS

Acute

Clinical manifestations of acute arsenic poisoning usually occur within the first few hours after ingestion or exposure; symptoms may occur as soon as 30 minutes after exposure. The earliest clinical features reflect multiorgan involvement, which is manifested often as acute gastroenteritis and is variably associated with encephalopathy, pancytopenia, hepatitis, cardiomyopathy, and dermatitis (Table 42-3).[10] Death from acute arsenic poisoning is usually caused by irreversible circulatory insufficiency. If the patient survives the initial illness recovery may be complicated by the development of

---

Table 42-3 Clinical Features of Acute Arsenic Intoxication

Gastrointestinal
  Metallic taste in the mouth
  Garlic odor on the breath
  Dysphagia
  Abdominal pain
  Vomiting
  Diarrhea
  Shock
Cardiac
  Decreased force of contraction
  Sinus tachycardia
  Ventricular dysrhythmia
  Nonspecific electrocardiographic changes
Neurologic
  Headache
  Muscle weakness
  Muscle cramps
  Peripheral neuropathy
  Paresthesia
  CNS depression
  Coma
Cutaneous
  Skin pigmentation changes
  Aldrich-Mees lines

---

nephritis, including hematuria, albuminuria, and glycosuria.

Gastrointestinal

Whatever the route of exposure, the presenting symptoms in most cases of acute arsenic poisoning are those of severe gastritis or gastroenteritis. Initially, the patient experiences a metallic taste in the mouth and a garlicky odor on the breath.[5] Burning and dryness of the mouth and throat, dysphagia, colicky abdominal pain, projectile vomiting, and profuse watery diarrhea or "rice-water stools" are also early manifestations and occur within hours of exposure. Shock develops rapidly as a consequence of dehydration and generalized vasodilation. Because the lesions are usually due not to local corrosion but to vascular damage from absorbed arsenic, the first symptoms may be delayed for several hours. These complaints are invariably followed by a constellation of features reflecting multiple organ involvement.

Cardiac

Arsenic is a myocardial toxin that produces decreased contractile force of myocardial fibers secondary to inhibition of oxidative phosphorylation. Cardiac toxicity includes sinus tachycardia and ventricular dysrhythmias.[8] Electrocardiographic changes include nonspecific ST segment changes, prolonged QT interval, and T wave inversion.[4]

Neurologic

Neurologic manifestations include pain in the extremities, headache, muscle weakness, CNS depression with coma, and polyneuropathies. The neuropathy is a late occurrence in the course of acute arsenic intoxication.[11] It usually appears between 1 and 2 weeks after a single ingestion and involves both sensory and motor nerve fibers. Sensory changes are usually the initial manifestation.[12] Paresthesias, aches, cramps, and tender muscles are common, and burning pain in the soles of the feet is a frequent complaint.[13] The abnormal sensations increase in severity, and the areas of numbness extend rapidly and symmetrically through the limbs distally to proximally. Symptoms of severe neuropathy become more intense over the course of 1 to 2 weeks, reach a maximum, and then take weeks and sometimes months to abate. The degree of recovery depends on the severity of the neuropathy. Complete recovery occurs in purely sensory and the mildest sensorimotor cases. Patients with severe degrees of motor disability take longer to recover, and permanent disability occurs in the most severe cases.[12]

A great decline in mortality has resulted in a relative increase in the incidence of arsenical neuropathy. This is because patients who previously would have died from the effects of fluid loss during initial acute gastrointestinal illness now survive to develop neuropathies and other disorders formerly seen only in those with chronic exposure.[13]

Cutaneous

Cutaneous involvement, including increased skin pigmentation, is considered a common characteristic of acute arsenic poisoning and may occur weeks after an acute ingestion. Transverse white striae in the nails (Aldrich-Mees lines) are often seen. These lines are considered an actual deposit of arsenic and usually take 5 to 6 weeks to appear over the lunulae, so that a gross estimation of the time of exposure can be made by the distance of the line from the base of the nail. Aldrich-Mees lines are nonspecific for arsenic poisoning; they have also been noted in association with thallium intoxication and various nontoxic clinical conditions (Table 42-4).

Chronic

Chronic arsenic poisoning (Table 42-5) is insidious and often requires multiple hospitalizations before the correct diagnosis is discerned.

Cutaneous

The cutaneous manifestations of chronic arsenic ingestion are characteristic but for the most part nonspecific. The earliest manifestation is persistent erythematous flushing caused by cutaneous capillary dilation (Table 42-4). Shortly thereafter, melanosis of nonexposed areas and hyperkeratosis occur. Desquamation of the skin

Table 42-4 Conditions Associated with White Nail Striae

Arsenic intoxication
Thallium intoxication
Trichinosis
Psoriasis
Leprosy
Malaria

Table 42-5 Clinical Features of Chronic Arsenic Intoxication

Cutaneous
   Aldrich-Mees lines
   Alopecia
   Brittle nails
   Desquamation of skin
   Facial edema
   Flushing
   Hyperkeratosis
   Melanosis of nonexposed areas
   Pruritus
Gastrointestinal
   Anorexia
   Cirrhosis of liver
   Diarrhea
   Jaundice
   Nausea
   Vomiting
Neurologic
   Ataxia
   Diplopia
   Muscular atrophy
   Muscular paralysis
   Optic neuritis
Hematologic
   Anemia
   Leukopenia
   Thrombocytopenia
Miscellaneous
   Cough
   Conjunctivitis
   Hoarseness
   Salivation

and brittle nails with classic Aldrich-Mees lines may occur. In addition, there may be patchy or diffuse alopecia and edema of the face, periorbital region, or ankles from localized transudation of intravascular fluid. Aldrich-Mees lines may not be seen in chronic arsenic poisoning unless acute episodes have been superimposed.

Neurologic

In advanced arsenic poisoning, neurologic symptoms are prominent. Although encephalopathies have been described, peripheral neuritis is more common. Prolonged poisoning eventually leads to muscular atrophy, paralysis, and ataxia. Although cranial nerves are usually spared in chronic arsenic intoxication, diplopia and optic neuritis with dimming or concentric loss of vision are occasionally encountered. The manifestations of arsenical encephalitis may be similar to those of Wernicke's syndrome and Korsakoff's psychosis because of blockade of thiamine-associated metabolic reactions. Peripheral neuropathies may present with a "glove-and-stocking" distribution of sensory loss.[11]

Hematologic

Chronic arsenic intoxication is also associated with severe hematopoietic disturbances.[5] Anemia and leukopenia are almost universal and are frequently accompanied by thrombocytopenia. The anemia is usually normochromic and normocytic. Interference with folate metabolism may result in mild megaloblastic changes. Karyorrhexis, or fragmentation of the red blood cell nucleus, is characteristic of arsenic poisoning, and typical "cloverleaf" nuclei may be seen.

Miscellaneous

Among late symptoms and signs of chronic arsenical poisoning are anemia, cirrhosis of the liver, and jaundice (which may also be noted after an acute ingestion). Chronic arsenic poisoning may also be characterized by pruritis, soreness of the mouth, inflammation of the conjunctiva and nasal mucosa, salivation, loss of appetite, nausea, vomiting, and diarrhea.[7,14]

ARSINE GAS

Arsine is the most dangerous form of arsenic and the most serious in terms of industrial hazard.[15] Arsine is a colorless, nonirritating gas that can produce poisoning at less than 30 parts per million (ppm), a concentration that is far less than that at which its faint smell of garlic is detectable.[16] Lewisite, a war gas, is an arsine derivative.

Arsine is liberated whenever hydrogen is generated in the presence of arsenic. Any ore contaminated with arsenic will also liberate arsine when treated with acid.[17] Most industrial instances of arsine poisoning have occurred among metallurgical workers from the action of water or acid on arsenic-bearing metals.[15] In addition, arsine gas may be encountered during electrolyte processes, the manufacture of zinc chloride and sulfate, and the smelting of metallic arsenical ore and in any setting where impure acids or metals are used.[17]

Mechanism of Toxicity of Arsine

Arsine inhibits tissue oxidation and particularly affects erythrocytes, causing intravascular hemolysis. The mechanism of toxicity may relate to the inhibition of glutathione, which is necessary for red blood cell integrity. Glutathione is a peptide composed of glutamic acid, cysteine, and glycine and contains sulfhydryl or thiol groups, and it is thought that an irreversible complex with the arsenic atom is formed, causing hemolysis of the mature red blood cell.[16]

Signs and Symptoms of Arsine Poisoning

The interval between exposure to arsine and the onset of symptoms is variable. There is usually a delay of 2 to 24 hours before manifestations of poisoning arise (Table 42-6).

Early symptoms of acute exposure may include headache, anorexia, nausea, vomiting, and paresthesia.[5] Abdominal pain, chills, and hematemesis are common, and hemoglobinemia may appear as early as 4 hours after acute exposure. Frank jaundice and tenderness of the liver and spleen appear after 24 hours in acute cases. As with other conditions exhibiting acute massive hemolysis, anuria or hemoglobinuric nephrosis may result. Pulmonary edema and myocardial damage may also ensue.

Table 42-6 Clinical Features of Arsine Intoxication

Gastrointestinal
  Abdominal pain
  Anorexia
  Hematemesis
  Jaundice
  Nausea
  Vomiting
Neurologic
  Headache
  Paresthesia
Miscellaneous
  Anuria
  Hemolysis
  Myocardial damage
  Nephrosis
  Pulmonary edema

Survivors of acute poisoning usually regain a normal state after about 2 weeks. If death occurs, it usually results from sudden myocardial failure or pulmonary edema.

DIAGNOSIS

Acute Arsenical Intoxication

Arsenous oxide is as radiopaque as barium, and an alert clinician sometimes can make the diagnosis of arsenic ingestion from the plain film of the abdomen obtained during the workup of a gastroenteritis.

In acute arsenic poisoning, a history of arsenic ingestion can occasionally be elicited. Particular difficulty may be encountered with pediatric patients or unsuspecting victims of homicide attempts.[7]

Chronic Arsenical Intoxication

Chronic arsenic intoxication is more difficult to diagnose than acute intoxication. It should be considered in any patient who presents with combinations of neuropathy, skin rash, hematologic disturbances, and gastrointestinal complaints.[7]

Intoxication with Arsine Gas

Arsine gas exposure produces a striking anemia of the hemolytic type.[18] Arsine poisoning should be considered in the setting of an unknown gas causing a systemic reaction that includes anemia and hemolysis. Typical findings of arsenic poisoning may not be noted.[15]

LABORATORY ANALYSIS

Analysis of body tissues, nails, and hair is important in diagnosing chronic arsenic intoxication. Hair analysis by neutron activation not only provides precise quantitation of arsenic concentration but also allows segmental analysis to determine when arsenic was ingested and the number of episodes. The analysis requires only a few hairs, and pubic hair is preferable because arsenic adsorption to exposed hairs may occur in an environment with elevated concentrations of atmospheric arsenic. In addition, arsenic persists longer in pubic hair because of its slower growth. Hair and nail samples containing more than 3 ppm of arsenic or 100 mg of arsenic per 100 g of specimen are diagnostic of arsenic intoxication.[7]

TREATMENT

After acute arsenic ingestion, residual arsenic should be removed from the stomach by emesis or gastric lavage and subsequent administration of activated charcoal and a cathartic (Table 42-7). Intravenous fluids are necessary to maintain intravascular volume and to prevent circulatory collapse. These fluids should be vigorously replaced.

Chelation Therapy for Arsenic Intoxication

Measurement of the urinary excretion of arsenic during chelation therapy is important. When the 24-hour urinary arsenic excretion rate decreases to less than 50 μg per 24 hours, further chelation therapy is not necessary.

Table 42-7 Treatment of Arsenic Poisoning

Acute poisoning
  Emesis or lavage
  Charcoal and cathartic
  Adequate intravenous volume replacement
  Dimercaprol
    2.5 to 3.0 mg/kg IM every 4 hours for 2 days,
      then
    2.5 to 3.0 mg/kg IM every 6 hours for 1 day, then
    2.5 to 3.0 mg/kg IM every 12 hours for 10 days
Chronic poisoning
  Dimercaprol
  Penicillamine (250 mg orally 4 times a day)

Acute Arsenical Intoxication

Dimercaprol is specific for arsenic, and treatment should be started as soon as possible after the diagnosis has been established; the earlier dimercaprol is administered, the greater the possibility of avoiding serious intoxication. The use of dimercaprol to treat acute arsenic poisoning has been shown to be effective in preventing the occurrence of peripheral neuropathy if administered within 18 hours of ingestion.

Dimercaprol markedly enhances the urinary excretion of arsenic without damage to the excretory organs. The recommended dosage is 2.5 to 3.0 mg/kg intramuscularly every 4 hours for the first 2 days, every 6 hours during the third day, and every 12 hours for the next 10 days or until recovery is complete.[7]

Chronic Arsenical Intoxication

The benefit of using dimercaprol to treat chronic arsenic poisoning is less certain than for acute poisoning, but a trial may be warranted because, once arsenic is bound to tissues, it is tightly held and cannot be displaced easily by chelators. Although dimercaprol may dramatically reverse the hematologic disturbance, it may have no effect on the neurologic lesions caused by arsenic poisoning.

Intoxication with Arsine Gas

Chelation therapy affords no protection against arsine intoxication.[17] Because of the marked binding of the arsenic atom with hemoglobin arsine is poorly dialysable, and dialysis is primarily directed toward management of the associated renal failure.[16] Survival of arsine poisoning depends on the degree of hemolysis and the course of the renal failure.[15]

Role of Other Antidotes

Penicillamine also appears to promote the urinary excretion of arsenic in both acute and chronic poisonings, but it is not approved for this purpose by the FDA.[4,19]

In a search for an effective antidote with fewer side effects than dimercaprol, a series of mercaptoalkanesulfonates was synthesized.[20] Dimercaptopropanesulfonic acid (DMPS) and dimercaptosuccinic acid (DMSA) were two of these compounds. Both DMSA and DMPS have been shown to be effective for arsenic poisoning, but they have not been shown to be of benefit for acute arsine poisoning.[21,22] These water-soluble compounds are effective orally. They are also not yet approved for use by the FDA.

REFERENCES

1. Fernando P: Attempted homicide with arsenic. *Clin Toxicol* 1979;14:575–577.

2. Petery J, Gross C, Victorica B: Ventricular fibrillation caused by arsenic poisoning. *Am J Dis Child* 1970;120:367–371.

3. Beckett W, Moore J, Keogh J, et al: Acute encephalopathy due to occupational exposure to arsenic. *Br J Ind Med* 1986;43:66–67.

4. Peterson R, Rumack B: D-Penicillamine therapy of acute arsenic poisoning. *J Pediatr* 1977;91:661–666.

5. Vaziri N, Uphan T, Barton C: Hemodialysis clearance of arsenic. *Clin Toxicol* 1980;17:451–456.

6. Done A, Peart A: Acute toxicities of arsenical herbicides. *Clin Toxicol* 1971;4:343–355.

7. Schoolmeester W, White D: Arsenic poisoning. *South Med J* 1980;73:198–208.

8. Petery J, Rennert O, Choi H, et al: Arsenic poisoning in childhood. *Clin Toxicol* 1970;3:519–526.

9. Tadlock C, Aposhian H: Protection of mice against the lethal effects of sodium arsenite by 2,3-dimercapto-1-propanesulfonic acid and dimercaptosuccinic acid. *Biochem Biophys Res Commun* 1980;94:501–507.

10. Kjeldsberg C, Ward H: Leukemia in arsenic poisoning. *Ann Intern Med* 1972;77:935–937.

11. Hessl S, Berman E: Severe peripheral neuropathy after exposure to monosodium methyl arsonate. *J Toxicol Clin Toxicol* 1982;19:281–287.

12. Lequensne P, McLeod J: Peripheral neuropathy following a single exposure to arsenic. *J Neurol Sci* 1977; 32:437–451.

13. Freeman J, Couch J: Prolonged encephalopathy with arsenic poisoning. *Neurology* 1978;28:853–855.

14. Greenberg C, Davies S, McGowan T, et al: Acute respiratory failure following severe arsenic poisoning. *Chest* 1979;76:596–598.

15. Hocken A, Bradshaw G: Arsine poisoning. *Br J Ind Med* 1970;27:56–60.

16. Coles G, Davies H, Daley D, et al: Acute intravascular hemolysis and renal failure due to arsine poisoning. *Postgrad Med J* 1969;45:170–172.

17. Fowler B, Weissberg J: Arsine poisoning. *N Engl J Med* 1974;291:1171–1174.

18. Levinsky W, Smalley R, Hillyer P, et al: Arsine hemolysis. *Arch Environ Health* 1970;20:436–440.

19. Kuruvilla A, Bergeson P, Done A: Arsenic poisoning in childhood: An unusual case report with special notes on therapy with penicillamine. *Clin Toxicol* 1975;8:535–540.

20. Lenz K, Hruby K, Druml W, et al: 2,3-Dimercaptosuccinic acid in human poisoning. *Arch Toxicol* 1981; 47:241–243.

21. Aposhian H, Carter D, Hoover T, et al: DMSA, DMPS, and DMPA as arsenic antidotes. *Fundam Appl Toxicol* 1984;4:S58–S70.

22. Graziano J, Cuccia D, Friedheim E: The pharmacology of 2,3-dimercaptosuccinic acid and its potential use in arsenic poisoning. *J Pharmacol Exp Ther* 1978; 20:1051–1055.

ADDITIONAL SELECTED REFERENCES

Aposhian H, Hsu C, Hoover T: D,L- and *meso*-Dimercaptosuccinic acid: In vitro and in vivo studies with sodium arsenite. *Toxicol Appl Pharmacol* 1983;69:206–213.

Donofrio P, Wilbourn A, Alberg J, et al: Acute arsenic intoxication presenting as Guillain-Barré–like syndrome. *Muscle Nerve* 1987;10:114–120.

Kerr H, Saryan L: Arsenic content of homeopathic medicines. *Clin Toxicol* 1986;24:451–459.

Levin-Scherz J, Patrick J, Weber F, et al: Acute arsenic ingestion. *Ann Emerg Med* 1987;16:702–704.

part XI

ENVIRONMENTAL TOXINS

chapter **43**

Rodenticides

Poisonings with various kinds of pesticides account for about 10% of all deaths caused by solid and liquid substances—a small but significant percentage of acute human poisonings. Since the mid-1940s more than 15,000 compounds, representing more than 35,000 different formulations, have been used as pesticides. The term pesticide is a general term that classifies these substances on the basis of their actions rather than chemically; the term encompasses insecticides, rodenticides, fungicides, herbicides, and fumigants.[1] Because pesticides are manufactured for the purpose of destroying organisms that are considered undesirable for one reason or another, it is not surprising that all pesticides are capable of producing harm to humans.[2]

Most pesticides are not pure compounds but complex mixtures containing various isomers, byproducts, and reactants. Either the active pesticidal ingredient or the solvent may cause toxicity. For example, liquid pesticides are formulated in petroleum distillates, such as kerosene, which may also have serious toxic potential apart from that associated with the pesticidal solute. Aspiration of the hydrocarbon may therefore be an additional hazard of the product.

Pesticide poisonings occur most often during the spring and summer months, when pesticides are used most frequently. Individuals who handle the concentrated pesticide, such as agricultural workers, formulators, loaders, and appliers, are at greatest risk.

Many of the noninsecticide pesticides are extremely toxic and have limited usefulness because of their toxicity. The rodenticides comprise a group of pesticides that are toxic and have rather wide application but are restricted by government regulations.

A rodenticide is any commercially available product designed expressly to kill mice, rats, squirrels, gophers, and other small rodents. Rodenticides contain various toxins ranging in potency from the highly toxic phosphorus, monofluoroacetate, *p*-nitrophenolurea, strychnine, thallium, arsenic, and zinc phosphide compounds to the less toxic hydroxycoumarins and indanediones (Table 43-1). There has yet to be an effective rodenticide developed that is nontoxic to humans.

PHOSPHORUS

Actions

Elemental phosphorus occurs in three forms: red, yellow or white, and black.[3] Red and black phosphorus are nonvolatile, insoluble, and nonabsorbable and therefore nontoxic. Yellow phosphorus, however, is a toxic compound that

Table 43-1 Rodenticides

Phosphorus
Monofluoroacetate
p-Nitrophenolurea
Strychnine
Thallium
Arsenic
Zinc phosphide
Hydroxycoumarins
Indanediones

causes severe local and systemic reactions.[1] (White phosphorus, when exposed to light, turns yellow; hence the names are synonymous.[4]) Yellow phosphorus is luminescent and highly flammable and spontaneously combusts in air. It is a general protoplasmic poison, causing damage to multiple organ systems including the gastrointestinal tract and cardiovascular, hepatic, and renal systems.[4] Toxicity is increased when phosphorus is in the form of fine particles or emulsions or is dissolved in organic solvents such as alcohol, fats, and oils.[5]

At one time yellow phosphorus was used in match tips, fireworks, and unlicensed medical remedies. Numerous fatalities resulted from ingestion of these compounds.[6] Matches that can be struck on any rough surface now contain either red phosphorus or phosphorus sesquisulfide together with potassium chlorate and glue.

Because of the increasing resistance of rodents to warfarin-containing substances (see below), yellow phosphorus has come back on the market as a rodenticide paste to be spread on crackers or bread. It may be present in concentrations of up to 5% (Table 43-2).[6]

Table 43-2 Selected Phosphorus-Containing Rodenticides by Trade Name

Blue Death Rat Killer
Patterson's Zinc Phosphide Rodent Bait
Stearn's Electric Brand Paste
Common Sense Rat Preparation
J-O Electric Paste
Rat-Nip
Senco Paste

Toxicity

Dermal Absorption

Phosphorus can be absorbed by all routes, including dermally and by inhalation.[4] Skin contact produces painful second- and third-degree chemical and thermal burns. Phosphorus absorbed through the skin may produce a sudden and marked reversal of the ratio of serum calcium to phosphorus.

Gastrointestinal Absorption

Classically phosphorus poisoning is divided into three phases (Table 43-3), although this description may not apply to many patients who ingest pesticide pastes.[7] The initial symptoms may be painful second- and third-degree burns that develop a few minutes to hours after exposure. A gastroenteritis may follow, resulting from local irritation and causing nausea, vomiting, diarrhea, phosphorescent vomitus, and intense abdominal pain.[5] Often a garlic odor can be detected from the vomitus. In this phase, acute cardiovascular collapse may result from direct action of phosphorus on the myocardium.[4,7] Many patients who ingest phosphorus paste may be asymptomatic when first seen in the emergency department, with the garlic odor and mucosal burns occurring in only a small percentage of cases.[1]

The next phase is a lull or symptom-free period that may last for several weeks; during

Table 43-3 Phases of Acute Phosphorus Poisoning

Phase 1
    Painful burns
    Gastroenteritis
    Phosphorescent vomitus
    Abdominal pain
    Garlic odor of vomitus
    Cardiovascular collapse
Phase 2
    Symptom-free period
Phase 3
    Gastrointestinal intoxication
    Hepatic intoxication
    Renal failure
    CNS intoxication

this time the patient appears to recover. The final phase represents systemic intoxication from the action of the absorbed phosphorus and involves the gastrointestinal tract, liver, heart, kidneys, and CNS. Death is usually attributed to irreversible shock, hepatic or renal failure, CNS or myocardial damage, or massive hematemesis.

Treatment

There is no antidote for acute yellow phosphorus poisoning.[7] Treatment is directed toward removing the toxin as soon as possible after ingestion, preventing its absorption from the gastrointestinal tract, and providing intensive supportive care to maintain vital signs.[1] Both the patient and clinician should be protected from further contact with the phosphorus to avoid burns of the skin and eyes. Cutaneous burns should be washed with copious amounts of water. If the phosphorus was ingested, gastric lavage with large quantities of potassium permanganate (1:5000) has been recommended to oxidize the phosphorus into the relatively harmless oxide.[5] Although some investigators recommend administration of copper sulfate solution, this is contraindicated.[5] Activated charcoal can adsorb phosphorus and thus should be administered.[8]

FLUOROACETATE DERIVATIVES

Actions

Monofluoroacetate (Compound 1080, SMFA) is a white, odorless, tasteless crystalline compound that looks like flour or baking soda; it is usually mixed with a black dye. Fluoroacetamide (Compound 1081) is a related fluoroacetic derivative that has actions similar to those of fluoroacetate but a somewhat slower onset of symptoms. Both compounds are highly effective poisons for all kinds of rodents but must be used with great caution because of their toxicity to other animals and humans. Because of their extreme toxicity they are sold only to licensed pest-control operators.[9]

Fluoroacetate occurs naturally as a constituent of a South African plant and is toxic when in-gested, inhaled as dust, or absorbed through open wounds (it is not absorbed through the intact skin).[9,10] Its action is related not to its fluoride content but to the fact that it is converted to fluorocitrate in the body, which then interferes with the Krebs cycle by acting as a potent competitive inhibitor for the enzyme aconitase in the tricarboxylic acid cycle that normally converts citrate to isocitrate. The effects are especially noted in the heart and CNS.[1]

Toxicity

Toxic symptoms are delayed for 2 to 3 hours after ingestion of fluoroacetate or absorption through broken skin because of the conversion of fluoroacetate to fluorocitrate. When symptoms begin they are usually severe (Table 43-4).[1,10]

General response to poisoning includes nausea and vomiting. CNS effects are usually agitation, a depressed level of consciousness, apprehension, seizures, and coma. The cardiovascular effects may include ventricular ectopy, bigeminy, supraventricular or ventricular tachycardia and ventricular fibrillation and may lead to death.[1]

Treatment

Treatment of fluoroacetate poisoning is mainly nonspecific and supportive. Contaminated clothing should be removed and the skin

Table 43-4 Symptoms of Fluoroacetate Poisoning

General
  Nausea
  Vomiting
Central nervous system
  Agitation
  Lethargy
  Apprehension
  Seizures
  Coma
Cardiovascular
  Supraventricular tachycardia
  Ventricular ectopy
  Bigeminy
  Ventricular tachycardia
  Ventricular fibrillation

washed with soap and water. Seizures can be controlled with diazepam. There is evidence that an extrinsic supply of acetate ions, such as from glycerol monoacetate, has antidotal effects by competitively blocking the conversion of fluoroacetate to fluorocitrate in the tricarboxylic acid cycle. Although no clinical trials have confirmed the efficacy of this treatment, it is still advocated for acute ingestion. Glycerol monoacetate (0.24 g/kg), sodium acetate (0.12 g/kg), and ethyl alcohol are recommended.[1] Another dosage regimen for glycerol monoacetate is to administer 0.5 mL/kg intramuscularly every 30 minutes for several hours and then a reduced dose for at least 12 hours. Monoacetin may also be administered in the same dosage. These compounds should be administered parenterally as soon as a definite diagnosis is made. Treatment can be expected to produce local edema, sedation, and vasodilation.[1]

p-NITROPHENOLUREA

Actions

p-Nitrophenolurea, also known as Vacor®, is a toxic, single-dose, quick-kill rodenticide. Vacor® was introduced in 1975 and was initially marketed as safe for humans.[11] The manufacturer has withdrawn the product from the market[12] because it has caused a significant number of deaths since it was introduced.

p-Nitrophenolurea is chemically related to alloxan and streptozocin, both of which are potent pancreatic β-cell toxins and have been used for a number of years to induce diabetes in experimental animals and to treat islet cell carcinoma.[12] All these substances, including Vacor®, appear to act by interfering with nicotinamide metabolism in pancreatic β cells, liver cells, and brain in rodents and humans, causing acute diabetes mellitus and autonomic dysfunction.[12] Ingestion of as little as a single 30-g packet of the yellow-green powder has caused death.[13]

Toxicity

Symptoms may be delayed in onset from 4 to 48 hours, which is the time necessary for enzyme interference to occur (Table 43-5).[11] Early symptoms may include nausea and vomiting, abdominal pain, and confusion. Later, the patient may complain of or exhibit chest pain, glycosuria, hyperglycemia, ketosis, seizures, and autonomic dysfunction.[1,9]

The autonomic dysfunction may involve both sympathetic and parasympathetic nerves and may be manifested by postural hypotension (which is an early feature), hypothermia, dysphagia, dystonia, impaired pupillary responses, impotence, bowel and bladder dysfunction, and motor and sensory neuropathy (Table 43-6).[14] This neuropathy frequently develops within the first day after ingestion and produces the greatest degree of long-term disability in most patients.[9,14] The neuropathic symptoms often progress over several days, and the greatest impairment usually occurs distally. A period of hypoglycemia may develop before hyperglycemia because of a sudden release of insulin stored in damaged pancreatic tissue. Late sequelae include cardiovascular collapse, respiratory failure, coma, and death. Death has been

Table 43-5 Symptoms of p-Nitrophenolurea Poisoning

Nausea
Vomiting
Abdominal pain
Confusion
Glycosuria
Hyperglycemia or hypoglycemia
Ketosis
Seizures
Autonomic dysfunction
Diabetic ketoacidosis

Table 43-6 Autonomic Dysfunctions Associated with p-Nitrophenolurea Poisoning

Postural hypotension
Hypothermia
Dysphagia
Dystonia
Impotence
Bowel and bladder dysfunction
Motor and sensory neuropathy

due to ketoacidosis, gastrointestinal perforation, cardiac dysrhythmias, and pneumonia.[12]

Long-term sequelae in the form of glucose intolerance and neurologic dysfunction have been frequent among the survivors of acute intoxication. Some individuals have permanent insulin-dependent diabetes and long-term problems associated with autonomic dysfunction.[13]

Treatment

Attempts at inducing emesis and catharsis may be ineffective because of the ileal and esophageal hypomotility produced by *p*-nitrophenolurea poisoning.[13] These measures are still recommended, however, if the ingestion is recent enough. There are no supporting data to suggest that ion trapping and forced diuresis are of benefit, nor is there evidence that dialysis or hemoperfusion is efficacious in treating *p*-nitrophenolurea ingestion.[14] The diabetes mellitus produced by Vacor® may be difficult to manage in many cases. Regular eating may be difficult for some individuals because of gastrointestinal hypomotility and in some cases because of severe anorexia.

Specific treatment consists of administering niacinamide (nicotinamide), which interferes with the toxin's ability to reduce intracellular synthesis of nicotinamide adenine dinucleotide. When administered within a few hours of ingestion, niacinamide can prevent the development of pancreatic destruction and disturbances in autonomic function. *N*-Methylniacinamide, niacin (nicotinic acid), and L-tryptophan, which are all precursors of nicotinamide adenine dinucleotide, have no effect on preventing depression of liver nucleotide concentration or on the development of diabetes mellitus. In addition, niacin should not be substituted for nicotinamide because the vasodilatory effects of niacin may add to the problems of blood pressure control.[5,14] Niacinamide (500 mg) should be injected intravenously and followed by 100 to 200 mg intravenously every 4 hours for 2 to 3 days. If signs of toxicity develop, the frequency of injection should be increased to every 2 hours at a dosage not to exceed 3 g/day in adults or 1.5 g/day in children. Diabetic ketoacidosis should be managed with insulin.[1]

Dihydroergotamine therapy, if instituted early in the course of an intoxication, has been shown to be of benefit to some patients with severe postural hypotension.[13,15]

STRYCHNINE

Actions

Strychnine and brucine are alkaloids derived from seeds of *Strychnos nux-vomica*; neither has any demonstrated therapeutic value.[16,17] Brucine poisoning is not a major toxicological problem, although this alkaloid may act as a local anesthetic. Strychnine was at one time a notorious agent in suicidal and homicidal poisonings and was included in various over-the-counter tonics, stimulants, veterinary preparations, cathartics, and laxatives.[18] It can still be found in a number of preparations.[19] Cases of strychnine poisoning are now rare and usually limited to accidental poisoning from strychnine-containing rodenticides (Table 43-7) or from substances of abuse that are cut with this alkaloid.[1]

Strychnine is readily absorbed from the gastrointestinal tract and mucous membranes of the nose and mouth; symptoms of intoxication appear as early as 10 to 30 minutes after ingestion.[20] Poisoning secondary to insufflation of strychnine mistaken for cocaine has been reported.[16] Although strychnine acts only on the CNS, it does not preferentially bind to that

Table 43-7 Selected Strychnine-Containing Rodenticides by Trade Name

Kilmice
Gopher Death
Mologen Mouse Lure
Rat-Seed
Hot Springs Buttons
Elroy Mouse Bait
Mo-Go
Mice Doom Pellets
Mouse Seeds
Pied Piper Kwik Kill
Sanaseed
Sweeney's Poison Wheat
Gopher Go
Mouse Nots

tissue. Strychnine is largely detoxified in the liver, and only a small amount is excreted unchanged in the urine.[21]

Strychnine is the prototype of chemicals that selectively block inhibitory neurons in the CNS, resulting in hyperexcitability.[22] It competitively blocks glycine, which is an inhibitory neurotransmitter at the postsynaptic receptor sites of ventral horn motor neurons of the spinal cord (Fig. 43-1).[20,23] Neuronal systems lacking specific synaptic inhibitory fibers are not excited by strychnine; thus the cardiovascular and gastrointestinal systems are not directly affected.[17,24,25]

Toxicity

The first signs of strychnine poisoning may be myoclonus and a slight twitching of the limbs that is followed by sudden convulsions involving all muscles (Table 43-8). The initial event can also be a generalized seizure without any prodrome. These seizures may be painful because the patient may be awake and aware of the surroundings. Convulsive activity may occur spontaneously or may be excited by minor sensory

Table 43-8 Signs and Symptoms of Strychnine Poisoning

Hyperthermia
Myoclonus
Opisthotonos
Rhabdomyolysis
Risus sardonicus
Seizures
Trismus

input such as auditory or tactile stimuli.[25] The body arches backward in hyperextension (opisthotonos) with the arms and legs extended and the feet turned inward.[26] The patient may exhibit trismus and facial contortions producing a characteristic fixed grinning expression (risus sardonicus).[16] Contraction of the muscles of the diaphragm together with spasm of the thoracic and abdominal muscles may arrest respiration.[25] The convulsions may recur repeatedly; each lasts from 30 seconds to 2 minutes and is followed by a 10- to 15-minute interval, during which the sensorium may be clear.[22] The seizures may be followed by a period of depression. Patients

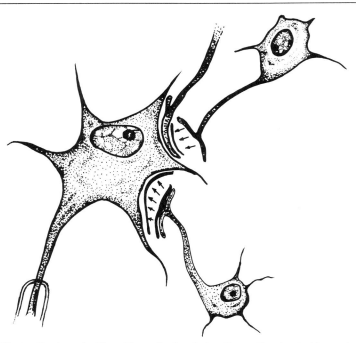

Figure 43-1 Blockade of Glycine Uptake at the Motor Neuron by Strychnine. *Source:* Reprinted with permission from *American Journal of Medicine* (1983;74:507–512), Copyright © 1983, Technical Publishing Company.

seldom survive more than five untreated seizures, although some have survived ten episodes.[19] Death may be from respiratory failure, medullary paralysis, or asphyxia during the convulsive activity. Depending on the length of the seizure, cyanosis may develop. If death does not result from seizures or associated conditions, recovery may be complete.[20,25]

Other problems associated with strychnine intoxication stem from the profound muscle spasms.[17] Lactic acidosis, hypoxia, and rhabdomyolysis may occur,[26] and whole body core temperature may be elevated. Acute renal failure may also ensue.

Laboratory Analysis

Strychnine can be detected by various laboratory methods,[17] especially colorimetry and ultraviolet spectrophotometry. The most specific method is gas chromatography with flame ionization. Serum strychnine concentrations can be measured, but they correlate poorly with symptoms.

Treatment

Treatment is directed toward establishing an airway to prevent asphyxia, controlling seizure activity to prevent trauma from involuntary movements, and decreasing any further absorption of the compound while treating the patient supportively.[1]

The preferred method of controlling strychnine-induced seizure activity is the use of intravenous diazepam with or without a short-acting barbiturate.[3,22,25] Diazepam is the drug of choice because it appears to act as a γ-aminobutyric acid agonist.[3,19,23] The barbiturates provide the same agonist activity as benzodiazepines and should have the same efficacy.[23,27] Neither the benzodiazepines nor the barbiturates antagonize the glycine receptor inhibition, and so that even in large doses these drugs may not be completely effective.[19]

If standard anticonvulsants do not control seizure activity, the patient should be pharmacologically paralyzed with pancuronium[16] to prevent the continued production of lactic acid and resultant metabolic acidosis and rhabdomyolysis, both of which are determining factors for long-term outcome.[26] Pancuronium is advocated because it is a nondepolarizing neuromuscular blocking agent.[21] Gastric lavage may then be performed and followed by administration of activated charcoal. An emetic should not be administered. Gastric emptying techniques are not advocated in the seizing patient because of the increased sensory stimulation. If respiratory depression occurs, respiration should be assisted or mechanically controlled.[26]

Because the limiting factor in strychnine excretion through the kidney is its metabolism by microsomal liver enzymes, forced diuresis is usually of no appreciable benefit in drug removal.[16,26] This is contrary to some reports that advocate diuresis for increasing excretion.[18] In addition, acidification of the urine may predispose a patient with rhabdomyolysis to acute tubular necrosis and renal failure because the excretion of myoglobin is decreased in an acid urine. In addition, peritoneal dialysis and hemodialysis appear to be of little benefit because of strychnine's rapid clearance from the blood.[19,25]

THALLIUM

Actions

Thallium is among the most lethal poisons and produces one of the highest incidences of long-term sequelae, mainly neurologic. Thallium was discovered in the mid-1800s by a scientist searching for another element, tellurium. Thallium was used until the early 1900s to treat diseases such as syphilis, ringworm, and dysentery and until the 1950s in some countries as a depilatory paste. In industry, thallium may be encountered as a byproduct of the production or use of various metals and alloys, jewelry and optical lenses,[28] thermometers, electronic equipment, and various pigments. Because of its high toxicity its use as a rodenticide is now restricted to government agencies, and it is available only by special permit.

In the United States acute thallium poisoning has most often been caused by ingestion of thallium-containing insecticides or rodenticides.

The latter are often prepared as wafers that are attractive to children as well as to rodents (Table 43-9).[29] Since the introduction of thallium sulfate (which is 60% to 80% thallium metal) as an effective odorless and tasteless rodenticide, suicidal and homicidal thallium poisonings have increased considerably.[30] Poisoning from industrial exposure is expected to increase as well because glass and pharmaceutical firms have begun using thallium in manufacturing processes.

Thallium is especially toxic in its bivalent state as sulfate, acetate, and carbonate salts. The sulfide and iodide compounds are poorly soluble and, therefore, much less toxic.[31] Thallium sulfate and other soluble salts are absorbed rapidly and completely through the intact skin and mucous membranes of the mouth and gastrointestinal tract.[29]

Mechanism of Action

The effects of thallium are thought to be due to its interference with the metabolism of compounds containing sulfhydryl groups, especially those of the mitochondrial respiratory chain. Protein synthesis (particularly incorporation of cysteine) is inhibited, which may account for the symptom of alopecia (through prevention of keratinization; see below).[29]

In addition, cell membranes cannot distinguish between potassium and thallium ions because thallium behaves much like potassium in the body. Thallous ion has an affinity for sodium-potassium adenosine triphosphatase that is 10 times greater than that of potassium. Thallium is therefore preferentially transported into cells. Because it is similar to potassium, it substitutes for potassium in many physiologic reactions and depolarizes membranes in nerve

Table 43-9 Selected Thallium-Containing Rodenticides by Trade Name

Senco Corn Mix
Martin's Rat Stop
GTA Rat Bait
Gizmo Mouse Killer
Zelio Paste

and heart, antagonizes the effect of calcium on the heart, and corrects the cardiac effects of hypokalemia.[29,30] Unlike lead and arsenic, thallium is soluble at physiological pH and therefore does not form complexes in bone.

Toxicity

Symptoms of thallium poisoning are mainly referable to the CNS and the gastrointestinal tract (Table 43-10).[29] The gastrointestinal symptoms may follow absorption of thallium by any route after a latent period of 12 to 24 hours.

Table 43-10 Signs and Symptoms of Thallium Poisoning

Gastrointestinal
  Abdominal pain
  Anorexia
  Nausea
  Diarrhea
  Gastroenteritis
  Gingival discoloration
Neurologic
  Tremor
  Paresthesia
  Bilateral polyneuropathy
  Irritability
  Delirium
  Coma
  Pseudobulbar paralysis
  Seizures
  Somnolence
  Facial palsy
Ocular
  Ptosis
  Strabismus
  Mydriasis
  Amblyopia
  Optic atrophy
Autonomic
  Fever
  Tachycardia
  Orthostatic hypotension
  Urinary retention
  Constipation
  Dysrhythmias
Miscellaneous
  Alopecia
  Interference with nail growth
  Lines in the gingiva
  Liver necrosis
  Renal tubular damage
  Psychosis

Symptoms may include abdominal pain, anorexia, nausea, diarrhea, and hemorrhagic gastroenteritis. Death may be secondary to respiratory paralysis or circulatory disturbances.[28]

General

In severe cases of thallium poisoning, delirium, seizures, coma, and death may occur but usually not earlier than 8 to 10 days after ingestion. More often the acute gastroenteritis subsides, and the patient has an asymptomatic period of 3 to 4 days.[31] This is gradually replaced by signs and symptoms referable to one or several systems. Intermittent intestinal colic, nausea and vomiting, diarrhea, stomatitis, excessive salivation, and gingival discoloration comparable to that of lead line may be noted. The gingival discoloration appears in some cases within 2 to 4 days of exposure and represents precipitated thallium in the gums at the base of the teeth.

Neurologic

Neuromuscular symptoms such as tremors, paresthesias, and frank polyneuritis has been described as bilateral painful legs, and increase gradually until the patient may be hardly able to bear weight. The paresthesias usually begin as painful symptoms suggesting involvement of the smaller peripheral nerves that conduct sensory rather than motor impulses. Motor neuropathy follows with weakness; stretch reflexes are preserved until relatively late.

Mental changes are also frequent and may include poor concentration, irritability, somnolence, and occasional frank delirium; these may ultimately progress to coma. In serious or fatal cases of thallium poisoning pseudobulbar paralysis due to peripheral neuritis of the cranial nerves is observed. In addition, paralysis of the ocular muscles, ptosis, strabismus, mydriasis, facial palsies, amblyopia, paralysis of the recurrent nerve, and optic atrophy accompanied by loss of vision have been noted.[30,31]

Alopecia

Alopecia, which is usually due to a metabolic disturbance in the hair follicle, may occur simultaneously with severe polyneuritis approximately 14 days after exposure to thallium. It usually involves the entire scalp except for a small strip in the frontal area. Axillary, pubic, and facial hair may also be spared. Typically, a black pigmentation appears in the root of the hair and extends over its entire width. This is said to be specific for thallium and may be seen with the aid of a microscope. By the third week there is usually nearly complete alopecia. If the patient recovers, normal growth usually ensues.[29]

Aldrich-Mees Lines

Growth of the nails is impaired for a certain period, resulting in the appearance in the third or fourth week of typical semilunar white lines across the nails that parallel the growth of the nail and move toward the free edge. This is similar to Aldrich-Mees lines seen in arsenic poisoning.[31]

Miscellaneous

Toxic psychosis and seizures that may proceed to status epilepticus, central necrosis of the liver, and damage to the renal tubular epithelium may also occur in thallium poisoning. Autonomic disturbances such as fever, tachycardia, labile blood pressure, orthostatic hypotension, urinary retention, constipation, xerostomia, and cardiac dysrhythmias also frequently occur.

Laboratory Analysis

Laboratory clues in diagnosis of thallium poisoning include slightly lowered serum potassium and a mild hypochloremic metabolic alkalosis due to the effects of thallium on the renal tubule.[29] Examination of hair by chemical means is not useful because, unlike other metals, thallium is not incorporated into the hair matrix. Thallium concentrations in urine can be determined, and because thallium is not a normal constituent of the body any concentration may be considered significant.

Treatment

There is no known substance that can neutralize thallium that is absorbed and fixed in the tissues, especially nervous system tissue. No treatment has been shown unequivocally to hasten excretion or to prevent death or permanent systemic damage. Thallium poisoning appears to be refractory to most antidotal agents, including chelating agents such as dimercaprol, calcium EDTA, and penicillamine. All antidotes proposed only neutralize the thallium in the intestinal tract and the percentage after reabsorption that is excreted into the colon. Both diphenylthiocarbazone (Dithizon®) and diethyldithiocarbamate (Dithiocarb®) have been suggested as antidotes because of their ability to form readily excreted complexes with thallium, but there has been only limited experience with their use in humans. Recently it has been shown that diethylthiocarbamate causes CNS toxicity by redistributing thallium to the CNS; it should therefore not be used until more information is available about its efficacy.[29]

Gastric lavage with 1% sodium iodine should be performed as soon as possible after the diagnosis is made because it may be useful in converting the soluble thallium sulfate into insoluble thallium iodide. Oral administration of prussian blue (potassium ferric ferrocyanide) takes advantage of the high concentration of thallium in gastric secretions and in bile. Prussian blue is not absorbed from the gastrointestinal tract, and at the alkaline pH in small bowel thallium is substituted for potassium in the crystal lattice of the complex and is excreted in the feces. Prussian blue should be administered as a colloidal solution at 250 mg/kg/day combined with 15% mannitol or 70% sorbitol.[28]

Prevention and correction of fluid and electrolyte disturbances are important considerations, particularly if diarrhea is severe. If tachydysrhythmias occur, use of lidocaine or propranolol may be indicated. Shock may require the parenteral administration of fluids or vasopressors.[29]

Peritoneal dialysis, hemoperfusion, and hemodialysis have so far not been shown to reduce significantly the total body load of thallium, although it is clear that hemoperfusion is more effective than dialysis in removing thallium from the blood compartment.[28,32]

ANTICOAGULANT COMPOUNDS

The first anticoagulant used as a rodenticide was bishydroxycoumarin, but warfarin (acetonylbenzylhydroxycoumarin) has been shown to be about 50 times more lethal to rodents. Warfarin is available commercially as a 0.5% powdered concentrate (Table 43-11). Common rats have appeared to show resistance to the regular warfarin rodenticides because of a reduction in the efficiency of vitamin K metabolism; this is a heritable factor.[33]

Reduction of the carbonyl group of warfarin and replacement of the terminal methyl group with various substituted phenyl groups produces compounds with increased anticoagulant activity.[34] These hydroxycoumarin derivatives are known as "superwarfarins" because of their long duration of action[35,36] and include bromadalone, brodifacoum, and difenacoum (Table 43-11).[33,37,38] All these compounds are available in supermarkets, drugstores, and hardware stores (Table 43-12).

The indanedione anticoagulants contain many compounds that also have a longer duration of action than warfarin and are also referred to as superwarfarin compounds. These, too, induce profound changes in coagulation parameters.[39] These include chlorophacinone, diphacinone, pindone, and valone (Table 43-11).[40,41]

Warfarin has caused human intoxication in connection with therapeutic overdosage, homicide attempts, suicide attempts, and accidental substitution.[1,42]

Table 43-11 Anticoagulant Compounds used in Rodenticides

Hydroxycoumarins
  Warfarin
  Coumachlor
Long-acting hydroxycoumarins ("superwarfarins")
  Warfarin-type
    Brodifacoum
    Bromadalone
    Difenacoum
  Indanedione-type
    Chlorophacinone
    Diphacinone
    Pindone
    Valone

Table 43-12 Hydroxycoumarin Rodenticides by Trade Name

Agicide rat and mouse bait
Black Flag rat and mouse killer
Black Jack mouse and rat killer
D-con
Hot Shot rat killer
Kelley's red mix
Parsons rat killer
Rat-kill
Ro-do
Speckman's Deth-rat
Vam-o
Voo-doo 42
Zord rodenticide

Mechanism of Action

All the anticoagulant rodenticides act by interfering with the synthesis of vitamin K. Vitamin K is essential for normal blood coagulation because it is a cofactor for the postribosomal synthesis of clotting factors II, VII, IX, and X[43]; suppression of the hepatic formation of prothrombin and of factors VII, IX, and X produces clotting defects. In addition, anticoagulant rodenticides cause direct capillary damage.

Warfarin and related compounds interfere with clotting factor synthesis by blocking the vitamin K–dependent γ-carboxylation of glutamic acid residues in precursors of clotting factors II, VII, IX, and X.[37] The warfarin receptor is thought to be associated with the enzyme vitamin K epoxide reductase. This enzyme is responsible for the continuous regeneration of vitamin K in the physiologically important vitamin K–epoxide cycle. During this cycle, vitamin K_1 is converted to a biologically inactive metabolite called vitamin K_1-2,3-epoxide. This epoxide is reduced back to the vitamin by a microsomal epoxide reductase. Because the coumarin anticoagulants inhibit the epoxide reductase step, they are referred to as indirect antagonists of vitamin K.[43]

Warfarin is hydroxylated to inactive compounds by the mixed-function oxidase enzymes in the hepatic microsomes. These compounds are then excreted in the urine.

The superwarfarins are 10 to 20 times more potent than warfarin because they have a greater affinity for vitamin K_1 epoxide reductase, interrupt the vitamin K_1–epoxide cycle at more than one site, and have considerably more anticoagulant ability than warfarin.[37] The result is greater prolongation of clotting and prothrombin times. For example, brodifacoum and difenacoum have the same mechanism of action as warfarin but are far more powerful anticoagulants because of this increased duration of anticoagulation effect.[38] The half-life of some of the long-acting anticoagulants may be as much as 10 times the average plasma half-life of warfarin (42 hours). In addition, they also have a larger apparent volume of distribution—approximately 6 times that of warfarin (0.17 L/kg).[44] Finally, there is a more sustained concentration of the long-acting preparations in the liver.[45]

Toxicity

Early after an overdose of a coumarin anticoagulant there are no discernible toxic signs and symptoms. Multiple doses of warfarin are usually required to cause alterations in anticoagulant activity; this does not appear to be true for the long-acting preparations. Bleeding may be the first manifestation of toxicity; if it is internal it may not be easily diagnosed. Later symptoms may consist of an upper gastrointestinal bleed, melena, epistaxis, cerebrovascular accident, easy bruising, and hematuria. Anemia, shock, and death may also occur.

The anticoagulant effect of warfarin can be expected to disappear within a few days. Some cases of long-acting anticoagulant poisoning have required 42 days of vitamin K and plasma product treatment before the coagulation tests returned to normal.[46]

Laboratory Analysis

The principal diagnostic test for warfarin intoxication is a markedly reduced prothrombin time.[47] Prolonged clotting and bleeding times may also be diagnostic indicators. With ingestion of the long-acting preparations prothrombin activity should be monitored for a much greater period of time than is normally required for warfarin poisoning.

Treatment

From a management perspective, all the anticoagulant rodenticides may be handled in the same way. Vitamin K specifically antagonizes the deficiencies associated with these anticoagulants, so that pharmacologic doses of vitamin K_1 will provide the additional substrate necessary to resume the vitamin K_1–epoxide cycle and continue the carboxylation process, thereby reversing the hypoprothrombinemia.

At present, there is no standard regimen for the administration of vitamin K_1 as an antidote to coumarin anticoagulant poisoning. In the initial phases of poisoning, phytonadione (emulsified vitamin K_1) is the preferred antidote rather than menadione or vitamin K_3.[48] This is because the liver must metabolize vitamin K_3 to vitamin K_1, and this organ may be inhibited. The dose of vitamin K_1 is 15 to 25 mg administered parenterally in an adult and 5 to 10 mg in a child. If the drug is administered intravenously, the dose should not exceed 1 mg/min. In a warfarin overdose the duration of action of vitamin K may be shorter than normal, and repeated administration may be necessary to restore clotting factor synthesis.

Because the long-acting preparations can be detected in the urine for prolonged periods of time, oral vitamin K therapy can be used and may be necessary for at least 2 to 3 weeks[37]; it may be required for as long as 1 year in some cases. Fresh frozen plasma may also be used as adjunctive treatment as necessary.[34]

Rapid administration of vitamin K_1 may be associated with side effects such as facial flushing, chest constriction, and cyanosis.

REFERENCES

1. Dipalma J: Human toxicity from rat poisons. *Am Fam Physician* 1981;24:186–189.

2. Mortensen M: Management of acute childhood poisonings caused by selected insecticides and herbicides. *Pediatr Clin North Am* 1986;33:421–445.

3. Maron B, Krupp J, Tune B: Strychnine poisoning successfully treated with diazepam. *J Pediatr* 1978; 78:697–699.

4. Simon F, Pickering L: Acute yellow phosphorus poisoning. *JAMA* 1976;235:1343–1344.

5. McCarron M, Gaddis G, Trotter A: Acute yellow phosphorus poisoning from pesticide pastes. *Clin Toxicol* 1981;18:693–711.

6. Marin G, Montoya C, Sierra J, et al: Evaluation of corticosteroid and exchange transfusion treatment of acute yellow phosphorus intoxication. *N Engl J Med* 1976; 284:125–128.

7. Talley R, Linhart J, Trevino A, et al: Acute elemental phosphorus poisoning in man: Cardiovascular toxicity. *Am Heart J* 1972;84:139–140.

8. Holt L, Holz P: The black bottle: A consideration of the role of charcoal in the treatment of poisoning in children. *J Pediatr* 1963;63:306–314.

9. Peters K, Tong T, Katz K, et al: Diabetes mellitus and orthostatic hypotension resulting from ingestion of Vacor rat poison: Endocrine and autonomic function studies. *West J Med* 1981;134:65–81.

10. Peters R, Spencer H, Bidstrup P: Subacute fluoroacetate poisoning. *J Occup Med* 1981;23:112–113.

11. Fretthold D, Sunshine F, Udinsky J, et al: Postmortem findings for a Vacor poisoning case. *Clin Toxicol* 1980;16:175–180.

12. Gallanosa A, Spyker D, Curnow R: Diabetes mellitus associated with autonomic and peripheral neuropathy after Vacor rodenticide poisoning: A review. *Clin Toxicol* 1981; 18:441–449.

13. Benowitz N, Byrd R, Schamberlan M, et al: Dihydroergotamine treatment for orthostatic hypotension from Vacor rodenticide. *Ann Intern Med* 1980;92:387–388.

14. LeWitt P: The neurotoxicity of the rat poison Vacor. *N Engl J Med* 1980;302:73–77.

15. Jennings G, Ester M, Holmes R: Treatment of orthostatic hypotension with dihydroergotamine. *Br Med J* 1979; 2:307.

16. Gordon A, Richards D: Strychnine intoxication. *JACEP* 1979;8:520–522.

17. Lambert J, Byrick R, Hammeke M: Management of acute strychnine poisoning. *Can Med Assoc J* 1981; 124:1268–1270.

18. Teitelbaum D, Ott J: Acute strychnine intoxication. *Clin Toxicol* 1979;3:267–273.

19. Blain P, Nightingale S, Stoddart J: Strychnine poisoning: Abnormal eye movements. *J Toxicol Clin Toxicol* 1982;19:215–217.

20. Edmunds M, Sheehan T, Van't Hoff W: Strychnine poisoning: Clinical and toxicological observations on a nonfatal case. *Clin Toxicol* 1986;24:245–255.

21. Sparagli G, Mannaioni P: Pharmacokinetic observations on a case of massive strychnine poisoning. *Clin Toxicol* 1973;6:533–540.

22. Herishanu Y, Landau H: Diazepam in the treatment of strychnine poisoning. *Br J Anaesth* 1972;44:747–748.

23. Baran R: Nail damage caused by weed killers and insecticides. *Arch Dermatol* 1974;110:467.

24. Sofola O, Odusote K: Sympathetic cardiovascular effects of experimental strychnine poisoning in dogs. *J Pharmacol Exp Ther* 1976;196:29–34.

25. Dittrich K, Boyer M, Wanke L: A case of fatal strychnine poisoning. *J Emerg Med* 1984;1:327–330.

26. Boyd R, Brennan P, Deng J, et al: Strychnine poisoning. *Am J Med* 1983;74:507–512.

27. Oliver J, Smith H, Watson A: Poisoning by strychnine. *Med Sci Law* 1979;19:134–137.

28. Lehmann P, Favari L: Parameters for the adsorption of thallium ions by activated charcoal and prussian blue. *Clin Toxicol* 1984;22:331–339.

29. Davis L, Standefer J, Kornfeld M, et al: Acute thallium poisoning: Toxicological and morphological studies of the nervous system. *Ann Neurol* 1980;10:38–44.

30. Moses H: Thallium poisoning. *Johns Hopkins Med J* 1978;142:27–31.

31. Moeschlin S: Thallium poisoning. *Clin Toxicol* 1980; 17:133–146.

32. Kennedy P, Cavanagh J: Spinal changes in the neuropathy of thallium poisoning. *J Neurol Sci* 1976; 29:295–301.

33. Jones E, Growe G, Naiman S: Prolonged anticoagulation in rat poisoning. *JAMA* 1984;252:3005–3007.

34. Chong L, Chau W, Ho C: A case of "superwarfarin" poisoning. *Scand J Haematol* 1986;36:314–315.

35. Breckenridge A, Cholerton S, Hart J, et al: A study of the relationship between the pharmacokinetics and the pharmacodynamics of the 4-hydroxycoumarin anticoagulants warfarin, difenacoum and brodifacoum in the rabbit. *Br J Pharmacol* 1985;84:81–91.

36. Stowe C, Metz A, Arendt C, et al: Apparent brodifacoum poisoning in a dog. *J Am Vet Med Assoc* 1983; 182:817–818.

37. Barlow A, Gay A, Park B: Difenacoum (Neosorexa) poisoning. *Br Med J* 1982;285:541.

38. Bachmann K, Sullivan T: Dispositional and pharmacodynamic characteristics of brodifacoum in warfarin-sensitive rats. *Pharmacology* 1983;27:281–288.

39. Park B, Scott A, Wilson A, et al: Plasma disposition of vitamin K_1 in relation to anticoagulant poisoning. *Br J Clin Pharmacol* 1984;18:655–662.

40. Lipton R, Klass E: Human ingestion of a "superwarfarin" rodenticide resulting in a prolonged anticoagulant effect. *JAMA* 1984;252:3004–3005.

41. Mroczek W, Martin M: Warfarin-induced necrosis of skin. *Ann Intern Med* 1975;82:381–385.

42. Fristedt B, Sterner N: Warfarin intoxication from percutaneous absorption. *Arch Environ Health* 1965;2: 205–208.

43. Bell R: Metabolism of vitamin K and prothrombin synthesis: Anticoagulants and the vitamin K–epoxide cycle. *Fed Proc* 1978;37:2599–2604.

44. Shearer M, Barkhan P: Vitamin K_1 and therapy of massive warfarin overdose. *Lancet* 1979;1:266–267.

45. Murdoch D: Prolonged anticoagulation in chlorphacinone poisoning. *Lancet* 1983;1:355–356.

46. Hadler M, Shadbolt R: Novel 4-hydroxycoumarin anticoagulants active against resistant rats. *Nature (London)* 1975;253:275–277.

47. Lacy J, Goodin R: Warfarin-induced necrosis of skin. *Ann Intern Med* 1975;82:381–382.

48. Bjornsson T, Blaschke T: Vitamin K_1 disposition and therapy of warfarin overdose. *Lancet* 1978;2:846–847.

chapter 44

Insecticides: Nicotine, Organochlorines, and Pyrethrins

Insecticides are pesticides used in the control of insects that may be either vectors of disease or destroyers of agricultural products.[1] Insecticides include nicotine, organochlorines, pyrethrins, the acetylcholinesterase inhibitors; the organophosphates, and carbamates.[2,3] This chapter is devoted to a discussion of nicotine as an insecticide and in tobacco[4]; the organochlorines, which for the most part have been banned; and the pyrethrins, which are generally considered a safe group of insecticides.[5] The acetylcholinesterase inhibitors are discussed in Chapter 45.

NICOTINE

Nicotine (methylpyridylpyrrolidine) is one of the most toxic and rapidly acting poisons. It has no therapeutic uses but was once widely employed as a horticultural insecticide in vapor or spray form. Although it occurs naturally in tobacco products, it is also available as a colorless, volatile, and strongly alkaline liquid.

Tobacco leaves contain 2% to 5% of the alkaloid *Nicotiana tabacum*.[6] The leaves are prepared as smoking and chewing tobacco and as snuff; tobacco has also been used in enemas and poultices.[7-9] The use of smokeless tobacco, which is usually applied between the cheek and gum, is becoming an increasingly widespread practice[10]; the nicotine from the tobacco is quickly absorbed through the oral mucosa into the bloodstream.[11]

Absorption

Nicotine is readily absorbed through the intact skin, respiratory tract, and mucous membranes (including the rectal mucosa). It is also incompletely absorbed through the gastrointestinal tract; absorption by this route is slow, so that metabolic activity may be able to keep pace with absorption.[9] Some cases of nicotine poisoning after dermal absorption have been due to careless handling of the compound when it was employed as an insecticide.[12] Poisonings have also occurred from tobacco enemas used in the treatment of intestinal parasitic infestation, in skin contact with tobacco infusions or poultices, and from inhalation of insect sprays.[13] A number of fatal poisonings have occurred in the last few years from "salads" prepared with wild flora that included wild tobacco.

Dosage of Nicotine in Tobacco and Nicotine Gum

One tobacco cigarette contains approximately 20 to 30 mg of nicotine,[14] although the usual dose absorbed from cigarette smoking is 1 to

2 mg. Cigars contain approximately 15 to 40 mg of nicotine. Cigarette butts contain approximately 25% of the original nicotine content. Orally ingested nicotine is less toxic than may be expected because the centrally mediated vomiting induced by the alkaloid usually causes emptying of the stomach before a fatal dose is absorbed and because there is a significant first-pass effect through the liver.[7]

Clove cigarettes contain larger amounts of nicotine, and poisonings have been reported from their use.[15]

Nicotine gum (Nicorette®), a relatively recent source of nicotine in the United States, has been used in Europe for more than 20 years.[10,16] The gum is composed of a gum base and a natural extract of the tobacco plant bound to an ion-exchange resin, which provides a controlled release.[17] One piece of gum contains 2 or 4 mg of nicotine. Because Nicorette® is in gum form, some patients may not realize that it is a medication.[9,11] Nevertheless if used inappropriately it is more dangerous than one ingested cigarette and produces blood nicotine concentrations equivalent to smoking half a cigarette per hour. In 30 minutes of chewing, 90% of the nicotine from the gum is released.[18] If the gum is accidentally swallowed the nicotine is poorly absorbed; the absorbed portion undergoes significant first-pass metabolism in the liver.[16]

Toxicity

Toxic effects from nicotine ingestion (Table 44-1) are usually rapid, and in severe cases death may occur within a few minutes; ingestion of small amounts of nicotine may lead to rapid or gradual onset of symptoms. Nicotine acts on autonomic ganglia and postsynaptic neurons by first stimulating and then depressing ganglia and nerve endings.[19] The mechanism of stimulation is a direct acetylcholine-like action on the ganglia that is followed quickly by a prolonged ganglionic blockade due to persistent depolarization.[7,10] A similar action occurs at the neuromuscular junction, causing total paralysis of skeletal muscles and subsequent respiratory failure.[14] This peripheral skeletal muscle paralysis does not affect all muscle groups simul-

Table 44-1 Features of Nicotine Poisoning

Gastrointestinal
  Emesis
  Salivation
  Diarrhea
Neurologic
  Weakness
  Headache
  Dizziness
  Hyperpyrexia
  Mydriasis
Dermal
  Pallor
  Diaphoresis
Cardiovascular
  Tachycardia
  Hypertension
  Cardiovascular collapse
Respiratory
  Respiratory failure

taneously or equally.[17] Respiratory failure from neuromuscular paralysis, which is one cause of death in nicotine overdose, usually occurs before central respiratory failure.[13] The CNS is affected initially by stimulation of the medullary centers and later by depression.[19] Nicotine also has a direct excitatory effect on smooth muscle leading to vasoconstriction and increased intestinal motility.[18]

Usually there is a spontaneous emesis as a result of stimulation of the chemoreceptor trigger zone; this may be accompanied by profuse salivation.[19] There is simultaneously a stimulation of both cholinergic and adrenergic postganglionic autonomic neurons, causing symptoms such as weakness, pallor from peripheral vasoconstriction, headache, dizziness, diaphoresis, prostration, and vomiting.[15] In addition, there may be profuse diaphoresis, abdominal pain, diarrhea, hyperpyrexia, and mydriasis. In small doses, nicotine may produce miosis.[15]

The cardiovascular responses are generally due to initial stimulation of sympathetic ganglia as a result of the release of norepinephrine. Tachycardia and hypertension may be observed. Hypotension may be followed by cardiovascular collapse and death.

Nicotine does not cause any irreversible changes, and complete recovery can be expected in the patient who has had cardiovascular and respiratory support. Some of the dose is metabolized, and the remainder is eliminated in the urine.[17]

Green tobacco sickness, an occupational illness of tobacco harvesters, is a self-limiting illness of short duration.[6,8] Although the cause is not known for certain, evidence suggests that nicotine is the most likely causative agent. Symptoms of this illness are similar to those of mild nicotine intoxication.[8,19]

Diagnosis and Laboratory Determinations

The diagnosis of nicotine poisoning is usually suggested primarily by the clinical history. Plasma nicotine concentrations are not clinically useful.[19] The ingestion of more than one cigarette, three cigarette butts, one cigar butt, or any amount of nicotine gum should be considered potentially serious.[17,20]

Treatment

Prompt treatment for acute nicotine intoxication is essential. If skin contact has occurred, the contaminated clothing should be removed and the skin thoroughly washed with soap and water. Cutaneous nicotine poisoning may be prolonged as a result of continued absorption despite skin decontamination. Physicians should anticipate this possibility and be prepared to give intensive care for at least 12 to 24 hours.

Emesis is usually a spontaneous event if a significant amount of nicotine is absorbed, so that emesis induction may not be necessary. If emesis has not occurred, the stomach should be emptied and activated charcoal and a cathartic administered. Hypotension may be treated with intravenous fluids and by placing the patient in Trendelenburg's position. If there is no response to these methods pharmacologic treatment may be necessary.[19]

Pharmacologic treatment may consist of atropine for parasympathetic excess and an α-blocking agent for increased sympathetic activity. Sympathomimetics may be required for symptomatic hypotension that cannot be corrected.

Table 44-2 Chlorinated Hydrocarbon Insecticides

Chlorinated ethane derivatives
Chlorophenothane (DDT)
Chlorinated cyclodienes
Chlordane
Dieldrin
Aldrin
Chlordecone (Kepone®)
Endrin
Isobenzan
Heptachlor
Trichlor
Isodrin
Hexachlorcyclohexanes
Lindane (Kwell®)

CHLORINATED HYDROCARBONS (ORGANOCHLORINES)

The chlorinated hydrocarbons were used extensively as insecticides from the mid-1940s until the 1960s and are now used only on a limited basis[21]; many have been banned or severely restricted. Those still available are methoxychlor, kethane, and lindane.

Organochlorine insecticides comprise chlorinated ethane derivatives, of which chlorophenothane (DDT) is the best known; chlorinated cyclodienes, including chlordane, aldrin, dieldrin, heptachlor, and endrin; and other hydrocarbons, including such hexachlorcyclohexanes as lindane, toxaphene, and mirex (Table 44-2).[21]

Actions

Organochlorines are lipid-soluble, low–molecular weight compounds with a wide range of toxicities. Their principal action is generalized stimulation of the CNS by altering the transport of sodium and potassium ions across axonal membranes. Slowing of the repolarization of nerve cell membranes then results in the propagation of multiple action potentials for each stimulus.[22]

All the chlorinated hydrocarbons have low water solubility, and because they are lipophilic they generally distribute in parallel with the tissue concentration of total lipid. They are not well absorbed through the skin. They are degraded slowly in the environment and have been shown to accumulate in fish and animals, making them an environmental hazard.[23] The widespread use of the organochlorine pesticides and other polyhalogenated hydrocarbons during the last 25 years has led to their ubiquitous presence in the environment.

Types of Organochlorine Insecticides

Chlorinated Ethane Derivatives (DDT)

DDT (trichloro-bis-*p*-chlorophenylethane), the prototype of the chlorinated hydrocarbons and of the chlorinated ethanes, was discovered during World War II and used with great success for controlling insect vectors of diseases such as typhus, malaria, and bubonic plague.[24] The compound is credited with making as important a contribution to human health as antibiotics.[25] Extensive agricultural use of DDT did not begin until the late 1940s, when the compound became available for civilian use and was found to be effective for the control of a wide range of insects of agricultural importance. DDT has a wide margin of safety when used properly, and despite its previous widespread use there is no documented, unequivocal report of a fatal human poisoning.[25] Nevertheless, because of the accumulation of DDT in the animal kingdom and the environment, in 1972 DDT was banned in the United States for all but essential public health use and for a few minor uses in protecting crops for which there are no effective alternatives. DDE (bis-*p*-chlorophenyldichloroethylene) is the principal metabolite stored in fat. Since 1951 there has been no progressive increase in human fat concentrations of DDT or DDE.[24]

DDT acts primarily on the CNS, cerebellum, and higher motor cortex. DDT does not penetrate the skin well, and the dry powders and aqueous solutions are also poorly absorbed from the gastrointestinal and respiratory tracts.

Chlorinated Cyclodienes

Most of the chlorinated cyclodiene insecticides have been banned in the United States except for a few restricted and specialized uses. They are still used in some countries, however,

and products containing them may still be found in American homes.

Seizures induced by the cyclodiene insecticides may be preceded by subjective complaints, but frequently they occur with no prodromal signs and symptoms. Prodromal signs that have been reported include headache, visual disturbances, dizziness, diaphoresis, insomnia, nausea, vomiting, and malaise.[23] An important difference between DDT and the chlorinated cyclodienes is that the latter are readily absorbed by intact skin.[26]

Chlordane. Commercial chlordane contains chlordane, heptachlor, and trichlor.[27,28] The results of studies involving humans indicate that chlordane is even more dangerous than DDT.[27] Chlordane was once widely used as an insecticide, but currently it is limited to professional underground application for termite control.[29] Chlordane and heptachlor were banned from public use in 1976.[30] Human chlordane poisonings were never common, but even though the agent is no longer available to amateur gardeners accidental poisoning still occurs.[26]

Like most halogenated hydrocarbon insecticides, chlordane is slowly metabolized and is excreted primarily in the feces.[31,32] Because of its storage in body fat, chlordane has a high degree of persistence and also a high potential for cumulative neurotoxicity. Chlordane is absorbed dermally and by inhalation and is less toxic than heptachlor, to which it is chemically closely related.[29]

Dieldrin, Endrin, and Isodrin. Dieldrin is the epoxide of aldrin, which is also used as an insecticide. The corresponding stereoisomers are endrin and isodrin. Endrin and isodrin are 2 to 3 times more poisonous than dieldrin and aldrin. Aldrin and dieldrin were banned in the United States as agricultural insecticides in 1974.[31] Especially when dissolved in oil, dieldrin is readily absorbed through the skin, respiratory mucosa, and the gastrointestinal tract. Dermal exposure results in systemic poisoning without skin irritation or local sensitization except secondary to the solvent or vehicle.[31]

Hexachlorcyclohexanes

Although there are four common isomers of benzene hexachloride, the one most often used as an insecticide is γ-benzene hexachloride (lindane), which is commercially available as Kwell®. γ-Benzene hexachloride is more properly called hexachlorocyclohexane because all the carbon double bonds in the benzene ring are saturated; benzene hexachloride is still used as a generic name for this compound, however. Lindane was formerly widely used as a crop insecticide, in home and garden sprays, and in products to control ectoparasites on livestock and pets. Although few human fatalities have occurred, many nonfatal poisonings have been reported.[32]

Lindane is absorbed by all routes including the intact skin. It is more acutely toxic than DDT, although symptoms of poisoning are similar for both compounds. Some individuals appear to be more susceptible to poisoning by lindane than by DDT, and violent tonic-clonic seizures have occurred in severe cases of acute poisoning. In addition, seizures and coma have been reported in children after prolonged topical use of lindane.[26]

Kwell® contains 1% lindane in a cream or lotion, which is intended principally for the treatment of scabies, and in a shampoo, which is intended for human and animal use in the treatment of head and pubic lice. When the toxicity of lindane is considered in the emergency department, it is important to distinguish between the topical form and the commercial-grade insecticide.[32]

Toxicity

The toxicity of the chlorinated hydrocarbons as a group varies widely. When absorbed systemically in significant quantities, any member of this group can produce paresthesias of the tongue, lips, and face; general malaise; headache; loss of appetite; nausea; vomiting; and abdominal pain (Table 44-3).[28] Neurologic manifestations include hyperexcitability, muscle fasciculations, and gross tremor, which may follow in rapid succession if the dose is sufficiently large. Seizures occur only with severe intoxication.[26] The chlorinated cyclodienes stimulate the CNS to a greater extent than DDT and tend to produce seizures before other, less serious signs of illness appear.[29] In addition, the

Table 44-3 Features of Poisoning with Chlorinated Hydrocarbon Insecticides

Paresthesia
Malaise
Headache
Nausea
Abdominal pain
Hyperexcitability
Muscle fasciculations
Seizures

chlorinated hydrocarbons sensitize the myocardium to epinephrine and may produce refractory ventricular dysrhythmias.

Treatment

Treatment for organochlorine poisoning consists of supportive therapy and decontamination. Therapy is directed toward efforts to remove the poison and to control the CNS effects, including tremors and convulsions. Sympathomimetics such as epinephrine should be avoided because they may sensitize the myocardium and cause resultant refractory dysrhythmias. Diazepam or phenobarbital may be used to control seizures.[32]

PYRETHRINS

Pyrethrum has been known and used as an insecticide for many years. Pyrethrins is a collective term that indicates naturally occurring insecticidal agents obtained from the flowers of the chrysanthemum plant [*Chrysanthemum (Pyrethrum) cinerariaefolium*] (Table 44-4). They can be prepared by drying and grinding the flowers to a powder. The powder may contain 1% to 3% of the active material. The pyrethrins are contained in most household insecticide sprays and powders.[33,34]

Pyrethrum comprises six active pyrethrins; of these, pyrethrin I is the most active for killing insects and pyrethrin II for rapid "knock-down."[33] These agents are toxic to houseflies, fleas, chiggers, mosquitoes, and the various body lice.[35] The pyrethrins are not miticidal and are therefore not effective for the treatment of scabies. Pyrethrins have low toxicity to humans.

They are rapidly metabolized and leave virtually no residuum in the atmosphere.[34] The pyrethrins are less toxic to mammals than all the other major classes of insecticide.[33,36]

Synthetic pyrethrins, called pyrethroids, are generally more effective at killing insects than the pyrethrins (Table 44-4). There are two classes of pyrethroids based on the chemical composition and clinical signs produced in poisoned animals.[37] Type I pyrethroids (permethrin and resmethrin) lack an α-cyano group; poisoning by these compounds is characterized by ataxia, hyperexcitability, seizures, and tremors. Type II pyrethroids contain the α-cyano group (fenvalerate, dellamethrin, and cypermethrin). Poisoning by these compounds may involve inhibition of γ-aminobutyric acid activity resulting in incoordination, seizures, excessive salivation, and coarse whole-body tremors.

Table 44-4 Pyrethrins and Pyrethroids

Allethrin
Barthrin
Bioallethrin
Bioresmethrin
Cyclethrin
Cypermethrin
Decamethrin
Dellamethrin
Dimethrin
Fenopropathrin
Fenvalerate
Flucythrinate
Fluvalinate
Jasmolin
Permethrin
Phenolthrin
Resmethrin
Tetramethrin
Transallethrin

Many times the pyrethrins have a synergist such as piperonylbutoxide added to the compound. Piperonylbutoxide is a synthetic piperic acid derivative that has little or no insecticidal activity[36] but that potentiates the pyrethrins by inhibiting the hydrolytic enzymes responsible for their metabolism. Piperonylbutoxide increases insecticidal activity by 2 to 10 times.

Toxicity

The belief that pyrethrins are nontoxic to humans appears to be well founded. Workers have handled the pure pyrethrins, and doses have been taken orally without ill effect.[33] Neither the natural nor the synthetic pyrethrins is significantly absorbed through intact skin. The main effect in sensitive individuals is an allergic reaction sometimes consisting of bronchoconstriction.[38] Dermatitis secondary to the pyrethrins usually occurring after chronic exposure has also been noted.[37] Paresthesias have been reported with the chronic use of one of the pyrethrins.[34] More severe systemic reactions have not been reported.[34,38] Asthma, vasomotor rhinitis, and anaphylaxis have also been reported.

Treatment

Treatment of pyrethrin exposure is usually not necessary unless it is directed toward the allergic response. Decontamination is usually all that is necessary. Antihistamines may relieve allergic signs and symptoms. If the patient is manifesting bronchoconstriction, a bronchodilator should be administered. Kerosene and naphtha, which are common solvents in pyrethrin sprays, are generally more hazardous than the pyrethrins, and treatment may have to be directed toward effects of exposure to these compounds.[38]

REFERENCES

1. Byard J: Mechanisms of acute human poisoning by pesticides. *Clin Toxicol* 1979;14:187–193.

2. De Palma A, Kwalick D, Zukerberg N: Pesticide poisoning in children. *JAMA* 1970;211:1979–1981.

3. Kline S, Bayer M: Insecticide poisoning. *Top Emerg Med* 1979;1:73–83.

4. Zavon M: Poisoning from pesticides: Diagnosis and treatment. *Pediatrics* 1974;54:332–336.

5. Hayes W: Epidemiology and general management of poisoning by pesticides. *Pediatr Clin North Am* 1970; 17:629–644.

6. Gehlbach S, Williams W, Perry L, et al: Nicotine absorption by workers harvesting green tobacco. *Lancet* 1975;1:478–480.

7. Manoguerra A, Freeman D: Acute poisoning from the ingestion of *Nicotiana glauca. J Toxicol Clin Toxicol* 1983; 19:861–864.

8. Gehlbach S, Williams W, Perry L, et al: Green tobacco sickness. *JAMA* 1974;229:1880–1883.

9. Mensch A: Nicotine overdose after a single piece of nicotine gum. *Chest* 1984;86:801–802.

10. Connolly G, Winn D, Hecht S, et al: The reemergence of smokeless tobacco. *N Engl J Med* 1986;314: 1020–1027.

11. Belanger G, Poulson T: Smokeless tobacco: A potential health hazard for children. *Pediatr Dent* 1983;5: 266–269.

12. Horan J, Linberg S, Hackett G: Nicotine poisoning and rapid smoking. *J Consult Clin Psychol* 1977;45: 344–347.

13. Battersby E, Cable J: Nicotine poisoning. *N Z Med J* 1964;63:367–368.

14. Garcia-Estrada H, Fischman C: An unusual case of nicotine poisoning. *Clin Toxicol* 1977;10:391–393.

15. Rosenberg J, Benowitz N, Jacob P, et al: Disposition kinetics and effects of intravenous nicotine. *Clin Pharmacol Ther* 1980;28:517–522.

16. Kozlowski L, Appel C, Frecker R, et al: Nicotine, a prescribable drug available without a prescription. *Lancet* 1982;1:334.

17. McNabb M, Ebert R, McCusker K: Plasma nicotine levels produced by chewing nicotine gum. *JAMA* 1982; 248:865–868.

18. Malizia G, Andreucci G, Alfani F, et al: Acute intoxication with nicotine alkaloids and cannabinoids in children from ingestion of cigarettes. *Hum Toxicol* 1983;2:315–316.

19. Saxena K, Scheman A: Suicide plan by nicotine poisoning: A review of nicotine toxicity. *Vet Hum Toxicol* 1985; 27:495–497.

20. Atland P, Rattner B: Effects of nicotine and carbon monoxide on tissue and systemic changes in rats. *Environ Res* 1979;19:202–212.

21. Sato A, Nakajima T: A structure-activity relationship of some chlorinated hydrocarbons. *Arch Environ Health* 1979;34:69–75.

22. Sanborn G, Selhorst J, Calabrese V, et al: Pseudotumor cerebri and insecticide intoxication. *Neurology* 1979;29:1222–1227.

23. Guzelian P, Vranian G, Boylan J, et al: Liver structure and function in patients poisoned with chlordecone. *Gastroenterology* 1980;78:206–213.

24. Kreiss K, Zack M, Kimbrough R, et al: Cross-sectional study of a community with exceptional exposure to DDT. *JAMA* 1981;245:1926–1930.

25. Wilson D, Locker D, Ritzen C, et al: DDT concentrations in human milk. *Am J Dis Child* 1973;125:814–817.

26. Rasmussen J: The problem of lindane. *J Am Acad Dermatol* 1981;5:507–516.

27. Kutz F, Strassman S, Sperling J, et al: A fatal chlordane poisoning. *J Toxicol Clin Toxicol* 1983;20:167–174.

28. Olanoff L, Bristow W, Colcolough J, et al: Acute chlordane intoxication. *J Toxicol Clin Toxicol* 1983; 20:291–306.

29. Aldrich F, Holmes J: Acute chlordane intoxication in a child: Case report with toxicological data. *Arch Environ Health* 1969;19:129–132.

30. Wang H, MacMahon B: Mortality of workers employed in the manufacture of chlordane and heptachlor. *J Occup Med* 1979;21:745–748.

31. Curley A, Garrettson L: Acute chlordane poisoning: Clinical and chemical studies. *Arch Environ Health* 1969; 18:211–215.

32. Morgan S, Stockdale E, Roberts R, et al: Anemia associated with exposure to lindane. *Arch Environ Health* 1980;35:307–310.

33. Casida J, Gammon D, Glickman A, et al: Mechanism of selective action of pyrethroid insecticides. *Annu Rev Pharmacol Toxicol* 1983;23:413–438.

34. Knox J, Tucker S, Flannigan S: Paresthesia from cutaneous exposure to a synthetic pyrethroid insecticide. *Arch Dermatol* 1984;120:744–746.

35. Smith D, Walsh J: Treatment of pubic lice infestation: A comparison of two agents. *Cutis* 1980;26:618–619.

36. Elliott M, Farnham A, Janes N, et al: Potent pyrethroid insecticides from modified cyclopropane acids. *Nature (London)* 1973;244:456–457.

37. Martin J, Hester K: Dermatitis caused by insecticidal pyrethrum flowers. *Br J Dermatol Syph* 1941;53:127–142.

38. Carlson J, Villaveces J: Hypersensitivity pneumonitis due to pyrethrum. *JAMA* 1977;237:1718–1719.

ADDITIONAL SELECTED REFERENCES

Arterberry J, Bonifaci R, Nash E, et al: Potentiation of phosphorus insecticides by phenothiazine derivatives: Possible hazard, with report of a fatal case. *JAMA* 1962; 182:110–112.

Benowitz N, Lake T, Keller K, et al: Prolonged absorption with development of tolerance to toxic effects after cutaneous exposure to nicotine. *Clin Pharmacol Ther* 1987; 42:119–120.

Curley A, Kimbrough R: Chlorinated hydrocarbon insecticides in plasma and milk of pregnant and lactating women. *Arch Environ Health* 1969;18:156–164.

Hayes W, Curley A: Storage and excretion of dieldrin and related compounds: Effect of occupational exposure. *Arch Environ Health* 1968;16:155–162.

Hruban Z, Schulman S, Warner N, et al: Hypoglycemia resulting from insecticide poisoning: Report of a case. *JAMA* 1963;184:590–594.

Maibach H, Feldmann R, Milby T, et al: Regional variation in percutaneous penetration in man. *Arch Environ Health* 1971;23:208–211.

Thomas C, Aust S: Free radicals and environmental toxins. *Ann Emerg Med* 1986;15:1075–1083.

Warren M, Conrad J, Bocian J, et al: Clothing-borne epidemic. *JAMA* 1963;184:94–96.

Wolfe H, Durham W, Walker K, et al: Health hazards of discarded pesticide containers. *Arch Environ Health* 1961; 3:531–537.

Young R, Jung F, Ayer H: Phorate intoxication at an insecticide-formulating plant. *An Ind Hyg Assoc J* 1979; 40:1013–1016.

chapter 45

Insecticides: Acetylcholinesterase Inhibitors

The acetylcholinesterase inhibitor insecticides comprise two distinctly different chemical groups that have the same basic mechanism of action but different toxicities. These two groups are the organophosphates and the carbamates.[1] The organophosphate insecticides are most often involved in serious human poisoning.[2-4] Formulations range from less than 1% to more than 95% of pure material. To date several thousand organophosphate compounds have been synthesized, and more than 100 different products are currently marketed.[5] Usually, organophosphates sold for household use are more dilute formulations (about 1% to 2%) compared to those sold for agricultural use (40% to 50%).[6]

Access to these types of insecticides is difficult to control because of their overwhelming availability. They are found in flea collars, ant traps, fly paper, and various sprays for domestic and garden use, and they are used commercially to a great extent.[7,8]

HISTORY

The organophosphates were produced during World War II when the Germans were unable to use nicotine as a pesticide and sought new compounds that could act as both insecticides and lethal gases.[1] Scientists developed refinements of the alkyl esters of phosphoric acid, which were the prototypical organic phosphates that proved to be more effective as insecticides than nicotine and also very effective nerve gas. The most toxic of the organophosphates have been stockpiled as nerve gas for possible use in chemical warfare.[9] Sarin and soman are two examples of these gases.[10,11]

CLINICAL USES OF ACETYLCHOLINESTERASE INHIBITORS

The carbamates have been used in the treatment of myasthenia gravis and glaucoma (Table 45-1).[7] Carbamate use has decreased for these conditions because of the narrow margin of safety between therapeutic and toxic doses.[5] The carbamates have also been used in the treatment of tachydysrhythmias and anticholinergic overdose.

Table 45-1 Clinical Uses of Acetylcholinesterase Inhibitors

Myasthenia gravis
Glaucoma
Supraventricular tachydysrhythmias
Treatment of anticholinergic poisoning

ACETYLCHOLINESTERASE INHIBITORS AS INSECTICIDES

Like the chlorinated hydrocarbons, the acetylcholinesterase inhibitors have increased the yield of agricultural produce and have helped control insect vectors of malaria and other diseases.[12] But unlike the chlorinated hydrocarbons, the acetylcholinesterase inhibitors are relatively rapidly hydrolyzed, and thus residues of these materials on food have not been a problem.[2] In addition, they do not accumulate in the environment or in the animal body. Because of these important properties, they have replaced DDT and other chlorinated hydrocarbons. They do, however, have acute toxic effects and have caused numerous fatalities in humans and animals.[13,14]

ABSORPTION

The organophosphate insecticides are absorbed by all routes, including the skin, gastrointestinal tract, conjunctiva, and respiratory tract. Clothing-borne epidemics have also been reported.[15] Absorption in most instances of occupational poisoning has been through the skin and respiratory tract. The oral route is seen in those individuals who purposefully ingest the compound.[16,17]

The carbamates are not appreciably absorbed through the intact skin and typically do not cause toxicity by this route.[18,19]

TYPES OF CHOLINESTERASE

There are two general types of cholinesterase in the human.[2] Most cholinesterase in the nervous tissue and erythrocytes is acetylcholinesterase, which is the "true" enzyme that has an almost specific affinity for the naturally occurring substrate acetylcholine. The nonspecific enzyme pseudocholinesterase is made in the liver and found in serum and has the ability to hydrolyze a wide range of naturally occurring and synthetic esters in addition to acetylcholine.[12,20] Although both may be affected by the acetylcholinesterase inhibitors and both can be measured by laboratory methods, only acetylcholinesterase is specific for organophosphate poisoning.[1]

MECHANISM OF NEUROTRANSMISSION

The acetylcholinesterase inhibitors are powerful inhibitors of carboxylic esterase enzymes, including acetylcholinesterase and pseudocholinesterase.[21,22] Acetylcholine is the neurotransmitter at the postganglionic parasympathetic nerve endings, preganglionic nerves to parasympathetic and sympathetic ganglia, somatic motor nerve endings to striated muscle, and certain synapses in the CNS (Fig. 45-1).[14,23] Normally, acetylcholine is released at the nerve ending, crosses to the neuroreceptor site, and effects an action potential.[19]

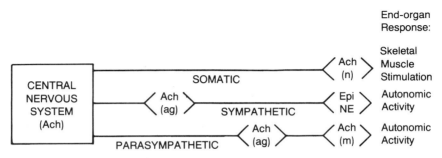

Figure 45-1 Mechanism of neurotransmission. Acetylcholine (Ach) in the central and peripheral nervous systems. Ach is the neurotransmitter at three peripheral sites: neuromuscular junction (n) and autonomic ganglia (ag) where nicotinic activity predominates; postganglionic parasympathetic receptors (m) where muscarinic activity predominates. In the CNS, nicotinic and muscarinic receptors are present. Norepinephrine (NE) acts at postganglionic sympathetic receptors, and epinephrine (Epi) is released from the adrenal medulla. *Source:* Adapted from *Principles of Clinical Toxicology* (pp 129–152) by TA Gossel and JD Bricker with permission of Raven Press, © 1984.

It is then released from the site and is hydrolyzed by the enzyme acetylcholinesterase. The breakdown of acetylcholine occurs by its binding to an anionic site on acetylcholinesterase.[4] The acetyl moiety next combines with an ester site on the enzyme and remains as the rest of acetylcholine cleaves off to form choline. Finally, the acetyl portion is rapidly hydrolyzed from the enzyme to form acetic acid and reactivated enzyme.[10,24]

Effect of Organophosphates on Neurotransmission

The organophosphates are similar in chemical structure to the cholinesterase molecule. These compounds interfere with the normal process of neurotransmission by inhibiting acetylcholinesterase as a result of firm binding of phosphate radicals from the organophosphate to the active (anionic) site of the enzyme.[22] A phosphorylated enzyme complex is then formed that has a much greater affinity for the enzyme than acetylcholine and results in an overabundance of acetylcholine at the neuroreceptor.[16,25] The overabundance initially stimulates and then paralyzes transmission in cholinergic synapses and nerve endings, sparing adrenergic synapses, and results in profound sustained stimulation of the autonomic nervous system, skeletal muscle, and CNS.[14,26] Without pharmacological intervention, the covalent binding of the phosphate radical to the active site of the cholinesterase transforms it to an inactive protein.[22]

Effect of Carbamates on Neurotransmission

The carbamates are also cholinesterase inhibitors similar in usage to the organophosphates; however, they do not contain a phosphate group and therefore have more reversible binding because the carbamate group can be cleaved off, although usually more slowly than the acetyl group of acetylcholine.[19] Carbamates cause carbamolation of the ester site of the enzyme and thus prevent the enzyme acetylcholinesterase from de-esterifying acetylcholine. This complex is unstable, and spontaneous reactivation of cho-

linesterase occurs fairly rapidly. These compounds generally have a shorter duration of action and lower toxicity than the organophosphates. In addition, they do not cross the blood-brain barrier well, so that central cholinergic effects are absent or minimal. For most carbamates, a wider range exists between toxic and lethal doses than for the organophosphates.[22]

Carbamates are often referred to as reversible cholinesterase inhibitors. This designation is not strictly correct because it implies that the carbamate is dissociated from the enzyme intact when in fact these compounds are covalently bound to the active site of the enzyme and are hydrolyzed in the same manner as acetylcholine.[1]

CHARACTERISTICS OF ACETYLCHOLINESTERASE INHIBITORS

Organophosphates

The organophosphates that are of greatest toxicity are primarily used as agricultural insecticides to increase crop yield and decrease vectors of disease (Table 45-2). They include tetraethylpyrophosphate (TEPP), which is a direct-acting, water-soluble insecticide. TEPP was the first organophosphate insecticide; it was developed in the early 1800s but was considered too toxic for use.

Parathion, a chemical ester of thiophosphoric acid, is commercially available as a 25% emulsion or water-wettable powder or dust and is another very toxic agricultural insecticide.[27–29] It is a yellow to dark-brown liquid of low vapor pressure that, because of its high toxicity, is not used in the home. It is one of the most commonly used agents in the United States and is responsible for a significant proportion of insecticide-related deaths. As little as one drop of concentrated material can be extremely dangerous.[27] Most occupational accidents involving parathion are ascribed to dermal exposure.[10] Although parathion is toxic, it is an indirect-acting compound that is converted by the liver to a more physiologically active and toxic form, paraoxon.[5]

Phorate, mevinphos, demeton, disulfoton, and guthion are other very toxic agricultural

Table 45-2 Organophosphate Pesticides in Decreasing Order of Toxicity

Highly toxic
 Tetraethylpyrophosphate (TEPP, Bladan®, Kilmite 40®, Tetron®, Kilmite®, Vapatone®)
 Phorate (Thimet®)
 Disulfoton (Di-Syston®)
 Paraoxon (Mintacol®)
 Parathion (Thiophos®, Etiolon®, Alleron®, Niagara Phoskil Dust®)
 Methylparathion (Dalf®, Penncap-M®)
 Demeton (Systox®)
 Mevinphos (Phosdrin®)
 Sulfotepp (Bladafum®, Dithione®)
 Methamidophos (Monitor®)
 Bomyl (Swat®)
 Guthion (Guthion®)
Moderately toxic
 Leptophos (Phosvel®, Abar®)
 Diazinon (Diazide®, Gardentox®, Spectracide®)
 Ethion (Nialate®)
 Fenthion (Baytex®, Entex®, Spotton®, Lysoff®)
 Coumaphos
 Acephate (Orthene®)
 Chlorpyrofos (Lorsban®, Dursban®)
 Dimethoate (Cygon®, Daphene®, Defend®)
 Phostex
 Crufomate
 Merphos (Folex®)
 Trichlorfon (Dipterex®, Dylox®, Neguvon®, Tugon®)
 Dichlorfenthion (Mobilawnr®, Bromexr®, Nemacider®)
 Fonofos (Dyfonate®)
 Dicrotophos (Bidrin®)
 Nalad (Dibrom®)
 Monocrotophos (Azodrin®)
 Phosphamidon (Dimercron®)
 Methidaton (Supacide®)
Mildly toxic
 Dichlorvos (DDVP, Vapona®, No-Pest Strip®)
 Temephos (Abate®, Abathion®)
 Chlorthion
 Malathion (Cythion®, Karbofos®, Malamar®)
 Ronnel (Korlan®, Trolene®, Viozene®)

Sources: Journal of the American Medical Association (1971;216:2131), Copyright © 1971, American Medical Association; *Recognition and Management of Pesticide Poisonings*, ed 3, by DP Morgan, US Environmental Protection Agency, 1982.

insecticides. Generally stored as powders or emulsions, they are diluted by the user as needed.

Organophosphates of intermediate toxicity include coumaphos, crufomate, and trichlorfon.

They are considered safe for use on domestic animals.[7]

Organophosphates of low toxicity are available for use in the home and garden and include malathion, which is one of the most widely used organophosphates. Malathion is also one of the least toxic organophosphate insecticides, being 100 to 1000 times less toxic than parathion.[28,29] Like parathion, malathion is oxidized by the liver to malaoxon, which has stronger cholinesterase-inhibiting activity. Another less toxic organophosphate is dichlorvos, which is marketed as Vapona® or DDVP and is incorporated into a plastic strip that slowly releases the vapor. DDVP is one of the few insecticides that have been tested directly on humans; it can be placed in the home and appears to be harmless when used as instructed.

Metabolism of Organophosphates

The metabolism of parathion is typical of the organophosphates. There are two major routes of parathion metabolism: (1) hydrolysis to diethylphosphorothioate and paranitrol, and (2) oxidation of the sulfur moiety to give paraoxon. Paraoxon is then hydrolized to diethylphosphate and paranitrophenol.[28]

Direct and Indirect Inhibitors

Some organophosphates are direct inhibitors of acetylcholinesterase, so that it is possible for them to produce local symptoms when absorbed from the eye, skin, or respiratory tract. Other compounds have only an extremely weak anticholinesterase action until they are transformed by the hepatic microsomal enzyme system to more toxic compounds.[15] Serious illness caused by skin exposure to indirect inhibitors is therefore frequently delayed for several hours until the drug is metabolized.[30] In massive poisoning, however, this lag may be absent.

Examples of direct inhibitors are TEPP and mevinphos, whereas parathion and malathion are examples of indirect-acting compounds.[31] In addition, parathion and other compounds can be photo-oxidized outside the body to the more toxic metabolite, which then may enter the body and cause immediate symptoms.

Carbamates

Carbamate insecticides range from the highly toxic aldecarb, carbofuran, and tirpate, to the intermediately toxic aminocarb, bendiocarb, Bux®, mimetan, and methomyl, to the minimally toxic fenethcarb, and carbaryl (Table 45-3).[18] The carbamates are characterized by both a brevity of action and a wide separation between the dose causing visible symptoms and the dose causing death.

Carbamates without insecticide activity have been used in medicine for many years (Table 45-4).[32] These include physostigmine for anticholinergic poisoning; pyridostigmine for myasthenia gravis; and neostigmine and edrophonium for paraoxysmal atrial tachycardia.[1,33] These agents have been replaced by other, more effective drugs.[19]

TOXICITY

Clinical Features

Most organophosphate insecticides have a characteristic garlic odor, and patients who have ingested or absorbed these compounds usually retain such an odor on the breath, vomitus, or feces for several days.[12] Organophosphates may be placed in another vehicle such as a hydrocarbon, in which case the hydrocarbon odor may be the primary odor.[34]

Clinical manifestations of intoxication with the acetylcholinesterase inhibitors may be grouped according to whether the effects are muscarinic (from an overstimulation of the parasympathetic nervous system), nicotinic (from ganglionic and myoneural junction stimulation), or due to the action on the CNS.[14] At low doses of organophosphates, muscarinic symptoms may predominate. In more severe intoxication, nicotinic and CNS symptoms may predominate. Acronyms have been devised for some of the signs and symptoms secondary to anticholinesterase inhibitor poisoning (Tables 45-5 and 45-6).

Gastrointestinal effects are usually the first symptoms to appear after ingestion of these agents (Table 45-7). Sweating and muscle fas-

Table 45-3 Carbamate Insecticides

Highly toxic
 Aldecarb (Temik®)
 Carbofuran (Furadan®)
 Tirpate
 Dimetilan (Snip Fly Bands®)
Moderately toxic
 Aminocarb (Matacil®)
 Bendiocarb (Ficam®)
 Befencarb (Bux®)
 Mimetan
 Methomyl (Lannate®, Nudrin®)
 Promecarb (Carbamult®)
 Methiocarb (Mesurol®, Draza®)
 Propoxur (Unden®)
 Primicarb (Aphox®, Rapid®)
Minimally toxic
 Fenethcarb
 Ambenonium
 Benzpyrinium
 Carbaryl (Sevin®)
 Demecarium

Table 45-4 Noninsecticide Carbamates

Edrophonium (Tensilon®)
Neostigmine (Prostigmin®)
Physostigmine (Antilirium®)
Pyridostigmine (Mestinon®)

Table 45-5 Muscarinic Effects of Organophosphate and Carbamate Insecticide Poisoning (Acronym: SLUG BAM)

S	Salivation, secretions, sweating
L	Lacrimation
U	Urination
G	Gastrointestinal upset
B	Bradycardia, bronchoconstriction, bowel movement
A	Abdominal cramps, anorexia
M	Miosis

Table 45-6 Nicotinic Effects of Organophosphate Insecticide Poisoning (Acronym: MTWtHF [days of the week])

M	Mydriasis, muscle twitching, muscle cramps
T	Tachycardia
W	Weakness
tH	Hypertension, hyperglycemia
F	Fasciculations

Table 45-7 Clinical Features of Organophosphate Intoxication

Muscarinic		Nicotinic	Central Nervous System
Mild	Moderate to Severe		
Anorexia	Abdominal cramps	Muscle twitching	Apprehension
Nausea	Diarrhea	Fasciculations	Restlessness
Chest tightness	Salivation	Cramps	Giddiness
Diaphoresis	Lacrimation	Weakness	Headache
	Urination	Mydriasis	Tremors
	Defecation	Tachycardia	Ataxia
	Wheezing	Hypertension	Seizures
	Miosis		Coma
	Increased secretions		
	Diaphoresis		

ciculations may be noted early after dermal exposure, and respiratory effects are first noted after inhalation.[2] Clinical evidence of intoxication generally becomes apparent within a matter of minutes to an hour after the exposure, with the exact time depending on the severity and route of exposure.[19] In mild intoxication, early complaints may be fatigue, headache, mild vertigo, weakness, loss of concentration, and blurred vision. Severe intoxication may result in muscular paralysis leading to sudden respiratory arrest[35]; symptoms leading to death may occur within 5 minutes. The symptoms of organophosphate poisoning may be delayed, especially if exposure is through skin application of an indirect-acting agent.[30] Compared to the organophosphates, the carbamates have a shorter duration of action and generally a lower toxicity, and although symptoms and signs of poisoning are similar there is a more rapid decline of effects.

Muscarinic Effects

The muscarinic effects are usually the first to appear and may occur within minutes after exposure. Symptoms include headache, anorexia, nausea, sweating, blurred vision, epigastric and substernal tightness, and heartburn. More severe muscarinic symptoms may include abdominal cramps, vomiting, dyspnea, diarrhea, salivation, lacrimation, profuse sweating, pallor, wheezing, micturition, defecation, increased bronchial secretion, bradycardia, car-

diac dysrhythmias, pulmonary edema, and miosis.[19]

Miosis is one of the most characteristic signs and is seen in the early stages of almost all cases of moderately severe poisoning.[14,36] Although miosis is often present, however, it is not a constant feature later in the exposure, and occasionally mydriasis may occur. Miosis develops as a consequence of marked parasympathetic stimulation of the iris, whereas mydriasis may be seen as a nicotinic effect of the organophosphates. Unilateral miosis by direct contact with a contaminated finger has also been noted.[32]

Nicotinic Effects

The nicotinic effects of anticholinesterase inhibitor poisoning (see Table 45-6) usually appear after muscarinic effects have reached moderate severity. These nicotinic effects may reflect a moderate to severe acute intoxication and may include muscle twitching and fasciculations.[16] These symptoms are often first noted in the eyelids but in serious poisoning are more prominent in larger muscles.[37] Muscle cramps and generalized and profound weakness may also be noted. These result from a depolarizing blockade of the neuromuscular junction. In addition, mydriasis, tachycardia, and hypertension may occur.[38] Transient hyperglycemia and glycosuria are not uncommon findings in severe organophosphate poisoning and may simulate diabetic ketoacidosis.[12,31,39] These nicotinic effects, as discussed earlier, have been attributed to stimulation of cholinergic preganglionic fibers to sympathetic ganglia and to the adrenal medulla as well as to a central increase in sympathetic vasoconstrictor tone.

Central Nervous System Effects

Organophosphates

In the CNS, acetylcholine receptors are distributed widely. With regard to organophosphate insecticide effects, the most important CNS locations are the respiratory and cardiovascular centers in the medulla.[39] CNS effects after organophosphate exposure are nonspecific and include anxiety, apprehension, restlessness, dizziness, giddiness, headache, tremors, ataxia, slurred speech, seizures, and coma.

Carbamates

Because the carbamates do not penetrate the CNS well, symptoms and signs are primarily muscarinic and nicotinic. If CNS symptoms do occur after carbamate poisoning, the possibility of a mixed intoxication or another cause should be strongly considered.[1,32]

Causes of Death

Death from poisoning with acetylcholinesterase inhibitors usually results from respiratory failure caused by a combination of factors, including an overstimulation of all three receptor types (Table 45-8). Bronchospasm, direct depression of the respiratory center with bradycardia and atrioventricular blocks, increased bronchial secretions, and decreased respiratory muscle strength all contribute.[16] As mentioned, respiratory muscle paralysis results from nicotinic activity and excessive pulmonary secretions, bronchoconstriction, and pulmonary edema are consequences of muscarinic activity,[19,21] and respiratory center depression appears to be a centrally mediated event.[18]

"Intermediate Syndrome"

An "intermediate syndrome" occurs 24 to 96 hours after poisoning, after the patient has

Table 45-8 Causes of Death in Acetylcholinesterase Inhibitor Exposure

Muscarinic activity
Excessive pulmonary secretions
Bronchoconstriction
Pulmonary edema
Nicotinic activity
Respiratory muscle paralysis
Central nervous system activity
Respiratory center depression

apparently survived the cholinergic phase of the overdose.[5,40] Symptoms noted during this phase have been attributed to involvement of respiratory muscles as well as of muscles in the proximal limbs and of neck flexors. Paralytic symptoms have lasted as much as 18 days. Because of the respiratory muscle involvement, apnea may ensue. This syndrome is not responsive to atropine or pralidoxime, and the patient may require ventilatory support.[4]

Delayed Neurotoxicity from Organophosphates

In addition to the intermediate syndrome, delayed neurotoxic effects of the organophosphates have also been reported 2 to 3 weeks after acute exposure and typically consist of a distal motor polyneuropathy.[41] The cranial nerves and respiratory muscles are spared.[4]

The mechanism of toxicity in delayed neurotoxicity is distinct from that in the acute phase. The delayed syndrome appears to involve phosphorylation and inhibition of the enzyme neurotoxic esterase.[41] Effects are not responsive to either atropine or pralidoxime. The incidence of delayed toxicity after organophosphate poisoning is low.[4]

LABORATORY DETERMINATIONS

A diagnosis of intoxication is based primarily on a history of exposure to an organophosphate 6 hours or less before onset of illness and clinical evidence of diffuse parasympathetic stimulation. Laboratory verification is based on depression of plasma and red blood cell cholinesterase to activities substantially lower than those before exposure (Table 45-9).[2,42] To detect a decrease in activity requires prior knowledge of a baseline activity measurement, however, which is unlikely.[43] In fact, the velocity of decline in cholinesterase activity is a more critical determinant than the absolute amount of the decline in predicting whether symptoms will manifest.

In actual practice it is not feasible for laboratory determinations to aid in the diagnosis, but blood should be drawn in a heparinized tube before treatment is instituted, and the red blood cells and plasma should be separated by centrifugation and then frozen if they must be kept for analysis. The laboratory may therefore aid in confirmation because treatment must often be initiated before laboratory results are available.[43]

Severe decreases in acetylcholinesterase activity are necessary before symptoms are seen. In acute poisoning, manifestations generally occur after more than 50% of red blood cell cholinesterase is inhibited; in mild poisoning, serum acetylcholinesterase activity is 20% to 50% of normal; in moderately severe poisoning, it is 10% to 20% of normal; and in severe poisoning, it is less than 10% of normal (Table 45-10).[12]

There are clinically significant differences between the two cholinesterases. Depression of red blood cell (true) cholinesterase is considered a specific response to the organophosphates, whereas pseudocholinesterase activity may vary in a number of different diseases or toxic states, such as infectious hepatitis, chronic gastritis, chronic pneumonia, and carcinoma of the stomach and kidney and in the malnourished elderly.[43] In actuality, inhibition of pseudocholinesterase does not contribute to the cholinergic poisoning syndrome.

If the red blood cell acetylcholinesterase has been completely and irreversibly inhibited by the organophosphates, recovery will take place at the same rate as new red blood cell regeneration (about 1% per day), whereas the enzyme in the plasma regenerates at a more rapid rate (approximately 25% in the first 7 to 10 days).[2,7] In severe poisoning, return to normal activity requires about 4 weeks for serum cholinesterase and about 5 weeks for erythrocyte cholinesterase.[14]

Table 45-9 Laboratory Determinations in Poisoning with Acetylcholinesterase Inhibitors

Red blood cell cholinesterase
Serum cholinesterase
Alkylphosphate metabolites
Electrocardiogram
Chest roentgenogram
Serum electrolytes

Table 45-10 Serum Acetylcholinesterase and Symptomatology

Percentage of Normal	Symptoms
> 50	No symptoms
20-50	Mild
10-20	Moderate
< 10	Severe

In addition to cholinesterase activity, diagnosis of some of the organophosphates can be confirmed by detecting the poison or one of the alkyl phosphate metabolites, such as paranitrophenol, in blood or urine. These methods are typically used for monitoring purposes in the industrial setting, but it is not likely that these tests would be available in an emergency setting.[18]

An electrocardiogram should be obtained to examine for evidence of heart blocks and a chest roentgenogram for evidence of atelectasis, aspiration, and pulmonary edema. Other laboratory findings that may be compatible with organophosphate poisoning but not diagnostic include hyperglycemia, hemoconcentration, leukocytosis, hypokalemia, acetonuria, and glycosuria.[5] Hyperamylasemia and proteinuria have also been noted.

TREATMENT

Exposure to the organophosphates and carbamates should be considered a medical emergency, and any patient with a diagnosis of insecticide poisoning should be hospitalized and kept under observation for at least 24 hours. Fatalities are usually the result of late recognition or inappropriate or insufficient therapy.[5]

Treatment should consist of cardiopulmonary resuscitation, if necessary, and removal of the individual from further exposure (Table 45-11). Clothing, including boots and shoes, should be disposed of in plastic bags, and the skin should be decontaminated with generous amounts of soap or detergent and water. If possible, it is best that the patient be taken to a separate area for showering and instructed to wash the hair thoroughly and to clean the fingernails and the umbilicus. To avoid contamination, clinicians should use gowns and gloves. Oxygen should be administered, and if the compound was orally ingested attempts should be made to retrieve the material with ipecac syrup or lavage and subsequent administration of activated charcoal. A cathartic may not be necessary, especially if the patient already has diarrhea. Careful attention must be paid to the removal of secretions and maintenance of a patent airway. If pulmonary edema occurs it should be treated vigorously.

If the patient is decontaminated outside the hospital facility, transportation to the hospital should be undertaken soon after decontamination is completed. Emergency department personnel should be notified in advance regarding the nature of the exposure so that proper arrangements can be made to avoid further contamination. The patient should be on a cardiac monitor because of the possibility of myocardial depression, heart block, or dysrhythmias. To avoid the possibility of respiratory arrest shortly after an overdose of organophosphates, patients should not be discharged from the hospital prematurely. If discharged, they should be informed to return if breathing difficulties appear.[5]

Contraindicated Drugs

Drugs contraindicated in the treatment of acetylcholinesterase inhibitor intoxication include morphine and succinylcholine, as well as the methylxanthines, phenothiazines, barbiturates, and loop diuretics (Table 45-12).

Antidotal Therapy

The pharmacologic management of organophosphates relies on the administration of atropine, which ameliorates the muscarinic and CNS manifestations, and of pralidoxime, which ame-

Table 45-11 Treatment of Poisoning with Acetylcholinesterase Inhibitors

Cardiopulmonary resuscitation (if necessary)
Decontamination
Cardiac monitoring
Oxygen
Suction
Atropine
Adult: 2 to 4 mg or more as needed
Child: 0.015 to 0.05 mg/kg
Pralidoxime
Adult: 1 g over 15 to 20 minutes (repeat as needed)
Child: 25 to 50 mg/kg

Table 45-12 Drugs Contraindicated in the Treatment of Acetylcholinesterase Inhibitor Poisoning

Barbiturates
Loop diuretics
Methylxanthines
Morphine
Phenothiazines
Succinylcholine

liorates the nicotinic and CNS manifestations.[2,16] Atropine should not be administered until cyanosis has been overcome because it may produce ventricular fibrillation in the presence of hypoxia.[14]

Atropine acts by binding competitively to the same site as acetylcholine but without depolarizing the postsynaptic membrane.[16] Nevertheless, it merely blocks certain actions of the acetylcholine already accumulated and does not reverse the fundamental biochemical lesion. The combination of both atropine and pralidoxime for organophosphate poisoning is more effective than either drug alone.

Poisoning with carbamate insecticides often does not require extensive treatment, and small doses of atropine may be all that is necessary.[44] Pralidoxime is not necessary for carbamate poisoning, but if a patient presents as an unknown acetylcholinesterase inhibitor exposure both atropine and pralidoxime should be administered because failure to administer pralidoxime can be lethal in an organophosphate poisoning.[22]

Patients who require treatment with these antidotes should be observed closely and continuously for not less than 24 hours. This is because serious and sometimes fatal relapses can occur as a result of continuous absorption of the poison when decontamination is incomplete or if the effects of the antidotes dissipate.

Atropine

Sufficient doses of atropine should be administered until muscarinic symptoms are relieved and signs of mild atropinization appear. Physicians unfamiliar with treating organophosphate poisoning tend to underdose with atropine; most fatalities occur as the result of underdosing. The dose of atropine may appear to be large, but the patient poisoned by cholinesterase inhibitors is well able to tolerate it, and failure to use the highest tolerable dose is far more serious than the effects of overdosage.[45]

Atropine sulfate should be administered to an adult at a dose of 2 to 4 mg intravenously and repeated every 2 to 5 minutes or until signs of atropinization appear. The pediatric dose of atropine is 0.015 to 0.05 mg/kg. Adequate atropinization is manifested by drying of secretions, dryness of the skin and mouth, mydriasis, flushing of the skin, and tachycardia. An important diagnostic clue is the failure of 1 to 2 mg of atropine to cause an anticholinergic effect. A mild degree of atropinization may need to be maintained for at least 48 hours; this should be titrated to the patient's physical signs. Although the average patient may need 40 mg of atropine per 24 hours, doses of more than 1 gram per day have sometimes been required. Cases have been reported in which patients received up to 30 g of atropine over a 5-week period.

An atropine drip has been used by some physicians when patients require massive amounts of atropine for reversal of symptoms. A concentration of 1 mg/mL (100 1-mL vials) of atropine has been infused without dilution and titrated to effect.[46]

Pralidoxime

Pralidoxime (Protopam®), an oxime, was one of the few drugs ever developed on the basis of a theory on how to correct a biochemical lesion.[47] At least three soluble salts of pralidoxime are in use in different countries. Pralidoxime chloride, pralidoxime methanesulphonate, and abidoxime (Toxogonin®) are identical in their action. In the United States, pralidoxime chloride is available and is probably safer than a number of other oximes studied.

Oximes are quaternary nitrogen-containing compounds that are thought to be unable to cross the blood-brain barrier and effect changes in the CNS. There is recent evidence, however, that this theory may not be correct.[14,25,47–49] The most striking support for the central action of the oximes comes from clinical observations of prompt recovery from coma and seizures after the administration of pralidoxime not attributable to improvement in other parameters.[14]

Pralidoxime is specifically adapted to reactivate acetylcholinesterase by removal of the phosphate group bound covalently to the ester site. In patients with acetylcholinesterase inhibitor poisoning, removal of the phosphate group completely restores normal activity of the enzyme and can produce clinical improvement within minutes.[1,16]

Dosage. Pralidoxime is administered intravenously in a dose of 1 to 2 g in 100 mL of 5% dextrose in water over a 15-minute period.[50,51] Recovery of consciousness and disappearance of toxic manifestations can occur within 10 to 40 minutes. The half-life of pralidoxime is 1 to 2 hours, and when manifestations recur in adult patients with severe poisoning pralidoxime should be infused at a rate up to 500 mg/ hour.[12,14] Treatment of severe poisoning with pralidoxime may require higher doses or continuous infusions.[51] Although there have not been any controlled studies to show the efficacy of continuous infusions, it has been suggested that the rate of 500 mg/hour be administered to a daily dose not to exceed 12 g in an adult. The initial pediatric dose of pralidoxime is 25 to 50 mg/kg.[2] Plasma concentrations of 4 μg/mL are normally seen at the time of reversal of anticholinesterase effects of organophosphates.[1]

Timing of Treatment. Treatment with pralidoxime is more effective if started early because the alkyl phosphate of the organophosphate gradually undergoes a secondary, irreversible reaction with the enzyme; this is known as *aging*. Inhibited acetylcholinesterase is not reactivated if it is already aged. This process of reversal is a time-dependent, nonenzymatic

Table 45-13 Side Effects of Pralidoxime

Dizziness
Blurred vision
Diplopia
Headache
Nausea
Tachycardia

cleavage of the phosphate bond of the enzyme complex[25] and is due to the loss of an alkyl or alkoxyl group.[26] Pralidoxime may therefore not be of benefit if given 36 to 48 hours after exposure to the insecticide.[51]

Oximes are only moderately effective when given alone, and because they act in a manner different from that of atropine the two drugs do not interfere with each other and can be administered at the same time. In addition, pralidoxime is most effective after a single exposure.

Side Effects. Side effects of therapeutic doses of pralidoxime have been minimal in normal subjects and practically nonexistent in individuals who have been poisoned.[14,44,50] Complaints have included brief episodes of dizziness, blurred vision, diplopia, headache, nausea, and tachycardia (Table 45-13).[51] The material is rapidly excreted from the body, chiefly in the urine.[51]

REFERENCES

1. Zweiner R, Ginsburg C: Organophosphate and carbamate poisoning in infants and children. *Pediatrics* 1988; 81:121–126.

2. Milby T: Prevention and management of organophosphate poisoning. *JAMA* 1971;216:2131–2133.

3. Davies J, Davis J, Frazier D, et al: Disturbances of metabolism in organophosphate poisoning. *Ind Med Surg* 1967;36:58–62.

4. Davies J: Changing profile of pesticide poisoning. *N Engl J Med* 1987;316:807–808.

5. Tafuri J, Roberts J: Organophosphate poisoning. *Ann Emerg Med* 1987;16:193–202.

6. Byard J: Mechanisms of acute human poisoning by pesticides. *Clin Toxicol* 1979;14:187–193.

7. Selden B, Curry S: Prolonged succinylcholine-induced paralysis in organophosphate insecticide poisoning. *Ann Emerg Med* 1987;16:215–217.

8. DePalma A, Kwalick D, Zukerberg N: Pesticide poisoning in children. *JAMA* 1970;211:1979–1981.

9. Namba T: Malathion poisoning. *Arch Environ Health* 1970;21:533–541.

10. Mortensen M: Management of acute childhood poisoning caused by selected insecticides and herbicides. *Pediatr Clin North Am* 1986;33:421–444.

11. Done A: "Nerve gases" in the war against pests. *Emerg Med* 1973;5:250–256.

12. Namba T, Hiraki K: PAM therapy for alkylphosphate poisoning. *JAMA* 1958;166:1834–1836.

13. Kopel F, Starobin S, Gribetz I, et al: Acute parathion poisoning. *J Pediatr* 1962;61:898–903.

14. Namba T, Nolte C, Jackrel J, et al: Poisoning due to organophosphate insecticides. *Am J Med* 1971;50:475–492.

15. Warren M, Conrad J, Bocian J, et al: Clothing-borne epidemic. *JAMA* 1963;184:94–96.

16. Namba T, Okazaki S, Taniguchi Y, et al: Inhibition by organophosphates and reactivation by oximes of tissue cholinesterase. *Naika Ryoiki* 1959;7:680–684.

17. Hayes W: Epidemiology and general management of poisoning by pesticides. *Pediatr Clin North Am* 1970; 17:629–644.

18. Lyon J, Taylor H, Ackerman B: A case report of intravenous malathion injection with determination of serum half-life. *Clin Toxicol* 1987;25:243–249.

19. Garber M: Carbamate poisoning: The "other" insecticide. *Pediatrics* 1987;79:734–738.

20. Arterberry J, Bonifaci R, Nash E, et al: Potentiation of phosphorus insecticides by phenothiazine derivatives: Possible hazard, with report of a fatal case. *JAMA* 1962; 182:110–112.

21. Ahlgren D, Manz H, Harvey J: Myopathy of chronic organophosphate poisoning: A clinical entity? *South Med J* 1979;72:555–558.

22. Becker C, Sullivan J: Prompt recognition and vigorous therapy for organophosphate poisoning. *Emerg Med Rep* 1986;7:33–39.

23. Durham W, Hayes W: Organic phosphorus poisoning and its therapy. *Arch Environ Health* 1962;5:21–47.

24. Kline S, Bayer M: Insecticide poisoning. *Top Emerg Med* 1979;1:73–83.

25. Lotti M, Becker C: Treatment of acute organophosphate poisoning: Evidence of a direct effect on the central nervous system by 2-PAM (pyridine-2-aldoxime methylchloride). *J Toxicol Clin Toxicol* 1982;19:121–127.

26. Fleisher J, Harris L: Dealkylation as a mechanism for aging of cholinesterase after poisoning with pinacolylmethylphosphonofluoridate. *Biochem Pharmacol* 1965;14: 641–645.

27. Fredriksson T: Percutaneous absorption of parathion and paraoxon: Decontamination of human skin from parathion. *Arch Environ Health* 1961;3:67–70.

28. Fredriksson T: Studies on the percutaneous absorption of parathion and paraoxon: Rate of absorption of parathion. *Acta Derm Venereol* (Stockh) 1961;41:353–362.

29. Healy J: Ascending paralysis following malathion intoxication: A case report. *Med J Aust* 1959;1:765–767.

30. Zavon M: Treatment of organophosphorus and chlorinated hydrocarbon insecticide intoxications. *Mod Treat* 1971;8:503–510.

31. Zadik Z, Blachar Y, Barak Y, et al: Organophosphate poisoning presenting as diabetic ketoacidosis. *J Toxicol Clin Toxicol* 1983;20:381–385.

32. Miller D: Neurotoxicity of the pesticidal carbamates. *Neurobehav Toxicol Teratol* 1982;4:779–787.

33. Gaines T: Acute toxicity of pesticides. *Toxicol Appl Pharmacol* 1969;14:515–534.

34. Tabershaw I, Cooper W: Sequelae of acute organic phosphate poisoning. *J Occup Med* 1966;8:5–20.

35. Brown H: Electroencephalographic changes and disturbance of brain function following human organophosphate exposure. *Northwest Med* 1971;70:845–846.

36. Sim V: Anticholinesterase poisoning. *Clin Pharmacol* 1974;9:146–148.

37. Fisher J: Guillain-Barré syndrome following organophosphate poisoning. *JAMA* 1979;238:1950–1952.

38. Dixon E: Dilatation of the pupils in parathion poisoning. *JAMA* 1957;163:444–445.

39. Ramu A, Drexler H: Hyperglycemia in acute malathion intoxication in rats. *Isr J Med Sci* 1973;9:635–639.

40. Senanayake N, Karalliedde L: Neurotoxic effects of organophosphate insecticides: An intermediate syndrome. *N Engl J Med* 1987;316:761–763.

41. Gadoth N, Fisher A: Late onset of neuromuscular block in organophosphate poisoning. *Ann Intern Med* 1978; 88:654–655.

42. Fournier E, Sonnier M, Dally S: Detection and assay of organophosphate pesticides in human blood by gas chromatography. *Clin Toxicol* 1978;12:457–462.

43. Coye M, Barnett P, Midtling J, et al: Clinical confirmation of organophosphate poisoning by serial cholinesterase analyses. *Arch Intern Med* 1987;147:438–442.

44. Green M, Reid F, Kaminskis A: Correlation of 2-PAM plasma levels after organophosphate intoxication. *Res Commun Chem Pathol Pharmacol* 1985;49:255–266.

45. Richards A: Malathion poisoning successfully treated with large doses of atropine. *Can Med Assoc J* 1964;91: 82–92.

46. LeBlanc F, Benson B, Gilg A: A severe organophosphate poisoning requiring the use of an atropine drip. *Clin Toxicol* 1986;24:69–76.

47. Holland P, Parkes D: Plasma concentrations of the oxime pralidoxime mesylate (P2S) after repeated oral and intramuscular administration. *Br J Ind Med* 1976;33:43–46.

48. Rosenberg P: In vivo reactivation by PAM of brain cholinesterase inhibited by paraoxon. *Biochem Pharmacol* 1960;3:212–215.

49. Firemark H, Barlow C, Roth L: The penetration of 2-PAM-C[14] into brain and the effect of cholinesterase inhibitors on its transport. *J Pharmacol Exp Ther* 1964;145: 252–265.

50. Calesnick B, Christensen J, Richter M: Human toxicity of various oximes. *Arch Environ Health* 1967;15: 599–608.

51. Thompson D, Thompson G, Greenwood R, et al: Therapeutic dosing of pralidoxime chloride. *Drug Intell Clin Pharmac* 1987;21:590–593.

ADDITIONAL SELECTED REFERENCES

Cavagna G, Locati G, Vigliani E: Clinical effects of exposure to DDVP (Vapona) insecticide in hospital wards. *Arch Environ Health* 1969;19:112–123.

Dressel T, Goodale R, Arneson M, et al: Pancreatitis as a complication of anticholinesterase insecticide intoxication. *Ann Surg* 1978;189:199–204.

Fredriksson T, Farrior W, Witter R: Studies on the percutaneous absorption of parathion and paraoxon: Hydrolysis and metabolism within the skin. *Acta Derm Venereol* (Stockh) 1961;41:335–341.

Goldin A, Rubinstein A, Bradlow B, et al: Malathion poisoning with special reference to the effect of cholinesterase inhibition on erythrocyte survival. *N Engl J Med* 1964;271:1289–1292.

Hruban Z, Schulman S, Warner N, et al: Hypoglycemia resulting from insecticide poisoning: Report of a case. *JAMA* 1963;184:590–594.

Levin H, Rodnitzky R: Behavioral effects of organophosphate pesticides in man. *Clin Toxicol* 1976;9:391–405.

Maibach H, Feldmann R, Milby T, et al: Regional variation in percutaneous penetration in man. *Arch Environ Health* 1971;23:208–211.

Maselli R, Jacobsen J, Spire J: Edrophonium: An aid in the diagnosis of acute organophosphate poisoning. *Ann Neurol* 1986;19:508–510.

Meller D, Fraser I, Kryger M: Hyperglycemia in anticholinesterase poisoning. *Can Med Assoc J* 1981;124: 745–748.

Muller F, Hundt H: Chronic organophosphate poisoning. *S Afr Med J* 1980;57:344–345.

Page L, Verhulst H: The oximes and organophosphate poisoning. *Am J Dis Child* 1962;103:185–190.

Sanborn G, Selhorst J, Calabrese V, et al: Pseudotumor cerebrii and insecticide intoxication. *Neurology* 1979; 29:1222–1227.

Sidell F: Soman and sarin: Clinical manifestations and treatment of accidental poisoning by organophosphates. *Clin Toxicol* 1974;7:1–17.

Victor S: Bell's palsy following organophosphate poisoning. *JAMA* 1978;239:1847–1848.

Wolfe, H, Durham W, Walker K, et al: Health hazards of discarded pesticide containers. *Arch Environ Health* 1961; 3:531–537.

Young R, Jung F, Ayer H: Phorate intoxication at an insecticide-formulating plant. *Am Ind Hyg Assoc J* 1979;40: 1013–1016.

Zavon M: Poisoning from pesticides: Diagnosis and treatment. *Pediatrics* 1974;54:332–336.

chapter 46

Herbicides

The dangers posed by herbicidal chemicals to organisms and the environment are considerable. Many of these chemicals were used during wartime and are now marketed for civilian use by farmers and homeowners for killing weeds and controlling brush. The most powerful of the herbicides are paraquat and the phenoxyacetic acid derivatives 2,4-dichlorophenoxyacetic acid (2,4-D) and 2,4,5-trichlorophenoxyacetic acid (2,3,4-T).

PARAQUAT AND DIQUAT

Paraquat (dimethylbipyridilium chloride, methylviologen) is a quaternary ammonium herbicide and the most important of a group of bipyridilium compounds used as herbicides (Table 46-1).[1] Other bipyridilium agents include diquat, difenzoquat, morfamquat, and chlormequat. These compounds are some of the most toxic poisons known to humans. Although the lung was once thought to be the target organ for the toxic effects of paraquat, it is now known that paraquat is a multisystem poison capable of causing toxicity also to the kidneys, liver, brain, heart, and muscles.[2]

Paraquat was first described in the latter part of the nineteenth century. It had been used as a redox indicator and was known as methylviologen until the 1950s, when it began to be marketed as an herbicide. It is now a widely used, rapidly acting contact herbicide that is inactivated by soil, particularly clay. The inactivation is due to the tenacious binding of the compound to the soil.

Paraquat appears to react within plant cells in conjunction with sunlight to generate superoxide radicals, which in turn destroy plant cellular membranes and desiccate the leaves. If sprayed plants are harvested before exposure to sunlight, desiccation does not occur and unaltered paraquat remains on the plant.[3]

Paraquat is used to control weeds and deep brush.[4] It has been used in many countries, including Vietnam, as a defoliant. Not long ago a government-sponsored aerial spraying program to destroy marijuana fields in Mexico was carried out. Mexican farmers, however, knowing that the action of paraquat depends on sunlight, began harvesting marijuana rapidly after spraying and wrapped the leaves in dark cloths for export to the United States. As a result there was great concern for a time that marijuana con-

Table 46-1 Bipyridilium Herbicides

Chlormequat
Diquat
Difenzoquat
Morfamquat
Paraquat

taminated with paraquat would cause poisoning in marijuana smokers. This has not been shown to occur, however.[4,5]

Diquat (ethylene bipyridilium), an analog of paraquat, is considered much less toxic.[6,7] It is also used as an herbicide and often is combined with paraquat.[6] Although poisoning by diquat is not as common, the signs and symptoms resemble those of paraquat but are milder.[7]

Diquat does not present the same pulmonary toxicity as paraquat, possibly because it does not accumulate in the lung. Because it is eliminated by the kidneys, it may cause renal damage leading to renal failure. A pre-renal component may add to this problem because of "third spacing" resulting in a decreased intravascular volume. Few fatalities have been associated with diquat intoxication.[7]

Absorption of Paraquat

Paraquat is highly toxic to humans. Lethal poisoning can occur by absorption through the skin, inhalation, and ingestion. Paraquat is poorly absorbed from the gastrointestinal tract, with less than 5% of an ingested dose typically being absorbed. Although the absorption of paraquat by this route may be incomplete it is nonetheless rapid, and symptoms of intoxication may be detected as early as 1 hour after ingestion. Because paraquat has an extremely low vapor pressure, the hazard of poisoning from inhalation is small.[8] Only small amounts of paraquat can be absorbed through unbroken skin, but broken skin can readily absorb the herbicide to cause severe or even fatal poisoning. This, however, is not a common mode of entry.[2]

Most serious poisonings have involved liquid concentrates, and most fatalities have occurred after ingestion of such preparations containing more than 25% paraquat. At this concentration, one or two mouthfuls may be fatal.[3]

Mechanism of Toxicity

Systemic toxicity in humans is thought to be mediated by the production of a superoxide anion, which through an intermediary reacts with lipids to form hydroperoxides that interfere with pulmonary surfactant function.[9,10] The result is cell damage producing inflammation, edema, and ultimately fibrosis. The formation of this toxic superoxide radical is more rapid under high oxygen tension, which is the proposed mechanism for the preferential site of paraquat toxicity in lung tissue.[11]

The herbicidal activity of paraquat is dependent on active photosynthesis, during which it competes with nicotinamide-adenine dinucleotide phosphate (NADP) for electrons furnished by a transfer system in the chloroplast. Toxicity is as a result of reduction by NADPH–cytochrome P-450 reductase (NADPH is the reduced form of NADP).[2] The addition of a single electron to paraquat produces methylviologen, a free-radical resonating structure with a blue color.[12] Methylviologen can react with molecular oxygen to regenerate paraquat ion and to yield such toxic and reactive products as hydrogen peroxide, superoxide anion, and peroxide anion.[11] Superoxide ions are also responsible for other membrane lesions and secondary necrosis of the upper digestive tract, the liver, the renal tubules, and the adrenal glands. The survival time in fatally poisoned patients is highly variable, with death occurring from a few hours to a month after ingestion.[2]

Paraquat also causes toxicity because the production of superoxide radicals initiates an arachidonic acid cascade that stimulates prostaglandin synthesis, leading to increased fluid flow into the intracellular space with subsequent pulmonary edema.[1]

Toxicity

Clinical Features

The major adverse effects of paraquat are corrosion of the gastrointestinal tract, pulmonary fibrosis, renal tubular necrosis, and hepatic necrosis (Table 46-2). Other lesions produced by paraquat include irritative dermatitis, nail damage, eye injury, and severe epistaxis.[5,8,10,13,14] Although caustic agents may result in mouth ulcers and many toxins produce hepatic or renal failure, the constellation of signs and

Table 46-2 Clinical Features of Paraquat Poisoning

Local
  Eye irritation
  Mucous membranes irritation
  Skin irritation
Gastrointestinal
  Burning sensation
  Ulceration
  Esophageal perforation
  Vomiting
  Abdominal pain
  Dysphagia
Respiratory
  Tachypnea
  Dyspnea
  Cough
  Cyanosis
  Pulmonary edema
  Pulmonary fibrosis
Renal
  Tubular necrosis
Hepatic
  Liver function test abnormalities
  Jaundice
Cardiac
  Conduction disturbances
  Myocarditis

symptoms of painful oral ulceration with subsequent hepatic and renal failure should alert the physician to the possibility of paraquat poisoning. Symptoms of paraquat ingestion depend largely on the amount consumed.

As mentioned above, death from paraquat poisoning usually occurs either within 1 to 5 days of ingestion or as long as several weeks after ingestion.[15]

Local Effects

The bipyridilium compounds may cause local skin lesions as a result of their corrosive nature. Dermal toxicity may also result from the effects of the wetting agent used for paraquat.[16] Paraquat may cause irritation of the eyes and mucous membranes, and partial-thickness burns of the skin have been noted.

Gastrointestinal Effects

Initial gastrointestinal manifestations of paraquat poisoning include an immediate burning and ulceration of the mouth, tongue, throat, and esophagus.[4] This is followed by vomiting, abdominal pain, dysphagia, and diarrhea. Esophageal perforation may occur. The initial phase of symptomatology may be followed by a latent period lasting up to 2 weeks, during which the patient appears to improve.

Respiratory Effects

Although paraquat causes multisystem damage, the highest tissue concentration is found in the lungs because there is active accumulation of paraquat in type II pneumocytes[1]; consequently there is more lung damage noted. Lung concentrations of paraquat may be 50 times higher than plasma concentrations. As discussed above, formation of the toxic superoxide radical causes membrane destruction and initiates an arachidonic acid cascade that stimulates prostaglandin synthesis, thereby leading to toxicity.[17]

Either the early or delayed appearance of respiratory distress or failure is characteristic of paraquat poisoning. Selective binding and persistence of paraquat in lung tissue is considered the cause of pulmonary fibrosis, which is generally the lethal complication and occurs at any time between 5 and 30 days after ingestion.[18] Massive doses of paraquat, however, may cause a fatal pulmonary edema and hemorrhage within 24 hours. The patient may develop dyspnea, tachypnea, and a nonproductive cough. As more damage develops, cyanosis is noted. Once symptoms are evident, the fibrosis progresses until death occurs secondary to the proliferative alveolitis; the alveolar walls become thickened, and the patient dies from asphyxiation.[16] The lethal amount of paraquat is relatively small, and death may result from progressive hypoxemia even with aggressive respiratory treatment.[16] The pathologic changes noted in the lung are identical to those from oxygen toxicity.

Renal Effects

Renal deterioration often begins 24 to 96 hours after paraquat ingestion. In most severe intoxications renal tubular necrosis develops. The renal disorder may be observed before the development of pulmonary fibrosis. Microscopically, tubular damage is noted in the kidneys.

Hepatic Effects

Hepatic insufficiency has been reported to occur within 24 to 48 hours of ingestion and may manifest as abnormalities in liver function tests. Jaundice may also be noted. The hepatic disorders may also be observed before the development of pulmonary fibrosis.

Cardiac Effects

Cardiac involvement may consist of conduction disturbances, epicardial hemorrhage, and myocarditis. Respiratory difficulties may then ensue.

Paraquat and Marijuana

Although there may be some degree of absorption of paraquat by inhalation, when paraquat is burned it is broken down to bipyridine. This compound has a toxicity similar to that of pyridine, which is a respiratory irritant present in tobacco smoke.[5] To date, there have been no documented cases of lung injury resulting from the use of paraquat-contaminated marijuana.

Laboratory Determinations

For patients with paraquat poisoning, serial chest roentgenograms should be obtained and arterial blood gases measured to determine the onset of pneumonitis. Renal output should be carefully monitored for signs of renal involvement. Liver function studies are necessary to monitor hepatic involvement. Measurements of serum paraquat concentration may be useful for prognostic purposes, but the diagnosis must be made quickly, before concentrations can be determined, to increase the likelihood of effective intervention. A qualitative colorimetric urine test is also available; this makes use of sodium dithionite and sodium hydroxide. Two milliliters of 1% sodium dithionite in 1N sodium hydroxide is added to 10 mL of urine. If the solution turns blue, the urine is positive for bipyridilium compounds.

Treatment

Treatment of paraquat intoxication is directed toward the removal of the material from the gastrointestinal tract and the prevention of further absorption by administering specific adsorbents. Initial treatment therefore consists of ipecac syrup or lavage, despite the corrosive nature of the compound.

Detoxification of Paraquat

Paraquat undergoes complete detoxification on contact with clay or earth, so that Fuller's earth (300 g of a 30% solution) or bentonite (200 to 500 mL of a 30% aqueous suspension) is an effective adsorbent; the addition of 20% mannitol or 70% sorbitol may accelerate the passage of contents through the gastrointestinal tract.[17,18] If neither of these adsorbents is available, then activated charcoal should be used. Many clinicians prefer activated charcoal because it is more readily available and can be administered more rapidly.[17] There is no strong evidence that multiple-dose activated charcoal is effective, however.[19]

Oxygen Therapy

It has been shown that lung damage from paraquat is enhanced by any concentration of oxygen. It is important, therefore, to give the patient hypoxic mixtures that protect the lung against damage from hyperoxygenation.[15,20,21] Early intubation and ventilation with positive-pressure breathing has been suggested as a method of administering low inspired oxygen tensions while facilitating adequate arterial oxygen pressure.[21]

Methods To Enhance Excretion

When first introduced, charcoal hemoperfusion was thought to be a major advance in the management of paraquat poisoning. Subsequent clinical experience has not always been associated with success, however.[12,22,23] Hemoperfusion may be of value in paraquat poisoning only if it can be instituted before toxic concentrations accumulate in the lung.[19,23] Paraquat has a large volume of distribution, and in most cases toxic concentrations are reached in the lungs before hemoperfusion can be started.[22] Further, forced diuresis, dialysis, and hemoperfusion appear to offer minimal success because only a small fraction of the compound is removed.[7,18] Dialysis is only useful if renal failure ensues.

Other Therapies

Some investigators have tried to prevent the pulmonary complications of paraquat intoxication by using immunosuppressants and by attempting to prevent the formation of superoxide radicals. Superoxide dismutase, which is an enzyme that destroys superoxide radicals, has not met with great success. Corticosteroids, fibrinolytic agents, and vitamin E (an antioxidant thought to be helpful as an oxygen scavenger) have all been tried but have not produced any beneficial results.[12]

2,4-D AND 2,4,5-T

2,4-D and 2,4,5-T are phenoxyl herbicide compounds that have been in use for more than 40 years in the United States.[24] These compounds are among the most widely used for weed control, especially broad-leafed plants. Many millions of pounds of these herbicides are used domestically on an annual basis by railroads, utility firms, paper manufacturers, and farmers to clear land of wild growth.[25]

Neither 2,4-D nor 2,4,5-T is absorbed appreciably through the intact skin, although 2,4,5-T appears to be more irritating on the skin and mucous membranes than 2,4-D. There does not appear to be any consistent pattern of toxic symptoms except in scattered cases, where a protracted peripheral neuropathy has been noted.

Clinical Manifestations and Treatment of Intoxication

Phenoxyacetic acid poisoning is surprisingly rare considering its widespread domestic use. Fatal self-poisoning is also rare, but there have been occasional reports of intoxication after overdose.[26]

Signs and symptoms of overdose may include fatigue, nausea, vomiting, anorexia, diarrhea, muscle fasciculations, ataxia, and peripheral neuropathy. Phenoxyacetic acid poisoning may also uncouple oxidative phosphorylation and produce pyrexia, hyperventilation, and hypoxemia. Hypersensitivity reactions involving respiratory complaints and dermatitis have also been reported.[25] Treatment is supportive and symptomatic.

Phenoxyacetic Acids and Dioxins

Although a thorough discussion of dioxins is beyond the scope of this book, recent reports concerning Agent Orange are worth mentioning. Over the last few years there has been great concern about the dioxins that have appeared as contaminants of 2,4,5-T.[24] If the reaction temperature during synthesis of 2,4,5-T is allowed to rise too high, dioxin is produced[27]; this does not occur with 2,4-D. Agent Orange, the defoliant used during the war in Vietnam, is an equal mixture of 2,4-D and 2,4,5-T contaminated with 2,3,7,8-tetrachlorodibenzo-*p*-dioxin. The long-term effects of this dioxin contaminant have given rise to a great deal of controversy. A number of lawsuits have been based on alleged adverse health effects from exposures to Agent Orange, including sterility, birth defects, disfiguring skin diseases, malignancies, and other illnesses.[27]

REFERENCES

1. Barabas K, Szabo L, Matkovics B: The search for an ideal antidote treatment in Gramoxone® intoxication. *Gen Pharmacol* 1987;18:129–132.

2. Thomas C, Aust S: Free radicals and environmental toxins. *Ann Emerg Med* 1986;15:1075–1083.

3. Smith L: Paraquat toxicity. *Philos Trans R Soc London Ser B* 1985;311:647–657.

4. Smith R: Spraying of herbicides on Mexican marijuana backfires on U.S. *Science* 1978;199:861–864.

5. Landrigan P, Powell K, James L, et al: Paraquat and marijuana: Epidemiologic risk assessment. *Am J Public Health* 1983;1:784–788.

6. McCarthy L, Speth C: Diquat intoxication. *Ann Emerg Med* 1983;12:394–396.

7. Williams P, Jarvie D, Whitehead A: Diquat intoxication: Treatment by charcoal hemoperfusion and description of a new method of diquat measurement in plasma. *Clin Toxicol* 1986;24:11–20.

8. Swan A: Exposure of spray operators to paraquat. *Chest* 1974;65(suppl):65–67.

9. Bus J, Aust S, Gibson J: Superoxide and singlet oxygen–catalyzed lipid peroxidation as a possible mechanism for paraquat toxicity. *Biochem Biophys Res Commun* 1974;58:749.

10. Conradi S, Olanoff L, Dawson W: Fatality due to paraquat intoxication: Confirmation by postmortem tissue analysis. *Am J Clin Pathol* 1983;80:771–776.

11. Bismuth C, Gardiner R, Dally S, et al: Prognosis and treatment of paraquat poisoning: A review of 28 cases. *J Toxicol Clin Toxicol* 1982;19:461–474.

12. Vale J, Crome P, Volans G, et al: The treatment of paraquat poisoning using oral sorbents and charcoal hemoperfusion. *Acta Pharmacol Toxicol* 1977;41(suppl): 109–117.

13. Baran R: Nail damage caused by weed killers and insecticides. *Arch Dermatol* 1974;110:467.

14. Wohlfahrt D: Fatal paraquat poisonings after skin absorption. *Med J Aust* 1982;1:512–513.

15. Fisher H, Clements J, Wright R: Enhancement of oxygen toxicity by the herbicide paraquat. *Am Rev Respir Dis* 1973;107:246–252.

16. Copland G, Kolin A, Shulman H: Fatal pulmonary intraalveolar fibrosis after paraquat ingestion. *N Engl J Med* 1974;291:290–292.

17. Meredith T, Vale J: Treatment of paraquat poisoning in man: Methods to prevent absorption. *Hum Toxicol* 1987; 6:49–55.

18. Hoffman S, Jederkin R, Korzets Z, et al: Successful management of severe paraquat poisoning. *Chest* 1983; 84:107–109.

19. Van de Vyver F, Guiliano R, Paulus G, et al: Hemoperfusion-hemodialysis ineffective for paraquat removal in life-threatening poisoning. *Clin Toxicol* 1985;23:117–131.

20. Brashear R, Sharma H, Deatley R: Prolonged survival breathing oxygen at ambient pressure. *Am Rev Respir Dis* 1973;108:701–704.

21. Rhodes M, Zavala D, Brown D: Hypoxic protection in paraquat poisoning. *Lab Invest* 1976;35:496–500.

22. Gelfand M, Winchester J, Knepshield J, et al: Treatment of severe drug overdosage with charcoal hemoperfusion. *Trans Am Soc Artif Intern Organs* 1977;23:599–604.

23. Mascie-Taylor J, Thompson J, Davison A: Hemoperfusion ineffective for paraquat removal in life-threatening poisoning. *Lancet* 1983;1:1376–1377.

24. Berwick P: 2,4-Dichlorophenoxyacetic acid poisoning in man. *JAMA* 1970;214:1114–1117.

25. O'Reilly J: Prolonged coma and delayed peripheral neuropathy after ingestion of phenoxyacetic acid weed-killers. *Postgrad Med J* 1984;60:76–77.

26. Cushman J, Street J: Allergic hypersensitivity to the herbicide 2,4-D in Balb/c mice. *J Toxicol Environ Health* 1982;10:729–741.

27. Tedschi L: Dioxin. *Am J Forensic Med Pathol* 1980; 1:145–148.

ADDITIONAL SELECTED REFERENCES

Siefkin A: Combined paraquat and acetaminophen toxicity. *J Toxicol Clin Toxicol* 1982;19:483–491.

Tungsanga K, Israsena S, Chusilp S, et al: Paraquat poisoning: Evidence of systemic toxicity after dermal exposure. *Postgrad Med J* 1983;59:338–339.

chapter 47

Hydrocarbons

Hydrocarbons are some of the most commonly used substances in industrialized society, and products containing hydrocarbons account for approximately 5% of all poisonings in children younger than 5 years of age.[1,2] The ubiquity of these agents in the household and the fact that many, particularly furniture polishes, are pleasantly scented and colored make them especially dangerous to young children, who often drink liquid hydrocarbons when left within reach by careless adults.[3]

Hydrocarbons are organic compounds that consist only of carbon and hydrogen molecules.[4] Hydrocarbon products are not pure substances but mixtures of saturated, unsaturated, ring, and straight-chain molecules.[5] The liquid forms comprise molecules containing 5 to 15 carbon atoms that are arranged in aliphatic (straight-chain), alicyclic, and aromatic (benzene-based) structures with varying amounts of sulfur, nitrogen, and oxygen impurities.[6,7]

Confusion has existed for many years as to the toxicity of hydrocarbons partly because the hydrocarbon products are not a single class of compounds but may contain other more toxic compounds as well. For instance, fuels such as gasoline, petroleum naphtha, and kerosene are among the most commonly ingested petroleum distillates; they carry a low systemic toxicity but are dangerous when their fumes are inhaled. Solvents and thinners, on the other hand, are more dangerous systemically because of their high content of benzene, toluene, xylene, and halogenated hydrocarbons. The toxicity of the various hydrocarbons must therefore be discussed in terms of the individual agents they contain (Table 47-1).[8]

TYPES OF HYDROCARBONS

Petroleum Distillates

Petroleum distillates (Table 47-2) are prepared by the fractionation of crude petroleum oil. All petroleum distillates are hydrocarbons, but not all hydrocarbons are petroleum distillates.[4] The petroleum distillates almost exclusively consist of the aliphatic hydrocarbons; in order of decreasing volatility the major fractions are petroleum ether, gasoline, mineral spirits, kerosene, fuel oil, lubricating oils, paraffin wax, and asphalt or tar.[8]

Mineral Seal Oil

Seal oil, which was originally obtained from seals and used primarily as fuel for lamps, is now obtained chiefly from petroleum; hence it is now called mineral seal oil to distinguish it from the animal seal oil. It is now almost exclusively used as a furniture polish.[3] Mineral seal oil is not absorbed from the gastrointestinal tract; the only problem associated with ingestion is the potential for aspiration pneumonitis.[5]

Table 47-1 Hydrocarbons and Their Uses

Product	Synonym	Use(s)
Benzene	Benzol	Paint thinner
Gasoline	Petroleum spirits	Fuel, paint thinner, glue thinner, high-performance fuel
Petroleum naphtha	Ligroin	Lighter fluid, high-performance fuel
VMP naphtha	Varnish naphtha	Paint thinner, varnish thinner
Turpentine	Pine oil	Paint thinner, shoe polish
Petroleum spirits	Mineral spirits, stodard solvent, white spirits	Paint solvent, dry cleaning agent, degreasing agent
Kerosene	Coal oil	Fuel, solvent, lighter fluid
Mineral seal oil	Signal oil, red furniture polish	Furniture polish
Fuel oil	Heating oil	Fuel
Petrolatum	Petroleum jelly	Laxative, ointment
Benzine	Petroleum ether	Dry cleaning agent, paint thinner, rubber solvent

Source: Adapted with permission from "Hydrocarbon Ingestion and Poisoning" by E Zieser in *Comprehensive Therapy* (1979;5:36), Copyright © 1979, Laux Publishing Company, Ayer, MA.

Table 47-2 Petroleum Distillates

Asphalt
Fuel oil
Gasoline
Kerosene
Lubricating oils
Mineral seal oil
Mineral spirits
Naphtha
Paraffin wax
Petroleum ether (benzine)

Naphtha and Petroleum Ether

Naphthas are mixtures of aliphatics and aromatics that are obtained in the distillation of coal tar or petroleum.[8] Petroleum naphthas include petroleum ether (more commonly known as benzine) and other compounds such as pentane and hexane. After ingestion, the major risk is that of aspiration pneumonitis.

Gasoline

Gasoline is the most commonly ingested distillate and consists of a mixture of aliphatic and acyclic hydrocarbons (mostly pentane and octane) but may also contain olefins, diolefins, cycloparaffins, and aromatic hydrocarbons in varying concentrations.[9,10] Additives may be present, such as tetraethyl lead and cresyl phosphates, but these do not pose a toxic hazard in acute ingestions.[11] Gasoline is probably not absorbed well from the gastrointestinal tract, but not enough data have been accumulated for this to be determined with any degree of certainty.[12] After ingestion, the major risk is that of aspiration pneumonitis.[13]

Kerosene

Kerosene or coal oil consists primarily of aliphatics and aromatics that may vary widely in composition.[14] It is used as a paint thinner, degreaser and cleaner, and fuel oil in lamps and stoves. It continues to be a popular vehicle for many insecticides and fungicides.[15] On prolonged or extensive contact with the skin, kerosene and its cogeners can produce epidermal necrolysis. After ingestion, the major risk is that of aspiration pneumonitis.[9]

Other Distillates

Turpentine

Turpentine (oil of turpentine, spirits of turpentine), an oleoresin distillate, is a mixture of various pine species, camphenes, and other complex terpenes of low volatility. It is commonly used in mixing oil-based paints and in removing paint stains. Turpentine is readily absorbed from the gastrointestinal tract, skin, and respiratory tract. In addition to the risk associated with aspiration, turpentine acts both as a local irritant and a CNS depressant.[16]

Coal Tar Derivatives

Coal tar derivatives, which include benzene, toluene, and xylene, are derived initially from the distillation of coal in the coking process and consist mainly of aromatic compounds. These compounds carry a greater risk of systemic toxicity than petroleum distillates.

The hydrocarbons most commonly ingested include petroleum solvents, dry cleaning fluids, spot removers, kerosene, lighter fluids, gasoline, and mineral seal oil (Table 47-2). The hydrocarbon derivatives are listed in Table 47-3.

ROUTES OF ABSORPTION

Hydrocarbons can be absorbed orally, through the skin, or by inhalation (Table 47-4). Each of these modes of absorption is associated with different sites of toxicity.[12] Ingestion is by far the most common route and may lead to chemical pneumonitis, CNS depression, and gastrointestinal irritation.[17] Direct skin contact may lead to dermatitis or contact burns. The inhalation of a hydrocarbon as a drug of abuse may lead to CNS dysfunction; cardiac, renal, and liver toxicity; and lead poisoning (see Chapter 33).[18,19]

PHYSICAL PROPERTIES OF HYDROCARBONS

The physical characteristics of the hydrocarbons can be described in terms of their viscosity, volatility, surface tension, and flammability. Viscosity is the most important property because it relates directly to the risk of pulmonary aspiration.[2,5]

Viscosity is the property describing the ability of a substance to flow and the friction produced during flow.[4] Surface tension is the force acting to maintain the integrity of a surface. The viscosity determines the likelihood of entry of a hydrocarbon into the lungs and the rate and extent of penetration into deep lung structures.[18]

Table 47-3 Other Hydrocarbon Distillates

Coal Tar
  Benzene
  Toluene
  Xylene
Oleoresin
  Turpentine

Table 47-4 Routes of Absorption of Hydrocarbons with Major Associated Medical Problems

Ingestion
  Chemical pneumonitis
  CNS depression
  Gastrointestinal irritation
Dermal contact
  Dermatitis
  Contact burns
Inhalation (see Chapter 33)
  CNS alteration
  Cardiac dysfunction
  Renal dysfunction
  Lead toxicity
  Liver dysfunction

A substance with low viscosity has less resistance to flow; consequently, even a small volume may be spread along the mucous membranes of the oral cavity and into the airway.[20,21] Low viscosity and surface tension therefore increase the aspiration hazard.[11]

The units of viscosity, Saybolt seconds universal (SSU), measure the time in seconds required for a sample liquid to flow through a calibrated orifice; the lower the viscosity, the less time required.[6] Substances with viscosities less than 45 to 60 SSU represent the greatest aspiration hazard; those with viscosities greater than 100 to 250 SSU have a minimal risk.[18]

Volatility is the ability of a liquid to evaporate rapidly and become a gas. The volatile hydrocarbons enter the CNS and other target organs most readily when absorbed by inhalation, ingestion, or, rarely, prolonged or extensive dermal contact.[4] Also, the most volatile hydrocarbons are the most flammable.

For toxicological purposes, the hydrocarbons can be divided into four categories on the basis of these properties (Table 47-5).[4]

Table 47-5 Properties of Hydrocarbons and Associated Toxicity

Properties	Example	Toxicity	
		Systemic	Pulmonary
Low viscosity, low volatility	Mineral seal oil	0	+ + + +
Intermediate viscosity, intermediate volatility	Gasoline, kerosene	+	+ + +
High volatility	Benzene, toluene, xylene, chlorinated hydrocarbons	+ + +	+
High viscosity, low volatility	Asphalt, tar, lubricating oils, mineral oil, fuel oil	0	0

Low Viscosity, Low Volatility

The first group comprises substances with low viscosity and insignificant volatility, making pulmonary complications the sole toxic complication. Mineral seal oil is the most commonly ingested product in this group. Systemic absorption of this compound is virtually nil.[11]

Intermediate Viscosity, Intermediate Volatility

The second group is low to intermediate in viscosity and intermediate in volatility. These agents cause aspiration pneumonitis and include gasoline, kerosene, and other similar mixed hydrocarbons.

High Volatility

The third group contains the highly volatile substances whose viscosity is not important to their toxicity. These agents are mainly the aromatic agents and are responsible for CNS and systemic poisoning. Examples are the aromatic hydrocarbons toluene, xylene, benzene, and some chlorinated hydrocarbons.

High Viscosity, Low Volatility

The fourth group of hydrocarbons poses no hazard to either the pulmonary system or the CNS because they are of low volatility and high viscosity. This group contains asphalt or tar, lubricating oils, mineral oil, and fuel oil.[20]

CLINICAL FEATURES OF INTOXICATION

Respiratory

Controversy has existed through the years as to whether the pulmonary insult from hydrocarbons is a result of systemic absorption or a direct effect of ingestion.[13] Evidence has now conclusively shown that the hydrocarbons are aspirated directly into the lungs during ingestion or subsequent emesis and that they do not cause lung damage after absorption through the gastrointestinal tract.[18]

Most patients brought to medical attention after hydrocarbon ingestion do not experience any pulmonary symptoms.[1] Only 10% to 25% of patients develop clinical or roentgenographic evidence of pulmonary involvement.[1] If aspiration does occur chemical destruction of surfactant may develop, resulting in severe ventilation and perfusion inequalities caused by alveolar and small airway closure. This leads to marked hypoxemia. Damage to the epithelial lining and pulmonary capillaries results in pathological findings such as interstitial inflammation, hyperemia, vascular thrombosis, hyaline membranes, and atelectasis.[22]

The accidental aspiration of liquids from the mouth occurs in just a few seconds, and usually the volume of liquid aspirated is self-limiting in a conscious individual. As soon as the liquid enters the lungs, normal physiological reflexes such as a momentary reflex cessation of breathing and the more active expulsive mechanism of coughing oppose further entry of the liquid. If symptoms occur after ingestion of the hydrocarbon, they are due to its being rapidly dispersed over the pharyngeal and glottic surfaces, with the more volatile components becoming gases on contact with the warm mucous membranes (Table 47-6).[23]

Initially, there may be a burning sensation in the mouth and throat that is followed by gagging, choking, coughing, and grunting respirations. These symptoms should be considered presumptive evidence of aspiration.[18] An initial cyanosis, which is often noted within minutes of aspiration, may be due to the replacement of alveolar gas by the vaporized hydrocarbon.[23]

Fever may occur 30 minutes to several hours after aspiration and bears no relation to the severity of the illness. It is part of the body's inflammatory response to a foreign substance rather than an indication of infection. Although infection may occur, its symptoms usually develop after the first 48 to 72 hours, with no particular organism predominating.[3] Acute epiglottiditis has also been reported with the presentation of severe sore throat, dysphagia, and progressive respiratory distress.[24]

When signs and symptoms of aspiration are present, they usually progress during the first 24 hours and then subside over the next 1 to 4 days. Should death occur it is attributable to pulmonary insufficiency and not CNS involvement.

Central Nervous System

In hydrocarbon poisoning CNS symptoms are rare.[7] When they do occur they may include lightheadedness, lethargy, dizziness, headache, nausea, weakness, and fatigue that can progress to confusion, excitement, visual disturbances, seizures, and coma (Table 47-7).[25]

Early theories regarding hydrocarbon poisoning tended to hold that CNS depression was a frequent and often serious complication of ingestion and that this was due to absorption into the systemic circulation.[2] It has been shown that, although systemic absorption does occur, patients must ingest large doses (more than 4 to 5 mL/kg) for CNS toxicity to occur.[18] The more likely mechanism for CNS dysfunction is hypoxia secondary to the pulmonary aspiration with subsequent respiratory damage.[26] In other words, when CNS symptoms occur they are secondary to hypoxia from the aspiration rather

Table 47-6 Respiratory Symptoms of Hydrocarbon Ingestion

Burning sensation in the mouth
Gagging
Choking
Cough
Grunting respirations
Cyanosis
Fever
Acute epiglottiditis (rare)

Table 47-7 Central Nervous System Symptoms of Hydrocarbon Ingestion

Lightheadedness
Lethargy
Dizziness
Confusion
Excitement
Headache
Visual disturbances
Seizures
Coma

than from any direct CNS toxicity from the hydrocarbon.[23] Although the aliphatic hydrocarbons typically produce CNS alterations secondary to hypoxia, the more volatile aromatic hydrocarbons such as benzene, toluene, and xylene are associated with a greater risk of systemic and CNS toxicity.[2] Hypoxia need not be present for CNS symptoms to appear with these aromatic compounds.

Gastrointestinal

Gastrointestinal effects of hydrocarbon poisoning, such as nausea, vomiting, abdominal pain, and diarrhea, are usually mild and are due to direct mucosal irritation.[4]

Cutaneous

Hydrocarbons in direct contact with the skin can cause dermatitis and burns. Dermatitis may manifest as comedones, acne, folliculitis, or photosensitivity.[4] Contact burns occur because of the fat-solvency properties of some of the hydrocarbons.[9,27] Burns that have been described with prolonged contact consist of erythema, with blister formation noted within 24 hours.[28] The burn is usually partial, and healing occurs in approximately 21 days, leaving behind a pink-stained area representing the dyestuffs in the hydrocarbon.[27]

In addition to local toxicity, certain hydrocarbons are readily absorbed through the skin and may cause toxic symptoms. Finally, the potential fire hazard posed by the hydrocarbons should always be considered; great care should be taken to avoid accidental ignition of hydrocarbons on the skin or clothing.[27]

Systemic

Systemic toxicity has been associated with some of the hydrocarbons or additives to hydrocarbon products (Table 47-8); symptoms are related to the chemical composition and volatility of the ingested substance. For example, the aromatics have a greater degree of systemic toxicity than the aliphatics. Ingestions of these substances should be treated differently from ingestions of fuels and furniture polishes because of this greater risk of systemic toxicity. The risk of aspiration for these compounds is relatively minor.[2]

Benzene

Benzene, also known as benzol, is an aromatic hydrocarbon obtained by fractional distillation of light oil of tar; it contains traces of carbon disulfide, phenol, toluene, xylene, and other substances.[11]

Benzene is widely regarded as the most dangerous hydrocarbon used in industry today.[6] It is rapidly absorbed upon ingestion, inhalation, or skin contamination and has a particular affinity for nerve tissue. Symptoms of intoxication may include marked excitatory effects with subsequent depression and respiratory failure. Chronic poisoning is much more common than acute poisoning and may result in hematologic abnormalities such as leukopenia, aplastic anemia, and acute myeloblastic leukemia (Table 47-9).[11] Because of its toxic potential, benzene has been banned as an ingredient in products intended for use in the home.[13]

Table 47-8 Hydrocarbons and Additives to Hydrocarbon Products That Cause Systemic Toxicity (Acronym: CHAMP)

C	Camphor
H	Halogenated hydrocarbons
	Tetrachloroethane
	Trichloroethane
	Carbon tetrachloride
	Freons
A	Aromatic hydrocarbons
	Benzene
	Toluene
	Xylene
	Aniline dyes
M	Metals
	Mercury
	Lead
	Arsenic
P	Pesticides (see Chapters 44 and 45)

Table 47-9 Symptoms of Benzene Intoxication

Aplastic anemia
Hepatic failure
Renal failure
Cardiac dysrhythmias
Respiratory depression
CNS depression

Toluene and Xylene

Toluene, which is a product of the distillation of coal tar, is used in industry in the manufacturing of paint, rubber, and plastic cements.[28] It has been described as causing a type I distal renal tubular acidosis and consequently carries a risk of causing systemic toxicity.[6] A potentially serious and sometimes life-threatening reaction to repeated toluene abuse is hypokalemic muscle paralysis secondary to renal tubular acidosis. Characteristic symptoms of toluene intoxication include hallucinations, combativeness, blurred vision, ataxia, slurred speech, and stupor (Table 47-10).

Toluene is metabolized by benzyl alcohol to benzoic acid and is excreted largely as hippuric acid. This may contribute to an anion gap metabolic acidosis in addition to the hyperchloremic metabolic acidosis secondary to the renal tubular acidosis.[28] The toxicity of xylene is similar to that of toluene.

Table 47-10 Symptoms of Toluene and Xylene Intoxication

CNS depression
Renal tubular acidosis
Cardiac dysrhythmias
Anion gap metabolic acidosis
Hypokalemia
Neuritis
Psychiatric disturbances
Bone marrow depression
Abdominal pain
Brain atrophy

Substances Added to Hydrocarbon Products

In addition to systemically toxic hydrocarbons, there are certain additives to hydrocarbon products for which the hydrocarbon acts only as the solvent. The toxicity of the additive is of concern in such materials.[4]

Camphor

Camphor can cause CNS stimulation and seizures (Table 47-11).

Metals

Metals attach to sulfhydryl groups in enzymes and cause multisystem organ failure (see Part X).

Aniline Dyes

Aniline dyes, which are manufactured from nitrobenzene, are sometimes added to hydrocarbons. Both aniline dyes and nitrobenzene can cause methemoglobinemia, hemolytic anemia, and CNS depression.

Halogenated Hydrocarbons

The halogenated hydrocarbons, such as carbon tetrachloride and trichloroethane, are in widespread use in both industry and the home and have potential multisystem toxicity (Table 47-12).[29,30] These hydrocarbons are excellent solvents for oils, waxes, and fats and are used as dry cleaning agents and surface degreasing compounds. In addition, they serve as vehicles for paints, varnishes, and other coatings. The most widely available halogenated hydrocarbon in household products is tri-

Table 47-11 Symptoms of Camphor Intoxication

CNS stimulation
Seizures
Circulatory collapse
Enteritis

Table 47-12 Symptoms of Intoxication with Halogenated Hydrocarbons

Cardiac dysrhythmias
Hepatitis
Nephritis
Gastroenteritis
CNS depression

Table 47-13 Laboratory Studies in Hydrocarbon Intoxication

Chest roentgenography
Bibasilar infiltrate
Atelectasis
Hemorrhagic bronchopneumonia
Pulmonary edema
Pleural effusion
Pneumothorax
Pneumomediastinum
Pneumatoceles
Arterial blood gases
Complete blood cell count
Serum electrolytes (for toluene or xylene poisoning)
Serum and urine metal concentrations
Methemoglobin concentration (for aniline or nitrobenzene poisoning)

chloroethane, which has replaced carbon tetrachloride in domestic solvents and cleaners.

LABORATORY DETERMINATIONS

Chest Roentgenography

Chest roentgenography is the single most important laboratory procedure in diagnosing hydrocarbon intoxication (Table 47-13); abnormalities usually appear by 12 hours after exposure.[2,4,31] The roentgenogram can be obtained in the acute phase and may be positive even within 30 minutes after an aspiration.[32]

Any pattern of infiltrate may be seen. Initially the roentgenogram may disclose fine, punctate, mottled densities in the perihilar areas that extend into the midlung.[23] Later, a patchy bibasilar infiltrate or atelectasis may be noted.[11] The roentgenographic abnormalities are most often bilateral, reach their maximum at 72 hours, and usually clear within a few additional days without residual abnormality.[33] The vast majority of patients with moderately severe to severe parenchymal disease show complete resolution of roentgenographic signs without complication.[10,34] Clinical symptoms usually correlate poorly with roentgenographic findings because the film may often be positive in the absence of respiratory symptoms.[11] In addition, resolution of the roentgenographic changes tends to lag behind clinical improvement.[32]

In addition to the signs of chemical irritation, hemorrhagic bronchopneumonia and pulmonary edema may be noted in the most severe cases.[23] Pleural effusion, pneumothorax, subcutaneous emphysema, pneumopericardium, pneumomediastinum, pneumatoceles, and cysts may form days after the aspiration of a hydrocarbon.[23,24]

Pneumatoceles are thought to result from overdistension and rupture of alveoli secondary to the intense inflammatory reaction in the bronchi.[34] They form after consolidation has cleared; this may be within days or weeks of aspiration. Most pneumatoceles contain fluid that is easily demonstrated on frontal and lateral views of the upright chest. They may appear as unexpected findings on chest roentgenograms without evidence of pneumothorax or empyema.[23,34]

Arterial Blood Gases

Arterial blood gases may be measured to ascertain the extent of hypoxemia. Values may reflect subtle abnormalities that may not be noted on the physical examination or radiographic studies.[32]

Complete Blood Cell Count

Although an acute leukocytosis is often noted early after an ingestion as a result of the irritant effect of the hydrocarbon, a persistent elevation in the white blood cell count after 48 hours is suggestive of bacterial superinfection. The degree of leukocytosis does not correlate well with severity of pneumonitis, nor does a normal white blood cell count exclude a pneumonitis.[33]

Miscellaneous

Serum electrolytes should be measured when chronic toluene ingestion or inhalation has occurred. Nitrobenzene and aniline cause a methemoglobinemia, so that methemoglobin concentrations should be measured. Serum and 24-hour urine concentrations of metals should be measured if these substances were ingested; values serve as a guide to chelation therapy.

With gas chromatography, quantitative hydrocarbon determinations from blood, urine, or expired air are possible. Such tests may help in the identification of the ingested substance but usually offer little help in clinical management and are therefore only necessary for forensic or medicolegal purposes.[4,11,35]

TREATMENT

There are three important points concerning hydrocarbon ingestion that must be kept in mind in treatment planning. First, the average volume that a child can swallow in one mouthful is less than 1 teaspoon (2.5 to 5 mL); for an adult the average volume is 3 teaspoons.[36] Second, it is rare for a patient to ingest more than two tablespoons of a substance.[1,4,14,37,38] Third, in general the patient who is asymptomatic at the time of initial evaluation remains asymptomatic regardless of the findings on the initial chest roentgenogram.

Supportive Care

Supportive care is the mainstay of treatment of hydrocarbon exposure (Table 47-14). If the airway is obstructed it should be cleared and suctioned. Supplemental oxygen is indicated in all hypoxemic patients. In severe intoxications, constant positive airway pressure in spontaneously breathing patients and positive end-expiratory pressure in ventilated patients prevents airway closure, thus improving the ventilation-perfusion ratios.[1] Because this therapy has

Table 47-14 Treatment of Hydrocarbon Exposure

Supportive care
Oxygen
Decontamination
Bronchodilators (theophylline)

Contraindicated measures
   Activated charcoal
   Emesis or lavage (in general)
   Prophylactic antibiotics
   Corticosteroids
   Oils

been associated with pneumothorax, however, it should be used with caution because these patients have lesions predisposing to pneumatoceles and pneumothorax.[39]

Decontamination

Decontamination may be necessary if there was any spillage of the material on the skin or clothes; this is done to prevent skin irritation and burns as well as to decrease cutaneous absorption. Exposed skin should be cleansed with water and soap.

Prevention of Absorption

The most important principle in the treatment of a patient with a hydrocarbon pneumonitis is prevention of further hydrocarbon aspiration. Because large volumes of hydrocarbons in the gastrointestinal tract can generally be tolerated without severe systemic changes, vomiting should not be induced nor should gastric lavage be attempted unless it is absolutely necessary.[18] There are differing reports as to the efficacy of activated charcoal, and although there is no contraindication to its use it is probably not necessary or wise to administer an agent that may cause emesis.[13]

Administration of Oils

In the past, the use of vegetable and mineral oils was suggested for hydrocarbon ingestion because they were thought to act as miscible agents to minimize the risk of absorption. Not only is this therapy ineffective, but it may increase the risk of lipoid pneumonitis, which is a nonfatal, low-grade, localized tissue reaction different and much less severe than a hydrocarbon pneumonitis.[11]

Gastrointestinal Emptying Procedures

For most hydrocarbon ingestions emesis or lavage does not improve the outcome, and neither is indicated for ingestions of the volatile hydrocarbons. In contrast, the systemic toxicity associated with aromatic hydrocarbons, additives to hydrocarbon products, and halogenated hydrocarbons requires that these substances be removed by gastrointestinal emptying procedures.

Indications

Emesis appears to be superior to lavage in decreasing the aspiration hazard,[2,11,37,40] although this is still an area of controversy. Emesis is indicated after the ingestion of benzene, toluene, halogenated hydrocarbons, camphor, heavy metals, pesticides, or any other systemically toxic ingredient[11] or if the dose of petroleum distillate ingested was greater than 4 to 5 mL/kg.

Contraindications

Emesis is not recommended if the patient has had a significant unprovoked emesis, is seizing, or lacks a gag reflex.[11] In addition, the ingestion of mineral seal oil, kerosene, petroleum naphtha, fuel oil, mineral, and lubricating oils, and mineral spirits in any quantity need not be retrieved.[2,8] Emesis is also contraindicated if the patient has ingested a high-viscosity, high–surface tension liquid such as grease, petroleum jelly, paraffin wax, tar, glues, or asphalt.

Use of Bronchodilators

Bronchodilators may be necessary if bronchoconstriction is present.[33] This condition occurs because of the direct irritant effect of hydrocarbons on the bronchioles. Bronchodilators such as theophylline may be beneficial in symptomatic patients.[4] Epinephrine and other sympathomimetics should be avoided if the patient has ingested a material that can sensitize the myocardium to catecholamines and cause ventricular fibrillation.

Use of Antibiotics

Fever that follows hydrocarbon aspiration is the result of tissue damage rather than infection.[33] Although the temptation is great to use antibiotics, they should not be used prophylactically because this may select out organisms that will be resistant to the antibiotic at a later time. The onset of fever after the first 48 hours may indicate secondary infection; treatment is then guided by appropriate bacterial cultures and Gram stain.[18,33]

Use of Corticosteroids

Corticosteroids in theory may be of benefit in the prevention of pulmonary reaction and subsequent edema, fibrosis, and hemorrhage, but controlled clinical studies have not demonstrated a therapeutic or prophylactic role.[41] In addition, corticosteroids have been shown to abolish the mononuclear response to pneumonitis and to decrease the protection against infection; they should therefore not be used.[1,15,23]

Recommendations for Admission

If the patient is asymptomatic with a normal chest roentgenogram, no hospitalization is necessary if symptoms do not occur within a 6-hour period of observation.[1] The same applies to the asymptomatic patient with an abnormal chest roentgenogram; a repeat roentgenogram is optional. The symptomatic patient, even with a normal chest roentgenogram, should be admitted if symptoms persist or worsen.[1] The asymptomatic individual who has ingested dangerous hydrocarbon additives should also be admitted.

REFERENCES

1. Anas N, Namasonthi V, Ginsburg C: Criteria for hospitalizing children who have ingested products containing hydrocarbons. *JAMA* 1981;246:840–843.

2. Zieserl E: Hydrocarbon ingestion and poisoning. *Compr Ther* 1979;5:35–42.

3. Shirkey H: Treatment of petroleum distillate ingestion. *Mod Treat* 1971;8:580–592.

4. Wasserman G: Hydrocarbon poisoning. *Crit Care Q* 1982;4:33–41.

5. Moriarty R: Petroleum distillate poisonings. *Drug Ther* 1979;9:47–51.

6. Geehr E: Management of hydrocarbon ingestions. *Top Emerg Med* 1979;1:97–110.

7. Wolfsdorf J: Kerosene intoxication: An experimental approach to the etiology of the CNS manifestations in primates. *J Pediatr* 1976;88:1037–1040.

8. Bratton L, Huddow J: Ingestion of charcoal lighter fluid. *J Pediatr* 1975;87:633–636.

9. Ainsworth R: Petro-vapor poisoning. *Br Med J* 1950;1:1547–1548.

10. Gurwitz D, Kattan M, Levison H, et al: Pulmonary function abnormalities in asymptomatic children after hydrocarbon pneumonitis. *Pediatrics* 1978;62:789–794.

11. Goldfrank K, Kirstein R, Bresnitz E: Gasoline and other hydrocarbons. *Hosp Physician* 1979;15:32–38.

12. Hansen K, Sharp F: Gasoline sniffing, lead poisoning, and myoclonus. *JAMA* 1978;240:1375–1376.

13. Arena J: Emergency treatment of hydrocarbon product ingestion. *JAMA* 1973;226:213–217.

14. Cachia E, Fenech F: Kerosene poisoning in children. *Arch Dis Child* 1964;39: 502–505.

15. Brown J, Burke B, Dajani A: Experimental kerosene pneumonia: Evaluation of some therapeutic regimens. *J Pediatr* 1974;84:396–401.

16. Harris W: Toxic effects of aerosol propellants on the heart. *Arch Intern Med* 1973;131:162–166.

17. Bass M: Sudden sniffing death. *JAMA* 1970; 212:2075–2079.

18. Boeckx R, Postl B, Coodin F: Gasoline sniffing and tetraethyl lead poisoning in children. *Pediatrics* 1977; 60:140–145.

19. Hayden J, Comstock B: The clinical toxicology of solvent abuse. *Clin Toxicol* 1976;9:169–184.

20. Gerarde H: Toxicological studies on hydrocarbons. *Toxicol Appl Pharmacol* 1959;1:462–474.

21. Panson R, Winek C: Aspiration toxicity of ketones. *Clin Toxicol* 1980;17:271–317.

22. Glaser H, Massengale D: Glue sniffing in children. *JAMA* 1962;181:300–303.

23. Campbell J: Pneumatocele formation following hydrocarbon ingestion. *Am Rev Resp Dis* 1970;101:414–417.

24. Grufferman S, Walker F: Supraglottitis following gasoline ingestion. *Ann Emerg Med* 1982;11:368–370.

25. Coulehan J, Hirsch W, Brillman J, et al: Gasoline sniffing and lead toxicity in Navajo adolescents. *Pediatrics* 1983;71:113–117.

26. Cohen S: The volatile solvents. *Public Health Rev* 1973;2:185–213.

27. Hunter G: Chemical burns of the skin after contact with petrol. *Br J Plast Surg* 1968;21:338–341.

28. Binns H, Gursel E, Wilson N: Gasoline contact burns. *JACEP* 1978;7:404–405.

29. Flowers N, Haran L: Nonanoxic aerosol arrhythmias. *JAMA* 1972;219:33–37.

30. Flowers N, Haran L: The electrical sequelae of aerosol inhalation. *Am Heart J* 1972;83:644–651.

31. Daeschner C, Blattner R, Collins V: Hydrocarbon pneumonitis. *Pediatr Clin North Am* 1957;4:243–249.

32. Dice W, Ward G, Kelley J, et al: Pulmonary toxicity following gastrointestinal ingestion of kerosene. *Ann Emerg Med* 1982;11:138–142.

33. Karlson K: Hydrocarbon poisoning in children. *South Med J* 1982;75:839–840.

34. Bergeson P, Hales S, Lustgarten M, et al: Pneumatoceles following hydrocarbon ingestion. *Am J Dis Child* 1975;129:49–54.

35. Dollery C, Dows D, Draffan G, et al: Blood concentration in man of fluorinated hydrocarbons after inhalation of pressurized aerosols. *Lancet* 1970;2:1164–1166.

36. Jones D, Work C: Volume of a swallow. *Am J Dis Child* 1961;102:427–429.

37. Press E, Done A: Solvent sniffing. *Pediatrics* 1967; 39:451–461.

38. Press E: Cooperative kerosene poisoning study: Evaluation of gastric lavage and other factors in the treatment of accidental ingestion of petroleum distillate products. *Pediatrics* 1962;29:648–662.

39. Gerarde H: Toxicological studies on hydrocarbons. *Arch Environ Health* 1963;6:325–341.

40. Ng R, Darawish H, Stewart D: Emergency treatment of petroleum distillate and turpentine ingestion. *Can Med Assoc J* 1974;111:537–538.

41. Marks M, Chicoine L, Legere G, et al: Adrenocorticosteroid treatment of hydrocarbon pneumonia in children: A cooperative study. *J Pediatr* 1972;81:366–369.

ADDITIONAL SELECTED REFERENCES

Baldachin B, Melmed R: Clinical and therapeutic aspects of kerosene poisoning. *Br Med J* 1964;2:28–30.

Eade N, Taussig L, Marks M: Hydrocarbon pneumonitis. *Pediatrics* 1974;54:351–356.

Kirk L, Martin K: Sudden death from toluene abuse. *Ann Emerg Med* 1984;13:68–69.

Law W, Nelson E: Gasoline sniffing by an adult: Report of a case with the unusual complication of lead encephalopathy. *JAMA* 1968;204:1002–1004.

Massengale O, Glaser H, LeLievre R, et al: Physical and psychologic factors in glue sniffing. *N Engl J Med* 1963; 269:1340–1344.

Polkis A, Burkett C: Gasoline sniffing: A review. *Clin Toxicol* 1977;11:35–41.

Reinhardt C, Azar A, Maxfield M, et al: Cardiac arrhythmias and aerosol "sniffing." *Arch Environ Health* 1971; 22:265–279.

Robinson R: Tetraethyl lead poisoning from gasoline sniffing. *JAMA* 1978;240:1373–1374.

Seshia S, Rajani K, Boeckx R, et al: The neurological manifestations of chronic inhalation of leaded gasoline. *Dev Med Child Neurol* 1978;2:323–324.

Sperling F: In vivo and in vitro toxicology of turpentine. *Clin Toxicol* 1969;2:21–35.

Streicher H, Gabow P, Moss A, et al: Syndromes of toluene sniffing in adults. *Ann Intern Med* 1981;94:758–762.

Talker S, Anderson R, McCartney R, et al: Renal tubular acidosis associated with toluene "sniffing." *N Engl J Med* 1974;290:765–768.

Taylor G, Harris W: Cardiac toxicity of aerosol propellents. *JAMA* 1970;214:81–85.

Taylor G, Harris W: Glue sniffing causes heart block in mice. *Science* 1970;170:866–868.

Valpey R, Sumi S, Corass M, et al: Acute and chronic progressive encephalopathy due to gasoline sniffing. *Neurology* 1978;28:507–510.

Young R, Grzyb S, Crismon L: Recurrent cerebellar dysfunction as related to chronic gasoline sniffing in an adolescent girl. *Clin Pediatr* 1977;16:706–708.

chapter 48

Plants

The ubiquity of poisonous plants in homes, fields, and gardens makes plant poisoning an ever-present potential health hazard. Phytotoxicology is the study of poisonings of humans and animals by plants.[1] As both medicinal agents and poisons, plants have been prominent in history, in the healing arts, in religious rituals, and as homicidal and suicidal agents.[2] The attractive appearance of many plants or plant parts often entices children and adults to sample them.[3] With the increasing popular interest in horticulture and health foods and the recent surge in outdoor camping activity, the number of cases of plant intoxication is increasing and is likely to continue to rise.

Plant ingestion may extend the treating physician beyond the limits of existing sources of medical knowledge, but emergency department staff should be able to recognize toxic house plants and should to some extent know the symptoms produced by their ingestion as well as appropriate treatment.[4] Although there are thousands of species of plants capable of producing moderate to severe and possibly fatal poisoning relatively few cases of serious intoxication occur in the United States, and these are associated with a limited number of plants.[5]

Poisonous plants may produce a wide range of clinical effects, some relatively minor and others severe enough to be fatal. The exact amounts required to produce toxic effects vary, depending on the type and part of the plant ingested, the age of the patient, and the season of the year. No botanical relationship exists to help localize toxicity in the plant kingdom.[3] Nearly all major groups of plants from algae and fungi through gymnosperms and angiosperms have ample toxic representatives scattered among them. Some plants poison if they are chewed or swallowed. Others poison by causing allergies, dermatitis, or mechanical injury.[4] Some plants are harmful if eaten or chewed at certain stages of their growth, and others are toxic at all stages. Parts of a plant can differ greatly in toxicity. A good example is rhubarb, which has a stalk that is commonly eaten but a leaf blade that is very toxic.[2]

Common or vernacular names are an entirely inadequate means of specifying plants, and without reliable determination of the botanical name the existing toxicological information concerning a given plant is unavailable for review. Definitive identification should be left to a professionally trained botanist. As an example, the common name ''hemlock'' may mean many different things. Water hemlock may cause seizures and is different from poison hemlock, which causes muscular paralysis.[1,3] Ground hemlock is another name for the native American yew and causes completely different symptoms. The hemlock tree, a conifer, is not considered poisonous. This chapter is not intended to provide detailed botanical classifications but to identify various classes of symptoms and signs caused by the various groups of plants.

A detailed history may be critical for distinguishing a potentially lethal ingestion from a mildly noxious exposure. Elements important in the history include onset of symptoms from time of ingestion, parts and amount of the plant consumed, initial symptoms, and method of preparation of the plant.

Patients poisoned by plant ingestion are asymptomatic in the great majority of cases. Rarely will a patient become mildly symptomatic.[6] Most patients present to the emergency department shortly after their symptoms begin, and in plant poisoning the presenting symptoms usually dictate the appropriate therapy because in most instances there is neither a specific treatment nor an antidote. The initial approach to management of any plant ingestion should be the same as that for any toxic ingestion. There is rarely a way to enhance the excretion of most ingested plants, so that there is typically no role for hemodialysis or hemoperfusion.[1]

In symptomatic patients, the important baseline laboratory tests are dictated on the basis of the type of plant ingested. Laboratory tests may include complete blood cell count; measurements of serum electrolytes, blood urea nitrogen, and serum creatinine; and urinalysis. If oxalate has been ingested, serum calcium and phosphorus measurements may be necessary. If a hepatotoxin is suspected, liver function and coagulation studies are recommended. For suspected cardiac glycosides, an electrocardiogram is necessary.[2]

The noxious chemicals in plants may be classified as alkaloids, glycosides, resins, phenols, alcohols, oxalates, and phytotoxins. Plants can also be grouped according to the symptoms produced on ingestion, which are based on the type of active compound in the plant or plant part. In this chapter plants are divided into the alkaloids, which include the belladonna group as well as the group associated with nicotine; the glycosides, which include the cardiac glycosides and cyanogenic glycosides; plants that cause direct skin injury on contact, such as those that contain oxalate; the gastrointestinal irritants; the hallucinogens; plants that cause seizures; plants that contain pressor amines; and plants that contain miscellaneous compounds.[3,4]

PLANTS THAT CONTAIN ALKALOIDS

Anticholinergic Alkaloids

The tropane alkaloids are often called belladonna alkaloids.[7] Plants that contain belladonna alkaloids produce their clinical effects by competitive inhibition of acetylcholine, whereby a dose-related blockade of the cholinergic nervous system develops. These plants may contain active ingredients such as atropine (hyoscyamine), scopolamine (hyoscine), stramonium alkaloids, and ecgonine compounds (Table 48-1).

The tropane alkaloids are rapidly absorbed from the gastrointestinal tract, mucosal surfaces, and respiratory tree.[8] The drugs are hydrolyzed in the liver and excreted in the urine. Young children are more sensitive to atropine poisoning than adults because of their lower tolerance to elevated body temperature, which may be caused by these agents.[9]

Datura species are the most commonly ingested anticholinergic plants. Common names include Jamestown weed, jimson weed, loco weed, devil's weed, and thornapple.[1] All parts of the plant are toxic. Jimson weed is widely distributed in fields and waste areas throughout the United States, especially in the south. The plant has white to purplish flowers and prickly seed pods. Adult poisonings are usually the result of ingesting tea made from the flowers, seeds, or leaves of jimson weed.[3]

Symptoms and treatment of anticholinergic poisoning are discussed in Chapter 7.

Solanine Alkaloids

The plant genus *Solanum* includes some 1500 species, and most contain the alkaloid solanine (Table 48-2). Some common plants that contain solanine include the potato (*Solanum tuberosum*) and the Jerusalem cherry (*Solanum pseudo-capsicum*).[10] The common

Table 48-1 Plants That Cause Anticholinergic Syndrome

Datura species (jimson weed)
Atropa belladonna (deadly nightshade)
Cestrum sp (jasmine)
Hyoscyamus niger (henbane)
Lycium haliamifolium (matrimony vine)

Table 48-2 Plants Containing Solanine

Solanum pseudo-capsicum (Jerusalem cherry)
Solanum tuberosum (potato)

Table 48-3 Nicotinelike Alkaloids

Common Name	Botanical Name	Alkaloid
Tobacco	*Nicotiana* sp	Nicotine
Golden chain tree	*Laburnum anagyroides*	Cytisine
Poison hemlock	*Conium maculatum*	Coniine

potato can cause intoxication from ingestion of leaves, all green parts of the plant, and the roots, which contain high concentrations of solanine. The Jerusalem cherry is a potted plant with attractive red berries that often appears in households during the Christmas season.

Solanine is a glycoalkaloid that when hydrolyzed by gastric acid yields a sugar and an alkamine.[6] The intact glycoalkaloid is an irritant to the mucous membranes and the gastrointestinal tract. The alkamine primarily affects the CNS, and the cardiovascular system.[1] Initial symptoms are burning of the mouth and oropharynx; gastrointestinal symptoms including nausea, vomiting, and diarrhea then develop. Neurologic symptoms include apathy, hallucinations, tremor, paralysis, and mydriasis.[5] Patients with solanine poisoning may also develop concomitant signs of anticholinergic poisoning. Most symptoms resolve within 24 hours, and deaths are rare.[2]

Nicotinelike Alkaloids

Plants containing nicotine, cytisine, and coniine all exert similar toxic actions. These are all pyridine or piperidine alkaloids; other substances of this type include lobeline, arecoline, and piperine (Table 48-3). The toxic effects of nicotine and treatment of intoxication are discussed fully in Chapter 44.

Fatalities from nicotine-containing plants have occurred with the ingestion of "salads" prepared from wild tobacco leaves (*Nicotiana*

sp). Symptoms can also occur from the ingestion of cigarettes, cigars, cigarette butts, snuff, and Nicorette® gum. The action of nicotine and its cogeners on neuroeffector junctions is rapid and variable. There is an initial stimulation of autonomic ganglia with a subsequent depression of transmission. Nicotine similarly affects the neuromuscular junction, with a stimulatory phase that is followed rapidly by paralysis.[3]

Cytisine poisoning is most commonly encountered in children who shell and eat the seeds from the pealike pods of the golden chain tree (*Laburnum anagyroides*).

Coniine, which is the principal alkaloid in poison hemlock, is a pyridine derivative similar to nicotine. Coniine poisoning usually results from eating of the parsleylike leaves or seeds of poison hemlock (*Conium maculatum*).[1] Poison hemlock is a European plant that was introduced into North America and grows in marshy areas; it should not be confused with water hemlock.[1] Poison hemlock and wild carrot both have a long, white, unbranched, turniplike taproot. The white flowers bloom in flat clusters and emit a strong odor of urine when crushed. The entire plant contains coniine, especially the seeds and roots. Poison hemlock eventually acts by depressing the CNS and bringing on paralysis. Death ensues when the muscles of respiration become paralyzed.[2]

Clinical Effects of Intoxication

Initial symptoms result from stimulation of autonomic ganglia. Clinical symptoms, however, are mixed because of the variability of the clinical response. Usually there is a spontaneous emesis within 15 to 30 minutes after ingestion. Initial parasympathomimetic signs change to sympathomimetic signs, and bradycardia, miosis, and hyperventilation may change to tachycardia and mydriasis. Seizures and hypotension may ultimately occur, along with respiratory failure.

Treatment

Treatment consists of supportive measures. It may be a mistake to treat the initial bradycardia with atropine because this naturally progresses to a tachycardia. If treatment of the bradycardia is necessary, temporary cardiac pacing may be indicated.

Purine Alkaloids

The purine alkaloids caffeine and theobromine are found in various plants. The derivative beverages may represent a toxic risk.[5]

Chapter 31 includes a discussion of caffeine toxicity.

PLANTS THAT CONTAIN GLYCOSIDES

Cardiac Glycosides

Plants that contain cardiac glycosides are the most widely used in standard medicine (Table 48-4). There are a number of varieties of these plants, including foxglove (*Digitalis purpurea*), oleander (*Nerium oleander*), and lily of the valley (*Convallaria majalis*).[11] Neither boiling nor drying affects the toxicity of these plants.

Glycosides in *Nerium oleander* include oleandrin, oleandroside, nerioside, and digitoxigenin. Yellow oleander contains thevetin and thevetoxin.[1] Oleander is a shrub that grows up to 20 feet in height. It is an extremely hardy plant and is popular because of the ease with which it is grown and its attractive red, pink, or white clusters of flowers. The entire plant is toxic; toxicity is also associated with smoke from burning cuttings and water in which the flowers are placed.[2] In addition to causing cardiac toxicity oleander also irritates mucous membranes, causing buccal erythema and burning of the mouth. Gastrointestinal effects include nausea, vomiting, increased salivation, abdominal pain, and diarrhea.[11]

Table 48-4 Cardiac Glycoside–Containing Plants

Digitalis purpurea (foxglove)
Nerium oleander (oleander)
Urginea maritima (squill)
Convallaria majalis (lily of the valley)
Thevetia peruviana (yellow oleander)

Several reports note a cross-reactivity between digitalis and oleander glycoside in radioimmunoassays, causing elevation of the reported digoxin concentration after ingestion of oleander. Because the amount of cross-reactivity is unknown, digitalis radioimmunoassay predicts only the presence of the glycoside, not the degree of toxicity.

A detailed discussion of signs, symptoms, workup, and treatment of the patient with cardiac glycoside intoxication is given in Chapter 15.

Andromedotoxin

Azaleas, rhododendrons, and laurels contain andromedotoxin, which has properties similar to those of the cardiac glycosides or veratrum alkaloids. All 250 species of azalea (*Rhododendron occidental*) are poisonous, although this is an area of controversy.[12] Andromedotoxin may cause hypotension and bradycardia. Other effects include salivation, nasal discharge, anorexia, vomiting, and diarrhea. These may progress to drowsiness, headache, seizures, paralysis, and coma.[6]

Symptoms of poisoning usually begin within 1 to 2 hours of ingestion. Initially there is local irritation of the mouth and emesis.[13] In contrast to poisonings with the pure cardiac glycosides, poisoning with these plants is associated with gastrointestinal manifestations and abdominal pain due to the presence of saponins and other irritants. Visual disturbances may also be noted. In a patient with a normal heart toxicity is generally manifested by conduction defects rather than by increased automaticity, and an electrocardiogram may show atrioventricular conduction defects and sinus bradycardia. Hyperkalemia may occur in severe ingestions because of interference with the normal cellular sodium-potassium transport mechanism.[11]

Cyanogenic Glycosides

Glycosides that yield hydrocyanic acid on hydrolysis are known as cyanogenic glycosides. The most important glycoside in this group is amygdalin, which is abundant in plants of the Rosaceae family. A full discussion of these glycosides is given in Chapter 20.

PLANTS THAT CONTAIN OXALATE

Many species of *Arum* contain calcium oxalate as a toxic ingredient. Other genera of plants that contain oxalates include *Monstera* (Swiss cheese plant), *Colocasia* (elephant's-ear), *Caladium*, and *Xanthosoma* (Table 48-5).[14] Oxalates can be in the form of insoluble calcium oxalate crystals, called rhaphides, or soluble sodium and potassium oxalate. The insoluble calcium oxalate is found in dieffenbachia and *Caladium* species.[15] Soluble oxalates are found in the leaves of rhubarb (*Rheum rhaponticum*) and other plants and may be rapidly absorbed through the gastrointestinal tract, causing systemic effects secondary to hypocalcemia.[16]

The dieffenbachia are both indoor and outdoor plants and resemble sugar cane or the banana plant. The dieffenbachia have a thick green stem with oval leaves up to 15 inches long.[14] Plants may grow 3 to 6 feet in height or more.[15] All parts of the diffenbachia are toxic, including the leaves, stem, and roots. The sap can produce corneal opacification if it comes in contact with the eye.[2,15]

Plants of the genus *Philodendron* are extremely popular houseplants because they require little light and attention. The tuber of *Colocasia antiquorum* (elephant's-ear) is processed into a starchy food called poi, but the green parts contain oxalates and cause significant irritation when ingested. Rhubarb is a coarse perennial plant the leaf blade of which contains soluble oxalate.[3]

Clinical Effects of Intoxication

Ingestion of calcium oxalate causes extreme irritation of the mucous membranes. Biting or

Table 48-5 Oxalate-Containing Plants

Arum sp
Philodendron sp
Dieffenbachia (dumbcane)
Caladium sp
Colocasia sp (elephant's-ear)
Rheum rhaponticum (rhubarb)
Arisaema triphyllum (Jack-in-the-pulpit)
Symplocarpus foetidus (skunk cabbage)

chewing plants containing these chemicals rapidly produces severe pain, salivation, swelling of the oropharynx, and speech difficulties.[13] Corrosive burns of the mouth, oropharynx, esophagus, and stomach may ensue. The airway may become obstructed as the tongue enlarges.

On occasion, systemic toxicity may occur.[11] This is especially true for the soluble oxalates as a result of their rapid absorption from the gastrointestinal tract. After absorption, the oxalate combines with calcium in blood to form calcium oxalate, which is excreted by the kidney.[13] This decreases the amount of ionized calcium in the body and may lead to tetany, fasciculations, or seizures. Acute renal failure may ensue as a result of obstruction of the renal tubules by the calcium oxalate crystals as well as by the chemical action of the oxalate ion. Oxalate crystals in the ureter, kidney, and bladder may also cause pain, oxaluria, oliguria, and hematuria.

Laboratory Analysis and Treatment

A measurement of serum calcium concentrations is indicated in all ingestions, although it is rare for the hypocalcemia to be a symptomatic problem. Symptomatic and supportive care is usually the extent of necessary treatment. A patent airway is the first concern, and patients should be observed for airway obstruction. Ice may be used to reduce swelling. A mixture of 2% viscous lidocaine with diphenhydramine elixir may be applied to the affected areas for local pain relief. Hypocalcemia should be treated by the parenteral administration of calcium gluconate or some other calcium salt. Neither antihistamines nor corticosteroids have been shown to be effective. If calcium oxalate crystals are present in the urine, maintenance of an adequate urine flow is mandatory.[2]

PLANTS CAUSING SEIZURES

The principal plants responsible for producing seizures as their primary toxic manifestation are water hemlock (*Cicuta* sp: beaver poison, wild carrot, wild parsnip, and cowbane) and chinaberry (*Melia azederach*); both are members of the carrot family.[17] Water hemlock is possibly the most toxic plant that grows in the United States.[1] It is found only in wet, swampy areas and is most often ingested by individuals who mistake it for wild parsnips because of the yellow oil that is produced when the plant is injured.[17] All parts of the plant are toxic, including the roots, leaves, and stems. The toxin has been called cicutoxin and is a highly unsaturated alcohol.

Symptoms begin within 15 to 60 minutes of ingestion and initially consist of muscarinic effects such as salivation, abdominal pain, diarrhea, and vomiting. This prodrome may be followed quickly by multiple grand mal seizures. Other CNS effects such as obtundation and respiratory distress may occur. Death may be secondary to the prolonged anoxia encountered with the tonic contractions.[17]

Treatment is symptomatic and supportive. Maintenance of a patent airway and seizure precautions should be the first priorities. Seizures may be controlled with diazepam. Vigorous fluid replacement with isotonic saline may be required.[1]

PLANTS THAT CONTAIN PHYTOTOXINS

Toxalbumins are phytotoxins, which are the most potent toxins in existence. The two most lethal plants containing toxalbumins are the castor bean and the jequirity bean (Table 48-6). The castor bean contains the toxalbumin ricin, and the jequirity bean contains abrin.[16]

The castor bean, which is obtained from a woody shrub that grows up to 15 feet in height, is white, black, and brown in a variegated pattern somewhat resembling a tick.[1] This bean is native to Asia and Africa but now grows in many uncultivated areas in the United States.[14] Ricin is composed of large protein molecules and

Table 48-6 Plants Containing Toxalbumins

Ricinus communis (castor bean)
Abrus precatorius (jequirity bean, rosary pea, precatory bean)
Hura crepitans (sandbox tree)
Jatropha sp (bellyache bush, Barbados nut)
Robinia pseudoacacia (black locust)

---

resembles bacterial toxins in its structure and antigenic ability. Ricin has both hemagglutinin and toxic hemolytic components.[14]

Jequirity beans are brought into the United States from Central and South America. The bean is small and red in color with a black "eye" at the hilus.[10] Because of its intense colors it has been used extensively in beadwork and jewelry in the West Indies. Recently jequirity beans have been used in necklaces, belts, moccasins and slippers, bead bags, and rosaries and for eyes in dolls.[11] In addition to abrin the jequirity bean contains an amino acid, abric acid, and glycyrrhiza.[10] The mature bean, if ingested whole, is innocuous because the hard outer shell is unaffected by digestive secretions.[13] Chewing destroys the shell and allows absorption of the toxin. The immature bean, whose shell is soft and easily broken, is equally poisonous.[2]

Clinical Effects of Intoxication

The toxic effects of abrin are considered due both to the red cell agglutination and to a direct toxic action on parenchymal cells. Ricin causes the same symptoms as abrin but does not cause local toxicity.[1] Recently there has been some question as to the actual toxicity of ricin.

Toxicity may be noted in two phases (Table 48-7). During the acute phase, which may last 2 to 24 hours, there is burning in the mouth and throat with subsequent gastroenteritis. Nausea, vomiting, and abdominal pain may also occur, and severe hemorrhagic gastroenteritis may ensue. Because of the fluid loss, severe dehydration may result in oliguria and cardiovascular collapse. During the second phase stupor, seizures, and death have been reported. Systemic symptoms involving the CNS and the cardiovascular system may begin

Table 48-7 Signs and Symptoms of Phytotoxin Poisoning

Acute Phase
  Burning in the mouth
  Burning in the throat
  Nausea
  Vomiting
  Abdominal pain
  Hemorrhagic gastroenteritis
Delayed Symptoms
  CNS
    Stupor
    Seizures
    Coma
  Cardiovascular
    Hypotension
  Retinal hemorrhage
  Scleral hemorrhage
  Hepatic necrosis
  Renal failure

Table 48-8 *Toxicodendron* Species Causing Dermatitis

T radicans (poison ivy)
T quercifolium, T diversiloba (poison oak)
T vernix (poison sumac)

after a delay of up to several days and may persist for as long as 10 days. Patients may develop hypotension, CNS hemorrhage, and retinal and scleral hemorrhages.[14] Hepatic necrosis and renal failure have also been described.[16] Because these beans are highly allergenic, they may cause dermatitis, urticaria, or anaphylaxis after skin contact.

Treatment

Treatment is supportive.[3] The patient who is symptomatic and appears to have local burns should be treated as for any caustic burn. Close monitoring of the electrocardiogram and fluid and electrolyte status is the mainstay of supportive care. Vigorous fluid replacement in severe cases may be required to keep up with fluid losses.[18]

PLANTS AFFECTING THE SKIN

There is a long list of plants that are capable of causing dermatitis in sensitized individuals, but the most frequent offenders are plants of the family Anacardiaceae, which contains species of *Toxicodendron* (Table 48-8).[19] These include plants with the common names of poison ivy,

poison oak, and poison sumac. At one time these plants were mistakenly classed in the genus *Rhus*.[18]

The *Toxicodendron* species are vigorous woody vines or shrubs that have a characteristic trifolate pattern. All these plants contain urushiol, an oil that acts as a hapten and elicits a type IV cell–mediated delayed hypersensitivity.[18]

Poison ivy is found throughout the United States and appears as a short ropelike vine or small shrub. In the western United States poison oak is an upright spreading shrub with oaklike leaves that are hairy on both sides; it grows as a low shrub in the eastern United States. Poison sumac is predominantly found east of the Mississippi River and grows as a tall shrub or tree up to 15 feet in height.

Mechanism of Toxicity

Urushiols are catechols with long carbon side chains; the differences among the urushiols in the various *Toxicodendron* species depend essentially on the length of the side chain.[4] Catechol molecules from the urushiol enter the skin and bind to surface proteins in the epidermis and dermis to form complete antigens. These "presenter" cells (catechol molecules that enter skin) transfer the antigen to T_4-inducer lymphocytes. After a second urushiol challenge, the lymphocytes elicit a cell-mediated cytotoxic immune response characterized by erythema, edema, and vesiculation.

The dermatitis associated with these plants results from a delayed hypersensitivity reaction; there is no reaction from the first exposure. Subsequent exposures may result in a reaction within 24 to 48 hours of contact, depending on the sensitivity of the individual. Some individuals never develop dermatitis despite frequent contact.[4]

Treatment

Treatment consists of immediately washing the exposed areas with soap and water. Although this does not prevent the dermatitis, it does prevent spread of the toxic chemical to other parts of the body. Drug therapy may involve the use of topical or systemic steroids.[3] The use of a potent topical steroid cream with an oral antipruritic agent may be all that is necessary in some individuals with minor, localized reactions. For severely affected patients a course of high-dose oral steroids in addition to an antipruritic is necessary. Typically a 10-day regimen of steroids is begun, with the dose being decreased every other day.[18] Attempts at oral desensitization with extracts from these plants have not been shown to be effective.[19]

PLANTS CAUSING GASTROENTERITIS

Most plant intoxications in the United States occur from the ingestion of plants containing gastrointestinal irritants. The onset of the irritant response is variable and depends on the chemical nature of the toxin.[13]

Although almost all plants may cause some degree of gastroenteritis, two groups of toxic chemicals are more specific for causing gastrointestinal irritation. These are (1) ilicin and (2) phytolaccine, phytolaccotoxin, and saponins.[3]

Ilicin

Ilicin is contained in holly berries (*Ilex* sp) and causes severe gastroirritation including nausea, vomiting, and diarrhea. Rarely, it may also result in stupor, narcosis, and CNS depression.

Phytolaccine, Phytolaccotoxin, and Saponins

Phytolaccine and phytolaccotoxin are two of the active compounds in pokeweed (*Phytolacca americana*)[20]; saponins and glycoproteins are also concentrated in the root. This shrublike plant is indigenous to the United States. Other names for pokeweed include pokeberry, Virginia poke, garget, and inkberry. The plant measures from 3 to 10 feet in height and has stout, reddish-purple branched stems. In the fall, the plant dies down to the ground, and in late summer and early fall it produces white to purplish flowers and round clusters of dark purple berries with red juice; these may be attractive to young children. Stains from these berries may be on the hands of an intoxicated individual.[3] Pokeweed root is often mistaken for horseradish, parsnips, or Jerusalem artichoke, and the shoots are sometimes substituted for asparagus. Native Americans have used the plant as an emetic and purgative, and the plant is still used today as a folk remedy for pruritus. Powdered pokeweed root is sold in health food stores as an herbal tea preparation.[20]

The effects of pokeweed intoxication may arise from ingestion of any or all plant parts, with the root having the largest amount of toxin. Intoxications have also been reported from liquid preparations of plant extracts and through skin contact with the plant itself. Although pokeweed can cause major gastrointestinal symptoms, it is safe for consumption if it is cooked twice in two different cooking waters.

The main toxic agents of pokeweed are the glycoside saponins and a glycoprotein mitogen known as pokeweed mitogen[3]; saponins are irritants when applied to the skin or mucous membranes.[13] The saponin glycosides are found throughout the plant kingdom, for example in English Ivy (*Hedera helix*), ginseng (*Panax ginseng*), and licorice (*Glycyrrhiza glabra*). After hydrolysis, saponin glycosides yield an aglycone, sapogenin (which is responsible for the toxicity), and a sugar that may enhance solubility and absorption.

Saponins may induce lysis of erythrocytes, causing hemolytic anemia. Most saponins are found in combination with other toxins, including gastrointestinal irritants and phytotoxins, which contributes to the widely varying clinical picture.[20]

As with many plant species, gastrointestinal symptoms predominate early after ingestion of pokeweed if it was not processed properly. Typically the patient complains of an initial burning sensation in the mouth and throat (Table 48-9).

Table 48-9 Clinical Effects of Pokeweed Intoxication

Gastrointestinal
   Burning in the mouth
   Burning in the throat
   Nausea
   Vomiting
   Hematemesis
   Abdominal pain
   Diarrhea
   Melena
Miscellaneous
   Weakness
   Decreased vision
   Respiratory depression
   Seizures
   Cardiac dysrhythmias
   Hypotension
   Diaphoresis

A severe hemorrhagic gastroenteritis associated with nausea, vomiting, hematemesis, abdominal cramps, diarrhea, melena, weakness, diaphoresis, and hypotension may ensue. In severe cases, there may also be neurologic symptoms such as decreased vision, respiratory depression, seizures, and cardiac dysrhythmias. Nonfatal cases usually resolve in 24 to 48 hours. Deaths have been reported.[20]

MISCELLANEOUS PLANT TOXINS

Poinsettia

The poinsettia (*Euphorbia pulcherrima*) is a member of a family that comprises more than 7000 herbs, shrubs, and trees. Although the family is morphologically diverse, the presence of latex or milky juice in these plants is common to all species. This latex is economically important as a natural rubber source.[21]

The poinsettia plant is an ornamental plant that is popular during the Christmas season. Its flowers are small and yellow[21]; it is the large colorful leaf that is responsible for the plant's popularity.[13] For many years the poinsettia was considered a poisonous plant that could be fatal if ingested, but it probably is not as toxic as some reports have indicated because little documentation of these serious effects can be found. The plant is capable of causing varying degrees of irritation of the local mucosa as well as gastroin-

Table 48-10 Clinical Effects of Mistletoe Poisoning

Gastrointestinal
   Gastritis
   Nausea
   Vomiting
   Diarrhea
Neurologic
   Hallucinations
   Delirium
   Coma
   Seizures
Cardiovascular
   Bradycardia
   Heart blocks

Table 48-11 "Nontoxic" Plants

African violet (*Saintpaulia*)
Aluminum plant (Pilea)
Aphelandia
Baby tears (Helxine)
Begonia (*Begonia*)
Blood leaf (Iresine)
Boston fern (*Nephrolepis exaltata bostoniensis*)
Ceropegia
Christmas cactus (Zygocactus)
Coleus (*Coleus*)
Copperleaf (*Abutilon*)
Corn plant (*Dracaena*)
Dandelion
Dracaena (*Dracaena*)
Dusty miller (cineraria)
False aralia (dizgotheca)
Gardenia
Gynura
Hawaiian ti (*Cordyline*)
Hibiscus
Jade plant (*Crassula arborescens*)
Lipstick plant (aeschynanthus)
Marigold (*Tagetes*)
Mother-in-law tongue (*Sansevieria*)
Palm
Peperomia (peperomia)
Prayer plant (*Maranta*)
Rosary vine (ceropegia)
Rose
Rubber plant (*Ficus elastica*)
Schefflera (brassaia)
Sensitive plant (*Mimosa pudica*)
Snake plant (*Sansevieria*)
Spider plant (anthericum)
Swedish ivy (plecthranthus)
Umbrella plant (*Cyperus alternifolius*)
Velvet plant (hoya)
Wax plant (hoya)
Weeping fig (ficus)
Zebra plant (aphelandia)

testinal distress. Treatment, if necessary at all, is symptomatic.[11]

Mistletoe

Mistletoe (*Phoradendron villasum*, *P flavescens*) is a woody perennial that usually grows on oak trees; it is also widely available during the Christmas season as an ornament. Its small white berries contain β-phenylethylamine and tyramine, which can act as pressor amines. Mistletoe extracts have been used in teas sold in health food stores and have also been used as illegal abortifacients. The teas are particularly toxic and have been associated with fatalities.

Gastrointestinal, neurologic, and cardiovascular effects may be noted from ingestion of mistletoe berries (Table 48-10). Gastrointestinal effects include gastritis and gastroenteritis. Neurologic effects have included hallucinations, delirium, coma, and seizures. Cardiovascular depression presents much like that associated with cardiac glycoside toxicity, with bradycardia and heart block noted.

Treatment is supportive and symptomatic. Intravenous fluids may be necessary for gas-

troenteritis, and diazepam may be required for seizures.[11]

Yew

The yew (*Taxus* sp) is a popular ornamental evergreen shrublike tree. Almost all parts of the yew are toxic, including its red berries. The yew contains taxine, which can cause cardiovascular effects, gastrointestinal complaints, neurologic problems, and respiratory depression. It may also cause erythema on the skin.

There is no specific treatment for taxine poisoning. Treatment is supportive and may include cardiovascular support in the form of intravenous fluids and antidysrhythmic agents.

"NONTOXIC" PLANTS

Although almost any substance taken in a large enough quantity may be toxic, there are a number of plants that when ingested mistakenly will result in little toxicity. Table 48-11 lists those plants that are associated with very little toxicity or are essentially nontoxic.

REFERENCES

1. Geehr E: Common toxic plant ingestions. *Emerg Med Clin North Am* 1984;2:553–562.

2. DiPalma J: Poisonous plants. *Am Fam Physician* 1984;29:252–254.

3. Spoerke D, Hall A, Dodson C, et al: Mystery root ingestion. *J Emerg Med* 1987;5:385–388.

4. Epstein W: The poison ivy picker of Pennypack Park: The continuing saga of poison ivy. *J Invest Dermatol* 1987;88:7s–11s.

5. Kingsbury J: Phytotoxicology: Part I: Major problems associated with poisonous plants. *Clin Pharmacol Ther* 1969;10:163–169.

6. Kingsbury J: Phytotoxicology: Part II: Poisonous plants and plant-caused emergencies. *Clin Toxicol* 1969; 2:143–148.

7. Bryson P, Watanabe A, Rumack B, et al: Burdock root tea poisoning. *JAMA* 1978;239:2157–2158.

8. Rhoads P, Tong T, Banner W, et al: Anticholinergic poisonings associated with commercial burdock root tea. *Clin Toxicol* 1985;22:581–584.

9. Bryson P: Burdock root tea poisoning. *JAMA* 1978;240:1586.

10. Hart M: Jequirity-bean poisoning. *N Engl J Med* 1963;268:885–886.

11. Yarbrough B: Plant poisoning: A comprehensive management guide. *ER Rep* 1983;4:19–24.

12. Klein-Schwartz W, Litovitz T: Azalea toxicity: An overrated problem? *Clin Toxicol* 1985;23:91–101.

13. Kunkel D, Spoerke D: Evaluating exposures to plants. *Emerg Med Clin North Am* 1984;2:133–144.

14. Rauber A, Heard J: Castor bean toxicity re-examined: A new perspective. *Vet Hum Toxicol* 1985;27:498–502.

15. Drach G, Maloney W: Toxicity of the common houseplant dieffenbachia. *JAMA* 1963;184:113–114.

16. Rauber A: Observations on the idioblasts of dieffenbachia. *Clin Toxicol* 1985;23:79–90.

17. Landers D, Seppi K, Blauer W: Seizures and death on a White River float trip—Report of water hemlock poisoning. *West J Med* 1985;142:637–640.

18. Epstein W: Plant-induced dermatitis. *Ann Emerg Med* 1987;16:950–955.

19. Marks J, Trautlein J, Epstein W, et al: Oral hyposensitization to poison ivy and poison oak. *Arch Dermatol* 1987;123:476–478.

20. Roberge R, Brader E, Martin M, et al: The root of evil—Pokeweed intoxication. *Ann Emerg Med* 1986;15: 470–473.

21. Edwards N: Local toxicity from a poinsettia plant: A case report. *J Pediatr* 1983;102:404–405.

ADDITIONAL SELECTED REFERENCES

Giannini J, Castellani S: A manic-like pyschosis due to Khat (*Catha edulis* Forsk.). *J Toxicol Clin Toxicol* 1982;19: 455–459.

Harrison T: Ergotaminism. *JACEP* 1978;7:162–169.

Haynes B, Bessen H, Wightman W: Oleander tea: Herbal draught of death. *Ann Emerg Med* 1985;14:350–353.

Millet Y, Jouglard J, Steinmetz M, et al: Toxicity of some essential plant oils: Clinical and experimental study. *Clin Toxicol* 1981;18:1485–1498.

Segelman A, Segelman F, Karliner J, et al: Sassafras and herb tea: Potential health hazards. *JAMA* 1976;236:477.

Siegel R: Ginseng abuse syndrome: Problems with the panacea. *JAMA* 1979;241:1614–1615.

Siegel R: Herbal intoxication: Psychoactive effects from herbal cigarettes, tea, and capsules. *JAMA* 1976;236: 473–476.

chapter 49

Mushrooms

Mycology, or the study of mushroom fungi which includes the study of mushrooms, was originated by the ancient Greeks, who sought to distinguish poisonous mushrooms from the edible varieties.[1] Today, the gathering and eating of mushrooms remains a popular pastime in Europe and has recently become popular in the United States, partly because of increased interest in "organic" foods.[2,3]

Of the approximately 2000 species of wild mushrooms as many as 50 to 100 may be considered toxic,[4,5] and of these many are widely distributed.[6] There are a few that should be regarded as lethal. Toxic and nontoxic species often grow in the same places and may resemble each other.[7] Mushroom species for the most part are not unique in appearance, and most of the popular edible varieties have one or more poisonous look-alikes. Even a trained mycologist may not be able to distinguish edible from poisonous mushrooms without a microscopic examination.[8]

Mushrooms are plant fungi; because they do not contain chlorophyll they must rely on dead organic material to survive.[9,10] The mushroom is the reproductive fruit of the mycelium; its relation to the mycelium is analogous to the relation of any fruit to the tree. Mature mushrooms eject spores that are dispersed by wind to establish new mycelia.

MUSHROOM IDENTIFICATION

In a suspected case of mushroom poisoning, identification of species by morphological characteristics is a formidable task because the appearance of the mushroom may be distorted, especially when parts are brought to the physi-

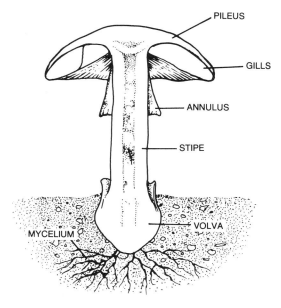

Figure 49-1 Parts of a mushroom. *Source*: Copyright © 1975 by Scientific American Inc. All rights reserved.

cian or after the mushroom has been ingested.[3,8] Attempts to identify the mushroom by collecting specimens from the same area are of little value because poisonous species frequently grow in immediate proximity to nontoxic ones.[6] Examination of fungus spores in the gastric contents may also be inconclusive.[8]

Mushroom Anatomy

The mushroom is comprised of the stipe or stalk; the pileus, or cap; and the gills, the vertical plates that radiate from the stalk on the underside of the cap (Fig. 49-1).[6] Although these names are the important parts of the mushrooms, in actuality it is not necessary for either the patient or the physician to know this. The physician will make the diagnosis and treatment decision on other criteria.

Examination of Spores

Examination of mushroom spores is also a task that will not yield practical information that a physician might utilize. Nevertheless, a procedure is outlined for those interested in spore identification. To prepare spores, the gastric juice is filtered through cheesecloth and then centrifuged. The heavier layer contains the spores and can be placed under a microscope with an oil-immersion lens.[2] Spores are generally the same size as a red blood cell.[6] The physician should then use a textbook or handbook of mycology for identification of spores, as that discussion is beyond the scope of this text.

Mushroom Identification and the ED Physician

The emergency department physician must therefore have access to a simpler approach than species identification to the patient who has ingested a potentially toxic mushroom.[5] This approach divides the toxic mushrooms into two major groups: those that cause symptoms immediately after ingestion, and those that cause delayed symptoms (Table 49-1).[8,11] Under these major groups mushrooms are divided into

Table 49-1 Toxicological Classification of Mushrooms

Delayed symptoms (more than 6 hours after ingestion)
   Group I—Cyclopeptide-containing species
   Group II—Monomethylhydrazine producers

Immediate symptoms (less than 6 hours after ingestion)
   Group III—*Coprinus* sp
   Group IV—Muscarine-containing species
   Group V—Ibotenic acid–containing species
   Group VI—Indole-containing species
   Group VII—Gastrointestinal irritants

at least seven groups on the basis of the type of toxin and the symptoms elicited.[7] Each group has a predictable target organ, incubation period, and clinical presentation.[4] A diagnosis and treatment regimen based on these criteria will be accurate more than 90% of the time.[2,11]

In general, the time of onset of symptoms from ingestion is inversely proportional to the overall severity of the mushroom ingested.[12] An immediate response is one in which symptoms appear from a few minutes to 6 hours after ingestion; a delayed response shows symptoms arising beyond this time limit.[7] The important considerations for mushrooms causing an immediate response are that poisoning is rarely serious and that treatment is conservative and symptomatic.[5] A fatal outcome from poisoning by these mushrooms is extremely rare and may be attributed to inadequate fluid and electrolyte management in young children.[11] Delayed symptoms from mushroom ingestion, appearing more than 6 hours after ingestion and generally after approximately 12 hours, are indicative of a serious poisoning with a potentially grave prognosis.[12]

Toxins may be identified by radioimmunoassay from a sample of the mushrooms or in gastric juice, stool, urine, or blood. Laboratory tests are rarely needed for institution of appropriate patient management, however.[4]

Severity of symptoms depends on the season, the maturity of the mushroom when picked and eaten, the location of the mushroom, the amount ingested, the method of preparation of the mushroom, and the age of the patient (Table 49-2).[3] There is no simple test for distinguishing the edible species from the poisonous ones.[5]

Table 49-2 Factors Influencing Severity of Symptoms of Mushroom Poisoning

Season of the year
Maturity of mushroom
Location of mushroom
Amount of mushroom ingested
Method of preparation
Age of patient

Table 49-3 Cyclopeptide-Containing Mushrooms

Amanita bisporigera
Amanita hydroscopica
Amanita ocreata
Amanita phalloides
Amanita suballiacea
Amanita tenuifolia
Amanita verna
Amanita virosa
Galerina autumnalis
Galerina marginata
Galerina venenata
Lepiota sp

Mushrooms that are considered lethal belong for the most part to the cyclopeptide-containing species. In fact, almost all deadly mushrooms are members of a single genus: *Amanita*. The distinguishing feature between the cyclopeptide mushrooms and all of the other groups that may produce symptoms but rarely produce death is that, with the cyclopeptides, the symptoms commence after 6 hours after ingestion. All of the other poisonous but not deadly mushrooms will have symptoms that commence before 6 hours after ingestion. Although this generalization is not absolute, it is a worthwhile guide to the consideration of mushroom toxicity.

MUSHROOMS WITH DELAYED ONSET OF SYMPTOMS

The mushrooms in groups I and II account for more than 95% of deaths associated with mushrooms.[8,11,12]

Group I—Cyclopeptide-Containing Mushrooms

Almost all of fatal mushrooms are species in the genus *Amanita*; these include *A phalloides* (destroying angel), *A virosa*, *A bisporigera*, and others (Table 49-3).[9,13] *Amanita phalloides* generally appears in late summer or fall and grows to a height of 3 to 8 inches.[14] The cap varies in color from light yellow to greenish-brown, and the stalk is usually lighter, from a light greenish-yellow to pure white. *Amanita virosa* is pure white throughout.

Members of the genus *Galerina* also cause severe toxicity, but these mushrooms are not as likely to be chosen for ingestion.[15]

Amanita phalloides was once thought to be strictly a European mushroom[8]; it was first positively identified growing wild in the United States in 1970.[3] It is now found in all areas of the United States but to a greater degree in the Western coastal states.[16] This mushroom may have been introduced into the United States by inadvertent transportation on the roots of imported ornamental trees.[2]

The principal toxins of this group are complex proteins containing cyclic heptapeptides, called phallotoxins, and cyclic octapeptides, called amatoxins.[17] These cyclopeptides consist of amino acids linked together by peptide bonds to form a continuous ring.[13] *Amanita* species contain both these toxins, whereas *Galerina* species contain only amatoxins. Amatoxins are believed to be the major toxins responsible for the symptoms and pathology due to ingestion of *Amanita phalloides* and related mushrooms.[16] Cooking, steaming, or drying do not materially affect the toxins in these species.[8]

Phallotoxins include phalloidin, phalloin, phallisin, phallacidin, phalacin, and phallisacin.[15] In vitro, the phallotoxins appear to disrupt hepatic cell membranes and to change the structure of the hepatic endoplasmic reticulum.[7] The phallotoxins are not well absorbed from the gastrointestinal tract and therefore contribute little to toxicity. The major contributing toxins are the amatoxins.[8]

Amatoxin is a collective term for a number of orally toxic cyclic octapeptides, of which five have been characterized. They have been designated as α-, β-, γ-, and ε-amanitin and amanin. The amanitins have a delayed toxicity that commences about 16 to 24 hours after mushroom ingestion.

Amatoxins are taken up by hepatocytes, in which their primary action is to inhibit nucleoplasmic RNA polymerase II, which in turn interferes with the synthesis of messenger RNA.[17] This effectively halts protein synthesis and causes cellular necrosis, which ultimately results in a severe acute hepatitis indistinguishable from acute viral hepatitis.[7] Amanitin is also a direct-acting nephrotoxin that produces necrosis of the distal and proximal convoluted tubules.[6,11] It appears that the effects of amatoxin are dose dependent, with low doses producing solely renal involvement and high doses producing hepatic damage. In other words, the target organ appears to be dependent on the quantity of mushroom toxins ingested.[2]

Clinical Effects

Because of the delayed onset of symptoms in poisonings with phallotoxic *Amanita* species, patients frequently may not associate their symptoms with the ingestion of the wild mushroom.[5] Therefore, a careful history of the patient's activities before the onset of symptoms is imperative.[7]

Symptoms of poisoning characteristically occur in three stages (Table 49-4). Although any type of eukaryotic cell can be damaged by amatoxin, the initial stage of the clinical picture is dominated by lesions of intestinal mucosal cells and the final stage by deterioration of liver cell function.[16] The hepatic destruction noted is similar to that seen in poisonings with substances such as acetaminophen and carbon tetrachloride, which are converted in the liver into toxic metabolites.[17]

Stage I. The first stage occurs abruptly 6 to 24 hours after ingestion. The patient may complain of abdominal pain and subsequent nausea, violent emesis, and diarrhea; occasionally hematochezia and hematuria are noted.[13] These symptoms are frequently accompanied by fever, tachycardia, hyperglycemia, hypotension, dehydration, and electrolyte imbalance.[9] If a large amount was eaten or if medical care is not provided, death may occur from fluid and electrolyte loss.[3] This can usually be avoided with

Table 49-4 Signs and Symptoms of Poisoning with *Amanita phylloides* Species

Stage I (6 to 24 hours)
Abdominal pain
Nausea
Emesis
Diarrhea
Hematochezia
Hematuria
Fever
Hyperglycemia
Tachycardia
Electrolyte imbalance
Stage II (24 to 48 hours)
Period of "recovery"
Stage III (3 to 5 days)
Hepatic dysfunction
Renal dysfunction
Myocardial dysfunction

vigorous intravenous therapy and other supportive measures.[8]

Stage II. During the next 24 to 48 hours there appears to be remission of symptoms in the face of progressive deterioration of hepatic and renal function.[5]

Stage III. The third stage occurs 3 to 5 days after ingestion of the mushroom and consists of increasing hepatocellular damage and renal impairment. This is noted by massive elevations in the liver function tests and the development of jaundice and hepatic coma. Because amatoxins enter liver cells more rapidly than other organ cell types, and because protein synthesis is active in liver cells, the hepatocyte is rendered vulnerable to the inhibitors of the transcription processes.[7] In addition, myocardiopathy and coagulopathy may be present, and seizures, coma, and death may occur. Death from *Amanita phylloides* species is usually the result of hepatic or renal failure or both and may occur 4 to 7 days after ingestion.[17]

Laboratory Analysis

Baseline laboratory data should be obtained. Depending on the certainty of the diagnosis, laboratory studies may include a complete blood cell count, serum electrolytes, blood urea nitrogen, glucose concentration, creatinine concentration, urinalysis, liver function tests,

Table 49-5 Laboratory Studies in Poisoning with
Amanita phylloides Species

Complete blood cell count
Serum electrolytes
Blood urea nitrogen
Blood glucose concentration
Serum creatinine concentration
Urinalysis
Liver function tests
Prothrombin time
Partial thromboplastin time
Platelet count
Fibrinogen concentration
Amatoxin radioimmunoassay

---

prothrombin time, partial thromboplastin time, platelet count, and fibrinogen concentration (Table 49-5).[8,11] Serum or urine should be saved and sent for radioimmunoassay of amatoxins to an appropriate referral center[16]; these tests are usually beyond the capabilities of most hospital laboratories.[17] A urine sample may show identifiable quantities of amatoxins within 90 to 120 minutes of ingestion.

Treatment

Treatment consists of supportive care and vigorous intravenous fluid replacement to correct fluid loss. Attention must also be directed toward correcting any metabolic and coagulation disturbances.[3] Although the cyclopeptide-containing mushrooms cause more than 95% of the deaths from mushroom poisoning, the overall survival rate is 75% to 80% with supportive therapy.[11,13]

There is no satisfactory treatment for the hepatorenal phase of amatoxin poisoning. Neomycin is not recommended because of the associated renal damage from amatoxin. Dietary protein should be restricted and parenteral vitamin K and fresh frozen plasma provided as necessary.[17]

Many treatment regimens have been advocated for poisonings with *Amanita phylloides* species, including thioctic acid, penicillin, cimetidine, silibinin, and extracorporeal methods. None of these has been shown to be of benefit, however.[11,13]

Thioctic Acid. Thioctic acid (α-lipoic acid) is a component of coenzymes in the Krebs cycle

that is necessary for oxidation of ketoacids such as pyruvate.[18] This agent has been advocated for mushroom poisonings since the 1960s, but there has been no well-designed clinical trial to document its efficacy.[2,13]

Penicillin. The proposed mechanism of action of intravenous penicillin is competition with amanitin for binding sites on serum proteins. This leaves more toxin free for renal excretion and less to be taken up into liver cells. This treatment has not been shown to be clinically effective, however.[5]

Cimetidine. Cimetidine produces a competitive inhibition of the cytochrome P-450 system by binding of its imidazole ring to the heme moiety on the cytochrome.[19] Although theoretically this compound may be protective or antidotal in poisonings with *Amanita phylloides* species, no clinical trials have shown this to be the case.[19]

Silibinin. Silibinin is a water-soluble preparation of silymarin and has been advocated in Europe as an antidote in poisonings with *Amanita phylloides* species. Silymarin is the active ingredient of the milk thistle; it is thought to inhibit the penetration of the amatoxins into liver cells.[13] There are not enough data to verify the benefit of silibinin, and it is not available in the United States.

Extracorporeal Methods. Both dialysis and hemoperfusion have been advocated in the past for poisonings with *Amanita phylloides* species, but there is no evidence that either procedure is protective. These procedures may actually worsen the patient's prospect of recovery, perhaps by unfavorably influencing the already-compromised coagulation pattern. Hemodialysis has been used successfully to treat renal failure but not to remove amanitin, which is poorly dialyzable.

Liver Transplantation. A relatively new treatment suggested for acute hepatic failure from poisonings with *Amanita phylloides* species is liver transplantation. This heroic measure may be offered to the patient with a deteriorating liver function in the face of optimal supportive care.[8]

Group II—Monomethylhydrazine Producers

The morels are one of the most highly prized of all edible mushrooms. Toxic *Gyromitra* species resemble this type of mushroom and are called "false morels." The morels have a cap resembling a pine cone that is textured with ridges and pits and is attached at the base of the mushroom.[20] *Gyromitra* species are called false morels because they have a wrinkled or saddle-shaped cap unattached at the base.[7] Distinguishing between these two types of mushrooms is difficult. Most poisonings have occurred in Europe, although there have been occasional poisonings reported in North America (Table 49-6).[2]

Mechanism of Toxicity

Mushrooms of the genus *Gyromitra* contain gryomitrin, which in most individuals is hydrolyzed to monomethylhydrazine after ingestion. Monomethylhydrazine acts as a competitive inhibitor of the coenzyme pyridoxal phosphate (vitamin B_6),[20] which serves as a coenzyme for many enzyme systems, including γ-aminobutyric acid, decarboxylases, deaminases, and transaminases. Inhibition of pyridoxal phosphate results in multiorgan dysfunction. Damage may extend to the liver, kidneys, CNS, and hematopoietic system.[7]

Clinical Effects of Intoxication

Because the toxic component of this group of mushrooms is highly volatile it is inactivated by cooking. If the mushroom is not cooked, then symptoms are typically delayed for 6 to 12 hours after ingestion. Whether or not the mushroom was cooked is an important part of the history.

Initially gastrointestinal symptoms predominate, with complaints of bloating, nausea, vomiting, diarrhea, cramping, and abdominal pain (Table 49-7). These symptoms are usually self-limited and resolve in 1 to 3 days.[20] Other symptoms may be noted subsequently; these consist of hemolysis (which may also occur early), hemoglobinemia, clinical anemia, jaundice, and hemoglobinuria. The mechanism of the hemolysis is unknown. There appears to be a direct effect on the mixed-function oxidase systems in the liver with subsequent hepatotoxicity.[15] Methemoglobinemia may also be noted. Because vitamin B_6 antagonists cause inhibition of the inhibitory neurotransmitter γ-aminobutyric acid, seizures are often noted in the symptomatic individual.[2]

Laboratory Analysis

Baseline laboratory studies should include a complete blood cell count, urinalysis, serum free hemoglobin concentrations, blood urea nitrogen, creatinine and glucose concentrations, liver function tests, serum electrolytes, arterial blood gas values, and a methemoglobin concentration (if necessary).[7]

Treatment

Although *Gyromitra* species have the potential to cause death, ingestion of these mushrooms is rarely fatal. None of the toxins in these species is related chemically to those of *Amanita phylloides* species. In addition, the symptoms of poisoning by these mushrooms are not the same as those of *Amanita* species.[12]

Table 49-6 Monomethylhydrazine Producers

Gyromitra ambigua
Gyromitra brunnea
Gyromitra caroliniana
Gyromitra esculenta
Gyromitra fastigiata

Table 49-7 Signs and Symptoms of *Gyromitra* Species Poisoning

Gastrointestinal
  Bloating
  Nausea
  Vomiting
  Diarrhea
  Abdominal pain
Hematologic
  Hemolysis
  Hemoglobinemia
  Anemia
  Jaundice
  Methemoglobinemia
Hepatotoxicity
Neurologic
  Seizures

Treatment consists of supportive care with replacement of any fluid and electrolyte losses. Large parenteral doses of pyridoxine may be necessary to counteract the antagonistic effects of the monomethylhydrazine. Pyridoxine hydrochloride at a dose of 2 to 5 g in an adult or 25 mg/kg in a child should be administered intravenously. The urine should be alkalinized to prevent hemoglobin deposition. Dialysis is not recommended except for frank renal failure.[20]

MUSHROOMS WITH IMMEDIATE ONSET OF SYMPTOMS

Mushrooms in groups III to VII (see Table 49-1) are rarely involved in major medical problems except for fluid and electrolyte changes, which may be severe.

Group III—*Coprinus* Species

Ingestion of mushrooms in the genus *Coprinus*, specifically *C atramentarius*, and of *Clitocybe clavipes* produces no symptoms unless alcohol is ingested while the toxic components of the mushroom are still in the body. These mushrooms are considered both common and palatable; a characteristic is that at maturity the gills dissolve into an inky black fluid.[7]

Mechanism of Toxicity

Many *Coprinus* species contain coprine, which is metabolized after ingestion to an acetaldehyde dehydrogenase inhibitor. Coprine is broken down to another active derivative, aminocyclopropanol, which acts like disulfiram.[1] This reaction prevents the metabolism of acetaldehyde to acetate, thus allowing accumulation of acetaldehyde. There is some evidence that this reaction is due to β-receptor stimulation.

Clinical Effects

The mushroom and alcohol need not be ingested at the same time, and because the toxin is not cleared from the body for several days an alcoholic drink during that period may precipi-

Table 49-8 Signs and Symptoms of *Coprinus*–Alcohol Interaction

Gastrointestinal
 Nausea
 Vomiting
Skin
 Diaphoresis
 Flushing
 Throbbing in neck veins
Cardiovascular
 Chest pain
 Palpitations
 Supraventricular dysrhythmias
 Hypotension
Neurologic
 Paresthesias
 Headache

tate the reaction. If no alcohol is ingested during that time, no toxic symptoms occur.[15]

Symptoms may commence 20 minutes to 2 hours after consuming alcohol. The patient may experience an increase in body temperature with flushing, nausea, vomiting, a feeling of fullness and throbbing in the neck veins, chest pain, palpitations, paresthesias in the hands and feet, diaphoresis, and headache (Table 49-8). Supraventricular dysrhythmias and hypotension have been reported in severe cases. No deaths have been reported.[7]

Treatment

Most symptoms of poisoning resolve spontaneously within 3 to 6 hours, and treatment is symptomatic and supportive. There are anecdotal reports of success with parenteral antihistamines and ascorbic acid.[12]

Group IV—Muscarine-Containing Species

Muscarine is a natural parasympathomimetic alkaloid first isolated from *Amanita muscaria*; this species contains clinically insignificant amounts of muscarine, however.[7] It was subsequently found that mushrooms of the genera *Inocybe* and *Clitocybe* (Table 49-9) can cause muscarine poisoning, with cholinergic effects that can be blocked by atropine.

Table 49-9 Muscarine-Containing Mushrooms

Clitocybe cerrusata
Clitocybe dealbata
Clitocybe nuulosa
Inocybe fastigiata
Inocybe geophylla
Inocybe rimosus

In the symptomatic individual, signs of cholinergic activity may be noted 15 minutes to 2 hours after ingestion and may last for 6 to 24 hours. The most common feature is diaphoresis, which may be accompanied by abdominal pain, nausea, vomiting, salivation, miosis, blurred vision, bronchoconstriction, bradycardia, and hypotension (Table 49-10). Although atropine provides prompt and specific treatment for symptoms of muscarinic mushroom poisoning, it is only necessary in the substantially symptomatic individual. The dosage of atropine is related to the severity of symptoms and should be titrated to clinical effect.[7]

Group V—Ibotenic Acid–Containing Species

The toxic ingredients in *Amanita muscaria* are ibotenic acid and muscimol (Table 49-11).[7] Ibotenic acid is a derivative of glutamic acid, and muscimol is a derivative of γ-aminobutyric acid. Ibotenic acid is an unstable compound, especially in the presence of an acid.[21] It acts as an insecticide; flies die on contact with *A muscaria*, hence the name fly agaric. Muscimol is several times more active than ibotenic acid and is formed by decarboxylation of ibotenic acid. Muscimol and related compounds have been characterized as an anticholinergic by some authorities and as a γ-aminobutyric acid antagonist by others.

Clinical Effects

Amanita muscaria and *A pantheria* ("the panther") are common mushroom species intentionally ingested for their psychoactive properties. *Amanita muscaria* is probably the most common poisonous mushroom ingested in the United States.[21] Symptoms may occur 30 min-

Table 49-10 Signs and Symptoms of Muscarinic Mushroom Poisoning

Diaphoresis
Abdominal pain
Nausea
Vomiting
Salivation
Miosis
Blurred vision
Bronchoconstriction
Bradycardia
Hypotension

Table 49-11 Ibotenic Acid–Containing Mushrooms

Amanita cothurnata
Amanita gemmata
Amanita muscaria
Amanita pantherina

Table 49-12 Signs and Symptoms of Poisoning by Ibotenic Acid–Containing Mushrooms

Euphoria
Dizziness
Ataxia
Visual disturbances
Mydriasis
Agitation
Myoclonus
Seizures
Coma

utes to 2 hours after ingestion and include euphoria, dizziness, ataxia, and drunken behavior (Table 49-12). With severe intoxication, visual disturbances, mydriasis, agitation, myoclonus, seizures, and coma may occur. Contrary to some reports, no clear pattern of cholinergic or anticholinergic effects is observed.[7]

Treatment

Treatment is supportive. Because vomiting is not a clinical feature, attempts should be made to empty the stomach. Unless severe anticholinergic symptoms and signs are present, physostigmine should not be administered. Barbiturates and benzodiazepines should also not be administered because they may exacerbate toxicity.[21]

Table 49-13 Genera of Mushrooms That Are Gastrointestinal Irritants

Agaricus
Boletus
Chlorophyllum
Entoloma
Gomphus
Hebeloma
Lactarius
Lycoperdon
Morchella
Naematoloma
Paxillus
Pholiota
Polyphorus
Ramaria
Russula
Scleroderma
Tricholoma
Verpa

Table 49-14 Signs and Symptoms of Ingestion of Gastrointestinal Irritant Mushrooms

Present
  Nausea
  Vomiting
  Diarrhea
  Abdominal pain
Absent
  Diaphoresis
  Delirium
  Hallucinations
  Hepatorenal damage

Group VI—The Indole-Containing Mushrooms

The principal hallucinogenic mushrooms come from three genera found largely in the Pacific Northwest, Florida, and Hawaii. These are *Psilocybe*, *Paneolus*, and *Gymnophilus*.[22]

The chemical nature of psilocybin, which is the toxic ingredient in these mushrooms, resembles that of 5-hydroxytryptamine and lysergic acid diethylamide.[1,23] Although early after ingestion there are symptoms of weakness and dizziness, this usually passes on to a euphoria and dreamlike state with visual perceptual distortions. Most symptoms resolve within 4 hours. Treatment is supportive.[22,24] A discussion of the clinical effects produced by these mushrooms and treatment of intoxication is given in Chapter 34.

Group VII—Gastrointestinal Irritants

The most common adverse reaction to eating mushrooms is gastrointestinal irritation. Little is known about the chemistry and pharmacologic activity of the mushrooms in this group.[10] It appears that the toxin produced may be somewhat destroyed by heat, although cooking the mushrooms does not ensure safety.[4]

Although the species encountered most frequently in this group is *Chlorophyllum molybdites*, many of the common "little brown mushrooms" found in the backyard are found in this group (Table 49-13).[10]

Clinical Effects

The onset of signs and symptoms generally begin within 2 hours of ingestion and consist of gastrointestinal irritation in the form of nausea, vomiting, diarrhea, and abdominal pain (Table 49-14). The profuse, watery diarrhea may lead to significant volume and electrolyte loss. The illness is self-limited, and most symptoms resolve in 3 to 4 hours.[4] A characteristic of mushrooms in this group is the absence of intense diaphoresis, delirium, hallucinations, and hepatorenal damage.

Treatment

Because symptoms are self-limiting, no specific treatment other than fluid and electrolyte replacement is necessary. The very young and the debilitated are most vulnerable to the fluid and electrolyte shifts and should be monitored closely. In some cases, fluid loss has been of sufficient magnitude to induce hypovolemic shock.[4]

SUMMARY

Although mushroom identification is a formidable task, even for the professional mycologist, it is not necessary for the emergency

Table 49-15 Summary of the Features of Various Types of Mushroom Poisoning

Toxin	Genus	Organ systems affected	Symptoms	Time of onset after ingestion	Possible antidote
Amanitin, phalloidin (cyclopeptides)	Amanita Galerina	Blood, liver, kidney, gastrointestinal tract	Hematuria, proteinuria, gastroenteritis, jaundice	6–24 hours	Supportive care
Monomethylhydrazine (gyromitrin)	Gyromitra	Blood, liver, kidney, gastrointestinal tract	Hemolysis, abdominal pain, liver and kidney failure, weakness	6–24 hours	Pyridoxine, 25 mg/kg IV
Coprine	Coprinus	Autonomic nervous system	With alcohol ingestion, disulfiram-like reaction	20 minutes–5 days	Supportive care
Muscarine	Clitocybe (Omphalotus) Inocybe	Autonomic nervous system	Salivation, lacrimation, excessive urination, diarrhea	20 minutes–2 hours	Atropine, 2 mg IV (as indicated)
Ibotenic acid, muscimol	Amanita	Central nervous system	Dry mouth, cycloplegia (anticholinergic effects), delirium, ataxia	20 minutes–2 hours	Physostigmine, 2 mg IV (only when indicated)
Psilocybin, psilocin	Psilocybe Panaeolus	Central nervous system	Hallucinations, hyperkinetic state (anticholinergic effects)	15–30 minutes	Supportive care

Source: From *Toxic and Hallucinogenic Mushroom Poisoning* by Gary Lincoff and DH Mitchell. © 1977 by Litton Educational Publishing Inc.

department physician to identify the exact mushroom that is causing toxic symptoms to diagnose the patient's condition and to plan a treatment regimen that will be successful most of the time. This regimen consists of knowing when symptoms began after ingestion of the mushroom as well as characterizing the symptoms present (Table 49-15). If symptoms began within 6 hours of ingestion it is unlikely that they will progress to serious toxicity, and the signs and symptoms present dictate treatment necessary.[12] For the most part, treatment consists of fluid and electrolyte replacement. For those mushrooms that present with symptoms 6 hours after inges-

tion and generally after 12 hours, there is a good possibility of a serious poisoning with a potentially grave prognosis. Because there are no effective antidotes available for poisonings with *Amanita phalloides* and related species, the management consists of the same fluid and electrolyte support as well as monitoring for signs of hepatic and renal involvement. When mixed ingestions are suspected early symptoms should be treated, and when the patient is asymptomatic he or she may be discharged with instructions to return if gastrointestinal symptoms arise again. Alternatively the patient may be instructed to return for daily liver function tests.[12]

REFERENCES

1. Hanrahan J, Gordon M: Mushroom poisoning. *JAMA* 1984;251:1057–1061.

2. Becker C, Tong T, Boerner U, et al: Diagnosis and treatment of *Amanita phalloides*–type mushroom poisoning. *West J Med* 1976;125:100–109.

3. Parish R, Doering P: Treatment of *Amanita* mushroom poisoning: A review. *Vet Hum Toxicol* 1986;28: 318–322.

4. Blayney D, Rosenkranz E, Zettner A: Mushroom poisoning from *Chlorophyllum molybdites*. *West J Med* 1980;132:74–77.

5. Page L: Mushroom poisoning. *West J Med* 1980;132: 66–68.

6. Litten W: The most poisonous mushrooms. *Sci Am* 1975;232:90–101.

7. DiPalma J: Mushroom poisoning. *Am Fam Physician* 1981;23:170–172.

8. Bivins H, Knopp R, Lammers R, et al: Mushroom ingestion. *Ann Emerg Med* 1985;14:1099–1104.

9. Mitchel D: *Amanita* mushroom poisoning. *Ann Rev Med* 1980;31:51–57.

10. Levitan D, Macy J, Weissman J: Mechanism of gastrointestinal hemorrhage in a case of mushroom poisoning by *Chlorophyllum molybdites*. *Toxicon* 1981;179–180.

11. Lampe K: Current concepts of therapy in mushroom intoxication. *Clin Toxicol* 1974;7:115–121.

12. Hanrahan J, Gordon M: Treatment of mushroom poisoning. *JAMA* 1984;252:3130–3133.

13. Floersheim G: Treatment of human amatoxin mushroom poisoning: Myths and advances in therapy. *Med Toxicol* 1987;2:1–9.

14. Kelner M, Alexander N: Endocrine hormone abnormalities in *Amanita* poisoning. *Clin Toxicol* 1987;25:21–37.

15. Lampe K, McCann M: Differential diagnosis of poisoning by North American mushrooms, with particular emphasis on *Amanita phalloides*–type intoxication. *Ann Emerg Med* 1987;16:956–962.

16. Pond S, Olson K, Woo O, et al: Amatoxin poisoning in Northern California, 1982–1983. *West J Med* 1986; 145:204–209.

17. Bartoloni F, Omer S, Giannini A, et al: *Amanita* poisoning: A clinical-histiopathological study of 64 cases of intoxication. *Hepato-Gastroenterol* 1985;32:229–231.

18. Plotzker R, Jensen D, Payne J: *Amanita virosa* acute hepatic necrosis: Treatment with thioctic acid. *Am J Med Sci* 1982;283:79–82.

19. Schneider S, Borochovitz D, Krenzelok E: Cimetidine protection against α-amanitin hepatotoxicity in mice: A potential model for the treatment of *Amanita phalloides* poisoning. *Ann Emerg Med* 1987;16:1136–1140.

20. Coulet M, Guillot J: Poisoning by *Gyromitra*: A possible mechanism. *Med Hypotheses* 1982;8:325–334.

21. Gilad E, Biger Y: Paralysis of convergence caused by mushroom poisoning. *Am J Ophthalmol* 1986;102: 124–125.

22. Curry S, Rose M: Intravenous mushroom poisoning. *Ann Emerg Med* 1985;14:900–902.

23. Peden N, Pringle S, Crooks J: *Hum Toxicol* 1982;1: 417–424.

24. Peden N, Bissett A, Macaulay K, et al: Clinical toxicology of magic mushroom ingestion. *Postgrad Med J* 1981;57:543–545.

ADDITIONAL SELECTED REFERENCES

Homann J, Rawer P, Bleyl H, et al: Early detection of amatoxins in human mushroom poisoning. *Arch Toxicol* 1986;59:190–191.

Schumacher T, Hoiland K: Mushroom poisoning caused by species of the genus *Cortinarium* fries. *Arch Toxicol* 1983;53:87–106.

Vesconi S, Langer M, Iapichino G, et al: Therapy of cytotoxic mushroom intoxication. *Crit Care Q* 1985;13: 402–406.

part XII

TOXINS IN FOOD

chapter 50

Sulfites and Monosodium Glutamate

Thousands of chemicals are used to preserve, color, and flavor foods and drugs. Reactions to foods or substances in foods may occur with disturbing frequency.[1] Many times, the reactions may go undiagnosed. There have been numerous reports of allergic reactions after the ingestion of food additives such as yellow dye and tartrazine, food preservatives and antioxidants such as sulfites, and flavor enhancers such as monosodium L-glutamate (MSG).[2] This chapter discusses the toxicity associated with the sulfites and MSG.

SULFITES

Sulfur dioxide and various sulfites have been used for centuries as preservatives, sanitizing agents, and selective inhibitors of growth of microorganisms in the food industry.[3,4] During Roman times sulfur wicks were burned to prevent further fermentation of wines and to inhibit the growth of yeast and mold.[3,5] Because ingestion of sulfites, even in large amounts, does not have apparent ill effects in normal individuals, they are listed on the FDA's schedule of substances generally recognized as safe.[6,7] Nevertheless, asthmatic patients are highly susceptible to bronchospasm following sulfite ingestion.[3] Recently the FDA has banned use of sulfites as preservatives in raw fruits and most vegetables.[5]

Uses

Sulfites prevent microbial spoilage and browning of foods and are also used as preservatives and antioxidants in a number of medications. Sulfites include potassium and sodium metabisulfite, potassium and sodium bisulfite, sodium sulfite, and sulfur dioxide (Table 50-1). All the sulfites contain sulfur in the 4^+ oxidation state and function as strong reducing agents.[8] The choice of a particular sulfite is made primarily on the basis of convenience because all are chemically equivalent, and a reaction reportedly provoked by a specific sulfite can generally be attributed to any of these closely related compounds.[3] The solid form, metabisulfite, is readily converted on hydration to the active component bisulfite, which under appropriate conditions can form sulfite or sulfuric acid.[8]

Table 50-1 Sulfites

Potassium metabisulfite
Potassium bisulfite
Sodium metabisulfite
Sodium bisulfite
Sodium sulfite
Sulfur dioxide

Table 50-2 Partial List of Foods That May Contain Sulfites

Alcoholic beverages (beer, cocktail mix, red wine, white wine)
Nonalcoholic beverages (colas, fruit drinks)
Baked goods (baking mixes, cookies, crackers, crepes, pie crust, pizza crust, soft pretzels, quiche crust, tortillas, waffles)
Coffee and tea, including instant tea
Condiments (olives, relishes, pickles, salad dressing mixes, wine vinegar)
Confections (brown sugar, raw sugar, powdered sugar)
Dairy analogs (filled milk)
Fish products (clams, crab, dried cod, lobster, scallops, shrimp)
Fresh fish (clams, crab, lobster, scallops, shrimp)
Fresh fruit (fruit salads, grapes, other)
Fresh vegetables (avocado salad, guacamole, cabbage, mushrooms, salad bars, tomatoes)
Gelatins/puddings/fillings (fruit filling, gelatin, pectin jelling agents)
Grain products (batters, breadings, corn starch, food starches, noodle/rice mixes)
Gravies/sauces (milk-based gravy, others)
Hard candy
Commercial jam and jelly
Nuts
Protein isolates
Processed fruits (dietetic fruit or juice, dried fruit, fruit juice, glacéed fruit, juice)
Processed vegetables (avocado mix, canned vegetables, dried vegetables, green vegetables, hominy, pickled vegetables, potatoes, spinach, vegetable juice)
Snack foods (apple bits, dried fruit, filled crackers, tortilla chips, trail mix, potato chips)
Soft candy (caramel, others)
Soups (canned soups, dry soup mix)
Sugar (white granulated)
Sweet sauces (corn syrup, dextrose monohydrate, fruit topping, glucose syrup, maple syrup, molasses, pancake syrup)

Source: Reprinted with permission from *Annals of Allergy* (1985;54:421), Copyright © 1985, American College of Allergists.

Sulfites in Foods

Sulfites can react with foods by reducing sugars, proteins, lipids, and their components to form combined sulfites. The antioxidant properties of sulfites keep fruits and vegetables looking fresh; oxygen is unavailable to promote bacterial growth, so that there is inhibition of enzyme-catalyzed oxidative discoloration and browning of these foods.[8] Because of this, their use in restaurant salad bars has increased in the last few years.

Sulfites are also used in many processed foods, including beer and wine, fruit drinks, baked goods, and dried fruits and vegetables (Table 50-2).[3] They are used in the processing of food ingredients such as gelatin, beet sugar, corn sweeteners, and food starches.[1] Sulfites are also used in industry as sanitizing agents for food containers and fermentation equipment.[6]

Sulfites in Medicine

Exposure to sulfites may also occur through many medications; thus sulfites may inadvertently be administered to sulfite-sensitive individuals.[7,8] Medications containing sulfites include adrenergic bronchodilator solutions, steroids,[9] antiemetics, cardiovascular preparations, antibiotics, analgesics, local anesthetics, psychotropic drugs, and intravenous solutions (Table 50-3). Because sulfites destroy thiamine, they are no longer used in thiamine-containing foods.[4,8,10]

Daily Intake of Sulfites

The average daily diet is estimated to contain from 2 to 15 mg of naturally occurring sulfites.[10] Dehydrated fruits and vegetables may contain up to 75 to 80 mg per serving, fruit

Table 50-3 Partial List of Medications That May Contain Sulfites

Nebulized bronchodilators
  isoetharine (Bronkosol)
  isoproterenol (Isuprel)
  metaproterenol (Alupent, Metaprel)
Cardiovascular drugs (parenteral)
  dopamine
  epinephrine (EpiPen Auto Injector, Anakit, etc)
  procainamide
  norepinephrine (Levophed)
  metaraminol (Aramine)
  isoproterenol
  methoxamine (Vasoxyl)
Psychiatric drugs (parenteral)
  chlorpromazine
  prochlorperazine
  imipramine (Tofranil)
  perphenazine (Trilafon)
  phenothiazines (eg, Torecan)
Analgesics
  codeine
  morphine
  acetaminophen (Tylenol, etc)
  pentazocine (Talwin)
  nalbuphine (Nubain)
  meperidine
  oxymorphone (Numorphan)
Peritoneal dialysis solutions
  Dialyte, Inpersol, etc
  Steroids, parenteral
    betamethasone
    dexamethasone
    prednisolone
    hydrocortisone
Miscellaneous
  otic preparations
  ophthalmic preparations
  liver injections
  ergoloid mesylates
  B complex
  edrophonium (Tensilon)
  sodium thiosulfate

Antiemetics (parenteral)
  metoclopramide (Reglan)
  promethazine (Phenergan)
  prochlorperazine (Compazine)
Antibiotics (aerosolized, parenteral)
  sulfonamides (Gantrisin, Bactrim, sulfadiazine,
    Septra, sulfacetamide)
  tetracyclines
  aminoglycosides (tobramycin, kanamycin,
    gentamicin, streptomycin)
IV Solutions
  Isolyte, Aminosyn, Travamin, Amigen, Inpersol,
    Ionosol, Alba-Dex, Intropin, ascorbic acid, Travert,
    FreAmine HBC, HepatAmine, parenteral nutrition,
    Travasol, etc
IV Contrast solutions
Local anesthetics
  mepivacaine (Carbocaine)
  chloroprocaine (Nesacaine)
  procaine (Novocain)
  bupivacaine (Marcaine)
  tetracaine (Pontocaine)
  lidocaine
  Mericaine
Muscle relaxants (parenteral)
  orphenadrine (Norflex)
  methocarbamol (Robaxin)
  tubocurarine

Source: Reprinted with permission from *Annals of Allergy* (1985;54:422), Copyright © 1985, American College of Allergists.

---

drinks up to 30 mg per serving, and sausages up to 60 mg.[3,7,11] Alcoholic beverages such as wine and beer may contain 5 to 10 mg per ounce. A single restaurant meal may contain more than 150 to 200 mg of sulfite.[6,8]

Metabolism

Sodium and potassium sulfites are stable salts. When added to water, they hydrolyze to sodium and potassium cations and bisulfite radicals. Acid pH, as in gastric contents, and increased temperature enhance these events.[1] The free bisulfite is then oxidized to sulfate by the enzyme sulfite oxidase and is excreted in the urine (Fig. 50-1). Sulfite oxidase is widely distributed in the body, with the highest activity found in the liver and kidney. Defects in sulfite oxidase activity may potentially be of importance in the pathogenesis of adverse reactions to sulfites.[3]

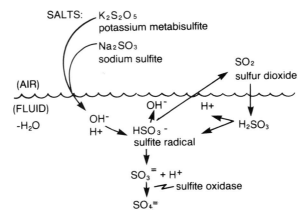

Figure 50-1 Sulfite chemistry. *Source:* Reprinted with permission from *Journal of Allergy and Clinical Immunology* (1984; 74:469–472), Copyright © 1984, The CV Mosby Company.

Sulfites are also formed during normal metabolism, particularly of cysteine.[12] Sulfite radicals are present in cells and plasma but are quickly converted by sulfite oxidase.[6]

Toxicity

The prevalence of sensitivity to sulfiting agents in the general population is unknown. Only a relatively small number of vulnerable individuals appear to develop systemic reactions to sulfites. The first documented report of a reaction to sulfites was in 1976. Since that time, sulfites have been reported to produce a wide spectrum of severe adverse reactions, including urticaria, angioedema, asthma, abdominal pain, and diarrhea.[1] Few reactions have been directly attributed to sulfites in drugs, which contain much smaller amounts of sulfites than foods.[8]

After exposure through inhalation, intravenous injection, or ingestion of sulfites the onset of symptoms is rapid, usually occurring within 2 to 15 minutes; onset tends to be more rapid when the sulfiting agents are ingested in solution. When sulfites are ingested in solid food the onset of symptoms is generally within 15 to 30 minutes, although some reactions to solid foods have occurred immediately.

A number of signs and symptoms have been ascribed to sulfite sensitivity (Table 50-4); besides those mentioned above, symptoms may include flushing, tingling, pruritus, tachypnea,

Table 50-4 Toxic Effects of Sulfites Noted in Sensitive Individuals

Minor
Abdominal pain
Conjunctivitis
Diarrhea
Dizziness
Dysphagia
Flushing
Nausea
Pruritus
Rhinitis
Swelling of the tongue
Tachycardia
Tachypnea
Tingling
Urticaria
Weakness

Major
Anaphylaxis
Bronchospasm
Loss of consciousness
Seizures
Death

wheezing, tachycardia, dizziness, and weakness. Rhinitis, conjunctivitis, and nausea[6] and dysphagia[10] have also been reported.[6] Swelling of the tongue may also occur in sulfite-sensitive individuals.[10] The most commonly reported reaction to sulfites is bronchospasm; this occurs most frequently in asthmatics. Bronchoconstriction has also occurred in asthmatics after inhalation of sulfite-preserved bronchodilator solutions. The most serious reactions from large amounts of sulfites are loss of consciousness, anaphylactic shock, CNS stimulation, seizures, and death.[8]

Mechanism of Toxicity

The mechanism of hypersensitivity to sulfites has not been fully explained, and it is likely that there are several mechanisms of toxicity. Some investigators have suggested an I_gE–mediated reaction, and in some cases an immunologic reaction may be involved. As mentioned above, there also appears to be a connection to sulfite oxidase deficiency in a small number of sensitive individuals. In addition, a cholinergic reflex mechanism has been suggested in view of the observation that many of the clinical manifestations reported with sulfite hypersensitivity are similar to those attributed to stimulation of the parasympathetic system. Stimulation of airway irritant receptors by inhaled sulfur dioxide has also been suggested as the mechanism for the immediate bronchospasm noted in some individuals.

Diagnosis

A history of an allergic reaction, anaphylaxis, or bronchoconstriction occurring during ingestion of food (particularly salads) or beverages in a restaurant provides a strong clue to the diagnosis of sulfite sensitivity.

Laboratory Confirmation

Cutaneous tests for immediate hypersensitivity to common foods may be negative in most sulfite-sensitive individuals. Confirmation of sensitivity to sulfites may be obtained through provocative challenges delivered by ingestion or inhalation of sulfites.

Treatment

There is no specific treatment for sulfite sensitivity reactions. Treatment is determined on the basis of the presenting symptoms (Table 50-5).

Table 50-5 Treatment for Sulfite Reactions

Prophylaxis
Cromolyn sodium
Nebulized atropine or cromolyn sodium
Asthma (as needed)
Epinephrine
Aminophylline
Antihistamines

Patients should be cautioned to avoid the use of foods and drugs containing sulfites.

Treatment of symptoms consists of the usual measures for asthma or anaphylaxis, including administration of epinephrine, aminophylline, and antihistamines, together with other appropriate support. Reactions to sulfites have been blocked with nebulized cromolyn sodium (Intal®) and nebulized atropine. A new drug, ketotifen (not yet available in the United States), has been shown to block metabisulfite-induced asthma.

MONOSODIUM GLUTAMATE

MSG is a widely used food additive; it is also on the FDA listing of substances that are generally recognized as safe.[13] MSG was discovered in the early 1900s when a chemist analyzed a seaweed that is commonly used as seasoning in Japanese cooking.[14,15] MSG now appears on the market as a flavor enhancer and is found in seasoned salts, soy sauce, bouillons, meat bases, and certain cooked or frozen foods.[16] It has also been suggested as the cause of the "Chinese Restaurant Syndrome," which is a benign, self-limiting process that has an excellent prognosis for immediate and rapid recovery.[13,17] Chinese Restaurant Syndrome is a misnomer because symptoms similar to those produced by MSG have been reported after ingestion of substances that contained MSG but were not Chinese foods or eaten in Chinese restaurants.[18]

Most MSG is prepared by fermentation of wheat, although 10% is obtained as a byproduct of sugar manufactured from sugar beets.[19]

Mechanism of Toxicity

Glutamate is a nonessential amino acid with a function as an amino carrier between L-ketoglutarate and glutamine.[20] L-Glutamic acid is present in large amounts in the CNS and has been suggested as a neurotransmitter. Glutamate is unique among amino acids by virtue of its direct utilization as an energy source by cerebral tissue.[14]

Glutamate appears to have minimal peripheral effects but has excitatory effects at central sites that affect cardiovascular control.[17] Glutamate also has numerous interactions with the tricarboxylic acid cycle and is an important precursor of glutathione and insulin as well as a critical source of urinary ammonium.[21] Glutamate is also a known precursor for synthesis of acetylcholine, and extracellular sodium ions enhance acetylcholine synthesis in ganglia.[18]

Pyroglutamate, which is formed from MSG when it is boiled, is similar to MSG but more readily crosses the blood-brain barrier.[14] Although both MSG and pyroglutamate have been shown to cause the Chinese Restaurant Syndrome, pyroglutamate provokes symptoms at lower concentrations than MSG, probably because of its greater permeation of the CNS.[13]

Currently it is thought that MSG produces a transient acetylcholinosis, which has signs and symptoms identical to those induced by acetylcholine.[22] This appears to account for the multiple symptoms affected by MSG toxicity. There may be a familial tendency toward development of this sensitivity.[23]

Toxicity

Symptoms related to MSG ingestion occur in a small percentage of the general public that is extremely sensitive to it.[21] Affected individuals experience symptoms within 15 to 45 minutes of ingestion. Effects may last for up to several hours, and spontaneous resolution has been noted.[11] Sometimes symptoms may not be noted for some hours after ingestion and may last for up to 2 days.[18,24]

As mentioned, signs and symptoms of toxicity appear to be similar to those induced by acetylcholine[21] and may include dizziness, facial flushing, heartburn, palpitations, burning in the chest, chest tightness, tightness of the scalp, frontal or temporal headache, nausea, abdominal pain, paresthesias and numbness over the

Table 50-6 Signs and Symptoms of MSG Reaction

Adults
Skin
    Flushing
    Scalp tightness
Neurologic
    Dizziness
    Headache
    Paresthesia
    Lightheadedness
Gastrointestinal
    Heartburn
    Burning in the chest
    Nausea
    Abdominal pain
    Thirst
    Chest tightness
Miscellaneous
    Palpitations
Children
Shivering
Shuddering
Irritability
Crying
Abdominal pain
Delirium

back of the neck, thirst, and lightheadedness (Table 50-6).[25] Other symptoms described in adults have been a feeling of pressure behind the eyes and diaphoresis.[23] In children, shivering and shuddering, irritability, crying, abdominal pain, and delirium have been described.[16,22]

Reaction most commonly occurs after eating food on an empty stomach. This is often when clear soup or broth is eaten as a first course because MSG is frequently added to clear soups and broths in considerable quantities to obtain a pleasantly strong meat flavor.[24] The rapid absorption of MSG under such circumstances may result in high serum concentrations that may overwhelm the blood-brain barrier, and trigger synthesis of acetylcholine.

Diagnosis

A thorough history and physical examination should be performed on all patients with signs and symptoms of MSG intoxication to rule out life-threatening disorders. Laboratory tests such as serum electrolytes, complete blood cell count, serum glutamate concentrations, or roentgenograms provide no additional information. There is no correlation between blood glutamate concentrations and the appearance of symptoms.[20]

Treatment

Normally MSG intoxication is benign and requires no treatment other than supportive care.[22]

In rare instances, patients may have cardiac symptoms that require electrocardiographic monitoring. In those instances a 12-lead electrocardiogram should be obtained. Dysrhythmias, if noted, should be treated with standard antidysrhythmic therapy. Occasionally bronchoconstriction may be noted and should be treated with the standard regimen, including β-specific nebulizers and intravenous xanthine derivatives.

REFERENCES

1. Mathison D, Stevenson D, Simon R: Precipitating factors in asthma. *Chest* 1985;87(suppl):50s–54s.

2. Swan G: Management of monosodium glutamate toxicity. *J Asthma* 1982;19:105–110.

3. Bush R, Taylor S, Busse W: A critical evaluation of clinical trials in reactions to sulfites. *J Allergy Clin Immunol* 1986;78:191–202.

4. Simon R: Sulfite sensitivity. *Ann Allergy* 1986;56: 281–292.

5. Stevenson D, Simon R: Sulfites and asthma. *J Allergy Clin Immunol* 1984;74:469–472.

6. Baker G, Collett P, Allen D: Bronchospasm induced by metabisulfite-containing foods and drugs. *Med J Aust* 1981;2:614–616.

7. Schwartz H, Sher T: Bisulfite sensitivity manifesting as allergy to local dental anesthesia. *J Allergy Clin Immunol* 1985;75:525–527.

8. Dalton-Bunnow M: Review of sulfite sensitivity. *Am J Hosp Pharmacol* 1985;42:2220–2226.

9. Koepke J, Christopher K, Chai H, et al: Dose-dependent bronchospasm from sulfites in isoetharine. *JAMA* 1984;251:2982–2983.

10. Jamieson D, Guill M, Wray B, et al: Metabisulfite sensitivity: Case report and literature review. *Ann Allergy* 1985;54:115–121.

11. Wolf S, Nicklas R: Sulfite sensitivity in a seven-year-old child. *Ann Allergy* 1985;54:420–423.

12. Napke E, Stevens D: Excipients and additives: Hidden hazards in drug products and in product substitution. *Can Med Assoc J* 1984;131:1449–1452.

13. Cochran J, Cochran A: Monosodium glutamania: The Chinese restaurant syndrome revisited. *JAMA* 1984;52:899.

14. Reif-Lehrer L: A questionnaire study of the prevalence of Chinese restaurant syndrome. *Fed Proc* 1977;36: 1617–1623.

15. Settipane G: Adverse reactions to sulfites in drugs and foods. *J Am Acad Dermatol* 1984;10:1077–1080.

16. Schaumburg H, Byck R, Gerstl R, et al: Monosodium L-glutamate: Its pharmacology and role in the Chinese restaurant syndrome. *Science* 1969;163:826–828.

17. Kerr G, Wu-Lee M, El-Lozy M, et al: Prevalence of "Chinese restaurant syndrome." *Research* 1979;75:29–33.

18. Ghadimi H, Kumar S, Abaci F: Studies on monosodium glutamate ingestion. *Biochem Med* 1971;5: 447–456.

19. Settipane G: The restaurant syndromes. *Arch Intern Med* 1986;146:2129–2130.

20. Kenney R, Tidball C: Human susceptibility to oral monosodium L-glutamate. *Am J Clin Nutr* 1972;25: 140–146.

21. Zautcke J, Schwartz J, Meuller E: Chinese restaurant syndrome: A review. *Ann Emerg Med* 1986;15:1210–1213.

22. Asnes R: Chinese restaurant syndrome in an infant. *Clin Pediatr* 1980;19:705–706.

23. Rubini, M: The many-faceted mystique of monosodium glutamate. *Am J Clin Nutr* 1972;24:169–171.

24. Wilkin J: Does monosodium glutamate cause flushing (or merely "glutamania")? *J Am Acad Dermatol* 1986;15: 225–230.

25. Yang W, Purchase E: Adverse reactions to sulfites. *Can Med Assoc J* 1985;133:865–880.

ADDITIONAL SELECTED REFERENCES

Bush R, Tasylor S, Holden K, et al: Prevalence of sensitivity to sulfiting agents in asthmatic patients. *Am J Med* 1986; 81:816–820.

Ghadimi H, Kumar S: Current status of monosodium glutamate. *Am J Clin Nutr* 1972;25:643–646.

Sauber W: What is Chinese restaurant syndrome? *Lancet* 1980;1:722–723.

Sher T, Schwartz H: Bisulfite sensitivity manifesting as an allergic reaction to aerosol therapy. *Ann Allergy* 1985; 54:224–226.

Twarog F, Leung D: Anaphylaxis to a component of isoetharine (sodium bisulfite). *JAMA* 1982;248:2030–2031.

chapter 51

Botulism

Botulism is an infrequent but devastating disease because the botulism toxin is one of the most dangerous toxins known.[1] The disease should be considered a true medical emergency. The causative organism, *Clostridium botulinum*, is an anaerobic, spore-forming, gram-positive, rod-shaped bacteria that is widely distributed in nature and is found mainly in the soil. These organisms elaborate the toxin, and a given strain of the organism produces only one toxin type.[2]

The term botulism is derived from the Latin word *botulus*, meaning ''sausage,'' because blood sausage was known for centuries to be associated with the symptom complex now recognized as botulism.[3] Clinically, botulism can be classified into three major types on the basis of the cause of the disease and the age of the patient.[1] These types are foodborne botulism, infant botulism, and wound botulism.[4] Further, there are seven serologically distinguishable toxins arbitrarily designated by the letters A through G. All are globular proteins approximately 150,000 daltons in molecular weight, and all act by the same mechanism. Most illness is caused by types A and B.[5] There is a distinct geographic distribution of these toxins in the United States.[1] Type A is evident primarily west of the Mississippi River, and type B is frequently seen in the eastern states. Type E is found predominantly in the Great Lakes region and in Alaska.[6]

Clostridium botulinum spores are resistant to heat, radiation, light, and drying. These spores germinate only under anaerobic and neutral or weakly acidic conditions if these are present for several days. Thus the ingestion of formed toxin, not simply of spores, is required in the foodborne or adult form of botulism. In infant botulism, the toxin is produced by incubation of the spores within the gastrointestinal tract.[5]

MECHANISM OF TOXICITY

Botulism toxin binds at the presynaptic clefts of cholinergic nerve terminals, blocking the release of acetylcholine at the neuromuscular junctions and peripheral autonomic synapses.[3] This results in the clinical manifestation of autonomic dysfunction and generalized paralysis. The toxin binds to all ganglionic and postganglionic parasympathetic synapses as well as neuromuscular junctions.[2] In the parasympathetic nervous system both preganglionic and postganglionic fibers are involved early, which results in severe autonomic dysfunction.[7]

On ingestion, botulism toxin is first transported across the intestinal wall into the serum. It then binds to a receptor on the surface of the presynaptic nerve membrane. The toxin or some part of it then crosses into the presynaptic terminal and combines with another internal receptor, which causes interference with acetylcholine release. This is an irreversible step leading to impairment of neurotransmitter release and resultant neuromuscular blockade. Although the presynaptic nerve can still propagate an impulse, there is no subsequent release of acetylcholine.

The effects of botulism toxin in some ways resemble those of curare except that the former acts presynaptically and its effects are only occasionally reversed by cholinesterase inhibitors.[3]

WOUND BOTULISM

Wound botulism is a rare clinical entity and results from an infection of a wound by *C botulinum* with subsequent in vivo production and systemic absorption of the toxin.[3,8] The incubation period is longer than for foodborne botulism.[4] Wound botulism has been associated with compound fractures, severe trauma, lacerations, puncture wounds, and hematoma.[3]

FOODBORNE BOTULISM

Botulism outbreaks are usually due to ingestion of tainted foods. Inadequate processing of non-acidic foods and home canning procedures are responsible in a great majority of cases; because spore germination is inhibited at low pH, acidic foods are less frequently contaminated.

Foodborne botulism most commonly results from eating uncooked preserved foods. Heating contaminated foods at 120°C for 30 minutes could inactivate the spores, but they may survive at boiling temperatures (100°C).[5]

Signs and Symptoms

Symptoms of botulism usually occur 12 to 36 hours after ingestion of contaminated food, although the incubation period can be as short as 4 hours or as long as 8 days (Table 51-1). Fever is usually not seen unless there is an infection from another source.

Gastrointestinal

Early symptoms of botulism include nausea, vomiting, abdominal cramps, and abdominal distension. These effects are due to the toxin's local action on the gastrointestinal tract. Constipation is common; diarrhea is rarely found.

Table 51-1 Signs and Symptoms of Foodborne Botulism

Gastrointestinal
- Nausea
- Vomiting
- Abdominal cramps
- Abdominal distension
- Constipation

Neurologic
- Eye
  - Blurred vision
  - Diplopia
  - Photophobia
  - Ptosis
  - Mydriasis
- Dizziness
- Dysarthria

Respiratory
- Respiratory failure
- Laryngeal obstruction

Neurologic

Systemic neurologic symptoms of botulism usually occur within 72 hours of gastrointestinal symptoms but may be delayed as long as 8 days. Early neurologic signs indicate a more severe infection and a worse prognosis.[9] Presenting neurologic symptoms are bulbar paralysis and a descending motor paralysis.[1] Various eye disorders may be early features and include blurred vision, diplopia, photophobia, ptosis, and mydriasis.[2] The highest cranial nerves are usually affected first, so that diplopia may be the first presenting symptom.[9] Dizziness and dysarthria may occur, and as the lower cranial nerves become involved the patient may complain of dysphagia and a dry mouth. The motor nerves are then involved, and peripheral muscle weakness progresses. When the muscles of respiration are affected, fatal dyspnea may result. There is no sensory involvement, and the patient may remain mentally clear; myotactic reflexes also remain intact.[2]

Cause of Death

The most serious effects of botulism are pulmonary infection or respiratory failure secondary to muscle dysfunction and bulbar paralysis. Although the most common cause of death is paralysis of the muscles of respiration, occasionally patients may succumb to sudden laryngeal obstruction or unexpected cardiac arrest.[1]

Diagnosis

The initial diagnosis of botulism is clinical and based on the history and physical examination. A correct diagnosis is difficult to make, and many times botulism is misdiagnosed in its early stages. Because most cases originate from tainted food, a careful history of ingestion of home-canned or home-prepared food should be sought. Definite diagnosis can be made by demonstration of toxin in serum or stool by the mouse inoculation test.[3]

Laboratory Analysis

Botulism toxin may be detected in serum provided that blood is collected soon after the onset of clinical symptoms. Serum (10 mL) should be obtained before treatment; but treatment should not be delayed while awaiting laboratory confirmation because this may require more than 24 hours.

Electromyography may help in the diagnosis by showing an increase in the abnormally small-amplitude muscle action potentials after repetitive nerve stimulation (staircase effect).[9] This is in contrast to findings in myasthenia gravis, in which repetitive nerve stimulation results in a decrease of the muscle action potentials.[7]

Routine studies including a complete blood cell count, serum electrolytes, calcium and magnesium concentrations, blood urea nitrogen, hepatic enzymes, lumbar puncture, and a chest roentgenogram are usually normal but may be altered by secondary dehydration or pneumonitis.

Treatment

General Measures

Treatment is supportive, and early intervention is indicated. Effective treatment comprises three stages: respiratory care, removal of the nonabsorbed enterotoxin, and possible antitoxin therapy.[2] Respiratory impairment may present the most serious, life-threatening consequence of botulism poisoning. Serial measurements of vital capacity are therefore indicated. Gentamicin and other aminoglycosides should be avoided if possible in a patient with botulism because there have been reports of potentiation of the neuromuscular blockade with such agents.

Guanidine

Because guanidine enhances release of acetylcholine from nerve terminals, its use has been suggested for treatment of botulism. Guanidine appears to be beneficial in patients with Eaton-Lambert syndrome, but clinical data have so far been inconclusive as to its effectiveness for botulism.

Antitoxin

The use of antitoxin to botulism toxin is still open to debate. It appears that antitoxin has relatively little effect on toxin types A and B but appreciable effect on type E. It does not reverse any neurologic damage that may have already occurred but may slow or halt the progression of the disease by binding to circulating toxin. Both a bivalent and a trivalent equine-derived antitoxin are available. The bivalent antitoxin contains 10,000 international units of antibody to types A and B, and the trivalent antitoxin contains antibody to types A, B, and E. Both are currently available from the Centers for Disease Control. Dosage is one vial every 4 to 5 hours and may be repeated for 4 to 5 doses.

The decision to administer antitoxin must be based on the risk of its side reactions compared to its potential benefit. The percentage of side reactions from all types of botulism antitoxin is significant. Acute reactions include urticaria, skin rash, and anaphylaxis. The necessary medications and equipment should be readily available for the treatment of any serious side effects.[8]

In instances in which the toxin type is unknown, the trivalent preparation is preferred. Before administering the antitoxin, inquiries should be made to determine whether there is a history of allergy, asthma, or hay fever. A skin test should be performed for horse serum sensitivity, and desensitization should be performed in the sensitive individual.

Human botulinogenic hyperimmune serum is under development but is not yet clinically available.

INFANT BOTULISM

Infant botulism was first described in 1976 and is now known to present with a diverse spectrum of clinical symptoms.[7] It is not a new disease but rather a newly recognized manifestation of an old disorder.[6,10]

Mechanism of Toxicity

No definitive food source can be implicated in most cases of infant botulism.[11,12] In this disorder the intestinal growth of the spores of *Clostridium botulinum* gives rise to subsequent systemic absorption of the toxin.[13] The spores germinate in the gastrointestinal tract and produce botulism toxin in vivo.[14] Most cases of infant botulism have been caused by either type A or B toxin, although recently a case caused by type F was reported.[13]

The age of onset of infant botulism ranges from 2 to 8 months, with peak incidence being at 2 to 4 months of age. Only infants less than 1 year of age appear to have multiplication of spores in the gastrointestinal tract.[6] Honey is the only food source that correlates strongly with infant botulism, and therefore honey should be avoided during this period of life because evidence suggests that a small percentage of all honey is contaminated by botulism spores, which cannot be destroyed.[15] The organism may survive passage through the infant stomach because of its alkaline pH and its relative lack of protease activity.[5]

Signs and Symptoms

The severity of illness in patients with infant botulism varies. The typical clinical syndrome is characterized by variable constipation with subsequent progressive weakness, hypotonia, cranial nerve dysfunction, and hyporeflexia (Table 51-2).[7]

Table 51-2 Signs and Symptoms of Infant Botulism

Gastrointestinal
  Constipation
Neurologic
  Diminished gag reflex
  Poor sucking ability
  Facial muscle weakness
  Ptosis
  Extraocular palsy
  Loss of head control
  Hyporeflexia
  Hypotonia
  Weakness

Gastrointestinal

Constipation is usually the first symptom, with the frequency of stool passage being less than 48 hours. Constipation may precede neuromuscular symptoms by as much as 3 weeks.

Neurologic

Cranial nerve dysfunction usually includes diminished gag reflex and poor sucking ability.[12] Other manifestations of motor cranial nerve dysfunction may include facial muscle weakness, ptosis, extraocular palsies, and sluggish pupillary light response.[11] Cranial nerves VII, IX, X, and XI are almost always involved, and nerves III, IV, and VI are less frequently affected. The infant may appear to be alert despite profound weakness[15]; this is characteristic of infant botulism. When the descending paralysis has affected bulbar musculature and has become generalized, loss of head control is prominent.[7]

Diagnosis

Because infants are unable to describe their symptoms, the onset of illness can only be detected by careful observation.[14] The differential diagnosis of infant botulism must rule out Guillain-Barré syndrome, metal encephalopathy, Reye's syndrome, sepsis, myasthenia gravis, tick paralysis, electrolyte imbalance, diphtheria, meningitis, and metabolic encephalopathy (Table 51-3).[15]

Electromyographic abnormalities are the only relatively specific finding in infant botulism

Table 51-3 Diseases To Rule Out in the Differential Diagnosis of Infant Botulism

---

Diphtheria
Electrolyte imbalance
Guillain-Barré syndrome
Metal encephalopathy
Meningitis
Metabolic encephalopathy
Myasthenia gravis
Reye's syndrome
Sepsis
Tick paralysis

---

short of isolating the spores. Brief, small-amplitude, overly abundant action potentials are noted.[8] In addition, as with the adult form of botulism, an incremental response to rapid, repetitive nerve stimulation is frequently noted. Routine laboratory studies including a complete blood cell count, serum electrolytes, and other tests will be normal unless secondarily affected by pneumonia or fluid and electrolyte shifts.[11]

Confirmation of the diagnosis of infant botulism requires isolation of the organism or demonstration of specific toxin in stool samples. In contrast to the foodborne type, only rarely is the serum positive for organisms or toxin.

Cause of Death

Death from infant botulism has been caused by pulmonary complications[7] including aspiration pneumonia, which results from the diminished gag reflex combined with weakness and incoordination of the muscles of deglutition.[15] Respiratory arrest secondary to manipulation for a lumbar puncture and ventilatory failure caused by paralysis of the muscles of respiration may also occur. There is suggestive evidence that infant botulism is the cause in some cases of sudden infant death syndrome.[11]

Treatment

Supportive Care

Current management of infant botulism consists of supportive respiratory and nutritional care, which should be meticulous. Patients should not be fed by mouth until they are able to gag and swallow. Nasogastric feedings may be necessary for adequate nutrition. Monitoring for apnea and bradycardia is essential in all patients.[7]

Cathartics

It has been argued that laxatives, cathartics, and enemas may decrease the concentration of intestinal organisms or toxin. Because these sick infants are generally in a precarious metabolic condition and because fluid or electrolyte disturbances may result from injudicious or repeated purgation, use of cathartics is not advocated.[8]

Antibiotics

Because penicillin has anticlostridial action it has been advocated for infant botulism.[14] There appears to be no protective effect noted after administration either orally or parenterally, however. Some investigators have suggested that lysis of the organisms by penicillin may make more toxin available for absorption.[10]

As with the adult form of botulism, aminoglycoside administration appears to worsen the muscle paralysis.

Antitoxin

The efficacy of antitoxin is even less clear in infant botulism than in adult botulism because antitoxin neutralizes only circulating toxin and not that bound to nerves. Circulating toxin has only rarely been found in patients with infant botulism, so that the benefit of antitoxin is minimal.[13]

Recovery

Once symptoms of infant botulism reach a nadir, the patient's condition usually persists unchanged for 2 to 3 weeks before slow recovery of strength occurs.[14] Toxin may be found in stool weeks to months after the patient has recovered.[13] Recovery from botulism implies establishment of new anatomical pathways at the synapse because toxin binding is apparently irreversible.[8]

REFERENCES

1. Sanders A, Seifert S, Kobernick M: Botulism. *J Fam Pract* 1983;16:987–1000.

2. Cherington M: Botulism: Ten-year experience. *Arch Neurol* 1974;30:432–437.

3. Hikes D, Manoli A: Wound botulism. *J Trauma* 1981;21:68–71.

4. Fullerton P, Gogna N, Stoddart R: Wound botulism. *Med J Aust* 1980;1:662–663.

5. Arnon S, Midura T, Damus K, et al: Honey and other environmental risk factors for infant botulism. *J Pediatr* 1979;94:331–336.

6. Aureli P, Fenicia L, Pasolini B, et al: Two cases of type E infant botulism caused by neurotoxigenic *Clostridium butyricum* in Italy. *J Infect Dis* 1986;154:207–211.

7. Arnon S: Infant botulism. *Annu Rev Med* 1980; 31:541–560.

8. Keller M, Miller V, Berkowitz C, et al: Wound botulism in pediatrics. *Am J Dis Child* 1982;136:320–322.

9. Merson M, Hughes J, Dowell V, et al: Current trends in botulism in the United States. *JAMA* 1974;229: 1305–1308.

10. Roland E, Ebelt V, Anderson J, et al: Infant botulism: A rare entity in Canada? *Can Med Assoc J* 1986;135: 130–131.

11. Brougnton R, Campbell J, Wilson H: Infant botulism. *South Med J* 1981;74:257–258.

12. Thompson J, Glasgow L, Warpinski J, et al: Infant botulism: Clinical spectrum and epidemiology. *Pediatrics* 1980;66:936–942.

13. Hoffman R, Pincomb B, Skeels M, et al: Type F infant botulism. *Am J Dis Child* 1982;136:270–271.

14. McCurdy D, Krishnan C, Hauschild A: Infant botulism in Canada. *Can Med Assoc J* 1981;125:741–743.

15. Brown L: Infant botulism and the honey connection. *J Pediatr* 1979;94:337–338.

chapter 52

Toxins Associated with Fish

Fish and shellfish are an increasing part of the diet of Americans, yet it has only been recently recognized that these animals are important causative agents in a number of neurologic and gastroenterologic disorders.[1] This chapter is limited to a discussion of ciguatera and scombroid poisoning, which are the most common disorders caused by fish or shellfish.[2,3] Disease arises from ingestion of a toxin known as ichthyosarcotoxin.[4,5]

CIGUATERA

Ciguatera is a serious and sometimes fatal disease caused by the ingestion of various tropical marine fishes.[6] It has been seen in islands of the Pacific and Caribbean Oceans.[2] The term ciguatera is a misnomer; it is derived from the Spanish word for a similar disease caused by a poisonous marine snail or mollusk known as cigua.[7] This animal is now known not to be a source of ichthyosarcotoxin.[4,8,9]

Toxicity from ciguatera is not confined to a single fish species but may result from ingestion of more than 400 species of herbivorous and carnivorous fish (Table 52-1). Migratory bottom-dwelling shore fish caught near reefs located between 35°N and 35°S latitudes are those that typically cause ciguatera.[1,5] Barracuda, jack, red snapper, grouper, and sea bass are commonly implicated in ciguatera.[10,11] The

entire fish or just the flesh or viscera may be toxic; the highest concentration is within the liver, intestines, and gonads.[6]

Although ciguatera affects persons residing in tropical and subtropical coastal regions of the world, importation of fish and fish products from these areas has made the problem of concern in many other locations where they may be sold.[4,8]

The chemical structure and mechanism of action of the ichthyosarcotoxin that causes ciguatera are not clearly defined.[6] The compound is relatively heat stable; therefore, cooking of the fish does not provide protection from illness.[2,9] It is also stable in gastric fluids. The toxin has been identified as a low–molecular weight lipid that is transmitted from fish to fish

Table 52-1 Fish Associated with Ciguatera

Amberjack
Barracuda
Coral trout
Eel
Emperor
Grouper
Kingfish
Paddletail
Parrot fish
Red snapper
Sea bass
Squirrel fish
Yankee whiting

through the food chain; it is thought to be produced by the dinoflagellate *Gambierdiscus toxicus*. The severity of poisoning is related to the size of the fish because large predator fish accumulate the toxin from eating smaller fish, which "graze" on the dinoflagellates.[5]

Toxicity

Toxicity appears to be dose related, with the worst reactions occurring in individuals who have had prior cases of ciguatera.[9,10] There is no uniformly reliable taste, appearance, or odor that distinguishes between contaminated and clean catch before ingestion. Sometimes animals, usually pets, are fed parts of a fish to determine whether it is contaminated; if symptoms of poisoning do not develop, the catch is considered fit for human consumption.[10] The disease is usually short-lived in most cases, and many patients do not seek medical attention. Although death is unlikely, signs and symptoms of the disease may be severe and produce long-term disability.[5]

More than 175 manifestations of symptoms have been noted in ciguatera (Table 52-2). Gastrointestinal symptoms usually occur early and are of short duration.[1] Neurologic manifestations may occur later in the course of the disease and may persist for weeks to months. Cardiovascular signs and symptoms may also be seen, with fairly profound hypotension and bradycardia noted.[4]

Gastrointestinal

Symptoms usually begin 2 to 6 hours after ingestion. Gastroenteritis with nausea, vomiting, diarrhea, and abdominal pain may appear initially.[7,12] These symptoms usually subside without therapy within a few hours.[11] Fever, diaphoresis, and sometimes bradycardia may accompany the gastrointestinal complaints.[6,8]

Neurologic

Typically the patient also complains of neurologic symptoms such as numbness and tingling, ataxia, and vertigo.[10] The neurosensory involvement is typically acral, affecting the perioral region and the distal extremities. Tingling of the mouth, tongue, or throat may therefore

Table 52-2 Signs and Symptoms of Ciguatera

Gastrointestinal
  Abdominal pain
  Diarrhea
  Nausea
  Vomiting
Neurologic
  Ataxia
  Paresthesia
  Temperature reversal
  Vertigo
Miscellaneous
  Arthralgia
  Bradycardia
  Death
  Diaphoresis
  Fever
  Hypotension
  Myalgia
  Respiratory paralysis
  Weakness

occur. In severe cases, a common complaint is that of "temperature reversal," that is, cold objects causing a burning sensation on contact with the fingertips, toes, or tongue.[2,11] This phenomenon usually develops 2 to 5 days after the ingestion.[3] Although the neurologic symptoms usually last no longer than a few days, they may occasionally recur for weeks or even months.[4]

Miscellaneous

Arthralgia, myalgia, and weakness are also commonly observed.[10] In extremely severe cases, there may be respiratory paralysis and death. Although ciguatera is not considered a fatal condition, there have been isolated reports of death.[6,8]

Mechanism of Action of Ciguatera Toxin

Ciguatera toxin demonstrates some anticholinesterase activity.[1,13] In addition, there appears to be an increase in the passive permeability of the nerve cell membrane to sodium with subsequent inhibition of action potential initiation.[12] This action may explain some of the neurologic manifestations noted.[4,9]

Differential Diagnosis

The differential diagnosis of acute ciguatera must rule out other marine poisonings, botulism, bacterial food poisoning, eosinophilic meningitis, organophosphate poisoning, and monosodium glutamate ingestion in sensitive individuals (Table 52-3).[3,10] Because many toxic marine ingestions share clinical manifestations and because laboratory assays for specific toxins may not be immediately available, an accurate and detailed history, physical examination, and brief laboratory evaluation must be relied on to make the diagnosis.[5]

Laboratory Analysis

The only widely recognized hematologic or biochemical abnormalities attributable to ciguatera that can be determined from laboratory tests are those secondary to the fluid and electrolyte disturbances associated with diarrhea and dehydration.[4] Results of electromyography are usually normal. In uncomplicated cases, electroencephalograms and results of lumbar puncture have also been normal.[13]

Efforts to establish the chemical identity of the heat-stable toxin and to develop assays for toxin in fish samples for use in outbreaks of ciguatera have met with only limited success.[1] Definitive identification requires the use of an animal bioassay, radioimmunoassay, or rapid enzyme immunoassay. Reliable screening tests are not readily available.[7,13]

Treatment

Treatment of ciguatera is supportive and symptomatic and consists of administration of antiemetic and antidiarrheal agents (as needed), fluids, and atropine when indicated for hypotension and bradycardia.[4] Atropine may have no effect on musculoskeletal or neurologic symptoms.[2] Pruritus may be relieved partially by H_1 histamine antagonists. Although calcium, corticosteroids, pralidoxime, and vitamin B complex have been suggested, they have not been demonstrated to be useful. Respiratory support

Table 52-3 Conditions To Rule Out in the Differential Diagnosis of Ciguatera

Other marine poisonings
Botulism
Bacterial food poisoning
Eosinophilic meningitis
Organophosphate poisoning
Monosodium glutamate sensitivity

is necessary for the rare case in which respiratory paralysis occurs.[7]

SCOMBROID POISONING

Scombroid fish poisoning is the only form of ichthyosarcotoxism in which toxin is formed by the action of bacteria on fish flesh. Worldwide, scromboid poisoning is the most common cause of toxicity resulting from the ingestion of fish.[7] It is also the only form of fish poisoning that is completely preventable with proper refrigeration and fish handling procedures.[14]

Fish Associated with Scombroid Poisoning

Most fish that have caused outbreaks of scombroid poisoning are members of the suborder Scombroidea. These are primarily found in tropical and temperate waters throughout the world. Commonly implicated species are tuna, mackerel, bonito, and skipjack.[14] Mahi-mahi or Pacific dolphin is a nonscombroid fish that has recently been associated with outbreaks of scombroid poisoning.

Mechanism of Toxicity

The flesh of fish causing scombroid poisoning contains a great deal of histidine. In the presence of certain bacteria and the proper conditions this histidine is broken down or decarboxylated to histamine, which causes symptoms when ingested. This bacterial enzymatic reaction occurs maximally at approximately 20°C and is prevented if bacterial growth is inhibited by adequate refrigeration.[14] Scombrotoxin is heat stable and is not destroyed by domestic or commercial cooking.

Although the exact nature of scombrotoxin is not known, it is believed to be made up of several substances that are histamine-related.[5] Saurine was once postulated as one of these substances, but current evidence indicates that the active substance is a histamine salt.[2]

Toxicity

Symptoms of scombroid poisoning may develop within minutes to hours of ingestion of tainted fish. The symptoms are the same as those of any histamine-mediated reaction and include urticaria, itching, dizziness, and abdominal cramps (Table 52-4). Flushing of the face, neck, and upper trunk is the most characteristic and consistent symptom of scombroid poisoning.[14] Nausea, vomiting, diarrhea, burning of the mouth and throat, and in more severe cases hypotension, bronchospasm, and respiratory distress may occur.

Laboratory Analysis

The diagnosis of scombroid poisoning is primarily clinical.[14] Blood histamine and urinary histamine metabolite concentrations are elevated in patients with scombroid poisoning, but meas-

Table 52-4 Signs and Symptoms of Scombroid Poisoning

Dermal
Urticaria
Pruritus
Flushing
  Face
  Neck
  Trunk
Gastrointestinal
Nausea
Vomiting
Diarrhea
Burning of the mouth
Abdominal cramps
Miscellaneous
Bronchospasm
Hypotension
Respiratory distress

urements of this kind are usually not necessary or easy to obtain.[2]

Treatment

Left untreated, symptoms of scombroid poisoning subside within 12 hours. Although fatalities have been reported, they are extremely rare. To avoid hypotension, intravenous fluid therapy may be initiated. Antihistamine administration results in rapid improvement.[5] In severe cases accompanied by bronchospasm, bronchodilators should be administered.[2]

REFERENCES

1. Cassanova M, Sanchez R, Marco R: Ciguatera poisoning. *Arch Neurol* 1982;39:387.

2. Dembert M, Strosahl K, Bumbarner R: Disease from fish and shellfish ingestion. *Am Fam Physician* 1981; 24:103–108.

3. Lawrence D, Enriquez M, Lumish R, et al: Ciguatera fish poisoning in Miami. *JAMA* 1980;244:254–258.

4. Bagnis R, Kuberski T, Laugier S: Clinical observations on 3009 cases of ciguatera (fish poisoning) in the South Pacific. *Am J Trop Med Hyg* 1979;28:1067–1073.

5. Halstead B: Current status of marine biotoxicology— An overview. *Clin Toxicol* 1981;18:1–24.

6. Chretien J, Fermaglich J, Garagusi V: Ciguatera poisoning: Presentation as a neurologic disorder. *Arch Neurol* 1981;38:783.

7. Hughes J, Merson M: Fish and shellfish poisoning. *N Engl J Med* 1976;295:1117–1120.

8. Russell F: Ciguatera poisoning: A report of 35 cases. *Toxicon* 1975;13:383–385.

9. Sims J: A theoretical discourse on the pharmacology of toxic marine ingestions. *Ann Emerg Med* 1987; 16:1006–1015.

10. Ho A, Fraser I, Todd E: Ciguatera poisoning: A report of three cases. *Ann Emerg Med* 1986;15:1225–1228.

11. Morris J, Lewin P, Hargrett N, et al: Clinical features of ciguatera fish poisoning. *Arch Intern Med* 1982; 142:1090–1092.

12. Rayner M: Mode of action of ciguatoxin. *Fed Proc* 1972;31:1139–1145.

13. Li K: Ciguatera fish poison: A cholinesterase inhibitor. *Science* 1965;147:1580–1581.

14. Dickinson G: Scombroid fish poisoning syndrome. *Ann Emerg Med* 1982;11:487–489.

part XIII

MISCELLANEOUS AGENTS

chapter 53

Phenytoin

Phenytoin is the most common anticonvulsant in use today. Although it is not a barbiturate, it is related to the barbiturates in chemical structure. Phenytoin is useful in the treatment of generalized tonic-clonic and partial-complex seizures. The primary site of action appears to be the motor cortex, where it inhibits the spread of seizure activity.[1] Phenytoin limits the development of maximal seizure activity from an active focus by stabilization of the excitable neuronal membrane.[2] It does this by interfering with the movement of ions across the cell membrane. Specifically, phenytoin decreases resting fluxes of sodium ions as well as sodium currents that exist during action potentials in chemically induced depolarization.[3] Although phenytoin is commonly advocated and used as an antidysrhythmic agent, it is not approved by the FDA for such use.

PHARMACOKINETICS

The pharmacokinetics of phenytoin are complicated and present a number of problems when dealing with toxicity. They are based on its limited aqueous solubility, dose-dependent elimination, and hepatic inactivation, all of which may be influenced by other drugs.

Phenytoin may be administered orally or intravenously. Oral absorption is slow and sometimes variable or incomplete. Oral phenytoin is absorbed most slowly from the stomach and more rapidly from the small bowel. Peak concentrations after a single oral dose may occur approximately 6 hours after administration.[4]

Although the drug has not been recommended for use in intravenous infusion because of the possibility that microcrystallization of phenytoin may occur, many clinicians suggest that intravenous infusions are feasible provided that appropriate precautions are taken.[5,6] The drug may be administered intravenously in normal saline no faster than 25 to 50 mg/minute to avoid such undesirable side effects as hypotension and cardiac dysrhythmias (Table 53-1). In neonates, the drug should be administered at a rate not

Table 53-1 Side Effects of Intravenous Phenytoin

Neurologic
  Nystagmus
  Ataxia
  Dizziness
Dermatologic
  Local burning
  Phlebitis
Cardiac
  Hypotension
  Bradycardia
  Cardiac dysrhythmias
  Increased PR interval
  Increased QRS complex duration
  Abnormalities of ST segment and T wave

exceeding 1 to 3 mg/kg/minute.[3] The intra-venous preparation of phenytoin is solubilized with 40% propylene glycol and 10% ethyl alcohol in addition to being adjusted to pH 12 with sodium hydroxide.[7-9]

Intramuscular administration is not suggested because absorption by this route is erratic and because plasma drug concentrations are unpredictable.[10] In addition, intramuscular phenytoin can cause tissue necrosis and sterile abscesses due to the high alkalinity of the solution.[6]

Some of the side effects that were previously recorded with intravenous phenytoin have been shown to be related to the solvent propylene glycol.[9] These effects are hypotension, disturbances of cardiac rhythm, prolongation of PR intervals and QRS complexes, and alterations of ST segments and T waves in the electrocardiogram.[8]

Elimination

Phenytoin is 90% protein bound, mainly to albumin. It has a volume of distribution of 0.6 to 0.7 L/kg.[11] Phenytoin is eliminated largely by parahydroxylation of one of the phenol rings to 5-hydroxyphenyl-5-phenylhydantoin, which is an inactive metabolite.[12] This mechanism is saturated at concentrations near the upper end of the therapeutic range.[3] Phenytoin therefore exhibits nonlinear Michaelis-Menten pharmacokinetics.[13] In low doses elimination appears to occur by a first-order process; with an increase in dose the plasma concentration increases disproportionately.[1] This change in kinetics from first-order to zero-order fits the Michaelis-Menten model of enzyme saturation.[12] Consequently, a small change in dose may cause a great change in the observed plasma concentration. As an example, the steady state plasma concentration may double or triple from a 10% increase in dose.[14]

At therapeutic concentrations phenytoin has a half-life of 7 to 24 hours; in healthy adults it averages 22 hours. As concentrations increase and the enzymes become saturated, the half-life also increases.[2] At concentrations greater than 30 μg/mL the half-life ranges from 72 to 120 hours.[11] Variations in half-life may be due to variations in hepatic function, enzyme self-induction, genetic factors affecting individual

Table 53-2 Drugs That Alter Phenytoin Serum Concentration

Increased Phenytoin Concentration
 Chlordiazepoxide
 Cimetidine
 Diazepam
 Dicumarol
 Dimercaprol
 Disulfiram
 Ethyl alcohol (acute)
 Isoniazid
 Phenothiazines
 Salicylates
 Trazodone
Decreased Phenytoin Concentration
 Carbamazepine
 Ethyl alcohol (chronic)
 Reserpine

---

differences in substrate saturation of the rate-limiting enzyme, and variations in dose dependency.

Drug Interactions

Various drugs may affect the serum concentration of phenytoin (Table 53-2).[15] Drugs that may decrease concentrations include chronically ingested alcohol, carbamazepine, and reserpine. Drugs that may increase concentrations include phenothiazines, diazepam, disulfiram, acutely ingested alcohol, salicylates, dicumarol, isoniazid, chlordiazepoxide, cimetidine, trazodone, and others. This may be due to the high protein binding by these drugs, which compete for binding sites on albumin and displace phenytoin or inhibit its metabolism by the liver.[12] Folic acid deficiency may result in an elevation of phenytoin in plasma because this cofactor is utilized in the metabolism of phenytoin.[4]

Adverse Reactions

Oral phenytoin can cause many uncommon adverse reactions (Table 53-3), including hematologic, reticuloendothelial, metabolic, gastrointestinal, neurologic, genitourinary, and cutaneous disorders (when chronically administered). Gingival hyperplasia is more common

Table 53-3 Adverse Reactions to Oral Phenytoin

Hematologic
  Thrombocytopenia
  Leukopenia
  Agranulocytosis
  Megaloblastic anemia
Cutaneous
  Morbilliform rash
  Stevens-Johnson syndrome
  Gingival hyperplasia
Gastrointestinal
  Nausea
  Vomiting
  Constipation

Table 53-4 Contributing Factors in Chronic Phenytoin Intoxication

Change in kinetics
Hypoalbuminemia
Chronic renal failure
Hepatic dysfunction
Genetic defect in phenytoin metabolism
Concomitant administration of other drugs

in young patients than in adults but has no predilection for either sex[1]; it never occurs in edentulous patients.[9] A period of 4 to 6 months is required for the changes to develop; if they are allowed to continue they reach a maximum in 9 to 12 months. This phenomenon disappears spontaneously after withdrawal of phenytoin.

Plasma Concentrations

Blood concentrations of phenytoin are usually measured as the total (bound and unbound) drug; therefore, medical disorders or drugs that displace or prevent phenytoin from binding with albumin may cause an increase in the free phenytoin fraction and may lead to intoxication even if the total amount of drug is within the therapeutic range.[2,16] Therapeutic plasma concentrations usually are in the range of 10 to 20 μg/mL.[17] Because the volume of distribution is relatively constant within the therapeutic range, it can be used to calculate appropriate doses for the attainment of desired serum concentrations.[18] In general, steady-state therapeutic plasma concentrations are achieved about 7 to 10 days after intiation of therapy with a daily oral dose of 300 mg in adults.[19,20] After intravenous administration, therapeutic plasma concentrations are attained within 1 to 2 hours.[12]

Because of the great variation in plasma concentrations that may occur, measurements should be performed when initiating therapy, changing the dose, or adding or deleting other drugs from the regimen.[21]

TOXICITY

Chronic phenytoin intoxication with typical therapeutic doses may result from several mechanisms (Table 53-4).[22,23] In patients with hypoalbuminemia, a large proportion of phenytoin remains unbound and therefore in active form.[24] In patients with chronic renal failure there is also a decreased ability to bind phenytoin.[25]

The mixed-function oxidases responsible for phenytoin metabolism are located in the central area of the liver lobules, and any damage to these areas can slow the rate of metabolism.[9] Phenytoin intoxication may therefore also result from hepatic dysfunction secondary to cirrhosis or hepatitis.[12] In addition, it may result from a genetic defect in phenytoin metabolism or, as stated above, from the inhibition of its metabolism by other drugs.[26] Intoxication may result from accumulation of the drug, which saturates the enzyme system and switches kinetics from first-order to zero-order.[17]

In therapeutic doses, phenytoin does not exhibit sedative properties. Overdose by the oral route gives rise to symptoms referable primarily to the cerebellum and vestibular systems; these are usually dose related. Because of the drug's long half-life, the major manifestations of intoxication may persist for 4 to 5 days after diagnosis.

Correlation between Serum Concentration and Toxic Effects

Most patients tolerate phenytoin blood concentrations less than 25 μg/mL (Table 53-5). Nystagmus on lateral gaze usually appears at 20 to 25 μg/mL. Ataxia and diplopia may occur at 30 μg/mL.[27] Although nystagmus and ataxia

Table 53-5 Phenytoin Serum Concentrations and Corresponding Toxic Effects

Concentration (micrograms per milliliter)	Symptoms
10 to 20	Therapeutic
20 to 30	Nystagmus, ataxia, diplopia
30 to 40	Dysarthria
40 to 50	Lethargy, drowsiness, asterixis
50 to 60	Stupor
> 60	Coma

Table 53-6 Non–Dose Related Toxic Effects of Phenytoin

Gastrointestinal
Nausea
Vomiting
Constipation
Neurologic
Confusion
Hemihyperesthesia
Hemiparesis
Choreoathetosis
Dystonia
Dysarthria
Generalized seizures

usually precede more severe symptoms, toxicity may remain unrecognized by the patient.[2] When the blood concentration exceeds 30 μg/mL dysarthria may be noted.[20] Concentrations greater than 40 μg/mL may cause lethargy, drowsiness, and, rarely, asterixis. Extreme lethargy and occasionally coma may occur with concentrations greater than 50 μg/mL.

Clinical Features

The common neurologic manifestations of phenytoin intoxication are nystagmus, ataxia, and dysarthria (Table 53-6). Non–dose related toxic effects appear in the gastrointestinal tract as nausea, vomiting, and constipation.[7] Blurred vision and a skin rash have also been noted.[9] Rarely, phenytoin may cause mental changes such as confusion and focal neurologic signs such as hemihyperesthesia and progressive hemiparesis.[28–31]

Movement disorders or choreoathetosis have also been described with phenytoin intoxication and are characterized by orofacial dyskinesia, hyperkinesis, limb chorea, ballismus, and dystonias.[32,33] Most cases of phenytoin-induced chorea have been associated with either markedly elevated phenytoin concentrations or preexisting brain damage, or both.[34,35] This type of movement disorder has also been reported in the acute administration of phenytoin at nontoxic doses.[36] A rare manifestation of phenytoin intoxication is generalized seizure activity, particularly when concentrations are high. Although seizures have occurred in this group of

patients, a causal relationship has never been demonstrated.[37]

Deaths from oral ingestion of an overdose of phenytoin are extremely rare; if death were to occur from oral administration it would be from progressive neurologic depression and coma, not from cardiac toxicity.[38] Most fatalities have been associated with intravenous preparations for the treatment of cardiac dysrhythmias.[39,40] The long duration of CNS effects and the potential for persistent neurologic sequelae exist.[41] Peripheral neuropathies have been described in patients receiving long-term phenytoin therapy, primarily in those with histories of phenytoin intoxication.[42] Degeneration of cerebellar Purkinje's cells in chronic phenytoin intoxication has also been documented.[2]

TREATMENT OF INTOXICATION

Treatment of phenytoin intoxication is nonspecific because there is no antidote. In the acutely overdosed patient, treatment consists of gastrointestinal emptying and subsequent administration of activated charcoal and a cathartic. Repeated oral doses of activated charcoal may be given, even though the efficacy of this regimen has not been established.[43] Generalized supportive care is usually all that is necessary. Ingestions of up to 300 mg/kg have been survived with conservative therapy.

Various adjunctive methods have been attempted to increase the clearance of phenytoin.[44] Hemodialysis, peritoneal dialysis, and forced diuresis have been shown to be of no value in the treatment of phenytoin intoxication.

Although the molecular size of phenytoin enables the drug to diffuse across a dialysis membrane, the protein binding appears to be a limiting factor. Charcoal hemoperfusion also does not result in significantly better clearance.[45] In addition, exchange transfusion has been of little value in treatment.[46]

The decision regarding when to recommence phenytoin therapy after an episode of acute intoxication depends on the availability of laboratory services for monitoring serum phenytoin concentrations.[12,47] If these services are available, therapy can begin again when serum concentrations are in the therapeutic range.

REFERENCES

1. Brown C, Kaminsky M, Feroli E, et al: Delirium with phenytoin and disulfiram administration. *Ann Emerg Med* 1983;12:310–313.

2. Cranford R, Leppik I, Patrick B, et al: Intravenous phenytoin: Clinical and pharmacokinetic aspects. *Neurology* 1978;28:874–881.

3. Rivey M, Schottelium D, Berg M: Phenytoin–folic acid: A review. *Drug Intell Clin Pharmacol* 1984;18:292–301.

4. Campbell W: Periodic alternating nystagmus in phenytoin intoxication. *Arch Neurol* 1980;37:178–180.

5. Bauman J, Siepler J, Fitzloff, J: Phenytoin crystallization in intravenous fluids. *Drug Intell Clin Pharmacol* 1977; 11:646–649.

6. Earnest M, Marx J, Drury L: Complications of intravenous phenytoin for acute treatment of seizures. *JAMA* 1983;249:762–765.

7. Atkinson A, Shaw J: Pharmacokinetic study of a patient with diphenylhydantoin toxicity. *Clin Pharmacol Ther* 1973;14:521–528.

8. Louis S, Kutt H: The cardiocirculatory changes caused by intravenous Dilantin and its solvent. *Am Heart J* 1967;74:523–528.

9. Olanow C, Finn A: Phenytoin: Pharmacokinetics and clinical therapeutics. *Neurosurgery* 1981;8:112–117.

10. Rosen M, Lisak R, Rubin I, et al: Diphenylhydantoin in cardiac arrhythmias. *Am J Cardiol* 1967;20:674–678.

11. Dodson W: Phenytoin elimination in childhood: Effect of concentration-dependent kinetics. *Neurology* 1980;30:196–199.

12. Adler D: Phenytoin. *Clin Toxicol* 1979;14:147–150.

13. Gugler R, Manion C, Azarnoff D: Phenytoin: Pharmacokinetics and bioavailability. *Clin Pharmacol Ther* 1975;19:135–142.

14. Albani M: An unusual case of phenytoin intoxication. *Neuropadiatrie* 1978;9:185–188.

15. Moling J, Posch J: Acute diphenylhydantoin intoxication. *Pediatrics* 1957;20:877–880.

16. Theodore W, Yu L, Price B, et al: The clinical value of free phenytoin levels. *Ann Neurol* 1985;18:90–93.

17. Leal K, Troupin A: Clinical pharmacology of antiepileptic drugs: A summary of current information. *Clin Chem* 1977;23:1964–1968.

18. Gill M, Kern J, Kaneko J, et al: Phenytoin overdose kinetics. *West J Med* 1978;128:246–248.

19. Kutt H, McDowell F: Management of epilepsy with diphenylhydantoin sodium. *JAMA* 1968;203:167–170.

20. Osborn H, Zisfein J, Sparano R: Single-dose oral phenytoin loading. *Ann Emerg Med* 1987;16:407–412.

21. Matthews C, Harley J: Cognitive and motor-sensory performances in toxic and nontoxic epileptic subjects. *Neurology* 1975;25:184–188.

22. Pruitt A, Zwiren G, Patterson J, et al: *Clin Pharmacol Ther* 1975;18:112–120.

23. Herberg K: Delayed and insidious onset of diphenylhydantoin toxicity. *South Med J* 1975;68:70–74.

24. Tibbs P, Bivins B, Rapp R, et al: Phenytoin-induced hypotension in animals receiving sympathomimetic pressor support. *J Surg Res* 1980;29:338–347.

25. Holcomb R, Lynn R, Harvey B, et al: Intoxication with 5,5-diphenylhydantoin (Dilantin). *J Pediatr* 1972; 80:627–632.

26. Selhorst J, Kaufman B, Horowitz S: Diphenylhydantoin-induced cerebellar degeneration. *Arch Neurol* 1972; 27:453–456.

27. Kuhn G: Serum theophylline and phenytoin levels: Can we afford to do them? Can we afford not to? *Ann Emerg Med* 1986;15:344–348.

28. Findler G, Lavy S: Transient hemiparesis: A rare manifestation of diphenylhydantoin toxicity. *J Neurosurg* 1979;50:685–687.

29. Parker W, Shearer C: Phenytoin hepatotoxicity: A case report and review. *Neurology* 1979;29:175–178.

30. Parker W, Gumnit R: Diphenylhydantoin toxicity: Dose-dependent blood dyscrasia. *Neurology* 1974;24:1178–1180.

31. Sandyk R: Transient hemiparesis—A rare complication of phenytoin toxicity. *Postgrad Med J* 1983;59:601–602.

32. Filloux F, Thompson J: Transient chorea induced by phenytoin. *J Pediatr* 1987;110:639–641.

33. Shuttleworth E, Wise G, Paulson G: Choreoathetosis and diphenylhydantoin intoxication. *JAMA* 1974;230:1170–1171.

34. Wilder B, Buchanan R, Serrano E: Correlation of acute diphenylhydantoin intoxication with plasma levels and metabolite excretion. *Neurology* 1973;23:1329–1332.

35. Wilder B, Ramsay E, Willmore L, et al: Efficacy of intravenous phenytoin in the treatment of status epilepticus: Kinetics of central nervous system penetration. *Ann Neurol* 1977;1:511–518.

36. Wilson J, Huff J, Kilroy A: Prolonged toxicity following acute phenytoin overdose in a child. *J Pediatr* 1979;95:135–138.

37. Bazemore R, Zuckerman E: On the problem of diphenylhydantoin-induced seizures. *Arch Neurol* 1974;31:243–249.

38. Laubscher F: Fatal diphenylhydantoin poisoning. *JAMA* 1966;198:194–195.

39. Gellerman G, Martinez C: Fatal ventricular fibrillation following intravenous sodium diphenylhydantoin therapy. *JAMA* 1967;200:161–162.

40. Fulop M, Widrow D, Colmers R, et al: Possible diphenylhydantoin-induced arrhythmia in hypothyroidism. *JAMA* 1966;196:168–170.

41. Dobkin B: Reversible subacute peripheral neuropathy induced by phenytoin. *Arch Neurol* 1977;34:189–190.

42. Damato A: Diphenylhydantoin: Pharmacological and clinical use. *Prog Cardiovasc Dis* 1969;12:1–15.

43. Mauro L, Mauro V, Brown D, et al: Enhancement of phenytoin elimination by multiple-dose activated charcoal. *Ann Emerg Med* 1987;16:1132–1135.

44. Spector R, Davidoff R, Schwartzman R: Phenytoin-induced ophthalmoplegia. *Neurology* 1976;26:1031–1034.

45. Baehler R, Work J, Smith W, et al: Charcoal hemoperfusion in the therapy for methsuximide and phenytoin overdose. *Arch Intern Med* 1980;140:1466–1468.

46. Larsen L, Sterrett J, Whitehead B, et al: Adjunctive therapy of phenytoin overdose—A case report using plasmapheresis. *Clin Toxicol* 1986;24:37–49.

47. Jacobsen D, Alvik A, Bredesen J, et al: Pharmacokinetics of phenytoin in acute adult and child intoxication. *J Toxicol Clin Toxicol* 1987;24:519–531.

ADDITIONAL SELECTED REFERENCES

Bridgers S, Ebersole J: Incidence of seizures with phenytoin toxicity. *Neurology* 1985;35:1767–1768.

Caracta A, Damato A, Josephson M, et al: Electrophysiologic properties of diphenylhydantoin. *Circulation* 1973;47:1234–1241.

Christiansen C, Kristensen M, Rodbro P: Latent osteomalacia in epileptic patients on anticonvulsants. *Br Med J* 1972;3:738–739.

Derby B, Ward J: The myth of red urine due to phenytoin. *JAMA* 1983;249:1723–1724.

Durelli L, Mutani R, Sechi G, et al: Cardiac side effects of phenytoin and carbamazepine: A dose-related phenomenon? *Arch Neurol* 1985;42:1067–1068.

Flowers F, Araujo O, Hamm K: Phenytoin hypersensitivity syndrome. *J Emerg Med* 1987;5:103–108.

Gallagher B, Baumel I, Mattson R, et al: Primidone, diphenylhydantoin and phenobarbital. *Neurology* 1973; 23:145–149.

Gerber N, Lynn R, Oates J: Acute intoxication with 5,5-diphenylhydantoin (Dilantin®) associated with impairment of biotransformation. *Ann Intern Med* 1972; 77:765–771.

Gharib H, Munoz J: Endocrine manifestations of diphenylhydantoin therapy. *Metabolism* 1974; 23:515–524.

Jones D, Helfer R: A teething lotion resulting in the misdiagnosis of diphenylhydantoin administration. *Am J Dis Child* 1971;122:259–260.

Kapur R, Girgis S, Little T, et al: Diphenylhydantoin-induced gingival hyperplasia: Its relationship to dose and serum level. *Dev Med Child Neurol* 1973;15:483–487.

Lindahl S, Westerling D: Detoxification with peritoneal dialysis and blood exchange after diphenylhydantoin intoxication. *Acta Paediatr Scand* 1982;71:665–666.

Marquis J, Carruthers S, Spence J, et al: Phenytoin-theophylline interaction. *N Engl J Med* 1982;307: 1189–1190.

Matzke G, Cloyd J, Sawchuk G: Acute phenytoin and primidone intoxication: A pharmacokinetic analysis. *J Clin Pharmacol* 1981;21:92–99.

Rodbro P, Christiansen C, Lund M: Development of anticonvulsant osteomalacia in epileptic patients on phenytoin treatment. *Acta Neurol Scand* 1974;50:527–532.

Rosenblum E, Rodichok L, Hanson P: Movement disorder as a manifestation of diphenylhydantoin toxicity. *Pediatrics* 1974;54:364–366.

Stilman N, Masdeu J: Incidence of seizures with phenytoin toxicity. *Neurology* 1985;35:1769–1772.

Tichner J, Enselverg C: Suicidal Dilantin poisoning. *N Engl J Med* 1951;245:723–725.

Vincent F: Phenothiazine-induced phenytoin intoxication. *Ann Intern Med* 1980;93:56–57.

Wallis W, Kutt H, McDowell F: Intravenous diphenylhydantoin in treatment of acute repetitive seizures. *Neurology* 1968;18:513–523.

Wit A, Rosen M, Hoffman B: Electrophysiology and pharmacology of cardiac arrhythmias: Part VIII: Cardiac effects of diphenylhydantoin: Part A. *Am Heart J* 1975;90:265–272.

Wit A, Rosen M, Hoffman B: Electrophysiology and pharmacology of cardiac arrhythmias: Part VIII: Cardiac effects of diphenylhydantoin: Part B. *Am Heart J* 1975;90:397–404.

Woodbury D: Phenytoin: Introduction and history. *Adv Neurol* 1980;27:305–313.

Zoneraich S, Zoneraich O, Siegel J: Sudden death following intravenous sodium diphenylhydantoin. 1976;91: 375–377.

chapter 54

Isoniazid

Since its introduction more than 30 years ago, isoniazid has been used worldwide as a synthetic antibiotic in the treatment of active pulmonary tuberculosis as well as prophylactically in patients with a positive tuberculin skin test.[1] Isoniazid intoxication is most commonly encountered in groups where tuberculosis is prevalent. The wide availability of the drug has led to a number of reports of accidental or intentional acute poisonings after excessive ingestion.[2]

PHARMACOKINETICS

Isoniazid (INH®, Niconyl®, Nydrazid®) is a hydrazide of isonicotinic acid.[3] It is absorbed rapidly from the gastrointestinal tract and from intramuscular administration. Plasma concentrations reach their peak 1 to 2 hours after oral administration and fall to 50% in 6 hours.[4] It is not substantially protein bound and diffuses into all body fluids. It is excreted mainly in the urine, partly unchanged and partly acetylated, and small amounts are excreted in the bile.[5] The primary route of isoniazid inactivation is by acetylation and dehydrazination.[6]

The plasma half-life of isoniazid in patients with normal renal and hepatic function ranges from 1 to 4 hours depending on the rate of metabolism. The rate of disappearance of isoniazid from serum is the determining factor in the manifestation of toxicity and varies greatly among individuals; this variability is genetically determined, resulting from a relative deficiency of the hepatic enzyme N-acetyltransferase. Individuals may be identified as having slow, intermediate, or rapid rates of acetylation[2]; the rate of acetylation is usually constant for each individual. Approximately 50% to 60% of Caucasians and Blacks have slow rates of acetylation.[7] Most Orientals and Eskimos have rapid rates of acetylation. Consequently, both a higher incidence and a more severe form of toxicity from isoniazid may be expected in Caucasian and Black individuals.[1]

Isoniazid has a comparatively wide margin of safety between therapeutic and toxic doses.[8] Side effects are not uncommon, but at small doses they are, for the most part, not severe (Table 54-1). Peripheral neuropathy is the most common neurologic manifestation and is usually preceded by paresthesia of the feet and hands.[9] Neurotoxic effects may be prevented or relieved with low doses of pyridoxine (vitamin B_6) during therapy. Psychotic and depressive reactions

Table 54-1 Side Effects of Isoniazid

Peripheral neuropathy
Paresthesia
Psychosis
Depression
Hepatitis

associated with suicidal manifestations have also been reported.[3] Severe and sometimes fatal hepatitis associated with isoniazid therapy has been reported and may develop even after many months of treatment.[10] This risk appears to be age related, older patients being at greatest risk.[5]

MECHANISM OF ACTION

The metabolic abnormalities and CNS alterations caused by isoniazid overdose are thought to be a result of alterations in the metabolism of pyridoxine, which consequently affects the production of γ-aminobutyric acid (GABA), an inhibitory synaptic neurotransmitter in the brain (Fig. 54-1).[11] Glutamic acid decarboxylase (GAD) is the enzyme that converts glutamic acid to GABA[12]; this enzyme requires pyridoxal-5'-phosphate, which is the active form of pyridoxine, as a coenzyme.[4] Large doses of isoniazid inhibit the utilization of pyridoxine and increase its urinary excretion through the formation of isoniazid-pyridoxine hydrazones that are rapidly excreted by the kidney.[12] It is thought that the intractable seizures seen with isoniazid intoxication are due to the inhibition of the GABA, which results in unopposed excitation.

At the molecular level, isoniazid interferes with nicotinamide adenine dinucleotide (NAD)–catalyzed reactions.[7] NAD is recognized as an essential component of the energy-producing reactions of glycolysis and the tricarboxylic acid cycle.[2] The introduction of isoniazid into the NAD molecule forms an inactive analog of NAD that seriously disrupts intermediary metabolism and inhibits the conversion of lactate to pyruvate.[13]

TOXICITY

Typically after ingestion of large amounts of isoniazid, the patient experiences a latent period of 30 minutes to 2 hours (Table 54-2).[8] Subsequently there is the gradual development of nausea, vomiting, blurred vision, visual hallucinations (which may include colored lights, spots, or strange designs), dizziness, slurred speech, dilated pupils, ataxia, tachycardia, and hyperthermia.[7] Within 90 minutes to 3 hours after

Figure 54-1 Mechanism of Interference of Isoniazid in Metabolism of γ-Aminobutyric Acid

Glutamic acid Glutamic acid
                decarboxylase γ-Aminobutyric acid
                (requires vitamin B_6)

Isoniazid + Vitamin B_6 ⟶ Isoniazid–pyridoxine hydrazone

Table 54-2 Signs and Symptoms of Isoniazid Intoxication

Gastrointestinal
  Nausea
  Vomiting
Neurologic
  Blurred vision
  Dizziness
  Slurred speech
  Mydriasis
  Ataxia
  Hallucinations
  Hyperreflexia or areflexia
  Stupor
  Seizures
  Coma
Metabolic
  Metabolic acidosis
  Hyperglycemia
  Glycosuria
  Hyperthermia
Miscellaneous
  Hypotension
  Cyanosis
  Tachycardia
  Pneumonitis
  Death

---

ingestion, which corresponds roughly to the time at which peak isoniazid serum concentrations are attained, the patient may suddenly lapse into stupor and may also develop sudden tonic-clonic generalized or localized seizures.[14] There may then be rapid progression to intractable coma, marked hyperreflexia or complete areflexia, severe hypotension, cyanosis, and death.

Metabolic alterations associated with isoniazid intoxication include severe metabolic acidosis, hyperglycemia, and glycosuria. In severe cases, pneumonitis and cardiorespiratory arrest may occur.[13]

The underlying cause of the metabolic acidosis in isoniazid intoxication is not entirely

Table 54-3 Laboratory Abnormalities in Isoniazid Intoxication

---

Hyperglycemia
Glucosuria
Ketonuria
Hyperkalemia (mild)
Elevated serum isoniazid concentration
Anion gap metabolic acidosis
Increased excretion of pyridoxine

Table 54-4 Laboratory Determinations in Isoniazid Intoxication

---

Arterial blood gas
Serum electrolytes
Blood urea nitrogen
Serum glucose concentration
Blood type and cross-match
Serum isoniazid concentration (if available)

Table 54-5 Treatment for Isoniazid Overdose

Medical observation (6 hours if asymptomatic)
Emesis or lavage
Charcoal and cathartic
Intravenous fluid therapy
    Hypotension
    Diuresis
Sodium bicarbonate (as necessary)
Pyridoxine (2 to 5 g IV)
Forced (alkaline) diuresis
Dialysis (if renal failure present)

---

understood. It has been suggested that the acidosis is related to the inhibition of the NAD, which consequently causes a buildup of lactic acid.[7] Another proposed mechanism is that the metabolic acidosis is due to the lactic acidosis secondary to the prolonged seizure activity.[13]

DIAGNOSIS

The diagnosis of isoniazid intoxication should be considered in patients presenting with unexplained seizures and metabolic acidosis.[15] Many times these seizures are unresponsive and refractory to conventional antileptic therapy.[2] Isoniazid as a cause of seizures should be considered in patients who have access to the drug and in anyone whose seizures are poorly controlled with the usual anticonvulsants and in whom isoniazid overdose could be suspected.[11]

LABORATORY ANALYSIS

Although there are numerous methods for determining isoniazid concentrations in blood or urine, there are few laboratories that are able to make such measurements except in experimental situations.[16,17] In a therapeutic situation, serum concentrations are usually between 1 and 7 μg/mL.[4] Blood concentrations of isoniazid are usually significantly higher in acute intoxications than those from therapeutic doses[6]; toxic blood concentrations are considered greater than 20 μg/mL.[18]

Laboratory tests usually reveal a severe metabolic acidosis, hyperglycemia, glycosuria, ketonuria, mild hyperkalemia, and increased urinary excretion of pyridoxine (Table 54-3).[17] Blood should therefore be drawn for arterial blood

gases, serum electrolytes, blood urea nitrogen, and glucose concentration. Blood should also be typed and cross-matched in the event that hemodialysis is required (Table 54-4).[12]

TREATMENT

Because of severe morbidity and high mortality rates, patients who are asymptomatic after isoniazid overdose should be observed medically for at least 4 to 6 hours (Table 54-5).[16] It may also be safer to assume that absence of symptomatology reflects a latent period rather than lack of a toxic response to isoniazid.[11]

Emergency treatment consists of attention to the airway, cardiorespiratory support, treatment of seizures, correction of the metabolic acidosis, enhancing excretion of the drug, and administration of pyridoxine.[14]

Supportive care includes emesis or gastric lavage with subsequent administration of activated charcoal and a cathartic. Intravenous fluids should be given both to control hypotension and to induce a diuresis. Sodium bicarbonate is usually not needed for the metabolic acidosis if seizure activity is stopped with adequate doses of pyridoxine.[18]

Pyridoxine

Therapeutic trials have shown the effectiveness of parenteral doses of pyridoxine to treat isoniazid intoxication, especially the associated seizure activity.[4] Pyridoxine is thought to prevent the effects of isoniazid on GAD activity and thereby to prevent a decrease in brain GABA. Large doses of pyridoxine are given intravenously on the basis of a suspected milligram-per-milligram equivalency of ingested isoniazid.[15] If the amount of isoniazid ingested is unknown, 5 g of pyridoxine (50 ml of a 10% solution) is given over 3 to 5 minutes and may be followed in 30 minutes by an additional 5 g.[14] Preferably pyridoxine therapy should be started in the latent interval between ingestion and seizure activity.

Pyridoxine is commercially available as 10-mL vials containing 1 g of pyridoxine each. The danger of pyridoxine overdosage is slight, and although chronic intoxication can occur[19] acute intoxication occurs only if massive amounts are administered.[14] Toxic effects of pyridoxine include tachypnea, postural reflex abnormalities, paralysis, and convulsions; these usually arise after more than 5 to 6 g/kg has been administered (Table 54-6).[11]

Animal studies suggest a synergistic effect of pyridoxine and diazepam in the suppression of isoniazid-induced seizures. Phenytoin and barbiturates do not appear to be effective for these seizures.[14] Phenytoin may even be toxic to patients with a high serum isoniazid concentration because isoniazid is a potent inhibitor of phenytoin metabolism by inhibition of the parahydroxylation of phenytoin. This may lead to excessive concentrations of phenytoin and associated toxic symptoms.[18]

Table 54-6 Side Effects of Pyridoxine (5 to 6 g/kg)

Tachypnea
Postural hypotension
Paralysis
Seizures

Bicarbonate

If seizure activity is allowed to continue before pyridoxine is given, a severe lactic acidosis can result.[4] This reverses when seizures abate. Also, because the lactic acidosis seen after seizures resolves spontaneously and because metabolic alkalosis may result from metabolism of excess lactate, the administration of large amounts of bicarbonate may be potentially harmful.[15]

Methods To Enhance Excretion

Forced diuresis has been shown to increase clearance of isoniazid.[4] In addition, isoniazid is dialyzable by either peritoneal dialysis or hemodialysis, although if adequate doses of pyridoxine are given dialysis does not seem to be required except in those patients who develop acute renal failure.[13,15]

REFERENCES

1. Byrd R, Nelson R, Elliott R: Isoniazid toxicity. *JAMA* 1972;220:1471–1473.

2. Cameron W: Isoniazid overdose. *Can Med Assoc J* 1978;118:1413–1414.

3. Terman D, Teitelbaum D: Isoniazid self-poisoning. *Neurology* 1970;20:299–304.

4. Coyer J, Nicholson D: Isoniazid-induced convulsions. *South Med J* 1976;69:294–297.

5. Bahri A, Chiang C, Timbrell J: Acetylhydrazine hepatotoxicity. *Toxicol Appl Pharmacol* 1981;60:561–569.

6. Holdiness M: Neurological manifestations and toxicities of the antituberculosis drugs. *Med Toxicol* 1987;2:33–51.

7. Chin L, Sievers M, Herrier R, et al: Convulsions as the etiology of lactic acidosis in acute isoniazid toxicity in dogs. *Toxicol Appl Pharmacol* 1979;49:377–384.

8. Sievers M, Herrier R, Chin L, et al: Treatment of acute isoniazid toxicity. *Am J Hosp Pharmacol* 1975;32:202–206.

9. Miller J, Robinson A, Percy A: Acute isoniazid poisoning in childhood. *Am J Dis Child* 1980;134:290–292.

10. Bailey W, Weill H, DeRouen T, et al: The effect of isoniazid on transaminase levels. *Ann Intern Med* 1974;81:200–202.

11. Wason S, Lacouture P, Lovejoy F: Single high-dose pyridoxine treatment for isoniazid overdose. *JAMA* 1981;246:1102–1104.

12. Sievers M, Chin L: Treatment of isoniazid overdose. *JAMA* 1982;247:583–584.

13. Bear E, Hoffman P, Siegel S, et al: Suicidal ingestion of isoniazid: An uncommon cause of metabolic acidosis and seizures. *South Med J* 1976;69:31–32.

14. Yarbrough B, Wood J: Isoniazid overdose treated with high-dose pyridoxine. *Ann Emerg Med* 1983;12: 303–305.

15. Cocco A, Pazourek L: Acute isoniazid intoxication—Management by peritoneal dialysis. *N Engl J Med* 1963; 269:852–853.

16. Brown A, Mallett M, Fiser D, et al: Acute isoniazid intoxication: Reversal of CNS symptoms with large doses of pyridoxine. *Pediatr Pharmacol* 1984;4:199–202.

17. Scott E, Wright R: Fluorometric determination of isonicotinic acid hydrazide in serum. *J Lab Clin Med* 1967;70:355–360.

18. Brown C: Acute isoniazid poisoning. *Am Rev Respir Dis* 1972;105:206–216.

19. Schaumburg H, Kaplan J, Windebank A, et al: Sensory neuropathy from pyridoxine abuse. *N Engl J Med* 1983;309:445–448.

Therapeutic Blood Concentrations of Selected Drugs

Drug	Therapeutic Range
Analgesics	
Acetaminophen	10.0–20.0 μg/mL
Ibuprofen	10.0–50.0 μg/mL
Indomethacin	0.5–3.0 μg/mL
Pentazocine	0.14–0.6 μg/mL
Propoxyphene	50–200 ng/mL
Salicylate	10.0–25.0 mg/dL
Antibiotics	
Amikacin	15–25 μg/mL (peak)
	10–15 μg/mL (trough)
Chloramphenicol	15–25 μg/mL (peak)
	10–15 μg/mL (trough)
Gentamicin	<12.0 μg/mL (peak)
	<2.0 μg/mL (trough)
Kanamycin	20–25 μg/mL (peak)
	4–6 μg/mL (trough)
Tobramycin	<12.0 μg/mL (peak)
	<2.0 μg/mL (trough)
Anticonvulsants	
Carbamazepine	4.0–8.0 μg/mL
Ethosuximide	40–100 μg/mL
Phenobarbital	15.0–40.0 μg/mL
Phenytoin	10.0–20.0 μg/mL
Primidone	5.0–12.0 μg/mL
Valproic acid	50–100 μg/mL
Antihistamines	
Brompheniramine	12.0–17.0 ng/mL
Chlorpheniramine	10.0–40.0 ng/mL

Drug	Therapeutic Range
Chlorphentermine	150.0–350.0 ng/mL
Cimetidine	0.2–2.5 µg/mL
Diphenhydramine	100–1000 ng/mL
Hydroxyzine	50.0–200.0 ng/mL
Methapyrilene	5.0–100.0 ng/mL
Antipsychotics	
Chlorpromazine	30.0–35.0 ng/mL
Haloperidol	5.0–20.0 ng/mL
Lithium	0.5–1.5 mEq/L
Mesoridazine	150–1000 ng/mL
Perphenazine	0.5 µg/dL
Prochlorperazine	100.0–500.0 ng/mL
Promazine	100.0–500.0 ng/mL
Promethazine	100.0–500.0 ng/mL
Thioridazine	100–150 µg/dL
Thiothixene	1.0 µg/dL
Trifluoperazine	80 µg/dL
β-Adrenergic blocking agents	
Atenolol	1.3 µg/mL
Propranolol	40.0–80.0 ng/mL
Benzodiazepines	
Alprazolam	8.0–37.0 ng/mL
Chlordiazepoxide	500–1000 ng/mL
Clonazepam	10.0–70.0 ng/mL
Clorazepate	300.0–1000.0 ng/mL
Diazepam	100.0–700.0 ng/mL
Flurazepam	10.0–140.0 ng/mL
Lorazepam	5.0–30.0 ng/mL
Oxazepam	200.0–500.0 ng/mL
Bronchodilators	
Dyphylline	5.0–15.0 µg/mL
Oxtriphylline	10.0–20.0 µg/mL
Theophylline	10.0–20.0 µg/mL
Cardiac drugs	
N-Acetylprocainamide	5.0–10.0 µg/mL
Amiodarone	0.5–3.0 µg/mL
Digitoxin	10.0–25.0 ng/mL
Digoxin	0.8–2.1 ng/mL
Diltiazem	100–200 ng/mL
Disopyramide	2.0–5.0 µg/mL
Flecainide	200–800 ng/mL
Lidocaine	1.2–5.0 µg/mL
Mexiletine	0.7–2.0 µg/mL
Procainamide	4.0–8.0 µg/mL
Quinidine	2.0–5.0 µg/mL
Tocainide	4.0–10.0 µg/mL
Verapamil	50.0–400.0 ng/mL

Drug	*Therapeutic Range*
Central nervous system stimulants	
Amphetamine	20–100 ng/mL
Caffeine	5.0–14.0 μg/mL
Diethylpropion	100.0–300.0 ng/mL
Methamphetamine	10.0–50.0 ng/mL
Pheniramine	20.0–200.0 ng/mL
Phenmetrazine	50.0–250.0 ng/mL
Metals	
Arsenic	0.0–20.0 ng/mL
Cadmium	0.01–0.02 μg/dL
Copper	10.0–150.0 μg/dL
Iron	50–150 μg/dL
Lead	0.0–25.0 μg/mL
Mercury	0.5 μg/mL
Miscellaneous	
Carbamezapine	3–13 μg/mL
Cyanide	0.05 μg/mL
Isoniazid	1.0–7.0 μg/mL
Metronidazole	3.0–15.0 μg/mL
Narcotics	
Codeine	10–120 ng/mL
Hydrocodone	10.0–40.0 ng/mL
Hydromorphone	10.0–30.0 ng/mL
Meperidine	50–500 ng/mL
Morphine	40.0–150.0 ng/mL
Oxycodone	50.0–100.0 ng/mL
Propoxyphene	100.0–400.0 ng/mL
Sedative-hypnotics	
Amobarbital	2.0–10.0 μg/mL
Butabarbital	7.0–15.0 μg/mL
Butalbital	2.0–5.0 μg/mL
Chloral hydrate	2.0–10.0 μg/mL
Ethchlorvynol	1.0–6.0 μg/mL
Glutethimide	5.0–15.0 μg/mL
Hexobarbital	2.0–5.0 μg/mL
Mephobarbital	5.0–15.0 μg/mL
Meprobamate	8.0–24.0 μg/mL
Methaqualone	1.0–8.0 μg/mL
Metharbital	10.0–30.0 μg/mL
Methyprylon	4.0–10.0 μg/mL
Pentobarbital	0.5–3.0 μg/mL
Phenobarbital	15.0–40.0 μg/mL
Secobarbital	0.5–5.0 μg/mL
Thiopental	1.0–5.0 μg/mL
Tricyclic antidepressants	
Amitriptyline	100–250 ng/mL
Amoxapine	50–400 ng/mL

Drug	Therapeutic Range
Desipramine	150–300 ng/mL
Doxepin	100–200 ng/mL
Imipramine	150–300 ng/mL
Maprotiline	150–400 ng/mL
Nortriptyline	50–150 ng/mL
Protriptyline	70–250 ng/mL
Trazodone	300–1600 ng/mL

Volumes of Distribution of Selected Drugs

Drug	Volume of Distribution (liters per kilogram)
Acebutolol	1.2
Acetaminophen	0.75–1.0
Acetylsalicylic acid	0.1–0.3
Acyclovir	0.71
Alprazolam	12.0
Alprenolol	3.0
Amantadine	6.0
Aminoglycosides	0.2–0.5
Amiodarone	66.0
Amitriptyline	15
Amobarbital	2.4
Amphetamines	0.6
Amphotericin B	4.0
Atenolol	0.56
Atropine	2.4
Benzodiazepines	3.0–10.0
Bromide	>40
Bromocriptine	3.5
Caffeine	0.75
Carbamazepine	1.4
Captopril	0.70
Chloral hydrate	0.75–0.90
Chloramphenicol	0.9
Chlordiazepoxide	0.3
Chlorpromazine	10.0–35.0
Chlorpropamide	0.47
Cimetidine	1.0–2.0
Clonazepam	5.0–10.0

Drug	Volume of Distribution (liters per kilogram)
Clonidine	2.0
Clorazepate	1.0
Cocaine	2.0
Codeine	3
Dapsone	1.5
Desipramine	35.0
Diazepam	1.0–2.0
Digitoxin	0.54
Digoxin	7.0–10.0
Diltiazem	5.0
Diphenhydramine	3.0–4.0
Diphenoxylate	4.6
Disopyramide	0.6
Doxepin	20.0
Ethambutol	0.8
Ethanol	0.6
Ethchlorvynol	3.0–4.0
Ethosuximide	0.9
Fenoprofen	0.08–0.1
Fentanyl	4.0
5-Fluorouracil	0.38
Flurazepam	22.0
Furosemide	0.2
Glutethimide	20–25
Halazepam	1.0
Haloperidol	18
Heparin	0.06
Ibuprofen	0.14
Indomethacin	0.3–0.9
Isoniazid	0.6
Ketamine	3.0
Labetalol	11.0
Lidocaine	1.5
Lithium	0.7–2.0
Lorazepam	1.3
Melphalan	0.63
Meperidine	4.5
Methadone	6.0–10.0
Methicillin	0.6
Methyldopa	0.29
Metoprolol	4.0–5.0
Metronidazole	1.1
Minoxidil	2.7
Morphine	3.0
Nadolol	2.0–3.0
Naloxone	3.0
Naproxen	0.09
Narcotics	3.0–5.0

Drug	Volume of Distribution (liters per kilogram)
Nicotine	2.6
Nifedipine	1.2
Nitrazepam	2.0
Nitroglycerin	3.3
Nortriptyline	18.0
Oxazepam	1.0–5.0
Oxyphenbutazone	0.14
Oxyprenolol	1.5
Pentazocine	5.0
Pentobarbital	1.0–2.0
Perphenazine	18.0–30.0
Phenobarbital	0.60–0.75
Phenothiazines	20.0–30.0
Phenylbutazone	0.02
Phenytoin	0.75
Pindolol	2.0
Practolol	1.6
Prazepam	4.5
Prazosin	0.6–1.0
Prednisone	1.0
Primidone	0.60
Procainamide	1.9
Propranolol	4.0
Protriptyline	22.0
Pyridostigmine	1.1
Quinidine	3.0
Rifampin	0.93
Salicylate	0.1–0.3
Secobarbital	1.5
Sotalol	0.7
Temazepam	15
Tetracycline	3.0
Theophylline	0.46
Thiopental	2.3
Timolol	1.5
Tocainide	3.0
Tolmetin	0.04
Triazolam	1.5–2.5
Valproic acid	0.13
Verapamil	4.0–6.0
Warfarin	0.1

Street Names of Abused Drugs

Amphetamines
Bam
Beans
Bennies
Black and whites
Black beauties
Black birds
Black cadillacs
Black dex
Black mollies
Blacks
Bombido
Bombita
Box cars
Brown and clears
Bumblebees
Cartwheels
Chalk
Chicken powder
Coast-to-coast
Co-pilots
Crank
Crink
Cris
Criss-cross
Cristina
Crossroads
Cross-tops
Crystal
Dex
Dexies

Dice
Diet pills
Double-cross
Eye-openers
Fives
Footballs
Green and clears
Hearts
Jelly babies
Jelly beans
Jolly beans
L.A.
LA turnabouts
Lid poppers
Lightning
Little bomb
Meth
Minnibennies
Nuggets
Peaches
Pep pills
Pink hearts
Powder
Reducing pills
Rhythm
Roses
Snow pellets
Snow seals
Speed
Splash
Spliven

Sweets
Thrusters
Wake-ups
Water

Barbiturates

Block busters
Blue
Blue and reds
Blue angels
Blue birds
Blue bullets
Blue clouds
Blue devils
Blue dolls
Blue heavens
Bombita
Christmas trees
Double-trouble
Downers
Downs
F-40
F-66
GBS
Golf balls
Goofballs
Goofers
Green dragons
Lay back
M and M's
Marshmallow reds
Mexican reds
Mexican yellows
Nebbies
Nemmies
Nimbies
Nimby
Nols
Oral pob
Peanuts
Phennies
Pink ladies
Pinks
Purple rocks
Rainbows
Red
Red birds
Red devils
Red dolls
Red lilies
Reds
Reds and blues

Seccy
Seggy
Sleepers
Sleeping pills
Stopped
Stumblers
T-birds
Tooies
Tooties
Yellow bullets
Yellow dolls
Yellow jackets
Yellows

Chloral hydrate

Chlorals
Coral
Green frog
Jellies
Jelly beans
Joy juice
Knock-out drops
Mickey Finn
Peter

Cocaine

Base
Baseball
Basuco
Bazooka
Bernice
Bernies
Big bloke
Big C
Big flake
Big rush
Blotter
Blow
C
Candy
Carrie
Cholly
Coke
Corine
Corrine
Crack
Crystal
Dama blanca
Dama blance
Dream
Dust
Flake
Free base

Gift of the Sun God
Gin
Girl
Gold dust
Gravel
Green gold
Happy dust
Happy trails
Hard stuff
Heaven dust
Heaven leaf
Her
Hit
Jam
Joy powder
Lady
Leaf
Line
Noise candy
Nose
Nose candy
Pasta
Pimp
Rock
Roxanne
Schmack
She
Snort
Snowbirds
Snowcones
Snow flake
Snow seals
Star dust
Star-spangled powder
Supercoke
Toot
White girl
White lady
Whites

Combinations

Black dust = phencyclidine, heroin, embalming fluid
Blue velvet = paregoric + antihistamine
Boat = phencyclidine, heroin, embalming fluid
C and H = cocaine + heroin
C and M = cocaine + morphine
Dynamite = marijuana + heroin
Fours and dor's = codeine + glutethimide
Four-way = LSD + STP + methedrine + cocaine

F-66 = amobarbital + secobarbital
H and C = heroin + cocaine
Killer weed = phencyclidine + marijuana
Loads = codeine + glutethimide
Love trip = mescaline + MDMA
MDA = LSD + cocaine + heroin
OJ = marijuana + opium
Pineapple = heroin + methylphenidate
Pink wedges = LSD + STP + strychnine + cocaine
R and R = Seconal + wine
Snowball = cocaine + heroin
Speedball = cocaine + heroin
T's and blues = pentazocine + tripelennamine
Turps = terpin hydrate with codeine
Whiz bang = cocaine + heroin

Ethchlorvynol

Jelly beans
Mr. Green Jeans
Pickles

Fentanyl-like drugs

China white
Super heroin

Hashish and tetrahydrocannabinol

Black Russian
Crystal tea
Fingers
Gram
Keif
Kif
Kristal tea
Krystal tea
Quarter moon
Soles
Tac
THC

Heroin

Big H
Big Harry
Bindle
Blanco
Bombido
Boy
Brown
Brown sugar
Buju
Bundle
Butu
Caballo
Caca

Carga
China white
Chinese red
Chiva
Crap
Deuce
Dirt
Dogie
Doojee
Doper
Dujie
Dynamite
Flea powder
Foolish powder
H
Hairy
Half bundle
Half load
Hard candy
Hard stuff
Harry
Harry Jones
Henry
Hessle
Horse
Joy powder
Lady Jane
Little bomb
Mexican brown
Mexican mud
Nickel bag
Nickel deck
Nitroglycerin tabs
Noise
Pack
Pee
Persian brown
Powder
Quill
Salt
Scag
Scat
Shil
Shit
Skag
Skid
Smeck
Spoon
Stuff
Tecata

Thing
TNT
White stuff
Lysergic acid diethylamide (LSD)
Acid
Animal
Barrels
Battery acid
Beast
Big D
Black acid
Blotter acid
Blotter cube
Blue acid
Blue barrels
Blue cheers
Blue heaven
Blue microdot
Blue mist
Brown dots
California sunshine
Chief
Chocolate chips
Coffee
Contact lens
Crackers
Cube
Cupcakes
D
Domes
Double dome
Electric Kool Aid
Flats
Four-way
Ghost
Grape parfait
Green single domes
Hawaiian sunshine
The Hawk
Haze
Heavenly blue
Lime acid
LSD
Lucy in the Sky with Diamonds
Mellow yellow
Microdot
One-way
Orange barrels
Orange cupcakes
Orange mushrooms

Orange sunshine
Owskey's acid
Owsley
Paper acid
Pearly gate
Pink wedge
Pink witches
Purple barrels
Purple dragon
Purple flats
Purple haze
Purple hearts
Purple microdot
Purple wedge
Red dragon
Royal blue
Sandoz
Smears
Squirrels
Star
Sugar
Sugar lump
Sunshine
Ticket
Trips
Twenty-five
Vodka acid
Wafer
Wedding bells
Wedge
White lightning
Window glass
Window pane
Window pane acid
Yellow
Yellow dimples
Yellow kimples
Zen

Marijuana
Acapulco gold
Ace
Ashes
Baby
Bad seed
Bhang
Black mote
Block
Bobo bush
Bomber
Boo

Brick
Broccoli
Bush
Butter
Butter flower
Can
Cannabis
Carmabis
Chiba-driba
Chicago green
Colorado cocktail
Columbian
Columbus black
Dagga
Dope
Doper
Dry high
Fine stuff
Fingers
Flower
Fu
Fuel
Gage
Ganja
Giggle smoke
Gold
Goof butt
Grash
Grass
Green
Griefo
Griffo
Guage
Hash
Hashish
Hashish oil
Hay
Hemp
Herb
Hot sticks
Indian Bay
Indian hat
Indian hemp
J
Jane
Jay
Jay joint
Jive
Jive stick
Joint

Joy smoke
Joy stick
Khat
Kick-stick
Killer weed
Kilo
Lid
Locoweed
Love weed
Mary
Mary Jane
Mexican Brown
MJ
Mohasky
Mojo
Mooters
Mootos
Mor-a-grifa
Mota
M.U.
Muggies
Muggles
Mutah
Panama gold
Panama red
Pat
Pod
Pot
Rainy-day woman
Reefer
Roach
Rope
Sativa
Seeds
Seeds and stems
Seeds and twigs
Smoke
Spilm
Spliff
Stack
Stick
Straw
Supergrass
Sweet Lucy
T
Tea
Texas stick
Thai stick
Twistum
Viper's weed

Weed
Yellow submarine
Ying gee

MDA, MDMA, DMT, and STP
Adam
AMT
Businessman's special
Businessman's trip
DET
DMT
DOB
DOM
Eve
Love drug
Love trip
Orange cupcakes
Serenity
Serenity, Tranquility, and Peace
Speed for lovers
Sweet tart
Syndicate acid

Methaqualone
AS
Citrexal
Disco biscuits
Love drug
Luding out
Luds
Paris 400
Q
Quads
Quas
714's
Soapers
Sopors

MPPP
New heroin
Synthetic demerol
Synthetic heroin

Nitrites
Ames
Amies
Amyes
Amys
Aymes
Boppers
Heart-on
Pearls
Poppers
Snappers

Opium
- Big O
- Hop
- Hophead
- Joy plant
- O
- OJ
- OP
- Pin yen
- Skee
- Tar
- Toys
- When-shee
- Yellow she baby
- Yellow shee
- Yen Shee Suey
- Zero

Peyote and mescaline
- Beans
- Big chief
- Button
- Cactus
- Cactus head
- Hikori
- Hukuli
- Hyatari
- Love trip
- Mesc
- Mescal
- Mescal beans
- Mescal button
- Mese
- P
- Pink wedge
- Seni
- Tops
- White light

Phencyclidine and ketamine
- Angel dust
- Angel hair
- Angel mist
- Crystal
- Crystal joint
- DOA
- Dust
- Dusted parsley
- Elephant tranquilizer
- Goon
- Green
- HCP
- Hog
- Horse tranquilizer
- K
- Kay jay
- Killer weed
- Kristal
- Kristal joint
- Love boat
- Lovely
- PCP
- Pits
- Purple
- Rocket fuel
- Sernyl
- Special-la-coke
- Super acid
- Super C
- Tic
- Wack
- White horizon

Psilocybin
- God's flesh
- Mexican mushroom
- Mushroom
- Simple simon

Index

Note: Italicized numbers indicate material found in tables, figures, or exhibits.

F

Fab therapy, 175-78
  as antidote, *11*
  dosage of, 177, *177*
  indications for, 176-77
  side effects of, 178
False aralia, *573*
Fastin, *370*
Febrigesic, *415*
Febrinol, *415*
Feco-T, *465*
Feldene, *445*, 449
Femiron, *465*
Fenamate derivatives, *445*, 449
Fenbufen, *445*, 449
Fenethcarb, *537*
Fenfluramine, trade names of, *370*
Fenoprofen, *445*, 449-50
  volume of distribution of, 628
Fenopropathrin, *530*
Fenoterol, *73*
Fentanyl
  as controlled substance, 319, *319*
  description of, 332
  naloxone and, *340*
  as opiate agonist, 326
  street names of, 332
  as synthetic narcotic, 326
  volume of distribution of, 628
Fentanyl-like drugs, street names of, 633
Fenthion, *536*
Fenvalerate, *530*
Fenyhist, *76*
Feosol, *465*
Feostat, *465*
FEP. *See* Free erythrocyte protoporphyrin
Fergon, *465*
Fer-In-Sol, *465*
Ferndex, *370*
Fero-Gradumet, *465*
Ferralet, *465*
Ferralyn, *465*
Ferric chloride test, 438-39
Ferrihemoglobin, 263
Ferrocholinate, percentage of iron in, *467*
Ferrous fumarate
  percentage of iron in, *467*
  trade names of, *465*
Ferrous gluconate
  percentage of iron in, *467*
  trade names of, *465*

Ferrous sulfate
  activated charcoal and, 24-25, *25*
  percentage of iron in, *467*
  trade names of, *465*
Ferrous-G, *465*
Fetus, carbon monoxide poisoning and, 231
Ficam, *537*
Ficus, *573*
Ficus elastica, 573
Fiorinal, *347*
Fire(s)
  as source of carbon monoxide, 223
  as source of cyanide, 242, *242*
First-order elimination, 58-59, *59*
First-pass effect, 58, *58*
Fischer test, 470-71
Fish
  ciguatera and, *605*
  scombroid poisoning and, 607
  toxins associated with, 605-08
Flashbacks, 407
Flecainide, therapeutic blood concentrations of, 624
Fleet enema
  dosages of, 28
  in treatment of iron poisoning, 471
Flexon, *77*
Flucythrinate, *530*
Flufenamic acid, *445*
Fluids and electrolytes
  balance, maintenance of
    in carbon monoxide poisoning, 233
  disorders
    pathophysiology of, *434*
  in salicylate poisoning, 433-34
Fluorescence polarization immunoassay, 47
Fluorescence spectroscopy, 49
Fluoroacetate poisoning, 513-14, *513*
Fluorocarbons, inhalation abuse and, 391, *392*
Fluorouracil, volume of distribution of, 628
Fluphenazine, 142, *142*, *143*
Flurazepam, *356*
  metabolite of, *38*
  therapeutic blood concentrations of, 624
Fluvalinate, *530*
Folex, *536*
Folic acid, 298
Fomac, *429*
Fonofos
  as moderately toxic organophosphate, *536*
Foodborne botulism, 600-02
  cause of death in, 600-01
  diagnosis of, 601

O